Case studies for complementary therapists: a collaborative approach

Case studies for complementary therapists: a collaborative approach

Kelly Galvin
BNat Dip Ed (Adult and Tertiary),
Course leader of Advanced Diploma of Naturopathy,
Holmesglen, Victoria

Madelaine Bishop
BHlthSc (Compl Med),
Adv Dip Naturopathy,
Grad Dip Clinical Acupuncture,
Cert IV in Workplace Training & Assessment,
Senior Clinic Supervisor and Lecturer in Clinical Practice and Nutrition,
Australian Institute of Holistic Medicine (AIHM), WA

ELSEVIER

ELSEVIER

Elsevier Australia. ACN 001 002 357
(a division of Reed International Books Australia Pty Ltd)
Tower 1, 475 Victoria Avenue, Chatswood, NSW 2067

Notice

This publication has been carefully reviewed and checked to ensure that the content is as accurate and current as possible at time of publication. We would recommend, however, that the reader verify any procedures, treatments, drug dosages or legal content described in this book. Neither the author, the contributors, nor the publisher assume any liability for injury and/or damage to persons or property arising from any error in or omission from this publication.

National Library of Australia Cataloguing-in-Publication Data

---

Galvin, Kelly.

Case studies for complementary therapists : a collaborative approach / Kelly Galvin, Madelaine Bishop.

9780729539555 (pbk.)

Includes index.

Communication in medicine.
Diagnosis—Management.
Therapeutics—Management.
Medical personnel—Relations.

Bishop, Madelaine.

610.696

Publisher: Sophie Kaliniecki
Developmental Editor: Neli Bryant
Publishing Services Manager: Helena Klijn
Project Coordinator: Natalie Hamad
Edited by Matt Davies
Proofread by Tim Learner
Cover and internal design by Avril Makula
Index by Annette Musker
Typeset by TNQ Books and Journals Pvt. Ltd.
Moved to Digital Printing 2016

Contents

Foreword

The move towards complementary healthcare has been escalating over four decades. This demonstrates a mainstreaming of what was once fringe alternative practice, and is being led predominantly by educated consumers from affluent Western nations. Many of the traditional medical practices of the West, having continued under the radar, are now resurgent. Meanwhile, developing nations attempt to maintain their traditional methods while modern Western medical technologies and practices are introduced. It is an era of rapid expansion of choice for individuals seeking healthcare that is safe, coherent, effective and, importantly, one that matches their worldview. These people aim to integrate the best of each approach; the word 'alternative' is now redundant.

Practitioners of medicine of any kind have a primary responsibility before any therapy is employed – that of diagnosis. To the Greeks, *dia-gnosis* meant a discerning of the truth between two possibilities, but in practice there are often many more possibilities for the cause of a patient's presenting problem. This complexity in the search for causation is central to the practice of medicine, and nowhere more so than in natural and complementary medicine (NCM). The holistic principles underlying these practices encompass the biological, psychological, social and environmental aspects of health, and a multitude of causes and effects can be found in the extended interview with a patient that is a feature of NCM practice.

So, the process is complex and the risks that something may be missed are high. Teaching and assessing this skill in students is difficult. Then along comes a resource that makes the educator's job so much more simple – this book. *Case Studies for Complementary Therapists: a collaborative approach* offers a clear, clinically oriented foundation for case taking and initial diagnostic workup for practitioners of NCM who often operate as a primary health system contact; people may present having had no other consult for their complaints.

The authors are experienced clinicians with extensive teaching experience that results in learning aids like mnemonics and decision-making trees that build a scaffolding for students to make sense out of the chaos. A feature of diagnosis in NCM is the search for issues that are at the centre of the individual's experience – so-called 'core' issues that invoke vital questions. What are the essential ingredients that matter? What binds this presentation together? What cannot be ignored to unlock the case and the inherent healing within? What are the seeds of origin of the dysfunction? This concept was profoundly elucidated by Hahnemann and his successors in homeopathic thought – that each individual must be treated as such; everything is core to their story, their perception and their unique expressions become the most vital pieces of information used to design a well-crafted and balanced management plan.

This book employs a logical framework in the art and science of diagnosis, and therefore will assist students and practitioners of NCM in becoming safer and more reliable members of the healthcare team. Other healthcare providers can build further trust that their referred patients will be managed with knowledge and expertise. The authors are to be commended.

Paul Orrock, RN, ND, DBM, DO, MAppSc(Research), GradCertHEd
Senior Lecturer, School of Health and Human Sciences,
Southern Cross University, Lismore, NSW, Australia

Foreword

This book is a valuable resource not only for students but also practitioners of complementary and alternative medicine (CAM). It will further develop their skills in case history taking, clinical diagnosis and case management. For students, the text is laid out in such a clear and structured way that it facilitates self-directed learning, strengthening all aspects of case taking as well as broadening the understanding of a range of treatment approaches. With the emphasis on integrative case management there is appropriate sensitivity to building confidence yet, at the same time, developing the awareness of symptoms and situations where referral to other healthcare providers is indicated. With the strengthening of regulation by the CAM professions, this book is also a valuable resource for self-directed continuing professional development that is likely to be a future requirement to ensure registration is maintained.

At the University of Westminster, with its extensive portfolio of bachelor's and master's degrees in CAM, the book will be an asset in developing the knowledge, understanding and clinical reasoning skills of students. The eclectic approach enables the book to be of value not only in countries where naturopathy encompasses both herbal medicine and nutritional therapy but also in the United Kingdom where they are practised as separate professions but there is a realisation of the importance of knowing more about each therapy. In busy teaching clinics, such as the Polyclinic of the University of Westminster, the book will be a valuable resource for group study or if patients do not attend their appointments. The inclusion of possible treatments and collaborative referral options enables the book to be a resource in mixed therapy teaching groups, where the importance of integrative case management is recognised.

Although treatment protocols are identified, the structured process of case analysis and decision making facilitate the development of the transferable and effective skills of clinical reasoning, no matter which CAM therapies are practised. The use of a simplistic case analysis framework ensures it can be effectively adapted for most models of CAM.

The wealth of the 35 fictional but realistic case studies that draw upon the clinical experience of the authors ensures the stories are true to life and within the realm of experience that most practitioners either would have or may meet in their practices. As the questioning protocols are clear and consistent, they are ideal for students or practitioners who have recently graduated and need their confidence strengthened through an approach that is resilient in the stressful situations of clinical practice.

Consistent with the approach of integrative case management, questions are included in each case to help the reader recognise symptoms and situations in which referral to other healthcare providers is indicated. The learning tools such as the 'apple' analogy and mnemonics provide a clear structure for the student to guide their learning of the skills of questioning and case analysis.

The inclusion of decision tables and referral flags and the emphasis on appropriate referral ensures readers will develop the knowledge and skills necessary for deciding on immediate referral for medical diagnosis, collaborative management or, if referral is not necessary, before CAM treatment can be started. The development of these skills has the potential to lead to holistic diagnosis and treatment options, as well as facilitating collaboration with mainstream medical and allied health practitioners. Such patient-centred approaches are essential if the interests of the patient are to be kept paramount.

In some countries, with the increasing likelihood of litigation, especially if an underlying pathology that may progress to disease is not detected by the CAM practitioner, there are implications with regard to not only the safety to continue to practice but also remaining registered with the professional body concerned. In addition, the development of the skills to discuss the perspectives and concepts with patients is likely to be a positive experience for all concerned, building confidence in the professionalism of the practitioner and increasing the likelihood of meeting the patient's needs.

This book is important because it provides a user-friendly resource for students and recent graduates, as well as for experienced practitioners who wish to satisfy continuing professional development self-directed study requirements. Written by practitioners, and informed by their own experiences in clinical practice, the book ensures the cases are realistic and relevant. The authors are to be congratulated for bringing together such a wide range of cases relevant for so many CAM practitioners to create such a valuable resource.

Brian Isbell, PhD, BSc, PGCHE, DO, MRN, MRSC, MSB
Head of the Department of Chinese Medicine and Complementary Therapies,
School of Life Sciences, University of Westminster, London, England

About the authors

Kelly Galvin
BNat (Southern Cross University), Dip Ed (Adult and Tertiary) (Murdoch University)
Course leader of Advanced Diploma of Naturopathy, Holmesglen (Victoria)

Kelly has been employed as a clinical supervisor and lecturer over the past decade at Southern Cross University (NSW), Australian Institute of Holistic Medicine (WA), University of Westminster (London) and now Holmesglen (Victoria).

In private practice, Kelly specialises in homeopathy, herbal medicine, nutrition, Bach flower essences, mind–body counselling, and hydrotherapy and massage techniques.

Madelaine Bishop
BHlth Sc (Compl Med) (Charles Sturt University), Adv Dip Naturopathy (AIHM), Grad Dip Clinical Acupuncture (AIHM), Cert IV in Workplace Training & Assessment (University of New England)
Senior clinic supervisor and lecturer in Clinical Practice and Nutrition, Australian Institute of Holistic Medicine (AIHM), WA

Madelaine has been employed as a lecturer and clinical supervisor for 12 years at the AIHM in Western Australia. Madelaine also works as a naturopathic educator, presenting seminars to a range of health professionals including medical practitioners, physiotherapists, dieticians and nursing practitioners.

Madelaine is in private practice in Jandakot, Western Australia, where she primarily utilises nutrition and herbal medicine along with acupuncture and homeopathy.

Dedications

Kelly:

For my husband, Matt, my son, Sam, and my mother, Louisa Galvin, for the infinite support, love and faith to actualise the dream.

In memory of my father, Simon Galvin, who wanted to publish a book of his own in life and passed on the bold inspiration.

Madelaine:

For my husband Mark, children James and Hannah, parents Hertha and John Saunders, and best friend Calee Dryga, for the love and support you gave me throughout the process of writing this book, and for being a constant reminder of what is really important in life.

For the Creator, with thanks for the abundant wealth of healing that can be found in the natural world.

Acknowledgements

'Whatever you can do, or dream you can do, *begin it*. Boldness has genius, power and magic in it.'

Johann Wolfgang von Goethe

We would like to thank everyone who has been so important throughout the process of developing *Case Studies for Complementary Therapists: a collaborative approach*. Special thanks to the respected peers in the global industry of healthcare who provided consistent encouragement for the concept of the book. Those people in the UK include: David Peters, Brian Isbell, Leon Chaitow, Roger Newman-Turner, Jill Rowley, Nicky Howard-Kemp, Hal Andrews and very special thanks to Stephanie Panayiotou. In Australia, thanks to Paul Orrock, Ian Howden, Sue Evans, Jon Wardle, Ruth Yuthok, Claire Modica, Sharon Adams and to Scott Little.

Our thanks for the consistent support provided through Elsevier, particularly by Sophie Kaliniecki, Sabrina Chew, Neli Bryant, Natalie Hamad and Matt Davies. Also, our sincere thanks to all the reviewers who contributed time and gave valuable feedback to our project.

We would like to extend our thanks to the students who have been involved with testing the concept of the case analysis formula provided in this textbook and for the relentless encouragement for us to produce a book. Particular thanks to students of the Australian Institute of Holistic Medicine in Perth, Southern Cross University in Lismore, University of Westminster in London and Holmesglen TAFE in Melbourne, who have contributed more than they realise to how the book was shaped.

A very special thanks to Deborah Sanderson who helped birth the initial curriculum material that provided the foundational concept of this book, and for her continued friendship and support throughout the years.

Finally, we would like to thank each other. Working together, mostly across continents and oceans, has been an absolute pleasure. It is rare to find a colleague with whom one can share a vision and work together with an effortless synergy to see it grow into a published work. We hope our readers gain as much benefit and enjoyment from reading this book as we did in writing it. We have been inspired by all those involved in the process and trust *Case Studies for Complementary Therapists: a collaborative approach* will become a tool for healing that will benefit the greater whole.

Kelly Galvin & Madelaine Bishop
Melbourne & Perth 2010

Reviewers

Catharine Avila
PhD (SCU), BSc Hons (Exeter University, UK), ND (NSW College of Natural Therapies and Traditional Chinese Medicine), MATMS
Lecturer, School of Health and Human Sciences, Southern Cross University, Lismore, NSW, Australia
Supervisor, Southern Cross University Health Clinic, Lismore, NSW, Australia

Brian Isbell
PhD, ND, Osteopath, BSc, MRSC, MSB
Head of Department, School of Life Sciences, University of Westminster, London, UK
Private practitioner, London, UK

Nicole Quaife
BHSci (Naturo)
Clinic Supervisor and Lecturer in Clinical Nutrition, Southern School of Natural Therapies, Melbourne, Victoria, Australia
Private practitioner, Hampton, Victoria, Australia

Andreas Syrimis
BSc (Hons) MSc, MCPP, MNIMH
Senior Lecturer, University of Westminster, University of East London,
Director of Admissions for NIMH, London, UK

P Spero Tsindos
ND (NSW Coll of Nat Med), MPH (Deakin), GCert Health promotion (Deakin), GCert Education (Higher Ed) (UQ)
Program Leader, Department of Occidental Medicine, Endeavour College of Natural Health, Victoria, Australia
Private practitioner, Victoria, Australia

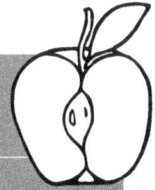

CHAPTER 1

Introduction

The purpose of this book is to help students and practitioners of complementary therapies extend their skills in clinical diagnosis and integrative case management. As complementary and alternative medicine (CAM) educators, we recognised our students' need for specific guidance in diagnosis and treatment prioritisation, along with the effective integration of a range of modalities into individualised holistic treatment programs. This style of case analysis was developed to provide students, teachers and practitioners with a framework within which they could effectively analyse and classify the extensive amount of information gathered in a CAM consultation [1]. We expect this book will be of particular benefit to CAM students and recent graduates who are seeking tools to enhance practice, particularly those who are learning or practising in countries in which CAM practitioners are not primary healthcare providers.

This book is intended to provide an insight into the initial consultation process, offering possible treatment and collaborative referral options for individual cases rather than dictating diagnostic analysis or treatment protocols for specific conditions, and it is not intended to be an instruction manual for treating all cases of specific conditions. Question suggestions have been provided to help the user collect the necessary information to develop a working diagnosis and treatment protocol for each individual case. Readers can then adapt questions, decision-making tools and therapeutic recommendations to suit the needs of their own clients.

Detailed explanations for specific treatment protocols and modalities are not included in each case because we have assumed our target readership has an understanding of basic CAM principles, herbal therapy and actions, along with nutritional and dietary protocols. Readers who are unfamiliar with these concepts are directed to the outline of the fundamental principles and practice of CAM in Chapter 2, and subsequently listed reference materials; these recommend some excellent resources.

The process of case analysis and decision making outlined in this book can help the user develop effective and appropriate treatment protocols within the time constraints of a busy clinic [1]. The case analysis format, together with the case studies in this book, have been used with great success in quite different CAM training institutions. Students found the decision-making framework extremely helpful, despite training within differing models of CAM. The inspiration to develop this book came from seeing how this method allowed student practitioners to collate facts and relate the information collected into an understanding of how the underlying issues connected to the presenting symptoms [5]. The case analysis framework is deliberately simplistic so it can be adapted for all models of CAM, and the analysis method presented can be used as a scaffolding on which varying levels of complexity can be formed into a holistic understanding of the general and specific needs of the individual client.

How to use this book

This book contains 35 fictional clinical case studies. While each case is fictional, we have drawn upon our clinical experience to make the stories realistic and truthful to the real-world experience of CAM practitioners. Each case is divided into different sections in order to more clearly outline the diagnostic and decision-making process.

The first section focuses on diagnostic analysis from a holistic perspective, taking into account both individual and common themes for specific disease conditions. The questioning protocols are focused on initial consultations; however, they can be adapted for use in subsequent consultations. It concludes with a decision table for referral, outlining referral flags, issues of significance and referral options with suggestions for further medical investigations. Additionally, a table of investigations for integrated holistic analysis is presented in Appendix B.

The three C's case analysis formula

CLINICAL QUESTIONS

Clinical questioning has been divided into three main sections called **the three C's**:
- **Complaint** – questions to define the client's presenting complaint. The aim is to *understand the complaint.*
- **Context** – questions to put the presenting complaint into context. The aim is to *understand the disease.* Questions on common contributing physical, dietary and lifestyle factors that may trigger the presenting complaint and lead to differential diagnosis considerations.
- **Core** – questions for holistic assessment to *understand the client.* Questions to reveal unique contributing emotional, mental, spiritual, metaphysical, lifestyle and constitutional factors for the individual client.

Although these categories have been set out in three chronological sections, it may be necessary to interweave the three lines of questioning throughout the consultation. How the questioning unfolds will depend upon the discretion of the practitioner, information-gathering priorities and rapport building with the client. The client may dictate which areas of information they wish to share, which will influence how the practitioner approaches questioning and information gathering. The examples of open and closed questions presented in this book have been designed to encourage confidence in the practitioner. Specific question examples may seem to extend beyond the level of qualification and jurisdiction of a non-primary practitioner. These questions have been included to help practitioners recognise symptoms and situations where referral to other healthcare providers is necessary. It is not our intention to encourage CAM practitioners to take over the role of primary healthcare professionals when that is beyond the scope of their training and professional boundaries. The purpose of these questions is to suggest ways in which CAM practitioners can elicit information that link the language of orthodox differential diagnosis into the observations and understandings acquired during the consultation process [7].

THE 'APPLE' ANALOGY

The three C's formula is woven into the clinical questions, case analysis, referral suggestions and treatment options for all cases studies presented in this book. To more

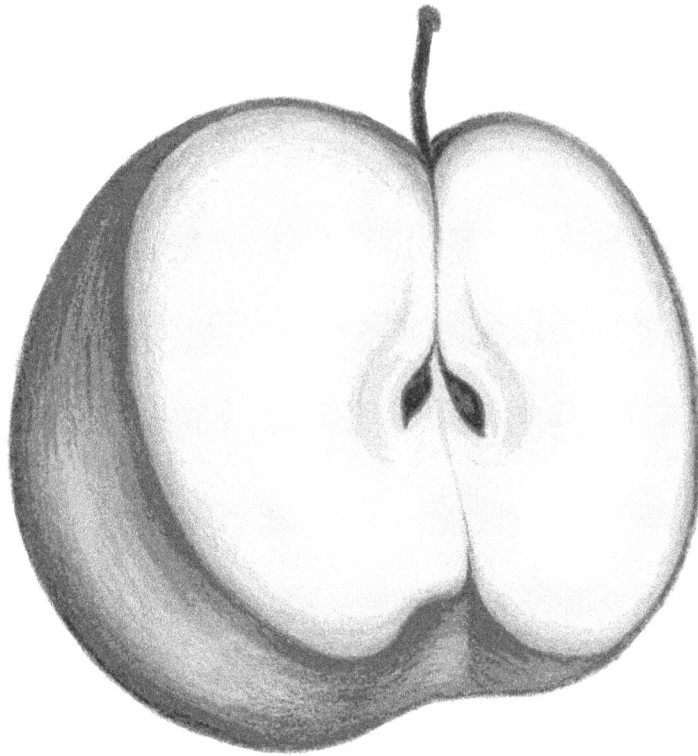

Figure 1 *Dissected apple showing the three layers corresponding to complaint (skin), context (flesh) and core (apple core)*

clearly illustrate this concept, we have likened the framework to the analogy of an apple, which consists of three distinct and purposeful layers.

1. The skin of the apple can be likened to the 'complaint', providing a first impression and surface information about why the client has come for help. This section shows us the cover that has developed as the underlying issues progress and manifest outwardly. For example, a feeling of fatigue is a 'complaint' symptom for which several reasons may need to be considered in order for it to be put into context.

2. The layers of physiological, environmental and lifestyle triggers of illness that are commonly shared or implicated in the development of conditions is the flesh of the apple, corresponding to the 'context'. This flesh is usually significant and helps identify the cause of complaint symptoms, which may be common to a number of different individuals. For example, if a group of people with low thyroid function experience fatigue, then the shared complaint symptom of fatigue can be understood within a common context for that disease process.

3. The underlying issues at the heart of the apple make up the core emotional and lifestyle triggers that are unique to each individual. The 'core' of an apple houses the seed in the same way that we house the seed of our illness. This is where an understanding of the metaphysical/spiritual/emotional influences on illness plays an important role, with consideration that physical manifestations of disease have an underlying energetic or emotional beginning [13, 18, 19]. If unique stressors for individuals are recognised as the seeds that can develop into illness, the core section

can be the gateway to understanding how to let go of the cycle of ill health and move towards wellness. The reasons an individual is vulnerable to compromised health are unique to that person and understanding those reasons is the key to holistic healing.

 By using the framework of the three C's formula it is possible to consider a case from a holistic perspective. If an individual is experiencing extreme stress due to their struggle to make life decisions based on their own values and beliefs rather than those of others (core), this stress may contribute to thyroid imbalance (context), thus causing the surface symptom of fatigue (complaint). In using this example we recognise the medical fact that hypothyroidism may cause fatigue and there is no biomedical evidence that hypothyroidism can result from the inability to make life decisions; however, chronic stress has been linked to the development and progression of a range of medical conditions including immune dysregulation [19]. It is therefore possible to see how chronic stress caused by an emotional conflict could trigger or worsen underlying immune-related thyroid dysfunction [19, 21]. We hope readers will be open to the concept of individual beginnings to common themes of illness. In offering this analogy as a suggested means of exploring individual cases, we are by no means suggesting this is the only way to perceive the causes of health imbalance in individuals with specific health conditions but rather suggesting that the three C's formula framework is useful in holistically analysing cases.

MNEMONICS

To further assist the reader we have developed mnemonics that guide the questions and case analysis. Mnemonics have been linked to the three C's case analysis formula and the 'apple analogy' explanation. The interweaving of these three tools allows the reader to follow the logic and flow of how the cases presented in this book have been analysed and treatment decisions have been determined. Question examples linked to mnemonics have been offered for each case as a working tool to help guide the the reader. We have intentionally included only a limited number of questions in each case and the reader is encouraged to refer to Appendix A for a more extensive list of clinical question examples. The reader can assume that in each case the practitioner would question the client extensively and cover all important/relevant body systems and symptoms. The extensive questions list in Appendix A list has been included to help guide readers with their own cases. To understand more thoroughly how the suggested mnemonics and questions can be incorporated into general case taking, one case example is provided at the end of Chapter 2 demonstrating more extensive questioning than has been applied to the other cases in this book.

The cases

Diagnosis

Each case in this book begins with a fictional case study including relevant medical investigations and physical examination history. We have deliberately limited information in the initial case presentation to allow readers to use their own diagnostic analysis skills to determine which specific questions are required to come up with a differential diagnosis list. To assist readers, a list of generic clinical questions is presented in Appendix A. A differential diagnosis list and working or confirmed diagnosis has also been provided. Although the title of each case provides the specific diagnosis, we encourage readers to go through the process of case analysis and come up with their

TABLE 1.1 **MNEMONIC KEY**		
SKIN OF THE APPLE	**FLESH OF THE APPLE**	**SEED OF THE APPLE**
COMPLAINT	CONTEXT	CORE
Understand the complaint	**Understand the disease**	**Understand the client**
'Outer layer' **O**nset **U**nderstanding the cause (client) **T**iming (duration, frequency) **E**xacerbating factors **R**elieving factors **L**ocation and radiation **A**ccount and description **Y**our practitioner impression **E**xamination and inspection **R**ating scale	**'Factors of disease'** **F**amily health **A**llergies and irritants **C**ancer and heart disease **T**rauma and pre-existing illness **O**bstruction and foreign body **R**ecreational drug use **S**urgery and hospitilisation **O**ccupational toxins and hazards **F**unctional disease **D**egenerative and deficiency **I**nfection and inflammation **S**upplements and side effects of medication and drugs **E**ndocrine/reproductive **A**utoimmune disease **S**tress and neurological **E**ating habits and energy	**'Seeds of health'** **S**upport systems **E**motional health **E**nvironmental wellness **D**aily activities **S**tress release **O**ccupation **F**amily and friends **H**ome life **E**ducation and learning **A**ction needed to heal **L**ong-term goals **T**ime to heal **H**as not been well since

own differential and working diagnoses before referring to the diagnostic information provided for each case.

Decision tables

Decision tables have been included in each case to help readers analyse and prioritise information and treatment options. The decision table format is designed to clearly present the specific holistic needs of the client while ensuring referral flags and issues of significance are properly addressed.

REFERRAL FLAGS AND ISSUES OF SIGNIFICANCE

'Referral' and 'issues of significance' flags are included in the decision table for referral to indicate symptom priority. Referral flags are symptoms that indicate the possibility of serious organic disease or the potential of harm to the client, and which require immediate referral to a primary healthcare practitioner [3]. 'Issues of significance' symptoms are not as urgent as referral flags but still need to be addressed. These symptoms may be benign but could also indicate more serious conditions and may require referral and collaborative case management at some stage.

Referral

Cases have been presented as either requiring immediate referral for medical diagnosis and collaborative management once diagnosis has been confirmed, or those that do not necessarily require immediate referral to a primary healthcare practitioner before CAM treatment is commenced. In the second instance, treatment recommendations are given and collaborative referral is recommended where appropriate. We have assumed that most readers of this book will be auxiliary practitioners rather than primary practitioners, and referral suggestions are based on this premise.

Treatment

The second section of each case provides holistic integrative treatment and lifestyle recommendations, with guidelines for managing the case in the context of the individual needs of the client. The decision table in this section is focused on assisting readers to formulate and prioritise a treatment program that reflects the complaint, context and core issues. Treatment suggestions have been presented in accordance with CAM principles starting with minimal active intervention and progressing through to greater levels of active intervention. In each case treatment recommendations cover commonly used CAM modalities beginning with recommendations for lifestyle and dietary interventions followed by physical treatment suggestions, and herbal and nutritional supplement suggestions. Treatment recommendations combine both evidence-based and traditional treatment approaches, which reflects the approach to treatment followed by many CAM practitioners [10, 24].

We believe the application of a Western scientific biomedical paradigm to some CAM modalities is not always helpful or even possible. A lack of scientific evidence for a specific CAM treatment or approach does not invalidate its use but can indicate the limitations of applying an evidence-based biomedical conceptual framework to certain CAM modalities and approaches [10, 12, 23, 25]. In such instances, for research to provide a truthful appraisal it must be done in a manner that incorporates and maintains the modality's underlying concepts and approaches to health and healing [8, 12, 22, 25, 26]. Traditional use can also be considered to be valid evidence based on the many years of use and traditional knowledge [9–11].

INTEGRATING CAM MODALITIES

In the experience of the authors, integrating more than one CAM modality into an individualised treatment program often brings superior results to using a single modality only. For example, nutritional therapy often combines well with herbal therapy and may be further augmented by incorporating a physical treatment modality. This type of integrative treatment approach has been used as the basis for the treatment recommendations in this book. Treatment suggestions are adapted to suit the needs of the individual client, taking into account factors such as financial status, likely compliance and the client's individual preference for particular treatments. A variety of options is offered in each case, but it is not necessarily assumed the client will take all of the supplements recommended. It should also be understood that if a particular treatment modality has not been included we are not implying it is not appropriate. The range of treatment modalities practised by CAM practitioners is wide and varied and we have therefore chosen to include treatment modalities that are common to most CAM practitioners. We strongly encourage individual students and practitioners to consider treatment options in these cases from the perspective of the modalities they are studying or practising. These treatment suggestions are based on the specific needs and circumstances of the client and are not intended to direct readers to follow prescribed herbal formulas and supplements for all similar cases they encounter in their own practice.

INTEGRATING CAM AND CONVENTIONAL MEDICINE

We acknowledge that several CAM modalities do not require orthodox medical diagnosis in order to effectively treat clients [4]; however, our book suggests a way this can be incorporated into healthcare management that provides benefits for both mainstream and complementary medicine. Integrating these aspects has the potential to enhance holistic diagnosis and treatment options along with providing an opportunity for positive collaboration with mainstream medical practitioners and allied health professionals [14–16]. Indeed, failure to detect underlying pathology may result in the progression of an illness into a more serious organic disease [3, 14]. As integration between CAM and mainstream medicine continues to unfold, mainstream medical practitioners are now more likely to train in areas of complementary medicine [16, 17, 20], and CAM practitioners may have additional training in an aspect of conventional medicine such as nursing, physiotherapy or medicine itself [3].

The referral recommendations in this book are not intended to fit every CAM model, and we recognise that CAM practice has various levels of primary care status globally, which will inevitably influence the priority of referral and which symptoms can be treated. We believe we are offering referral suggestions that include the varied legal and professional boundaries of CAM practitioners by encouraging referral that embraces the concept of open support from allied health professionals. These cases do not set out the definitive way to approach case management; rather, we present the idea of referral within the context of professional boundaries that focuses on the best interests of the client, who may want to be better 'informed' from a variety of perspectives regarding diagnosis and treatment options [7]. Achieving this balance can be difficult, and effective cross-referral and collaborative case management is reliant on the willingness of all health professionals to be open to different paradigms of health [3, 7].

We define collaborative referral as a referral from one healthcare practitioner to another, with the intention of shared care within the different areas of knowledge and expertise of each practitioner. We define cross-referral as referral from one healthcare practitioner to another when the referring practitioner discontinues care and effectively hands over treatment of the client to the other practitioner.

Because fundamental paradigms and methodology can differ so significantly, clients and practitioners may find diagnostic and treatment information from a range of perspectives confusing and conflicting [3, 4]. However, discussing the various perspectives and concepts with clients can be a positive experience for both the client and the practitioner if open communication is achieved [3]. Often genuine clarity comes with inner debate, reflection and questioning, and personal growth can be embraced through illness [9]. We believe that through this process clients can gain a clearer understanding, which can inform their personal choices as they make decisions about treatment and their journey towards wellness. Therefore, collaboration between healthcare practitioners can provide clients with a much more effective outcome [2, 7] and increases the likelihood of meeting all of the client's needs [2]. Holistic healthcare is far more than using a variety of CAM modalities but involves collaboration and cooperation between all of a client's healthcare practitioners [2, 6]. It is encouraging to note that recent Australian research has revealed medical practitioners are now more open to accepting the role of CAM practitioners in overall healthcare [3, 6].

The diagnostic and decision-making framework in this book can help readers become more confident in making sound treatment decisions by means of thorough analysis of the client's case history and individual needs. This is an area of weakness for some CAM practitioners, as highlighted by a 2005 La Trobe University report [3] that identified a number of risk areas for Australian naturopathic and Western herbal medicine practitioners. These risk areas include: poor prescribing; failure to recognise contraindications; inappropriate dosage and duration of therapy; lack of understanding of drug/nutrient/herbal interaction; failure to detect underlying pathology; misdiagnosis; failure to refer; and failure to disclose or offer informed consent [3]. This could be considered the responsibility of the practitioner and, in response to these concerns, we hope our book will offer students and practitioners effective tools to ensure higher standards of clinical care and treatment.

References

[1] M. Lloyd, R. Bor, Communication skills for medicine, third edn, Churchill Livingstone, Edinburgh, 2009.

[2] S. El-Hashemy, Naturopathic standards of primary care, CCNM Press, Toronto, 2008.

[3] P. McCabe, Tertiary education in naturopathy and western herbal medicine, in: V. Lin, A. Bensoussan, S. Myers, et al (Eds.), The practice and regulatory requirements of naturopathy and western herbal medicine, School of Public Health, La Trobe University, Melbourne, 2005. Available from <www.health.vic.gov.au/pracreg/naturopathy.htm> [accessed 18 October 2008].

[4] T. Jagtenberg, S. Evans, Global Herbal Medicine: A Critique, The Journal of Complementary Medicine 9 (2) (2003) 321–329.

[5] K. Ashcroft, L. Foreman-Peck, Learning and the reflective practitioner, in: Managing Teaching and Learning in Further and Higher Education, Falmer Press, London, 1994.

[6] D.M. Southern, D. Young, D. Dunt, N.J. Appleby, R.W. Batterham, Integration of primary healthcare services: perceptions of Australian general practitioners, non-general practitioner health service providers and consumers at the general practice-primary care interface, Evolution and Program Planning 25 (1) (2002) 47–59.

[7] D.H. Jeroen, A.A. Van Wijngaarden, R.H. de Bront, Learning to cross boundaries: The integration of a health network to deliver seamless care, Health Policy 79 (2–3) (2006) 203–213.

[8] S. Butelow, T. Kenealy, Evidence-based medicine: the need for a new definition, Journal of Evaluation in Clinical Practice 6 (2) (2000) 85–92.

[9] S. Mills, K. Bone, Principles & Practice of Phytotherapy; Modern Herbal Medicine, Churchill Livingstone, Edinburgh: London, 2000.

[10] L. Braun, M. Cohen, Herbs & Natural Supplements: An evidence based guide, second edn, Elsevier, Sydney, 2007.

[11] Guidelines for Levels and Kinds of Evidence to Support Indications and Claims For Non-Registerable Medicines, including ComplementaryMedicines, and other Listable Medicines. Therapeutic Goods Administration of Australia, 2001. Retrieved 16 March 2010. http://www.tga.gov.au/docs/html/tgaccevi.htm

[12] R.L. Nahin, S.E. Straus, Research into complementary and alternative medicine: problems and potential, British Medical Journal 322 (2001) 161–164.

[13] D.J. Tataryn, Paradigms of health and disease: a framework for classifying and understanding complementary and alternative medicine, Journal of Alternative & Complementary Medicine 8 (6) (2002) 877–892.

[14] M. Cohen, Practitioners and 'regular' doctors: Is integration possible? Medical Journal of Australia 180 (2004) 645–646.

[15] I.H. Kerridge, J.R. McPhee, Ethical and legal issues at the interface of complementary and conventional medicine, Medical Journal of Australia 181 (3) (2004) 164–166.

[16] D.K. Owen, G. Lewith, C.R. Stephens, Can doctors respond to patients' increasing interest in complementary and alternative medicine?, British Medical Journal 322 (2001) 154–158.

[17] M. Pirotta, M. Cohen, V. Kotsirilos, S.J. Farish, Complementary therapies: have they become accepted in general practice?, Medical Journal of Australia 172 (2000) 105–109.

[18] J.K. Kiecolt-Glaser, R. Glaser, Depression and immune function: Central pathways to morbidity and mortality, Journal of Psychomatic Research 53 (2002) 873–876.

[19] S. Cohen, D. Janicki-Deverts, G.E. Miller, Psychological Stress and Disease, JAMA 298 (14) (2007) 1685–1687.

[20] S. Levine, M. Weber-Levine, R. Mayberry, Complementary and alternative medical practices: Training, experience and attitudes of a primary care medical school faculty, Journal American Board of Family Practice 16 (4) (2003) 318–326.

[21] M.F. Prummel, T. Strieder, W.M. Wiersinga, The environment and autoimmune thyroid diseases, European Journal of Endocrinology 150 (2004) 605–618.

[22] A.F. Long, Outcome Measurement in Complementary and Alternative Medicine: Unpicking the Effects, Journal Altern Complement Med 8 (6) (2002) 777–786.

[23] S.A. Gaylord, J.D. Mann, Rationales for CAM Education in Health Professions Training Programs, Acad Med 82 (2007) 927–933.

[24] H.L. Eastwood, Complementary therapies: the appeal to general practitioners, Medical Journal of Australia 173 (2000) 95–98.

[25] M.R. Tonelli, T.C. Callahan, Why Alternative MedicineCannotBeEvidence-based,AcadMed76 (2001) 1213–1220.

[26] J. Sarris, J. Wardle, Clinical Naturopathy, an evidence-based guide to practice, Elsevier, Australia, 2010.

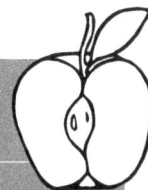

CHAPTER 2

The principles and practice of CAM

Principles of CAM

Within the field of complementary medicine there are many different modalities; however, all these modalities have a similar understanding of the importance of addressing the root cause of disease and supporting the body's inherent mechanisms of repair and recovery. Complementary medicine can be defined as a group of therapeutic and diagnostic disciplines that do not have the same theories and methods of teaching and provision as conventional biomedical healthcare [9, 15]. Commonly known CAM systems include Western herbal medicine, naturopathy, Chinese medicine, Ayurveda and homeopathy [15]. Other forms of therapy that come under the umbrella of CAM can include kinesiology, reflexology, reiki, flower essence therapy and aromatherapy [15]. Examples of complementary therapies commonly used in conjunction with conventional medicine include massage and nutritional therapy [15].

Holism is a fundamental principle in all CAM modalities. The term holism can have several meanings and, in the realm of healthcare, it refers to therapy that takes into account the understanding that illness is a manifestation of imbalance or disharmony in body, mind, emotion and often spirit [9]. The term 'integrative medicine' implies that complementary therapies are integrated into the structure of mainstream medicine [6], combining science, art, philosophy and medicine [8]. All aspects of lifestyle, including environment, diet, physical fitness, emotional stability, emotional awareness, sense of faith, belonging and meaning and purpose in life, are taken into consideration when forming an understanding about a person's health from a CAM perspective [9]; the notion of 'energy' is a shared understanding [9]. Integrative medicine can also be practised by CAM practitioners when they combine two or more CAM treatment modalities to form an individualised holistic treatment program. The term 'integrative medicine' therefore refers to more than just combining mainstream medicine with CAM therapies that have a biomedical science evidence base [15, 20].

There are many different treatment modalities used by CAM practitioners. Which treatment modality(ies) a practitioner recommends will depend on their training, experience and consideration of clients' individual needs and preferences. In CAM there is not necessarily only one 'right' way to treat a particular condition. This is because the aim of CAM treatment is to support the vital force and allow the body to heal itself, and there are often a number of ways this can be accomplished.

The principles listed below are the foundational principles of naturopathy. These principles, however, are relevant to all CAM modalities as the fundamental concepts of holism, addressing the root cause of illness and supporting the body's natural healing forces, are common to all. We have chosen to use the term CAM rather than naturopathy because it is more inclusive of a wide range of disciplines, and the target readership of this book includes practitioners from a range of disciplines in both CAM and conventional medicine.

Foundation principles

- **The healing power of nature** and **identify and treat the causes** [8, 10, 12, 17]. This principle acknowledges the body's innate ability to heal and self-repair and, therefore, the aim of treatment is to encourage the body's own capacity to heal by identifying and removing obstacles to optimal health [8, 9, 12, 15]. Treatment focuses on removing the causes of ill health rather than suppressing or eliminating symptoms to maintain health [7, 9, 12, 15]. Illness is considered a process of growth and, wherever possible, not to be suppressed. The aim of treatment is to establish optimal conditions for healing by supporting and mobilising the action of the body's innate self-healing abilities [10, 12, 69].

- **First do no harm.** This concept is inherent within the history of natural therapies and relates to the use (wherever possible) of restorative therapies that do not interrupt the self-adapting capacity of the body [7, 15, 72]. This principle also encompasses the importance of immediately attending to acute or emergency situations and, where necessary, repairing weakened tissues requiring more complex intervention by healthcare professionals from a range of disciplines [8, 10, 12, 69]. Doing 'no harm' therefore may include identifying situations requiring referral to other health professionals and following up on these in collaborative management. Additionally, 'doing no harm' includes practitioners becoming aware of personal agendas that may influence their decisions or hinder a therapeutic relationship with the client, and ensuring they always keep the best interests of their client clearly in mind [33].

- **The therapist as teacher.** The therapist teaches and guides through the process of healing [8, 10, 12, 69]. Illness is not to be feared but embraced as a learning process that can lead to growth for both the client and the practitioner [33, 69]. As a teacher, the therapist helps the client become self-regulating in maintaining their health, rather than just directing specific treatment without providing an understanding of why their health came to be compromised in the first place. This form of education focuses on the personal growth of the client [22] and recognises the life experiences that have shaped the client's learning goals and health outcomes [23, 24]. Helping clients understand the concept of growth through illness requires good rapport and communication between client and practitioner [69].

- **Treat the whole person.** Disease is a manifestation of imbalance in the body–mind state that can arise in the physical body from a range of causes including genetic, nutritional, environmental, emotional and trauma factors [9, 12, 66]. CAM treatment protocols aim to be client centred rather than disease oriented. This often requires therapy that holistically addresses all areas of imbalance in the whole person, not merely dealing with a single aspect of the symptom picture [15, 19].

- **Prevention.** Healthy lifestyle, good nutrition, clean air, spiritual wellbeing, light, rest, exercise, a sense of community, meaningful service or work and family are all part of promoting positive health [8, 10, 12, 15]. Prevention also includes identifying and removing factors that disturb health and wellbeing on all of these levels [10, 12, 18, 69]. This may involve removing sources of toxicity, such as poor lifestyle or dietary habits, allergies/intolerances/sensitivities, chemical or heavy metal toxicity or emotional toxicity, or enhancing neuro-muscular and skeletal integrity and enhancing emotional and mental health [10]. Prevention is about inspiring clients to choose a healthier lifestyle and helping them establish a beneficial way of living [10, 69].

The practice and role of CAM professionals

The role of CAM professionals and the legal and professional boundaries for primary diagnosis and healthcare by CAM practitioners varies between countries [68, 69]. In Australia and the United Kingdom (UK) CAM practitioners do not practise as primary healthcare providers and therefore need to work alongside medical practitioners to ensure appropriate medical diagnosis and management occurs within the framework of a holistic healthcare program [8, 13, 15]. In Canada and the United States (US), naturopaths practise as primary healthcare providers and therefore have a greater degree of autonomy and responsibility in diagnostic and treatment procedures [8, 15, 69, 71]. The modalities used by Australian naturopaths can be different from those used by British naturopaths. In the UK herbalists prescribe herbal liquid and tablet formulations, and naturopaths focus primarily on physical therapies and dietary treatment. In Australia naturopaths are likely to prescribe herbal and nutritional supplements along with physical therapies and dietary treatment [15].

The consultation process

Accurate information gathering is essential for a meaningful holistic diagnosis and treatment program. Integral to this process is the ability to ask questions in a way that elicits relevant information from the client. Effective information-gathering techniques are both an art and a skill, informed by an understanding of the **when**, **what** and **why** of clinical questioning [5]. Knowing **when** and **how** to question clients is influenced by the type of questions asked, consultation time, the individual needs of the client and the development of client–practitioner rapport [2, 5, 37]. Knowing **what** questions to ask ensures practitioners gain a relevant and thorough understanding of the client as they work towards a diagnosis; understanding **why** particular questions should be asked ensures practitioners have sufficient perspective for holistic case analysis and treatment recommendations. Integration of different questioning skills provides opportunities to recognise and understand potential physical, mental and emotional imbalances along with referral flags within each case. Skilful case taking therefore allows practitioners to holistically consider underlying reasons for the manifestation of disease, as well as negotiating treatment options and identifying where cross-referral to allied health professionals is necessary [2]. Ideally, a consultation is a journey in which both practitioner and client participate, understanding that the process is far more than just coming to an understanding of presenting symptoms [39]. It is in fact a process in which information is gathered in a professional, ethical and empathetic manner [2, 5] giving the client freedom to communicate their unique story and current problem in order for the practitioner to guide them towards meaningful treatment options and space for healing [5].

BUILDING RAPPORT

To ensure the consultation process is thorough and meaningful it is essential for rapport to occur between practitioner and client. The process of building rapport begins the moment the client enters the consultation room. It is therefore important for the practitioner to ensure they have let go of previous activities and are fully 'present' before commencing the consultation process [1]. Warmly introducing yourself and showing the client where to sit can help ease apprehension and help the client to feel more relaxed and secure [1, 49, 51]. Advising the client at the start of the consultation how much time it will take is also recommended so they are aware of how long they have to share their story [1].

During the case-taking process there will be times of active questioning, and perhaps also times of silence or reflective listening to allow the client time and space to fully explain their circumstances or consider suggestions. The practitioner may need to summarise or paraphrase the client's explanation in order to clarify information and they may also need to offer non-verbal cues and encouragement to help the client explain their story [1–3, 5, 38, 40–44, 51]. Non-verbal communication skills include knowing how to face a client, to make eye contact (where culturally and individually appropriate), to maintain an open posture and to use an appropriate tone of voice to sustain a relaxed atmosphere conducive to good communication [1, 5, 11, 45]. In this manner practitioners are not merely 'taking' information from the client but are actually 'receiving' a history from the client through both verbal and non-verbal communication, resulting from a positive rapport with the client [1, 70]. This process requires flexibility and openness on the part of the practitioner, along with professional honesty and confidence [1–3, 5, 38, 40–44, 51, 70].

An Australian survey conducted in 2005 revealed that one major aspect of satisfaction consumers have with CAM is that there is time for discussion and being listened to, along with a positive quality to the therapeutic relationship that develops [15]. Building rapport and offering empathy can often improve client adherence to treatment regimens for the long-term benefit of the client and the client–practitioner relationship [41, 70]. During a consultation it may be appropriate for the practitioner and client to alternate between asking and answering questions to promote a dialogue based on trust [5, 70]. This interplay and 'therapeutic conversation' can encourage empathy to develop, which inevitably gives the practitioner insight into the client's unique perspective and therefore helps them to better understand the client [5, 39, 70].

Building rapport also requires an awareness of cultural sensitivities. While the underlying principles of CAM practice require practitioners to consider each client as an individual, it is important to understand the individual needs of a client within their cultural or social context [1, 5]. When building rapport with clients, it is important for practitioners to understand that clients from cultures different from their own may respond differently to situations or questions from clients from their own background. The practitioner therefore needs to understand both the cultural background of each client and the personal culture of each individual.

If a client has hearing, speech or cognitive difficulties it is important that the practitioner does not make assumptions about what the client is trying to convey [1]. Alternative methods of communication, such as sign language, pointing to written words or symbols or using an interpreter, can be very helpful to ensure good communication and rapport [1, 49, 50]. It may be necessary to repeatedly confirm that the client understands questions and treatment options to ensure their consent is informed [1]. To help clients with hearing difficulties more easily lip read, the practitioner should sit in good light so their face can be clearly seen, remain still, not put objects in their mouth while talking, have minimal facial hair around the mouth and maintain good eye contact and an open facial expression [51]. If a client doesn't communicate in a language the practitioner can understand it may be necessary to seek assistance from an interpreter. It is wise for practitioners to be aware of the availability of interpreter services in their local area.

OPEN AND CLOSED QUESTIONING

During the initial stages of taking a case history, open-ended questions often allow practitioners to gain an overall impression of the client and begin to establish rapport [1, 2, 4, 45, 71]. Once this rapport has been initiated, the client is more likely to accept more challenging and probing questions [11, 39]. As the practitioner thoroughly investigates the client's condition, they will need to ask both open and closed questions in order to gain both the wider perspective and the specific detail required [2, 11, 71].

Specific or 'closed' questions are often required to obtain the information necessary to arrive at a specific working diagnosis or to determine whether there are red flags that warrant referral to other health practitioners [1, 2, 4]. These specific questions allow the practitioner to gain information not easily elicited from the client's own description [2, 6]. This line of questioning often concentrates on matching symptom pictures to common themes of organic disease [4, 11, 39]. However, relying solely on closed questioning will not elicit all necessary information, and it is the practitioner's responsibility to know what questions to ask to obtain all relevant information [2]. Diagnostic summaries that rely solely on closed questioning inevitably miss relevant holistic information and result in a case history that is too narrow [2]. Practitioners may need to explain to the client why closed questions are necessary so the client is able to place them in the context of their particular health issues [1, 11, 39]. Clients with speech impairments may have difficulty in easily answering open questions and in such situations the practitioner will need to direct the questioning in such a way that short answers are all that is necessary. Some clients may find speaking freely disconcerting or uncomfortable and prefer the practitioner to take the major role in the questioning process [1]. On the other hand, incorporating client-centred open questions into the consultation can result in spontaneous sharing of important information from the client. By expressing themselves in this manner, clients may experience an improvement in their overall emotional health and reduced manifestation of disease, lessening the need for diagnostic tests and cross-referral [1, 2, 46]. Open questions help practitioners to gain a broad perspective of how the client's state of imbalance developed [1, 2, 39]; opening up conversation in this way can be extremely useful to the practitioner allowing them time to listen while they consider what other information-gathering tools may be required [2].

Allowing time for a question to be answered thoroughly is necessary to gain an accurate history [1], and practitioners may find this challenging as they try to keep within the consultation time while still ensuring they arrive at a working diagnosis, develop a treatment program and identify situations requiring cross-referral [1, 51]. Because people take different amounts of time to answer questions it is important to allow the client sufficient time to frame their response. One of the aims of using open questions is for the client to feel they have conveyed their whole story [71]. Following open questions with closed questions to elicit specific information helps the practitioner to gather all relevant information [49]; concluding a consultation with specific questions and then summarising the information helps ensure accurate information has been gathered while maintaining consistency with the client's story [49]. General examples outlined in this chapter offer examples of how specific (closed) and open questions can complement each other in a clinical situation.

CAM DIAGNOSIS

There are two main factors in clinical diagnosis from a CAM perspective. The first is the understanding that each client is an *individual* and the reasons why physical or emotional imbalance manifests in the way it does must be understood from a unique perspective [2, 3]. The second factor is that physiological and mental manifestations of organic disease have common and specific symptomatic themes, which can be identified with effective case analysis [2, 4]. These symptomatic themes are recognised through effective questioning, thorough physical examination and utilisation of appropriate diagnostic tools. The aim of CAM diagnosis is to develop an *individualised* treatment program that is formulated with an understanding of the individual within the context of a disease process rather than by the disease diagnosis alone [5, 70, 72].

Using the three C's formula

Complaint

The first line of questioning in clinical case taking has the specific purpose of gathering information about the **presenting complaint(s)**. This information reveals the location, timing, pattern, aggravating and ameliorating factors and provides a clear description, rating and the overall character of the complaint [1, 2, 49]. Because the client may have more than one presenting complaint it may be necessary to go through this process more than once [2]. The presenting complaint that is most important to the client may not be the one the practitioner wants to explore later in the consultation [1], and the client may disclose additional complaints during the consultation process. By organising information in this way it is easier to come up with an overall working diagnosis and links to symptoms requiring referral are easier to identify. This first stage of a consultation is often when factual information is gathered, which can provide an opportunity for the client to relax and become accustomed to the consultation environment [45]. The way in which subsequent dealings and rapport with a client progresses is often influenced by the first consultation [1, 2, 50], so inappropriately worded comments or questions in an initial consultation may prevent the client from communicating core issues later on [2, 5, 45]. Attentive listening by the practitioner allows the client to offer all necessary information without hesitation. Such information may be critical in correctly determining a working diagnosis and identifying situations requiring referral and it will be difficult to achieve full therapeutic benefit for the client without it [1, 72].

Context

The second line of questioning focuses on investigating the range of symptoms that place the presenting complaint into context to understand the disease process. This line of questioning involves considering what is influencing the presenting complaint and draws upon knowledge of generic body systems and common lifestyle factors that may be causing or aggravating the presenting complaint [2]. For example, a client may present with abdominal pain that has several possible causes or reasons for development. Questions at this stage may be very specific to place the symptom of abdominal pain into context such as: 'Is your abdominal pain better for taking antacids or from sitting up?' (peptic conditions).

The context section focuses on a general body systems review that will enable a concise differential diagnosis to be considered. In the case-questioning and analysis we are most interested at this point with what common themes could trigger the complaint for anyone who may present with the complaint symptoms. The common disease processes are considered and focused upon. This allows relevant information to be elicited that may point towards potential referral situations, and ensures the client is properly informed about their health concern and is appropriately referred if necessary [1]. It is helpful to summarise to the client what information has been gathered through context questioning to ensure the line of enquiry and information gathered is relevant [1, 2].

Core

The third line of questioning relates to the core and holistic information concerning the individual client. It is equally important to focus on underlying emotional issues that may be contributing to the symptoms the client is experiencing. Questioning at this level may involve exploring information about family, friends, support networks, bereavements, shock or trauma, as well as specific behaviour integral to the development of the health imbalance [2, 50, 71].

People may experience disease symptoms without the presence of underlying pathology when symptoms have arisen from a bereavement, shock or trauma [2]. Likewise, individuals with the same disease diagnosis can experience quite different symptoms or 'illness' [2]. While CAM practitioners may not be qualified counsellors, the task of gathering a perspective of illness from each client is important [2, 6, 72]. A client may engage in a therapeutic consultation during a 'crossroads' in their life, hoping to find ways to change their future direction. This process may result in an aggravation of symptoms initially, such as the return of symptoms previously experienced, or even the development of new symptoms [8]. In these situations practitioners can facilitate time and space for their client to reconnect with the possibilities of a new beginning and the potential for personal growth [5]. Moods and emotions pervade all aspects of human behaviour and it is therefore necessary to understand the influence of mental and emotional conditions on the development and progression of the client's present state of health. This understanding also allows the practitioner to know how to help foster a healthier outcome for the future [5, 6]. For this reason it is essential to understand the wider context of the client's life.

The core section of questioning provided in this book is intended to acknowledge that all clients are unique and individual people and not merely a collection of symptoms [5, 6]. Practitioners who are sensitive to and understand the relevance of this line of questioning may choose to follow the client's agenda during the consultation, not assuming or reading information into the core section that is not true for the client [5]. The openness, trust and empathy that can develop between practitioner and client during the exploration of the core line of questioning creates an environment in which key information can be revealed [69, 72]. This area of questioning may reveal one or more emotional or mental health issues that practitioners would be wise to recognise and refer to appropriately qualified allied health professionals. This encourages integration and the possibility of working collaboratively for the optimal healthcare management of the client.

CAM treatment

Treatment or helping is not something 'done to' clients by CAM practitioners but is a collaborative effort between the practitioner and client [5, 6]. The CAM practitioner's aim is to ensure the client is asked clearly what they want, what they need and what they are willing to change [5]. The intrinsic motivation of the client is 'found' rather than 'created' and the client is encouraged to make choices for themselves [25–27]. Some clients are self-motivated and well informed while others may require structure, boundaries and direction so they can establish self-regulating preventative strategies that lead them towards long-term good health [25–27].

The goals of a CAM treatment program are therefore far more than simply achieving an improvement or elimination of troublesome physical symptoms [5, 15, 69]. While addressing the presenting complaint is important, programs should also help clients understand how and why the complaint developed in the first place and help them discover their personal potential, helping them work towards their desired lifestyle and optimum health both in the present and into the future [5, 72]. Individualised treatment programs also take into account the client's lifestyle as well as their financial, emotional and physical circumstances [5]. They are presented in a time and manner that is appropriate to the individual, ensuring they are not overwhelmed or disempowered [6]. The basis of treatment recommendations and expected outcomes are discussed [6] and if more than one treatment solution is available it may be appropriate to give clients an informed choice of their preferred option [6, 67]. At other times practitioners will need to direct clients towards important treatment recommendations, particularly in situations that require immediate medical collaboration [6]. This approach therefore requires flexibility and ongoing evaluation [5].

In keeping with the understanding of the innate intelligence of the vital force and *vis medicatrix naturae,* there may be times when the decision is made to not actively treat [7] but rather to respect the body's innate ability to self-heal without intervention. In some situations the consultation process may be healing enough [8]. Readers may be more familiar with the terms 'homeostasis' or 'general adaptation syndrome' to describe the body's innate self-healing force [8].

NEGOTIATING TREATMENT

Arriving at a mutually acceptable treatment program is essential for optimal client compliance. In order to gain insight into the client's expectations practitioners can ask questions such as 'What were you hoping I could do for your symptoms?' [1, 2, 50, 72], 'How do you hope I can help you with this?', 'What type of treatment were you expecting?' or 'What type of treatment approach were you hoping for?' [1, 2, 5, 6, 72].

If the client is uncertain or unclear about their expectations it will be necessary for the practitioner to give their opinion regarding their treatment options and the most appropriate course of action, clearly explaining the reasons for these recommendations [1, 6, 71]. Ways of suggesting treatment can include statements and/or questions such as 'Perhaps we could try this type of treatment plan first', 'One possibility is...', 'Sometimes I find that...' or 'How would you advise a friend in your situation?' [6]. This allows the client to participate in treatment decisions while the practitioner negotiates a specific therapeutic contract or treatment plan with them [6, 50]. It is also important to be honest about any uncertainties you may have as a practitioner about cultural sensitivities. 'I'm not always sure about cultural factors I need to be aware of so would you let me know if there is anything you don't understand or if there is anything specific I can do to help you be more confident about your treatment program?' [1]. Providing well-written and easily understandable information on the treatment program [1, 11, 71], explaining potential unexpected outcomes, outlining clearly how many visits may be required, summarising treatment priorities and asking the client if they understand the treatment plan all helps to ensure the highest potential of compliance can be reached [1, 71]. If the practitioner is clear about the intent and direction of therapy and/or prescribed treatments, it is more likely the client will understand and participate in the process [6].

Ending consultations

The closing phase of a consultation is the time to summarise the client's story and check for accuracy [11]. Ideally practitioner and client should feel they have both participated in the process of information gathering and arriving at a holistic understanding of the client's condition [11, 45, 72]. Phrases that can be used to finalise a consultation include:
- 'I would like to make sure I have understood you correctly. Today you shared that ...'[1]
- 'Do you feel you have told me enough or is there anything specific you would like to let me know before we finish?'
- 'Now that I understand more about your physical symptoms and how you are feeling, let's talk about the practical ways we can work together to help you.' [2]
- 'Thank you for sharing information with me because it has helped me understand your situation much better. Our time is up for today.'

Referral

At times it is necessary for practitioners to refer their clients to other healthcare professionals, particularly when situations requiring immediate cross-referral have been identified. Firm opening statements may be necessary to ensure the client understands the importance of the referral. At times the student or practitioner may find it difficult to confidently communicate their recommendation for referral. Examples of how to suggest to clients that they would benefit from a referral may include 'I have known cases where a counsellor has been very helpful' [6], 'I strongly advise…', 'My advice to you is…' or 'There is no doubt in my mind…' [6]. It is important the client understands the need for the referral and that the CAM practitioner and CAM therapies may still form part of their overall healthcare in conjunction with other health professionals [70]. One way to recommend referral could be 'I will write a referral letter to your GP/allied health professional explaining the symptoms you described today and ask them for a copy of the results of any investigations. Would you call me after your appointment and let me know what was discussed?' [2].

It is equally important to explain the importance of referral to a child, especially after they have developed a positive therapeutic rapport with the CAM practitioner. It may be appropriate to use wording such as 'I was just telling your parents about someone I would like you to meet and who I think would be very keen to meet you. She knows all about bad dreams and how to get rid of them. Would you like to meet her tomorrow?' [1].

Confidentiality

Clients who convey sensitive information during a consultation need to know their information will be kept confidential. In situations where you believe a client has physical or mental health issues beyond the scope of your professional expertise, it may be necessary to refer them to another healthcare provider who can help them. If a client communicates that they have a notifiable disease, is a danger to themselves or may harm others (e.g. issues surrounding child abuse, sexual abuse, domestic abuse or suicidal tendencies) it will be necessary to explain to the client that you must not be the only healthcare provider who knows this information [1, 51]. In some circumstances practitioners have a legal and professional duty of care to report or act upon such information [11, 51], for example, where it is discovered the client has been the victim of abuse. It may be helpful to the client if the practitioner initially explores why they feel unable to share this information with other health professionals or their general practitioner [1]. After they have shared the information with a CAM therapist, the client may begin to feel more confident in sharing it with another therapist. Provided that confidential information is received respectfully by practitioners, the opportunity to open doors to successful and voluntary collaborative referral in the future is more likely to occur.

Record keeping and informed consent

Some clients share their health history in ways that are difficult to record in notes. For example, recording answers to open questions may be difficult compared with answers to closed questions [1]. Consultation sheets that help direct questioning and facilitate easy recording of case notes are helpful (see Appendix B). It is extremely important that practitioners are confident and comfortable in recording case histories because case notes are not only a summary of information elicited during a consultation but are also legal documents [1, 50]. For this reason it is vital that case notes have clear headings, are organised, are concise, are easily interpreted, provide summarised information and only convey necessary personal client identification in the event they are misplaced [1, 50].

Because clients have legal access to their case notes, it is wise to ensure nothing is written that the practitioner would not want the client to see [50]. Practitioners should be aware of the legal requirements in their state or country regarding client record keeping, mandatory reporting, privacy legislation, etc. [68].

Clients should give informed consent before undertaking any procedures, treatments or taking prescriptions [1, 15, 68]. Although it is not always possible for a client to be 'truly informed', there are a number of ways practitioners can help the client make informed decisions. Assessing potential literacy, language or competency barriers to informed consent is essential [1, 51], and judging whether the client has demonstrated competency to give informed consent may need to be done by more than one health professional. For informed consent to be valid the client must be able to understand information about their condition and treatment options, remember the information, weigh up treatment options and believe the information is relevant to them [51, 67, 68]. Providing clearly written information to the client (if appropriate) that explains the recommended treatments or medicines is a good start. Determining the client's prior knowledge of any therapy from the outset is also helpful, as is offering specific information and instructions for the client to read at home. Providing a list of helpful telephone numbers and links to research literature or websites may be appreciated by the client. Ideally 'informed consent' is an educational process and not just an act of the client signing their name to a procedure [51]. Providing a copied treatment form for the client to sign and keep, offering suitable visual or audio information and suggesting avenues for further education on a proposed therapy may all help to ensure the client's implicit understanding for the management of their health condition [1, 51]. One way this can be suggested is by expressing 'First I will explain what treatment/medicines I am recommending and give you information to take home and read. Then we can discuss how I think this can help you. Finally, I will talk with you about potential effects of the treatment and try to answer any questions you may have' [1]. Essentially the way in which information is conveyed can have a significant effect on the client's satisfaction with and their compliance to a treatment protocol.

Interviewing children

Consultations between children and practitioners can be positive and rewarding experiences for all concerned when both the child and the parent are involved in the process. Effectively interviewing children requires specific skills and questioning techniques. Communication ability, knowledge of paediatric stages of development and appropriate questioning techniques for children at different ages are all important [1]. Checking periodically that the child understandings the meaning of questions helps ensure their answers are genuine [45].

Children have limited attention spans and can be easily bored, so it is important that the consultation process is not excessively long. If children are bored and irritable then parents are more likely to be distracted. In such situations it may be better to conduct the initial consultation over two shorter sessions than in one long session.

Positive communication between practitioners and children is integral to achieving a holistic understanding for diagnosis and treatment. Even though the accompanying adult can offer specific information and may communicate the majority of information to the practitioner, it is important to gain insight into the child's perspective and experience of their condition [14]. Communication with children should happen in ways appropriate to their level of understanding and communication, and practitioners should ensure children feel comfortable and at ease [1, 14]. Sitting at the child's level and arranging furniture so they feel comfortable can help achieve positive communication and rapport. Not talking down to children is important to make them comfortable and at ease [1]. Toys and activities appropriate for the child's age and stage of development help keep them occupied and entertained, and make their experience more positive. Toys and games offered to children should be safe and appropriate for their age and hygiene must be maintained to minimise the risk of cross-infection [1]. Allowing children to handle equipment after the practitioner has used it, having spares for children to play with or by using equipment on parents, siblings or toys can help reduce their anxieties or apprehension about the consultation and examination process.

Including children in the consultation process requires sensitivity to both verbal and non-verbal cues; questions should be prioritised and kept as brief as possible. Children should be given breaks and activities throughout the session to ensure they don't become overwhelmed or distressed by the questioning process [45]. It is also important to observe the way children and parents/caregivers relate to each other during the consultation process – this can provide valuable insights into the family dynamic and the emotional and mental state of the child.

Children may have significant anxieties or fears about medical appointments, particularly if they have seen many different healthcare practitioners. If a child is distressed or anxious it is important for the practitioner to continue to talk in a calm and reassuring voice to maintain a sense of calmness and balanced energy [1]. Allowing them to be held by their parent may also be helpful in such situations. Using terminology the child is familiar with to describe their symptoms helps the child understand what you are asking and helps them more easily explain their problem [1]. Playing games involving open and closed questions is another way to gather necessary information without making the child feel pressured or uncomfortable [14, 45]. Younger children may respond well to using a favourite toy to role play their symptoms [1], and may be more comfortable if you include their toys in the examination [1, 14]. Examples of how this can be done include 'Let's look at teddy's tummy to see where it hurts', 'Can I look in Panda's eyes too?', 'What do you think dolly needs to feel better?', 'Can you show piggy how wide you can open your mouth?' [1]. Providing drawing or art material can also be very helpful because some children will be more easily able to communicate through a drawing. Asking a child to draw a picture about when they are feeling unwell and then asking them to tell you about their picture can provide significant insight into symptoms and underlying causes or concerns [14].

Challenging consultations

From time to time practitioners may experience clients showing signs of anxiety, anger, aggression or distress during consultations. It is wise to ensure your practice environment is close to other people/practitioners and your consultation space not isolated. In the event of a challenging consultation experience, there are strategies that can assist the practitioner to guide the consultation in a productive direction. In such situations it may be necessary to stay calm and spend time with the client to help calm and defuse their distress [1]. However, the safety and duty of care from a CAM practitioner does not include staying in a dangerous situation with a client and it is within professional boundaries to discontinue a consultation if necessary [1]. Overall, if a tense situation presents with a client the aim is to initially actively listen, summarise what the individual is trying to convey, be specific about your intentions as a practitioner, offer reassurance and acknowledge the emotion they are experiencing is understandable [1, 49, 50, 73]. Maintaining empathy and not interrupting the client's flow of expression [73, 74], being non-judgemental, keeping a safe physical distance [75] and making sure there are no objects nearby that could be used as a weapon is also very important [1]. The crucial aspect to focus on in these situations is helping the client understand they have choices while remembering as a practitioner you also have a choice about how long you want the consultation process to continue. Ensuring the client feels they have been heard and understood can help to de-escalate difficult situations [73, 74], but, in doing this, practitioners should ensure they don't make agreements or promises that can't be kept. Maintaining a calm and composed appearance, speaking calmly and quietly, avoiding excessive eye contact and maintaining even breathing may help defuse a tense situation [1, 75]. Recognising signs of anxiety or anger, such as sweating, flushing, trembling, rapid and changing speech, loss of eye contact, impatience and dramatically changing body language, can help the practitioner to modify their questioning approach in response to the client and ensure the consultation process remains positive and productive [1, 75]. It is helpful to have a protocol in place to deal with such situations, which can include placing office furniture to allow the practitioner easy access to the door, signals to alert others that help is needed and emergency numbers on speed dial [75].

Professional boundaries

Primary healthcare management has been defined as 'the provision of a patient's overall healthcare management including the monitoring of all treatments in progress with other providers as appropriate' [11]. Co-treatment is defined as the 'treatment of a patient in concert with the doctor providing primary care management of the patient' [11], and consulting treatment as the provision of 'a second opinion or ancillary care for a patient whose primary care management is being provided by another doctor' [11]. In countries where CAM practitioners do not practise as primary healthcare providers, they must be aware of the legal and ethical boundaries that control the practice of CAM in their state or country [68]. Practitioners should also be aware of the implications of laws relating to the legal boundaries of their healthcare practice, client privacy, disclosure of information, mandatory reporting, freedom of information, occupational health and safety and so on [68]. It is essential for practitioners to maintain up-to-date knowledge of all legislation that affects their practice and the ongoing professional education requirements of their professional association [68].

While there are differences in the roles and practice of CAM throughout the world, there is much that is common to all. All CAM practitioners who follow the fundamental principles of CAM look for information to provide insight not only into the primary diagnosis of organic disorders but also to explore all possible obstacles to the self-regulating capacity of an individual, which may include underlying emotional aspects of disease [7]. CAM practitioners generally take more time to consult with clients than conventional medical practitioners, which allows for the gathering of a wider spread of information [2], helping the practitioner recognise underlying or associated symptoms requiring referral to other healthcare professionals.

One particularly important aspect of the CAM consultation is the involvement of clients in the decision-making and treatment process [15, 68]. Many health consumers interested in CAM therapies are 'information seekers' who may come from a background of internet searching and self-prescribing [15]. To ensure clients have realistic expectations about what CAM therapies can accomplish, it is important for practitioners to be clear with clients about the role of the CAM practitioner [11, 13].

Reflective practice and self-care

Self-care as a practitioner and exercising reflective practice is extremely important and encourages healthy personal and professional relationships to develop [55, 58]. Setting aside time for self-questioning and assessment can enable the CAM practitioner to continually engage in personal growth and develop professionally [29]. This is particularly important for final-year and newly graduated students who may have a self-concept that is connected to their new identity as a CAM practitioner. During this period of applying their new knowledge in practice, anxiety can be prominent and assumptions that were previously taken for granted regarding people, health and illness are challenged [25, 28, 29, 55]. Reflective practice is a tool students and professionals can use to develop skills and knowledge and link theory into practice [29, 60]. In this way learning can develop through experience and conscientious reflective practice and evaluation for future action can be honestly assessed [29]. This enables the student or practitioner to be less reactive during the process of implementing a therapeutic process with a client [29, 59, 60]. In essence, this practice tool assists the integration of professional knowledge with reflection to gain a professional response arising from an authentic and conscious state of mind and emotion [56]. Using reflective practice process in daily practice can help practitioners develop new courses of action, explore various ways of problem solving, gain personal and professional development, build knowledge through experience and resolve uncertainty [55]. This process is part of lifelong learning [57] and taking time every week to engage in a reflective exercise and record these stages in a workplace diary can be a valuable key to professional development [58]. The six reflective stages are: selecting an incident to reflect upon (positive or negative); observing and describing the experience; analysing the scene (including roles other people played in the incident); interpreting the incident (including identifying the purpose of reflection); exploring alternatives for how the experience could be different; and identifying possible future action [29]. Professional associations can play an important part in the process of reflective practice by outlining requirements for professional practice and conduct, and providing new members with mentoring schemes.

Reflective questions for the CAM practitioner may include [29]:
• What did I do in the consultation?
• During the consultation what feelings did I notice come to the fore?
• Why did I do that in the consultation?
• What may have triggered those initial feelings that surfaced while taking the consultation?
• How could I have done that differently?
• What situations in consultations do I try to avoid?
• How did I know what to do in the consultation?
• What assumptions am I making about a client?
• What have I learned from doing it that way in the consultation?
• What do I need to do to deal with these feelings?
• What have I learned to do in the future?
• What tools or skills can I use to help me not react so emotionally during a consultation?

After progressing through the reflective process, the next step is to implement reflective practice by undertaking the action that has been decided upon [29]. This will include identifying what is to be achieved, how this will be done, when and where this practice will take place and who is going to be involved [29].

Self-care for practitioners encompasses a personal effort to practise general holistic principles in their own life. This may include time for family, friends, creative outlets, exercise, good dietary habits, rest and having clear professional boundaries [62–65]. If a CAM practitioner is clear on their professional role, then there is more scope for their clients to accept this. With strongly defined boundaries, it is easier for practitioners to determine the amount of energy to give to their role [61]. Furthermore, when this confidence in self-care and self-boundaries is obvious in a practitioner, clients are more likely to follow their lead, resulting in a more positive therapeutic process [62].

References

[1] M. Lloyd, R. Bor, Communication skills for medicine, third edn, Churchill Livingstone, Edinburgh, 2009.

[2] J. Silverman, S. Kurtz, J. Draper, Skills for Communicating with Patients, second edn, Radcliff Publishing, Oxford, 2000.

[3] U. Chugh, N. Agger-Gupta, E. Dillmann, D. Fisher, P. Gronnerud, J.C. Kulig, S. Kurtz, A. Stenhouse, The case for culturally sensitive healthcare: a comparative study of health beliefs related to culture in six north east Calgary communities, Citizenship and Heritage Secretariat, Alberta, Calgary, 1994.

[4] J. Jamison, Differential Diagnosis for Primary Care, second edn, Churchill Livingstone Elsevier, London, 2006.

[5] G. Egan, The skilled helper. A problem-management and opportunity-development approach to healing, seventh edn, Brooks/Cole, Pacific Grove CA, 2002.

[6] R. Neighbour, The Inner Consultation: how to develop an effective and intuitive consulting style, Radcliff Publishing, Oxon, 2005.

[7] P. Orrock, in: L. Chaitow, E. Blake, P. Orrock, M. Wallden, P. Snider, J. Zeff (Eds.), Naturopathic Physical Medicine: Theory and Practice for Manual Therapists and Naturopaths, Churchill Livingstone, Philadelphia, 2008.

[8] L. Chaitow, E. Blake, P. Orrock, M. Wallden, P. Snider, J. Zeff, Naturopathic physical Medicine: Theory and Practice for Manual Therapists and Naturopaths, Churchill Livingstone Elsevier, Philadelphia, 2008.

[9] D. Peters, L. Chaitow, G. Harris, S. Morrison, Integrating Complementary Therapies in Primary Care, Churchill Livingstone, London, 2002.

[10] J.E. (C) Pizzorno, M.T. Murray, H. Joiner-Bey, The Clinicians Handbook of Natural Medicine, second edn, Elsevier, 2008.

[11] S. El-Hashemy, Naturopathic Standards of Primary Care, CCNM Press, 2008.

[12] R. Newman-Turner, Naturopathic Medicine, Thorson's, Wellingborough, 1990.

[13] Medical Practitioners Act of Western Australia, 2008. Retrieved 6 November 2009 from http://www.slp.wa.gov.au/pco/prod/FileStore.nsf/Documents/MRDocument:12955P/$FILE/MedPrctnrsAct2008_00-b0-00.pdf?OpenElement

[14] S. Docherty, M. Sandelowski, Focus on Qualitative Methods Interviewing Children, Research in Nursing & Health 22 (1999) 177–185.

[15] P. McCabe, Tertiary Education in Naturopathy and Western Herbal Medicine, in: V. Lin, A. Bensoussan, S. Myers, P. McCabe, M. Cohen, S. Hill, G. Howse (Eds.), The Practice and Regulatory Requirements of Naturopathy and Western Herbal Medicine, School of Public Health, La Trobe University, Melbourne, 2005. Available from <www.health.vic.gov.au/pracreg/naturopathy.htm> accessed 18 October 2008.

[16] T. Jagtenberg, S. Evans, Global Herbal Medicine: A Critique, The Journal of Complementary Medicine 9 (2) (2003) 321–329.

[17] H.A. Baer, Why is the Australian Government Interested in Complementary Medicine? A Case Study of Economic Rationalism, Complementary Health Practice Review 12 (2007) 167 (DOI:10. 1177/1533210107306134).

[18] J.L. Zeff, The process of Healing: A unifying Theory of Naturopathic Medicine, Journal of Naturopathic Medicine 7 (1) (1997) 122–125.

[19] H. Lindlar, Philosophy of Natural Therapeutics, CW Daniel Co Ltd, Saffron Walden, 1993.

[20] National Centre for Complementary and Alternative Medicine 2002, What is complementary medicine? <http://nccam.nih.gov/health/whatiscam/#3> accessed 26 November 2009.

[21] C.J. Bonk, D.J. Cunningham, Searching for learner-centred, constructivist and sociocultural components of collaborative educational learning tools, in: C.J. Bonk, K.S. King (Eds.), Electronic collaborators: learner-centred technologies for literacy, apprenticeship, and discourse, L. Erlbaum Associates, New Jersey, 1998.

[22] M.A. Wolf, Older adults: learning in the third age. Information series no 358, Eric Clearinghouse, Columbus, Ohio, 1994.

[23] M. Tennant, P. Pogson, Learning and Change in the Adult Years, Jossey-Bass, San Francisco, 1995.

[24] C.E. Kennedy, Adulthood, in: C.J. Titmus (Ed.), Lifelong education for adults: an international handbook, Pergamon, Oxford, 1989.

[25] K. Ashcroft, L. Foreman-Peck, Learning and the reflective practitioner, Managing Teaching and Learning in Further and Higher Education, Falmer Press, London, 1994.

[26] G. Foley, Understanding Adult Education and Training, second edn, Allen & Unwin, St Leonards, NSW, 2000.

[27] J. Biggs, Western misperceptions of the Confucian-heritage learning culture, in: D. Watkins, J. Biggs (Eds.), The Chinese Learner: Cultural, Psychological, and Contextual influences, Comparative Education Research Centre and Melbourne: Australian Council for Educational Research, Hong Kong, 1996.

[28] R. Burns, The Adult Learner at Work: A Comprehensive Guide to the Context, Psychology and Methods of Learning for the Workplace, Business and Professional Publishing, Chatswood, NSW, 1995.

[29] M. Jasper, L. Wigens (Eds.), Beginning Reflective Practice. Foundations in Nursing and Healthcare, Nelson Thornes, Cheltenham, UK, 2003.

[30] D.M. Southern, D. Young, D. Dunt, N.J. Appleby, R.W. Batterham, Integration of primary healthcare services: perceptions of Australian general practitioners, non-general practitioner health service providers and consumers at the general practice-primary care interface, Evolution and Program Planning 25 (1) (2002) 47–59.

[31] D.H. Jeroen, A.A. Van Wijngaarden, R.H. de Bront, Learning to cross boundaries: The integration of a health network to deliver seamless care, Health Policy 79 (2–3) (2006) 203–213.

[32] S. Butelow, T. Kenealy, Evidence-based medicine: the need for a new definition, Journal of Evaluation in Clinical Practice 6 (2) (2000) 85–92.

[33] S. Mills, K. Bone, Principles & Practice of Phytotherapy; Modern Herbal Medicine, Churchill Livingstone, Edinburgh: London, 2000.

[34] L. Braun, M. Cohen, Herbs & Natural Supplements: An evidence based guide, second edn, Elsevier, Sydney, 2007.

[35] Guidelines for Levels and Kinds of Evidence to Support Indications and Claims For Non-Registerable Medicines, including Complementary Medicines, and other Listable Medicines, Therapeutic Goods Administration of Australia, 2001, retrieved 16 March 2010. http://www.tga.gov.au/docs/html/tgaccevi.htm.

[36] R.L. Nahin, S.E. Straus, Research into complementary and alternative medicine: problems and potential, British Medical Journal 322 (2001) 161–164.

[37] M. Stewart, Towards a global definition of patient-centered care, BMJ 322 (2001) 444–445.

[38] S. Kurtz, et al., Marrying content and process in clinical method teaching; enhancing the Calgary-Cambridge guides, Acad Med 78 (2003) 802–809.

[39] C. Goodwin, Conversation Organisation: interaction between speakers and hearers, Academic Press, New York, 1981.

[40] J. Ruusuvouri, Looking means listening: co-ordinating displays of engagement in doctor-patient interaction, Soc Sci Med 52 (2001) 1093–1108.

[41] G.M. Gazda, F.R. Asbury, F.J. Balzer, W.C. Childers, R.E. Phelps, R.P. Walters, Human Relations Development. A manual for educators, Allyn and Bacon, Boston, MA, 1995.

[42] D. Tuckett, M. Boulton, C. Olson, A. Williams, Meetings Between Experts: an approach to sharing ideas in medical consultations, Tavistock, London, 1985.

[43] S. Ackerman, M. Hilsenroth. A review of therapist characteristics and techniques positively impacting the therapeutic alliance, Clinical Psychology Review 23 (2003) 1–33.

[44] S.L. Hatcher, T.K. Favourite, E.A. Hardy, R.L. Goode, et al., An analogue study of therapist empathetic process: Working with difference, Psychotherapy: theory, Research, Practice, Training 42 (2005) 198–210.

[45] D.M. Keats, Interviewing; a practical guide for students and professionals, Open University Press, Philadelphia, 2000.

[46] M. Stewart, J.B. Brown, A. Donner, I.R. McWhinney, J. Oates, W.W. Western, J. Jordan, The Impact of Patient-Centred Care on Patient Outcomes, Jounal of Family Practice 49 (2000) 796–804.

[47] R. McCabe, et al., Engagement of patients with psychosis in the consultation; conversation analytic study, BMJ 325 (2002) 1148–1151.

[48] R. Berkow, A.J. Fletcher, M.H. Beers, The Merck Manual, sixteenth edn, Merck Research Laboratories, Rathway, NJ, 1993 (later edition).

[49] N.J. Talley, S. O'Connor, Pocket Clinical Examination, third edn, Churchill Livingstone Elsevier, Australia, 2009.

[50] G. Douglas, F. Nicol, C. Robertson, Macleod's Clinical Examination, twelfth edn, Churchill Livingstone Elsevier, Edinburgh, 2009.

[51] P. Kumar, C. Clark, Clinical Medicine, sixth edn, Elsevier Saunders, London, 2005.

[52] P. Glasziou, Evidence-Based Diagnosis in Primary Care, Churchill Livingstone Elsevier, 2008.

[53] R.H. Seller, Differential Diagnosis of Common Complaints, fifth edn, Saunders Elsevier, Philadelphia, 2007.

[54] R.D. Collins, Differential Diagnosis in Primary Care, fourth edn, Lippincott Williams & Wilkins, Philadelphia, 2008.

[55] S.D. Brookfield, Becoming a critically reflective teacher, Jossey-Bass, San Francisco, 1995.

[56] R. Bairbre, Reflection in action. Developing reflective practice in Health and Social services, Ashgate Publishing Limited, Hampshire, UK, 2006.

[57] J. Hay, Reflective Practice and Supervision for Coaches, Open University Press, Berkshire, UK, 2007.

[58] N. Chapman, S. Dempsey, H.M. Warren-Forward, Workplace diaries promoting reflective practice in radiation therapy, Radiography 15 (2) (2009) 166–170.

[59] L. Crawford, P. Morris, J. Thomas, M. Winter, Practitioner development: from trained technicians to reflective practitioners, International Journal of Project Management 24 (8) (2006) 722–733.

[60] A. Manning, P. Cronin, A. Monaghan, K. Rawlings-Anderson. Supporting Students in Practice: An exploration of reflective groups as a means of support, Nurse Education in Practice 9 (3) (2009) 176–183.

[61] E.L. Teasdale, Workplace Stress, Psychiatry 5 (7) (2006) 251–254.

[62] J.D. Quick, A.B. Henley, J. Campbell Quick, The Balancing act: At work and at home, Organizational Dynamics 33 (4) (2004) 426–438.

[63] J.D. de Jong, P. Heiligers, P.P. Groenewegen, L. Hingstman, Why are some medical specialists working part-time, while others work full-time? Health Policy 78 (2–3) (2006) 235–248.

[64] G.A. Adams, Relationships between time management, control, work-family conflict, strain, Journal of Occupational Health Psychology 4 (1999) 72–77.

[65] R. Ilies, K.M. Schwind, D.T. Wagner, M.D. Johnson, D.S. DeRue, D.R. Ilgen, When can employees have a family life? The effects of daily workload and affect on work-family conflict and social behaviours at home, Journal of Applied Psychology 92 (5) (2007) 1368–1379.

[66] D.J. Tataryn, Paradigms of health and disease: a framework for classifying and understanding complementary and alternative medicine, Journal of Alternative & Complementary Medicine 8 (6) (2002) 877–892.

[67] I.H. Kerridge, J.R. McPhee, Ethical and legal issues at the interface of complementary and conventional medicine, Medical Journal of Australia 181 (3) (2004) 164–166.

[68] M.H. Cohen, Legal and ethical issues in complementary medicine: a United States perspective, Medical Journal of Australia 181 (3) (2004) 168–169.

[69] P. Poorman, L. Kim, P. Mittman, Naturopathic medical education: where conventional, complementary and alternative medicine meet, Complementary Health Practice Review 7 (2) (2001) 99–108.

[70] V.F. Keller, J.G. Carroll, A new model for physician patient communication, Patient Education and Counselling 23 (2004) 131–140.

[71] P. Maguire et al., Helping cancer patients disclose their concern, European Journal of Cancer 32A (1) (1996) 78–81.

[72] W. Weston, J. Brown, M. Stewart, Patient-Centred Interviewing Part I: Understanding Patients' Experiences, Canadian Family Physician 35 (1989) 147–151.

[73] P. Maguire, C. Pitceathly, Managing the difficult consultation, Clinical Medicine 3 (2003) 532–537.

[74] J. Halpern, Empathy and patient-physician conflicts, Society of General Internal Medicine 22 (2007) 696–700.

[75] I.P. Sempowiski, R.J. Brison, Dealing with office emergencies: Stepwise approach for family physicians, Canadian Family Physician 48 (2002) 1464–1472.

Example of complete case analysis format: chronic candidiasis

Case history

Thirty-year-old Karishma Singh has come to the naturopathic clinic because she feels there is something not quite right with her body. She has been taking the oral contraceptive pill for one year and no longer feels good about taking it. Since Karishma started taking the pill she has experienced recurrent vulval itch and irritation and a discharge she describes as 'curdy, like white cottage cheese'. Her doctor confirmed a diagnosis of chronic vaginal *Candida* infection and recommended she use a cream from the chemist. The cream clears up the itch and discharge but does not prevent it from returning. When the symptoms of discharge and itch are particularly bad, Karishma explains that a pain/discomfort on urination is also experienced, which she forgot to tell her doctor. Karishma tells you she has been advised to have a cervical smear; however, she has never had one and is very nervous, so has not followed up yet. Her doctor wanted to do a pelvic examination but she refused and has only allowed an abdominal physical examination at this stage.

Karishma tells you she has not spoken to her GP yet regarding her digestion, which she feels has not been very good lately. She often feels bloated and is having problems with flatulence. Her bowel can go from diarrhoea to constipation within a few days and since she has been taking the pill her digestive symptoms seem to have gradually worsened. When you ask her about her stools she tells you they are usually a light brown colour when formed and watery brown when loose, and usually don't float. She has not noticed any blood or mucus in them.

Karishma has been with her partner, Dev, for seven years and is thinking she would like to try for a baby soon. They both feel the time is right to settle down and become parents, and because of this she is keen to stop taking the pill. After all, they managed to use condoms for contraception for six years before she tried the pill. She would like your help to get her body back into shape before she starts to try for a baby.

Karishma works in public relations and needs to dress well for her job. She wonders whether the pantyhose she wears each day are aggravating her symptoms because she feels better on the weekends when she doesn't wear them. Karishma hasn't noticed whether anything in her diet affects her symptoms, but she does crave sweets and chocolate and always has a pack of lollies in her bag to help with her sugar cravings and to keep her energy levels up.

Karishma and Dev would both like to see her symptoms cleared up permanently because they have significantly curtailed their sexual activity over the past year. They both realise if they want to get pregnant they need to sort this problem out!

The following table suggests some sample questions you might ask as a practitioner [1–13].

TABLE 2.1 **COMPLAINT**	
Analogy: Skin of the apple Using the mnemonic 'OUTER LAYER'	**Complaint:** Define the presenting complaint and symptoms. *Vaginal discharge*
AREAS OF INVESTIGATION AND EXAMPLE QUESTIONS	**CLIENT RESPONSES**
Onset	One year ago.
Understanding the cause (client)	Since taking the oral contraceptive pill (OCP).
Timing (duration, frequency) *How long does the discharge last and how often does it occur?*	*I have discharge every day unless I use cream from the doctor, which clears it up for a while. It comes back if I stop using it.*
Exacerbating factors	Pantyhose, which she wears on weekdays, may be aggravating her symptoms.
Relieving factors	Cream prescribed by her GP clears up the itch and discharge but does not prevent it from coming back again.
Location and radiation	Recurrent vulval itch and irritation.
Account and description *Describe the odour of the discharge.*	Feels like an itch and irritation and a discharge like 'curdy, like white cottage cheese'. *No strong odour.*
Your practitioner impression	Karishma is feeling nervous about sharing such intimate information regarding her symptoms. It seems that Karishma is holding back some information.
Examination and inspection	Refused a pelvic examination with her doctor but allowed an abdominal physical examination. No tenderness on palpation or bulky uterus or bladder was observed.
Rating scale *On of a scale of 1 to 10 how uncomfortable is the discharge?*	*It's an 8 out of 10 most days if I'm not using the cream, with 10 being the worst it can be. With the cream it is about a 3 out of 10.*

TABLE 2.2 **CONTEXT**	
Analogy: Flesh of the apple Using the mnemonic 'FACTORS OF DISEASE'	**Context:** Put the presenting complaint into context to understand the disease. Common contributing physical, dietary and lifestyle factors that may trigger the presenting complaint and differential diagnosis considerations.
AREAS OF INVESTIGATION AND EXAMPLE QUESTIONS	**CLIENT RESPONSES**
Family health history *Have any family members experienced serious illness or similar symptoms to you?*	*My mother often experiences bloating and has had an abnormal cervical smear in the past.*
Allergies and irritants *Is the vaginal itching worse after using soaps, bath oils, bubble baths, douches, perfume, lubricants or antifungal creams?* (chemical vaginitis, vulvodermatoses)	*The itching is usually better after having a bath. I do not usually use many chemicals in the bath or on my skin.*
Cancer and heart disease *Do you experience any bleeding during or after intercourse?*	Has been advised to have a cervical smear. *No, I've never had any bleeding other than menstrual blood that I know of.*
Trauma and pre-existing illness *Have you experienced illness in the past that has been concerning or ongoing?* *It would help me make an assessment of how to help you if I could understand more about your sexual relationships. Do you mind me asking you some more personal questions around your sexual history?* When have built up a therapeutic rapport: *Do you use any sex toys or insert foreign objects into your vagina that may have contributed to your urinary symptoms?*	*I have been very healthy up until I began taking the pill a year ago.* *I feel comfortable with you.* *We are not that adventurous!*
Obstruction *Have you ever experienced severe abdominal pain and fallen pregnant while taking the pill?* (ectopic pregnancy)	*No, I've taken the pill correctly.*
Recreational drug use *Do you or your partner have a history of recreational drug use, smoking or drinking alcohol?*	*No, neither Dev nor I smoke or take drugs. We do not drink alcohol either for religious reasons.*
Surgery and hospitilisation *Have you ever been pregnant or had any abortions?*	*No. Dev and I have been very careful with contraception over the years.*
Occupational toxins and hazards *Has there been any new building where you work over the past year?*	*I get to travel a bit with my work and go in and out of different environments. The building where I spend most of the time is in need of a lick of paint though!*
Functional disease	Feels bloated and is having problems with flatulence. Bowel can go from diarrhoea to constipation within a few days.

▶

Degenerative and deficiency diseases *How would you rate your energy levels and have you ever had conditions such as anaemia in the past?*	My energy levels drop significantly in the afternoon and can be about 5 out of 10. My GP has suggested having some blood tests to check my iron levels but I'm a bit scared of needles.
Infection and inflammation *Has Dev experienced similar symptoms to you, such as discharge or itching of genital region?* (STD spread of infection) *Do you wipe from the back to front when going to the toilet?* (recurrent vaginal infections spread from anus to vagina)	No blood or mucus in stools. No. Dev doesn't have any symptoms. I don't take much notice of the way I wipe myself. Is there a proper way?
Supplements and side effects medication/drugs *Have you been prescribed any specific medication such as penicillin, ampicillin or sulfa drugs while you have experienced vaginal itching?* (medication causes of vulva itching)	No. The only medication I've been on is the pill.
Endocrine/reproductive/sexual health	On the OCP. Would like to try for a baby soon.
Autoimmune disease *Is there any family history of coeliac disease?*	Not that I know of.
Stress and neurological *Can you tell me more about why you don't feel comfortable with your doctor giving you a pelvic examination?*	I've never had one before and don't understand what's involved.
Eating habits and energy and exercise	Would like your help to get her body back into shape. Craves sweets and chocolate and always has a pack of lollies in her bag to help with her sugar cravings and keep her energy levels up.

TABLE 2.3 **CORE**	
Analogy: Core of the apple with the seed of ill health Using the mnemonic 'SEEDS OF HEALTH'	**Core:** Holistic assessment to understand the client; contributing emotional, mental, spiritual, metaphysical, lifestyle and constitutional factors that are unique to the individual
AREAS OF INVESTIGATION AND EXAMPLE QUESTIONS	**CLIENT RESPONSES**
Support systems *What support do you need most at the moment?*	Your support, my GP and of course Dev.
Emotional health *Do you have any significant fears or anxieties at the moment?*	I'm really worried that this discharge will not go away and affect my chances of becoming pregnant.

▶

Environmental wellness *How much time do you spend watching TV, being on the computer or speaking on your mobile phone?*	*A lot of time for all of those that you mentioned. My work requires me to be on the computer and phones all the time and I like to relax by watching movies with Dev in the evening.*
Daily activities *Describe your lifestyle.*	*Well … I am really busy. I get up early to go to work in the city, I have family commitments and then I need to make time for Dev so our relationship can be nurtured. I feel like I am on the go most of the time.*
Stress release	She and her partner would like symptoms cleared up permanently because they have significantly curtailed their sexual activity over the past year.
Occupation *Tell me about your job.*	*I love my job. I love being busy and working with people. I like being in a team too. I have worked in PR for nearly five years now.*
Family and friends *Do you have time to relax with family or friends?*	*We have a large family circle and enjoy a lot of social time. Sometimes I need some space of my own away from family actually!*
Home life *Are you happy where you are living at the moment?*	*Yes, we are looking to buy in the next year or so to expand if we get pregnant.*
Education and learning *Do you feel like you understand enough about your contraception options?*	*No. I would really like some guidance with this because I get embarrassed about asking this sort of thing with my GP.*
Action needed to heal *What do you think is the most important aspect of your life that needs changing?*	*For Dev and I to be able to have more physical intimacy in our relationship.*
Long-term goals *Tell me more about how you feel about trying to have a baby in the future.*	*I think about it all the time right now. Dev seems keen too.*
Time to heal *How long have you abstained from sexual intercourse to assist the healing of your symptoms?*	*We can go a whole month or so without having sex. This gets frustrating for us both.*
Has not been well since *Describe a time you can remember when you felt extremely healthy.* *What was the trigger that changed your state of health?*	*I felt great about two years ago when I was not on the pill, exercising more and having more time with Dev.* *When Dev wanted to stop using condoms and I went on the pill so we could have more sexual freedoms! That didn't turn out so well after all.*

TABLE 2.4 **KARISHIMA'S SIGNS AND SYMPTOMS**	
Pulse	65 bpm
Blood pressure	130/85
Temperature	35°C
Respiratory rate	16 resp/min
Body mass index	23
Waist circumference	77 cm
Urinalysis	No abnormality detected (NAD)

TABLE 2.5 **RESULTS OF MEDICAL INVESTIGATIONS** [4, 6, 13]	
TEST	**RESULTS**
Urine test for beta-HCG (β-HCG)	NAD – this test is more sensitive than a urine test for pregnancy
Oral examination for leukoplakia: *Candida albicans*, lichen planus, nutrient deficiency, alcohol abuse, smoking; precancerous lesions	No sign of oral leukoplakia
Abdominal inspection: guarding, rebound tenderness, palpation, abnormal pulsations (auscultation)	No sign of appendicitis, pancreatitis, kidney swelling, enlarged liver, bowel obstruction, perforated ulcer

TABLE 2.6 **DIAGNOSTIC CONSIDERATIONS THAT HAVE BEEN RULED OUT** [1–3, 11, 12]	
CONDITION AND CAUSES	**WHY UNLIKELY**
OBSTRUCTION	
Intestinal obstruction: (bowel cancer, adhesions, hernias, faecal impaction with overflow); abdominal distension	No vomiting or weight change, no significant abdominal pain reported; abdominal physical examination indicated no obstruction
INFECTION AND INFLAMMATION	
Pancreatitis	No glucose in the urine
Gastritis	No fever
Cystitis	Urinalysis NAD
Glomerulonephritis (advanced kidney infection)	Urinalysis NAD (would show protein and possibly macrocytic blood and low specific gravity), no hypertension, no fever
Pyelenophritis (upper urinary tract infection)	Urinalysis NAD (no leucocytes present), no fever

▶

Renal calculi	Urinalysis NAD
Viral liver infection: retrovirus, hepatitis; diarrhoea, stools pale	No significant abdominal discomfort or weight loss reported; no history or signs of jaundice and symptoms of tiredness, nausea, fatigue or weight loss
Bacterial infection: e.g. *Yersinia enterocolitica*, *Escherichia coli*, *Shigella*, *Staphylococcal enterocolitis*, ileocaecal tuberculosis (TB); diarrhoea is the main symptom	Usually self-limiting and acute in duration between 1 and 10 days depending on bacterial toxin; violent vomiting can be associated; no symptoms of blood in diarrhoea and nausea; no fever
Parasitic intestine infection: giardia, amoebiasis; diarrhoea, stools become very pale	Stools do not float indicating no mucus; loss of appetite is not a dominant symptom; no nausea, abdominal discomfort, blood in diarrhoea or headache symptoms
ENDOCRINE/REPRODUCTIVE/SEXUAL HEALTH	
Pregnancy: can occur while taking the OCP; may give symptoms of thrush, digestive complaints, feeling that 'something is different' in the body	Urine pregnancy test negative – may be advised to follow up with blood test
Diabetes: vaginal discharge, thrush, itching, diarrhoea, abdominal bloating, craving sugar	No glucose in the urine
Pelvic inflammatory disease/salphingitis: vaginal discharge, sexually active	Karishma's menstrual cycle is regular, vaginal discharge is not purulent and offensive, no backache or lower abdominal pain reported; no period pain; unsure at this stage if there is pelvic pain; no fever; no pain on sexual intercourse reported; physical exam will indicate whether pain on motion of cervix; further investigation may still be warranted to rule out pelvic inflammatory disease (PID) caused by less symptomatic organism such as chlamydial PID [56]

TABLE 2.7 **CONFIRMED DIAGNOSIS 2**	
CONDITION	**RATIONALE**
Candidiasis (moniliasis, *Candida albicans*)/ vaginitis	Vaginal discharge can be curdy (most common in yeast infections), recurrent and chronic episodes; symptom of vulvovaginal itching (most common in *Candida* infection); symptoms worse after wearing pantyhose; Karishma has sweet cravings and feels tired; symptoms of bloating and alternating diarrhoea with constipation is experienced with a history of taking the OCP [53]; *Candida* is a common cause of vaginal discharge in adult women; physical exam may indicate vulval inflammation

Case analysis

TABLE 2.8 **POSSIBLE FURTHER DIFFERENTIAL DIAGNOSIS** [1–12]		
Not ruled out by tests/investigations already done		
CONDITION AND CAUSAL FACTORS	**WHY POSSIBLE**	**WHY UNLIKELY**
ALLERGIES AND IRRITANTS		
Lactose intolerance	Diarrhoea, abdominal pain	No indication that symptoms become worse with diet
CANCER AND HEART DISEASE		
Cervical cancer	Vaginal discharge, symptoms worse with sexual intercourse; mother has history of abnormal cervical cells	Need to ask if pain/blood is experienced on intercourse; vaginal discharge can appear with blood
Uterine cancer	Vaginal discharge	Usually brown discharge
TRAUMA		
Sexual abuse	Vaginal discharge, unwilling to allow physical pelvic examination	No sign of psychological trauma at this stage; need more sensitive investigation
FUNCTIONAL DISEASE		
Irritable bowel syndrome	Bloating, constipation and diarrhoea; watery stools; no mucus or blood in stools	Need to determine if Karishma experiences any abdominal pain and if pain is relieved by passing a bowel motion
Functional diarrhoea	Chronic diarrhoea, anxiety and uncertainty about bowel function; usually symptoms occur without abdominal pain; usually there is no bleeding, weight loss or ongoing fatigue	Bowel motions are usually watery and occur first thing in the morning with no more passing during the day; defecation may only occur after eating food
DEGENERATIVE AND DEFICIENCY		
Causal factor: **Bile acid malabsorption:** due to conditions such as Crohn's disease, coeliac disease, increased small intestine transit, diabetic diarrhoea, postinfective gastroenteritis	Under-diagnosed cause of chronic diarrhoea; when the terminal ileum fails to reabsorb bile salts it causes diarrhoea and increases colonic motility	No significant abdominal discomfort or weight loss reported

INFECTION AND INFLAMMATION		
Bacterial vaginosis: increase in aerobic bacteria (*Gardnerella vaginalis*) and decrease in lactobacilli [54, 57]	Vaginal discharge; common cause of vaginal discharge in adult women; common during the reproductive years	Odour of the discharge is not offensive (cheesy or fishy), watery and grey-white; discharge is usually homogeneous; itching is not a prominent symptom; no increased frequency of urination reported; usually no symptoms of vaginal inflammation
Trichomoniasis: a flagellated protozoon that causes vaginitis and urethritis, predominantly sexually transmitted; *Trichomonal vaginitis* often associated with gonococcal or *Bacteroides cervicitis* [54, 57]	Vaginal discharge, local irritation and itching; common cause of vaginal discharge in adult women; can produce vaginitis with coexisting urethritis that causes pain on urination; sexually active; common in women of child-bearing age	Vaginal discharge is usually frothy, profuse, white-greyish green, smelly discharge; increased frequency of urination not reported
Genital herpes: common cause of cervicitis	Vaginal discharge (more uncommon); more common in women aged under 35 years; can get secondary infection of *Streptococcus* or *Candida*; sexually active	Herpetic lesions are painful and can affect not only vulva but also thighs, buttocks, vagina and cervix; lesions extremely painful
Vulvar dermatoses: dermatitis, psoriasis, lichen sclerosus [53]	Vaginal itching	Need to determine whether the itching is predominantly vulvar (more common in dermatitis and eczema) or vulvovaginal (more common in *Candida*)
Parasites: scabies, lice, pinworms	Vaginal itching	No discharge usually associated
Causal factor: **Hygiene:** poor anal to vulvar hygiene, retained tampons, dirty condoms or foreign objects	Vaginal itching and discharge	Discharge is usually smelly; Karishma is not sure how she wipes
ENDOCRINE/REPRODUCTIVE/SEXUAL HEALTH		
Vulvovaginitis/vaginitis: *Candida albicans*, *Trichomonas*, chemical reaction/allergy to vaginal sprays, douches or bubble baths, chemical irritants, tight nylon panties, mixed bacterial infection, foreign bodies	Vaginal discharge, vaginal itching; pain on urination	There may be internal pain on urination; need to determine whether Karishma experiences any external pain on urination; need to determine whether Karishma experiences pain on intercourse (usually more common in vulvar disease rather than vaginitis); further investigation allows for definitive diagnosis [50]

Urethritis: *Chlamydia trachomatis, Mycoplasma, D streptococci, Trichomonas, Candida albicans,* gonorrhoeal, herpes urethritis, masturbation, foreign body, horseback or bike riding	Vaginal discharge, sexually active; no blood or pyuria in urine; pain on urination	Need to determine whether Karishma's pain on urination is felt as internal pain and worse at beginning of urine stream
Acute cervicitis: *Chlamydia trachomatis, Neisseria gonorrhoea,* herpes simplex virus [57]	Vaginal discharge can be produced by cervicitis without vaginal infection	Need to determine if pain is experienced on intercourse and associated with purulent discharge; physical exam will indicate whether there is pain on motion of cervix
Chronic cervicitis	Vaginal discharge	Usually profuse discharge with lumbosacral backache
Gonorrhoea	Vaginal discharge can be produced by gonorrhoea without vaginal infection; sexually active	Itching is not a common symptom; need to determine whether Karishma has had any recent rectal infections, pain on walking or climbing stairs; physical exam will indicate whether there is pain on motion of the cervix; vaginal discharge usually yellow in colour
Chlamydia	Vaginal discharge; can produce vaginitis with coexisting urethritis that causes pain on urination; sexually active	Need to establish if mucopurulent cervicitis is occurring; increased frequency of urination not reported; physical exam will indicate whether pain on motion of cervix; vaginal discharge is usually yellow in colour
Endometriosis	Vaginal discharge	Usually brown discharge with associated abdominal and pelvic pain
Physiologic leukorrhoea	Vaginal discharge; discharge is usually profuse, thick, greyish white and has no odour	Must occur in the absence of yeast infection or *Trichomonas*; itching is not usually associated; more common in girls beginning their menarche
SUPPLEMENT INTAKE AND SIDE EFFECTS		
Supplement or food additive abuse: excess vitamin C or magnesium	Diarrhoea	No weight loss reported; has said she is not taking any supplements or herbal remedies

▶

Medication dysbiosis reaction (e.g. *Pseudomembranous colitis*)	Diarrhoea and vaginal thrush symptoms caused by recent medication use; Karishma is taking the OCP	Karishma has not recently taken antibiotics (resulting in fungal overgrowth), laxatives, antihypertensives, nonsteroidal anti-inflammatory drugs (NSAIDs)
AUTOIMMUNE DISEASE		
Coeliac disease	Fluctuation between constipation and diarrhoea, feels bloated; mother has experienced bloating and digestive symptoms	No indication symptoms become worse with diet; no abdominal pain reported; no known family history of coeliac disease
STRESS AND NEUROLOGICAL		
Causal factor: **Emotional stress**	Diarrhoea alternating with constipation	Karishma is feeling anxious about the effect of her symptoms on her intimate relationship with Dev and feels under pressure to clear them up to have a baby

Working diagnosis

KARISHMA AND CANDIDIASIS

Karishma is a 30-year-old woman with symptoms of vaginal discharge that are curdy and white in appearance and are associated with vulval itch, irritation and pain on urination when symptoms are at their worse. A cream prescribed by her doctor for thrush helps clear up the vaginal discharge and itch for a period of time and then returns. Karishma has experienced a change in her digestion since being on the oral contraceptive pill and experiences more bloating, flatulence with alternating diarrhoea and constipation. Karishma and her long-term partner, Dev, would like to begin planning a family and are seeking guidance for how to clear the vaginal symptoms up permanently and reach optimal health for fertility.

Karishma has presented with symptoms of candidiasis, a vulvovaginal fungal infection with *Candida albicans*, which is extremely common for young women [53]. Any organ of the body can be infected by *Candida albicans*; however, vaginal infection and oral thrush are the most common. Predisposing factors include pregnancy, taking the oral contraceptive pill, diabetes, antibiotic use and being immune compromised [54, 55]. In women the dominant symptom is vulval irritation with vaginal discharge. Normal vaginal discharge depends on the stage of menstrual cycle the woman is in. Discharge can present as thick whitish discharge from vaginal wall, thick cervical discharge at time of ovulation or thinner cervical discharge before and after ovulation; normal volume can range from 60 mL to 700 mL for different women. The vaginal discharge associated with *Candida* can be thick, 'curdy' in character resembling cottage cheese, with no particular offensive odour [57]. It is possible to experience recurrent episodes of *Candida* symptoms causing the condition to become chronic in nature. Examination shows swelling and irritation of the vulvae with skin that can be broken and very sore. Pain on urination may be an additional symptom experienced when vulval irritation has become severe.

General references used in this diagnosis: 2, 3, 11, 12, 53

TABLE 2.9 **DECISION TABLE FOR TREATMENT PRIOR TO REFERRAL**		
COMPLAINT	**CONTEXT**	**CORE**
Treatment for the presenting complaint and symptoms *Vaginal discharge*	Treatment for all associated symptoms	Treatment for mental, emotional, spiritual, constitutional, lifestyle issues and metaphysical considerations
TREATMENT PRIORITY	**TREATMENT PRIORITY**	**TREATMENT PRIORITY**
• Lifestyle recommendations to manage acute symptoms and reduce recurrence • Physical therapy recommendations to manage acute symptoms and reduce recurrence • Dietary recommendations to reduce overgrowth of *Candida* • Herbal tonic or tea to reduce overgrowth of *Candida albicans* **NB:** Herbal tonic must not be taken if Karishma is pregnant • Nutritional supplements to restore microbial balance in the bowel	• Dietary recommendations to improve general health and digestive health • Herbal therapy to improve and normalise digestive function • Nutritional supplements to promote general health, vitality and digestive health	• Physical therapy recommendations to help reduce Karishma's stress • Herbal tonic or tea with nervine action • Herbal, nutritional and lifestyle treatment recommendations to alleviate symptoms so intercourse is not uncomfortable for Karishma; this will help reduce her stress and anxiety about the impact of her symptoms on her intimate relationship with Dev

TABLE 2.10 **DECISION TABLE FOR REFERRAL** [1–3, 5–12]		
COMPLAINT	**CONTEXT**	**CORE**
Referral for presenting complaint	Referral for all associated physical, dietary and lifestyle concerns	Referral for contributing emotional, mental, spiritual, metaphysical, lifestyle and constitutional factors
REFERRAL FLAGS	**REFERRAL FLAGS**	**REFERRAL FLAGS**
• Chronic vulval irritation and vaginal discharge • Recurrent thrush	• Symptoms have worsened since use of the OCP	• Unwillingness to allow a pelvic exam to be performed
ISSUES OF SIGNIFICANCE	**ISSUES OF SIGNIFICANCE**	**ISSUES OF SIGNIFICANCE**
Nil	• Digestive problems may be affecting absorption of nutrients • Sugar cravings	• Symptoms affecting sexual health and intimacy with partner
REFERRAL DECISION	**REFERRAL DECISION**	**REFERRAL DECISION**
• Referral for medical investigations to rule out pathologies such as bacterial vaginosis or a sexually transmitted infection (STI) [50]	• Dietary assessment and potential food allergy/intolerance evaluation	• Medical counselling on educating about procedures of having cervical smear and genital examination and exploring reasons for refusal

TABLE 2.11 **FURTHER INVESTIGATIONS THAT MAY BE NECESSARY** [1–6, 12]	
TEST/INVESTIGATION	**REASON FOR TEST/INVESTIGATION**
FIRST-LINE INVESTIGATIONS:	
Serum test for β-HCG	More sensitive than a urine test to test for pregnancy
Pelvic and genital examination [51]	Appearance of labia, vulva, entire vagina, cervix, vaginal discharge should be inspected; cervical manipulation for masses or points of tenderness; scabies, contact dermatitis; bulky uterus indicates uterine cancer; vulval inflammation more often in *Candida* than in bacterial vaginosis
Cervical smear [57]	Determine whether *Candida*, trichomoniasis, bacterial vaginosis
High vaginal swab (HVS) [51, 52, 55, 57]	*Candida* and *Streptococcus*
Wet mount findings: saline and potassium hydroxide [51, 57]	Candidiasis (hyphae or spores), bacterial vaginosis (clue cells), trichomoniasis (protozoa, white blood cells), physiologic leukorrhoea (lactobacillus)
Vaginal secretion pH [51]	*Candida* (moniliasis < 4.5), bacterial vaginosis (> 4.7), trichomoniasis (> 6.0), physiologic leukorrhoea (< 4.5)
Nucleic acid amplification tests (NAATS) with urine or vaginal swab [14]	Gonorrhoea, chlamydia (often simultaneous infection)
Endocervical and urethral swab [57]	Chlamydia and gonorrhoea
Hay-Ison criteria: gram-stained slide of vaginal secretions from posterior fornix [57]	Bacterial vaginosis
Tzanck smear	From genital lesion to diagnose genital herpes
IF NECESSARY:	
Stool test	Parasites, occult blood, infection, cancer
Fasting blood glucose test	Eliminate possibility of diabetes
Antigliadin antibody blood test and/or jejunal biopsy	Coeliac disease
Elimination food diets	Investigate food allergies and intolerances

Confirmed diagnosis

Karishma has candidiasis, vulvovaginitis and dysbiosis from long-term use of oral contraceptive pill.

PRESCRIBED MEDICATION

• Oral flucazanole plus antifungal pessaries

TABLE 2.12 **DECISION TABLE FOR TREATMENT (ONCE DIAGNOSIS IS CONFIRMED)**		
COMPLAINT	**CONTEXT**	**CORE**
Treatment for the presenting complaint and symptoms	Treatment for all associated symptoms	Treatment for mental, emotional, spiritual, constitutional, lifestyle issues and metaphysical considerations
TREATMENT PRIORITY	**TREATMENT PRIORITY**	**TREATMENT PRIORITY**
• Continue with lifestyle and physical therapy recommendations to manage acute symptoms and reduce recurrence • Continue with dietary recommendations to reduce overgrowth of *Candida* • Continue with herbal tonic or tea to reduce overgrowth of *Candida albicans* • Continue with nutritional supplements to restore microbial balance in the bowel **NB:** Collaborative management with Karishma's GP is essential to ensure optimal treatment outcomes	• Alternative contraception options • Continue with dietary recommendations to improve general health and digestive health • Continue with herbal therapy • Continue with nutritional supplements • Preconception care program to improve Karishma's general health and prepare her for a healthy pregnancy • Nutritional supplements as part of Karishma's preconception care program **NB:** It would be beneficial for Dev to come to the clinic for a consultation so a specific preconception program can be drawn up for him as well [38]	• Continue with physical therapy recommendations to help reduce stress • Continue with herbal tonic or tea with nervine action • Continue with treatment to alleviate symptoms that are impacting on Karishma's intimate relationship with Dev

Treatment aims

- Provide symptom relief from the vaginal itch and soreness and prevent recurrence of thrush infection.
- Heal and restore inflamed and irritated vulval and vaginal mucosa [17].
- Reduce overgrowth of *Candida albicans* yeast and normalise bowel flora [15, 16].
- Address any related syndromes such as small intestinal bacterial overgrowth and leaky gut syndrome [15, 16].
- Identify and remove/treat potential causative or aggravating factors (e.g. oral contraceptive pill, use of nylon pantyhose, dietary factors, impaired immune function, blood-sugar disorder] [15, 16, 54].
- Support Karishma's immune function [15, 16].
- Improve upper digestive tract function [15].
- Assess and modify Karishma's diet to reduce or eliminate foods that promote the overgrowth of *Candida* [15, 16] and identify and eliminate allergic substances [15, 16, 54].
- Ensure blood-sugar levels are balanced [16, 21].

- Discuss contraceptive alternatives to the oral contraceptive pill with Karishma, and commence a preconception care program [18], ensuring the recurrent candidasis is brought under control prior to achieving pregnancy [32].

Lifestyle alterations/considerations

- Discuss the possibility of alternative forms of contraception with Karishma [15].
- Encourage Karishma to avoid taking antibiotics [15, 54].
- Encourage Karishma to wear cotton underpants and avoid wearing pantyhose and using soap on her vulval region [15, 16, 58].
- Re-innoculate vagina with *Lactobacillus rhamnosus* and *Lactobacillus gasseri* once treatment to kill *Candida* in the vulvovaginal area has been completed [33]. Probiotics can be applied via a pessary or mixed into yoghurt [33].
- Treat Dev topically with an antifungal cream [16, 32] to help prevent reinfection.
- Karishma and Dev should abstain from sexual intercourse until treatment of active vaginal infection has been completed [32].

Dietary suggestions

- Avoid foods high in simple carbohydrates, sugar and *trans* fats. Reduce consumption of saturated fats [15, 16, 22].
- Encourage Karishma to eat a nutrient-dense, antioxidant-rich whole-food diet to enhance her general health and immune function [15].
- She may find benefit from avoiding foods with a high yeast or mould content (such as cheese, alcohol, peanuts, dried fruit, yeasted bread and mushrooms) [15, 16].
- Encourage Karishma to minimise consumption of dairy foods because high lactose consumption may promote growth of *Candida albicans* [15].
- Encourage Karishma to regularly include omega-3-rich foods in her diet – they enhance adhesion of probiotics to the intestinal wall [34].
- Karishma could try to include 2–5 g of fresh garlic (bruised or crushed) in her diet each day. Garlic has antifungal and antioxidant properties, which are beneficial to her [16, 19].
- Encourage Karishma to eat a low glycaemic index/glycaemic load (GI/GL) diet to help balance her blood-sugar levels [21, 23].
- Identify and manage food allergies or intolerances [15, 16].
- Encourage Karishma to include soluble fibre in her diet each day to help promote the growth of healthy bowel flora [16, 31].

Physical treatment suggestions

- Acupuncture may be helpful to enhance Karishma's fertility through its effects on uterine blood flow [36].
- Massage therapy may help relax Karishma and reduce her stress levels [37].
- Hydrotherapy: vaginal douche with acidophilus yoghurt, diluted apple cider vinegar, tea tree oil, slippery elm, thyme and witch hazel for *Candida* [46]. Take a sitz bath with apple cider vinegar and oatmeal for 10–15 minutes for at least three days in a row for *Candida* [46]. An alternating hot (3 min) and cold (1 min) shower locally to the abdomen for bloating and digestive symptoms [46, 49]. To tone the abdomen apply a cold-wet compress, covering the abdomen with a dry towel and elastic bandage wrapped around the trunk at night for at least three months [46]. Take hot shallow baths and/or hot foot baths for stomach bloating [46]. Try constitutional hydrotherapy [47, 48].

TABLE 2.13 **HERBAL FORMULA (1:2 LIQUID EXTRACTS)**		
HERB	FORMULA	RATIONALE
Golden seal *Hydrastis canadensis* (cultivated/plantation source)	30 mL	Anti-inflammatory [42]; mucous membrane trophorestorative [19, 42]; antimicrobial [19, 43]; vulnerary [44]; traditionally used for digestive disorders [45]
Pau d' Arco *Tabebuia avellanedae*	60 mL	Immunostimulant [20, 44]; antifungal [20, 44]; antibacterial [20, 44]; antiparasitic [20, 44]
Gentian *Gentiana lutea*	10 mL	Bitter digestive stimulant [19, 44]; inhibits *Candida* overgrowth [15]
St Mary's thistle *Silybum marianum*	60 mL	Liver tonic [19, 20]; antioxidant [19, 20]; anti-inflammatory [19]; improves digestive function [19, 20]
Chamomile *Matricaria recutita*	40 mL	Antifungal [19, 20]; anti-inflammatory [19, 20]; helps relieve flatulence [19]; nervine [19, 20]
Supply:	200 mL	Dose: 5 mL 3–4 times daily

Tea tree oil (*Melaleuca alternifolia*)
Pessary or a tampon saturated with a 20% emulsified solution of tea tree oil can be inserted intravaginally each night to treat active vaginal *Candida* infection for a period of 5–7 days [19]; anti-fungal [19, 20]; antibacterial [19, 20]

Chaste tree (*Vitex agnus castus*) tablet equivalent to 2 g dried fruit daily or 2.5 mL liquid extract first thing in the morning [19]; helps to normalise hormonal balance following use of the OCP [19, 20]; to be used to assist Karishma's cycle to normalise once she ceases taking the OCP

TABLE 2.14 **HERBAL TEA**		
Alternative to herbal liquid if Karishma prefers a tea		
HERB	FORMULA	RATIONALE
Calendula flowers *Calendula officinalis*	1 part	Antifungal [19, 44]; anti-inflammatory [19, 44]; immunomodulator [19]; antioxidant [19]
Golden seal root *Hydrastis canadensis* (cultivated/plantation source)	1 part	See above
Chamomile flowers *Matricaria recutita*	2 parts	See above
Pau d' Arco bark *Tabebuia avellanedae*	2 parts	See above
Decoction: 1 tsp per cup – 1 cup 3 times daily		

TABLE 2.15 **NUTRITIONAL SUPPLEMENTS**	
SUPPLEMENT AND DOSE	**RATIONALE**
Saccharomyces boulardii 1 g daily [24]	Inhibits bowel concentrations of *Candida albicans* [24]
High-potency practitioner-strength **probiotic supplement** containing human strain organisms including *Lactobacillus acidophilus*, *Lactobacillus rhamnosus*, *Lactobacillus plantarum* and *Lactobacillus fermentum* [27–29] Dose as recommended by manufacturer	Probiotic supplementation is effective in treating and preventing overgrowth of *Candida albicans* in the intestinal tract [25, 28, 29] and helps strengthen the body's natural resistance to *Candida albicans* [26, 28]
High-potency practitioner-strength **multivitamin, mineral and antioxidant supplement** providing therapeutic doses of vitamins and minerals [15, 16]; ensure it includes a therapeutic dose of chromium to support normal blood glucose levels [19, 21] Dose as recommended by manufacturer	To support general health and enhance nutrient status; part of a preconception care program [30, 38, 39]
Omega-3 fish oil 1000 mg capsule twice daily [35]	Omega-3 oils help probiotics to adhere to mucosal surfaces [34]; an important part of a preconception care program due to the role of omega-3 fatty acids in reducing the risk of premature birth [40, 41] and enhancing fetal growth [40]

References

[1] R.H. Seller, Differential Diagnosis of Common Complaints, fifth edn, Saunders Elsevier, Philadelphia, 2007 383–392.

[2] P. Kumar, C. Clark, Clinical Medicine, sixth edn, Elsevier Saunders, London, 2005, pp. 91–92, 127–128, 214, 1283–1284.

[3] J. Jamison, Differential Diagnosis for Primary Care, second edn, Churchill Livingstone Elsevier, London, 2006 pp. 317–319.

[4] N.J. Talley, S. O'Connor, Pocket Clinical Examination, third edn, Churchill Livingstone Elsevier, Australia, 2009, p. 104.

[5] R.D. Collins, Differential Diagnosis in Primary Care, fourth edn, Lippincott Williams & Wilkins, Philadelphia, 2008 p 448.

[6] G. Douglas, F. Nicol, C. Robertson, Macleod's Clinical Examination, twelfth edn, Churchill Livingstone Elsevier, Edinburgh, 2009, pp. 94, 245, 404, 405.

[7] J. Silverman, S. Kurtz, J. Draper, Skills for Communicating with Patients, second edn, Radcliff Publishing, Oxford, 2000.

[8] R. Neighbour, The Inner Consultation: how to develop an effective and intuitive consulting style, Radcliff Publishing, Oxon, 2005.

[9] D. Peters, L. Chaitow, G. Harris, S. Morrison, Integrating Complementary Therapies in Primary Care, Churchill Livingstone, London, 2002.

[10] M. Lloyd, R. Bor, Communication Skills For Medicine, third edn, Churchill Livingstone Elsevier, Edinburgh, 2009.

[11] A. Polmear (Ed.), Evidence-Based Diagnosis in Primary Care, Churchill Livingstone Elsevier, Edinburgh, 2008 pp. 274–283.

[12] R. Berkow, A.J. Fletcher, M.H. Beers, The Merck Manual, sixteenth edn, Merck Research Laboratories, Rathway, N.J, 1993 (later edition).

[13] K.D. Pagna, T.J. Pagna, Mosby's Diagnostic and Laboratory Test reference, third edn, Mosby, USA, 1997 (later edition) pp. 846–859.

[14] E. Van Dyck, M. Ieven, S. Pattyn, L. Van Damme, M. Laga, Detection of Chlamydia trachomatis and Neisseria gonorrhoeae by Enzyme Immunoassay, Culture and Three Nucleic Acid Amplification Tests, Journal of Clinical Microbiology, vol. 39, (No 5) (May 2001) 1751–1756.

[15] J.E. Pizzorno, M.T. Murray, H. Joiner-Bey, The Clinicians Handbook of Natural Medicine, second edn, Churchill Livingstone, St Louis, 2008.

[16] H. Osiecki, The Physician's Handbook of Clinical Nutrition, seventh edn, BioConcepts Publishing, Eagle Farm, 2006.

[17] R. Berkow, A.J. Fletcher, The Merck Manual, sixteenth edn, Merck Research Laboratories, Rathway, N.J, 1992.

[18] H.D. Reynolds, Preconception Care; An Integral Part of Primary Care for Women, Journal of Nurse-Midwifery 43 (6) (1998) 445–458.

[19] L. Braun, M. Cohen, Herbs & Natural Supplements: An evidence based guide, second edn, Elsevier, Sydney, 2007.

[20] S. Mills, K. Bone, Principles & Practice of Phytotherapy: Modern Herbal Medicine, Churchill Livingstone, Edinburgh: London, 2000.

[21] G. Donders, H. Prenen, G. Verbeke, R. Reybrouck, Impaired tolerance for glucose in women with recurrent vaginal candidiasis, American Journal of Obstetrics and Gynecology 187 (4) (2002) 989–993.

[22] S.L. Vargas, C.C. Patrick, G.D. Ayers, W.T. Hughes, Modulating Effect of Dietary Carbohydrate Supplementation on Candida Albicans Colonisation and Invasion in a Neutropenic Mouse Model, Infection and Immunity 61 (2) (1993) 619–626.

[23] A. Akpan, R. Morgan, Oral Candidiasis, Postgraduate Medical Journal 78 (2002) 455–459.

[24] L.V. McFarland, P. Bernasconi, Saccharomyces boulardii: A Review of an Innovative Biotherapeutic Agent, Microbial Ecology in Health and Disease 6 (1993) 157–171.

[25] R.D. Wagner, C. Pierson, T. Warner, M. Dohnalek, J. Farmer, L. Roberts, M. Hilty, E. Balish, Biotherapeutic Effects of Probiotic Bacteria on Candidiasis in Immunodeficient Mice, Infection and Immunity 65 (10) (1997) 4165–4172.

[26] S. Payne, G. Gibson, A. Wynne, B. Hudspith, J. Brostoff, K. Tuohy, In Vitro Studies on Colonization Resistance of the Human Gut Microbiota to Candida albicans and the Effects of Tetracycline and Lactobacillus plantarum LPK, Current Issues in Intestinal Microbiology 4 (2003) 1–8.

[27] M.S. Sanders, T.R. Klaenhammer, The Scientific Basis of Lactobacillus acidophilus NCFM functionality as a Probiotic, Journal of Dairy Science 84 (2001) 319–331.

[28] M.E. Falagas, G. Betsi, S. Athanasiou, Probiotics for prevention of recurrent vulvovaginal candidiasis: a review, Journal of Antimicrobial Chemotherapy 58 (2006) 266–272.

[29] P. Cadieux, J. Burton, G. Gardiner, I. Braunstein, A. Bruce, C.Y. Kang, G. Reid, Lactobacillus Strains and Vaginal Ecology, Journal of the American Medical Association (15) (2002) 1940–1941.

[30] A.E. Czeizel, Prevention of congenital abnormalities by periconceptional multivitamin supplement, British Medical Journal 306 (1993) 1645–1648.

[31] M. Blaut, Relationship of probiotics and food to intestinal microflora, European Journal of Nutrition 41 (S1) (2002) I11–I16.

[32] B. Foxman, The Epidemiology of Vulvovaginal Candidasis: Risk Factors, American Journal of Public Health 80 (3) (1990) 329–331.

[33] S. Coudeyras, G. Jugie, M. Vermerie, C. Forestier, Adhesion of Human Probiotic Lactobacillus rhamnosus to Cervical and Vaginal Cells and Interaction with Vaginosis-Associated Pathogens, Infectious Diseases in Obstetrics and Gynaecology (2008) 549–640.

[34] P.E. Kankaanpaa, S.J. Salminen, E. Isolauri, Y.K. Lee, The influence of polyunsaturated fatty acids on probiotic growth and adhesion, FEMS Microbiology Letters 194 (2) (2001) 149–153.

[35] H. Osiecki, The Nutrient Bible, seventh edn, AG Publishing, Eagle Farm, 2008.

[36] R. Chang, P.H. Chung, Z. Rosenwaks, Role of acupuncture in the treatment of female infertility, Fertility and Sterility 78 (6) (2002) 1149–1153.

[37] C.A. Moyer, J. Rounds, J.W. Hannum, A Meta-Analysis of Massage Therapy Research, Psychological Bulletin 130 (1) (2004) 3–18.

[38] F. Naish, J. Roberts, The Natural Way to Better Babies, Random House, Sydney, 1996.

[39] C.L. Keen, M.S. Clegg, L.A. Hanna, L. Lanoue, J.M. Rogers, G.P. Daston, P. Oteiza, et al., The Plausibility of Micronutrient Deficiencies Being a Significant Contributing Factor to the Occurrence of Pregnancy Complications, The Journal of Nutrition 133 (2003) 1597S–1605S.

[40] P. Saldeen, T. Saldeen, Women and omega-3 Fatty acids, Obstetrical Gynecological Survey 59 (10) (2004) 722–730.

[41] A.P. Simopoulos, The importance of the ratio of omega-6/omega-3 essential fatty acids, Biomedicine and Pharmacotherapy 56 (2002) 365–379.

[42] M. Predny, J. Chamberlain, Goldenseal (Hydrastis canadensis): An annotated bibliography. Gen Tech Rep SRS-88, US Department of Agriculture, Forest Service, Southern Research Station, Asheville, NC, 2005 Retrieved 7 September 2009 from http//www.sfp.forprod.vt.edu/.

[43] F. Scassocchio, M.F. Cometa, L. Tomassini, M. Palmery, Antibacterial activity of Hydrastis canadensis extract and its major isolated alkaloids, Planta Med 67 (6) (2001) 561–564.

[44] S. Mills, K. Bone, The Essential Guide to Herbal Safety, Churchill Livingstone, St Louis, 2005.

[45] British Herbal Medicine Association, British Herbal Pharmacopoeia, BHMAA, 1983.

[46] D.D. Buchman, The complete book of water healing, Contemporary Books, McGraw-Hill Companies, New York, 2001.

[47] W. Boyle, A. Saine, Lectures in Naturopathic Hydrotherapy, Eclectic Medical Publications, Oregon, 1988.

[48] L.M. Watrous, Constitutional hydrotherapy: from nature cure to advanced naturopathic medicine, Journal of Naturopathic Medicine 7 (2) (1997) 72–79.

[49] E. Blake, in: L. Chaitow, E. Blake, P. Orrock, M. Wallden, P. Sinder, J. Zeff (Eds.), Naturopathic Physical Medicine: Theory and Practice for Manual Therapists and Naturopaths, Philadelphia, Churchill Livingstone Elsevier, 2008.

[50] A. Cleveland, Vaginitis: finding the cause prevents treatment failure, Cleveland Clin J Med 67 (2000) 634–646.

[51] K.K. Fox, F.M.T. Behets, Vaginal discharge: how to pinpoint the cause, Postgrad Med 98 (1995) 87–104.

[52] E. Jungmann, A.M. Johnson, G. Ridgway, et al., How useful are high vaginal swabs in general practice? Results of a multicentre study, Int J STD AIDS 15 (2004) 238–239.

[53] B. Welsh, A. Howard, K. Cook, Vaginal itch, Australian Fam Physician 33 (2004) 505–510.

[54] H. Mitchell, Vaginal discharge – causes, diagnosis and treatment, BMJ 328 (7451) (2004) 1306–1308.

[55] B.R. Rowe, M.N. Logan, I. Farrell, et al., Is candidiasis the true cause of vulvovaginal irritation in women with diabetes mellitus? J Clin Pathol 43 (1990) 644–645.

[56] I. Simms, F. Warburton, L. Westrom, Diagnosis of pelvic inflammatory disease: time for a rethink, Sex Transm Infect 79 (6) (2003) 491–494.

[57] L. French, J. Horton, M. Matousek, Abnormal vaginal discharge: using office diagnostic testing more effectively, J Fam Pract 53 (10) (2004) 805–814.

[58] G. Fisher, Treatment of vaginitis and vulvitis, Australian Prescriber 24 (3) (2001) 59–61.

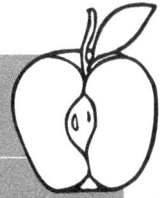

CHAPTER 3

Gastrointestinal system

Peptic ulcer

Case history

Forty-year-old Dan Noble has come to the clinic for help with digestive discomfort. Dan has been experiencing episodic problems with heartburn and uncomfortable burning or gnawing sensations in the centre of his abdomen that seem to occur about an hour after eating. Sometimes Dan also experiences heartburn or discomfort at night when he is in bed. When he gets a particularly bad episode he initially feels a sharp pain that then seems to become more like a dull ache after a while; it may last a couple of hours. The pain will often come on when he is hungry and before he eats a meal. He hasn't had any recurrent vomiting or diarrhoea accompanying his symptoms but sometimes feels a bit nauseous. He does remember vomiting one time when he had a bad episode and it relieved the symptoms of pain. He thought he must have had a stomach bug.

Dan finds that if he eats something his symptoms usually improve, although his appetite on the whole has decreased significantly. When symptoms are bad he gets a feeling of fullness very quickly after eating. He went to his local pharmacy and was given a bottle of antacid liquid, which does improve his symptoms.

Dan tells you he is the principal of a small independent school. He loves his job, but things have been quite stressful for the past couple of years because the school has been undergoing some major changes as they implement new policies and procedures for both teaching and administrative staff, as well as undertaking a new building program. He feels his stress levels have been quite high in the past but are now lessening because the new buildings have now been completed and staff seem to have adjusted to the changes.

Dan has been experiencing the symptoms on and off for about six months, but they seem to be getting worse and occurring more frequently. His wife tells him he is stressed and has lost weight so has suggested he might be able to get herbal or nutritional supplements to help with his stress.

When you ask Dan about other symptoms he tells you he sometimes gets tension headaches, particularly if he's had a busy week. He usually takes aspirin or ibuprofen, which work well for him. Apart from the stomach problems and occasional headaches Dan says he feels pretty good most of the time. He drinks 5–6 cups of coffee a day and more if things are particularly busy and he needs to keep going. He also often works through his lunch break and eats when he can, which is often on the run. Dan has noticed if he eats spicy foods he is more likely to experience the stomach problem, so he usually avoids it. Dan doesn't drink alcohol during the week, but will relax on the weekends with a bottle or two of red wine.

Dan realises he needs to manage his stress better and is hoping that reducing his stress will improve his digestive symptoms.

TABLE 3.1 **COMPLAINT** [1–11]	
Analogy: Skin of the apple	**Complaint:** Define the presenting complaint and symptoms; understand the complaint *Abdominal discomfort*
AREAS OF INVESTIGATION AND EXAMPLE QUESTIONS	**CLIENT RESPONSES**
Location and radiation *Does the pain always stay in the same area?*	Centre of his abdomen *Yes. It never seems to move to anywhere else.*
Your practitioner impression	Dan appears tense and uncomfortable; he shuffles in his seat. He appears physically and emotionally uncomfortable. Seems lacking in vitality.
Rating scale *On a scale of 1 to 10 how would you rate the abdominal discomfort, with 10 being as bad as can be?*	*When I get a sharp pain it is 8 out of 10 and when there is the dull ache it is about 6 out of 10.*

TABLE 3.2 **CONTEXT**	
Analogy: Flesh of the apple	**Context:** Put the presenting complaint into context to understand the disease
AREAS OF INVESTIGATION AND EXAMPLE QUESTIONS	**CLIENT RESPONSES**
Cancer and heart disease *Do you experience indigestion that is usually only related to physical activity?* (angina)	*No. I can often feel it when I am lying still.*
Functional disease *So would you say your indigestion is not related to physical activity?* (heartburn, oesophageal reflux)	*I can get the pain when I am still or when I am moving but most often when I am not moving.*

TABLE 3.3 **CORE**	
Analogy: Core of the apple with the seed of ill health	**Core:** Holistic assessment to understand the client
AREAS OF INVESTIGATION AND EXAMPLE QUESTIONS	**CLIENT RESPONSES**
Daily activities *How often does the abdominal discomfort disturb you during the night?*	*If I don't take the antacids I can be up most nights for a week and then it will settle down a bit.*

▶

▶ Action needed to heal	
What do you think is important to do for your symptoms to clear up in the short term?	*Coming today to see you to help with the stomach pain and stress levels. Maybe have more medical tests to find out what the pain actually is because it doesn't seem to be going away in a hurry.*

TABLE 3.4 **DAN'S SIGNS AND SYMPTOMS**	
Pulse	90 bpm
Blood pressure	120/75 sitting
Temperature	37°C
Respiratory rate	14 resp/min
Body mass index	21.5
Waist circumference	80.8 cm
Urinalysis	No abnormality detected (NAD)

Results of medical investigations

No medical investigations have been carried out yet.

TABLE 3.5 **UNLIKELY DIAGNOSTIC CONSIDERATIONS** [2, 7, 8, 10, 11, 54]	
CONDITIONS AND CAUSES	**WHY UNLIKELY**
CANCER AND HEART DISEASE	
Congestive heart failure	Blood pressure within normal limits; urinalysis NAD
Cluster headaches: common to begin in males between the ages of 40 and 60; no family history associated with cluster headaches	Extremely severe headaches, stabbing and burning; usually unilateral and pain behind eye radiating to the front of the face
INFECTION AND INFLAMMATION	
Kidney infection	Abdominal pain usually is lower and will radiate to lower back and groin rather than upper abdomen and shoulder; no urine crystals and red blood cells
Sinus headache: headache worse on waking in the morning	No upper respiratory symptoms mentioned, no frontal facial pain reported; need to check if dull ache is aggravated by bending
ENDOCRINE/REPRODUCTIVE	
Diabetes: delayed gastric emptying and complains of early fullness, nausea, bloating	Urinalysis NAD

Case analysis

TABLE 3.6 **POSSIBLE DIFFERENTIAL DIAGNOSIS**		
Not ruled out by tests/investigations already done [2, 7–11, 55, 57, 59, 61, 65]		
CONDITIONS AND CAUSES	WHY POSSIBLE	WHY UNLIKELY
CANCER AND HEART DISEASE		
Angina: brought on by physical activity and emotion; will be relieved by nitroglycerin	Burning sensation in chest, fast pulse	Usually not related to eating or abdominal symptoms; acute onset of symptoms; pain relieved by lying down
Gastric tumour: can have history of *Helicobacter pylori* (*H. pylori*) infection [67]	Pain relieved by food or antacids nausea; early satiety, weight loss, lack of appetite	May present with diarrhoea; no mention of blood or mucus in stools, abdominal distension or frequent vomiting; pain made worse or relieved by food
OBSTRUCTION AND FOREIGN BODY		
Acute gallstone pancreatitis: pain in the abdomen that is radiating, nausea, decreased appetite; commonly caused by gallstones that block the pancreatic drainage; often associated with alcoholic binges	Pain in upper abdomen	Upper abdominal pain usually radiates to the lower back; usually associated with significant fever, nausea, vomiting and change in bowel motions; will usually have lower abdominal symptoms such as flatulence
OCCUPATIONAL TOXINS AND HAZARDS		
Causal factor: **Sick building syndrome**	Headaches worse after working several days in a row; new buildings recently constructed	No upper respiratory complaints or fatigue reported
Causal factor: **Eye strain**	Headaches will generally occur after several days at work	Unusual unless work requires close vision or eyeglasses are not appropriate
FUNCTIONAL DISEASE		
Causal factor: **Intestinal gas:** from decreased motility and overgrowth of bacteria	Indigestion	More common in the elderly, vague symptoms of abdominal discomfort; will have lower abdominal symptoms such as flatulence
Causal factor: **Gas entrapment:** hepatic or splenic flexure syndrome	Can have abdominal discomfort that is referred as chest pain	Made worse by bending over
Causal factor: **Duodenal loop distention**	Indigestion, nausea	Specific to right upper quadrant pain, or pain in the right shoulder

▶

▶

Causal factor: **Hiatus hernia**	Heartburn, indigestion when associated with oesophagitis	Heartburn is a rare symptom of hiatus hernia unless accompanied by oesophagitis
Functional gastrointestinal disorder	Can have indigestion symptoms made worse by stress	No reports of diarrhoea alternating with constipation; symptoms would be vague and non-specific if a functional disorder; usually continuous pain with no significant weight loss; will have lower abdominal symptoms such as flatulence
Heartburn: not usually related to physical activity, brought on by oesophageal spasm [53]	Burning sensation in the chest, felt when lying down, caffeine frequently causes symptoms; pain related to meals and made worse by lying down	Pain would be intermittent over several minutes and recur over long periods; pain would radiate to the neck, jaw, arms and back; pain would be felt after heavy meals and bending over; certain foods can cause and relieve heartburn
Non-ulcer dyspepsia: may have *H. pylori*; pain or discomfort in the centre of the chest/upper abdomen [53, 56, 58]	Upper abdominal pain, feeling full quickly after eating, lack of appetite, nausea, belching, vomiting, bloating, burning sensation in chest or abdomen	No difficulty swallowing or vomiting mentioned by Dan; symptoms at night rare with non-ulcer dyspepsia; pain is usually worse after eating and not usually relieved by antacids with non-ulcer dyspepsia; diffuse abdominal pain is more common than precise location
Reflux-dyspepsia Oesophageal reflux (gastro-oesophageal reflux disease, GORD; gastroesophageal reflux disease, GERD)/peptic oesophagitis/spasm: pain not brought on by exercise; may be precipitated by gastric juices, bile and duodenal juices and eating in general; treatment for *H. pylori* is not useful for reflux dyspepsia [64, 66]; more likely diagnosis if hiatus hernia present; it is possible to have symptoms of epigastric pain without heartburn and reflux in GORD/GERD [52, 55, 56]	Tightness in chest, lack of appetite, becomes full quickly; common cause of heartburn symptoms that are relieved by antacids and made worse by lying down or bending over; will have chest pain; waterbrash symptoms signifies reflux; belching	In reflux, dyspepsia pain may radiate to the back, arms and neck; usually no nocturnal pain; can get nocturnal asthma and cough; common in pregnant women; chest and upper abdominal pain will be worse on stooping and after large meals; heartburn will be experienced more frequently than once every fortnight and acid regurgitation more than once a week; will have excess belching; possible to have overlapping condition with peptic ulcer; may have associated symptoms of asthma or chronic cough

▶

Dysmotility dyspepsia: caused by delayed gastric emptying rather than gastric hypersecretion; indigestion always brought on by eating; no *H. pylori* present [56]	Upper abdominal pain, nausea, early fullness, can be affected by stress; symptoms of heartburn reported	Symptoms often continuous, vomiting more than once every second month, hunger after feeling full quickly, heaviness after eating fatty foods or milk, bloating and distension in the abdomen; need to check if have any food intolerances
Causal factor: **Aerophagia**	Belching, heartburn symptoms, oesophageal reflux, functional GI disease	
DEGENERATIVE AND DEFICIENCY		
Ulcer-like dyspepsia Peptic ulcer: gastric/ stomach ulcer, duodenal ulcer, oesophageal ulcer; abdominal pain may be relieved by meals; can have overlapping symptoms of heartburn; will have *H. pylori* infection; risk factors are age 40 years and over, cigarette smoking, use of NSAIDs, family or past medical history of ulcer disease [56, 65]	Can point to where burning epigastric pain is in the abdomen and show clearly where it is radiating to; gnawing pain; associated symptoms of nocturnal abdominal pain, nausea, decreased appetite, early satiety, weight loss; symptoms have periodicity like an ulcer and be pain-free for several weeks; can develop from chronic anxiety, tension; abdominal pain relieved by small amount of specific foods or antacids; vomiting can provide relief from pain; taking aspirin and ibuprofen for tension headaches; no significant reflux	May have vomiting on onset and previous history of ulcer disease; can have haematemesis (vomiting of blood); a common sign with a peptic ulcer is a fear to eat, but not with a duodenal ulcer; possibly has concurrent reflux dyspepsia with ulcer dyspepsia
Cervical arthritis	Headache at the base of the head/neck area	No specific neck pain reported
Anaemia: organic dyspepsia; pernicious anaemia (B12 deficiency) can cause indigestion and may develop from atropic gastritis and be linked to persistant infection with *H. pylori* bacteria in the stomach	Eating fewer meals, weight loss	Need to assess mineral absorption, variety of food groups, quantity of meals; usually associated with a long history of indigestion
INFECTION AND INFLAMMATION		
Causal factor: ***H. pylori:*** improved by bismuth salts or antibiotics	Causes bloating, pain in the stomach; involved in peptic ulcer disease, gastric tumour	Not in oesophageal reflux or dysmotility functional dyspepsia

Gastritis: inflammation of stomach lining that can be made worse by aspirin, NSAIDs, corticosteroids, antibiotics, antiasthma agents; atropic gastritis from autoimmune destruction of parietal cells leading to lack of intrinsic factor and potentiating lack of B12	Abdominal pain, indigestion, burning; loss of appetite, sense of fullness, nausea; vomiting can provide relief from pain; taking aspirin and ibuprofen for tension headaches	Pain will be worse after eating in gastritis; often associated with alcoholism; vague indigestion is more common in gastritis rather than specific location
Giardia	Can present with upper abdominal symptoms such as nausea, bloating and persist for months	Symptoms will be persistent symptoms rather than episodic and may have diarrhoea
Chronic appendicitis	Upper abdominal intermittent pain, nausea, vomiting on one occasion	No constipation or fever
Cholecystitis: chronic and acute gall bladder inflammation	Symptoms can be vague gastrointestinal disturbance; biliary colic, right abdominal pain	The pain of gallstone colic/cholecystitis does not have periodicity like an ulcer; specific to right upper quadrant pain, or pain in right shoulder; will have lower abdominal symptoms such as flatulence
Hepatitis	Pain in upper abdomen that is radiating; nausea; loss of appetite	No increased diarrhoea or lower abdominal symptoms mentioned
Crohn's disease	Abdominal pain; lesions can be from mouth to anus; weight loss, abdominal pain, low-grade fever and nausea; inflammation is deep and patchy	No blood or mucus in stools; no diarrhoea mentioned or recurrent episodes of watery bowel motions during day and night; no fever
SUPPLEMENTS AND SIDE EFFECTS MEDICATION/DRUGS		
Causal factor: **Drug ingestion:** NSAIDs, antibiotics, potassium or iron supplements, alcohol, corticosteroids, theophylline derivatives, isoproterenol, anticholinergics	Heartburn and indigestion, can cause *H. pylori* negative gastritis, lower esophageal pressure; taking aspirin and ibuprofen for his tension headaches increases the risk of developing a peptic ulcer	
ENDOCRINE/REPRODUCTIVE		
Pancreatic disorders: chronic pancreatitis, vipoma (endocrine pancreatic tumour), Zollinger-Ellison syndrome	Symptoms of abdominal pain, episodes of pain, fatty diet; Zollinger-Ellison syndrome can present like a peptic ulcer (without *H. pylori* infection) with pain at night, nausea and lack of appetite	Symptoms of diarrhoea and steatorrhoea usually present; rare condition; will be from a long history of indigestion and often related to alcohol abuse

▶

STRESS AND NEUROLOGICAL DISEASE		
Migraine headache: severe painful headaches; often unilateral and located in the front and temporal regions of the head	Stress can exacerbate, can have indigestion and nausea as a complaint	Dan's headaches not aggravated by or related to sound or light; migraine headaches usually improve upon waking and after sleep; no indication of nausea and vomiting associated with headache
Causal factor: **Stress** [25, 26]	Headaches, heartburn, indigestion	
EATING HABITS AND ENERGY		
Causal factor: **Food intolerance amine/ salicylate sensitivity**	Headaches, drinking red wine, dairy; may be delayed sensitivity; salicylate sensitivity or overload can cause gastritis	Need to ask more regarding if the headaches are after eating particular foods that usually trigger migraine headaches
Causal factor: **Dehydration**	Lack of water in the diet, dull headaches, drinking excess tea and coffee, drinking alcohol	

TABLE 3.7 **DECISION TABLE FOR REFERRAL** [2, 7, 8, 10, 12]		
COMPLAINT	**CONTEXT**	**CORE**
Referral for presenting complaint	Referral for all associated physical, dietary and lifestyle concerns	Referral for contributing emotional, mental, spiritual, metaphysical, lifestyle and constitutional factors
REFERRAL FLAGS	**REFERRAL FLAGS**	**REFERRAL FLAGS**
• Can point to where the upper abdominal pain is • Initial sharp pain in the upper abdomen that then becomes dull • Indigestion symptoms becoming worse and more frequent • Episodic upper abdominal pain	• Dan has experienced weight loss	• Increased stress
ISSUES OF SIGNIFICANCE	**ISSUES OF SIGNIFICANCE**	**ISSUES OF SIGNIFICANCE**
• Indigestion that is worse at night and better with eating • Symptoms of indigestion worse with spicy foods • Improves with antacids • Vomiting improved symptoms on one occasion	• Lack of appetite • Building changes in work environment • Tension headaches • Excess caffeine in diet	• Changes in the work environment • Stress with managing staff and building changes
REFERRAL DECISION	**REFERRAL DECISION**	**REFERRAL DECISION**
• Medical assessment for upper abdominal pain [60]	• Dietary assessment	• Stress management

TABLE 3.8 **FURTHER INVESTIGATIONS THAT MAY BE NECESSARY** [2, 6–10, 11, 13, 54]	
TEST/INVESTIGATION	REASON FOR TEST/INVESTIGATION
FIRST-LINE MEDICAL INVESTIGATIONS:	
Abdominal inspection: guarding, rebound tenderness, palpation, abnormal pulsations (auscultation)	Signs of appendicitis, pancreatitis, kidney swelling, enlarged liver, bowel obstruction, perforated ulcer; positive Murphy's sign for inflamed gall bladder; hiatus hernia signs, swallowed air; mid-epigastric tenderness in gastric and peptic ulcer
Full blood count	Anaemia, inflammation, allergies
C-urea breath test	*H. pylori*
IgG antibodies	*H. pylori*
CRP (C-reactive protein)	When CRP is high it can indicate a bacterial infection
Stool test	Occult blood in stool may indicate ulcer or carcinoma, *H. pylori*
IF NECESSARY:	
Oesophageal motility studies	Cardiospasm, reflux oesophagitis
Bernstein test (dilute hydrochloric acid in the distal oesophagus)	Produce symptoms of oesophagitis
Oesophageal pH monitoring	Reflux oesophagitis GORD/GERD; may not determine oesophagitis
Endoscopy [60, 62]	Confirmation of peptic ulcer, gastric tumour, non-ulcer dyspepsia; may not always define GORD/GERD or *H. pylori*
GI radiographs	Oesophageal reflux, gas entrapment, gall bladder disease
Gastroscopy	Gastritis
Serum gastrin levels	To confirm or rule out Zollinger-Ellison syndrome and gastrinoma
Serum amylase	Pancreatitis
Small-bowel follow through	Exclusion or confirmation of Crohn's disease

Confirmed diagnosis

DAN AND PEPTIC ULCER

Dan is a 40-year-old man presenting at the clinic for help with digestive discomfort, which has come and gone over the past six months. When his symptoms are bad he experiences heartburn, a gnawing pain in the centre of his chest, a sharp pain that can become dull and lasts for a couple of hours and occasional nausea. Dan can experience symptoms before eating but will become full very quickly. He has an overall lack of

TABLE 3.9 **DECISION TABLE FOR TREATMENT (ONCE DIAGNOSIS IS CONFIRMED)**		
COMPLAINT	**CONTEXT**	**CORE**
Treatment for the presenting complaint and symptoms	Treatment for all associated symptoms	Treatment for mental, emotional, spiritual, constitutional, lifestyle issues and metaphysical considerations
TREATMENT PRIORITY	**TREATMENT PRIORITY**	**TREATMENT PRIORITY**
• Dietary recommendations to reduce the inflammation and irritation of gastric mucosa • Dietary recommendations to identify and eliminate specific dietary triggers • Lifestyle recommendations to avoid potential triggers for ulcer formation and eliminate likely triggers such as aspirin and NSAIDs • Dietary recommendations to soothe and heal the ulceration, reduce acute symptoms and help prevent the recurrence of peptic ulcers • Physical therapy recommendations to help relieve and treat the symptoms • Herbal tea, powder and tonic with anti-inflammatory, anti-ulcer, mucoprotective and healing properties • Nutritional supplements with anti-inflammatory, healing, mucosal strengthening, anti-ulcer and *H. pylori*-inhibiting effects • Probiotic supplementation to help inhibit *H. pylori*, reduce inflammation and antibiotic side effects **NB**: Tests to monitor Dan's vitamin and mineral levels should be done after 6 weeks and again after 8–12 weeks to ensure levels stay within normal range; dosage can be adjusted if necessary based on test results	• Recommendations to improve Dan's diet and lifestyle • Recommendations for Dan to exercise regularly • Recommendation for Dan to take time out to eat his lunch slowly and in a quiet place • Nutritional supplement recommendations to improve Dan's general health and increase levels of essential nutrients	• Recommendation for Dan to review his work–home life balance and delegate or offload work where possible • Recommendation for Dan to take up recreation activities outside of work to help reduce stress • Recommendation for Dan to use stress-management techniques • Herbal powder and tonic with adaptogenic, tonic and nervine action • Herbal tea with nervine action • Recommendation for a regular massage to reduce stress • Nutritional supplement to help support Dan's stress response

appetite and has lost weight recently. Dan says he is definitely burping more often and his symptoms can be worse when he is lying down at night. During the consultation Dan reveals that although he loves his job as a principal of a small school, he has experienced excessive stress with changes in procedures and staff as well as building renovations. He takes aspirin or ibuprofen regularly for tension headaches and has been drinking up to six cups of coffee a day and sometimes skips meals.

Dan required immediate referral and was diagnosed with a **peptic ulcer**, a condition involving the development of an ulcer near the acid-bearing area of the stomach, duodenum, oesophagus or jejunum. Epigastric pain that a person can point to is a key feature of peptic ulcers.

Peptic ulcers can be single or multiple open sores affecting the mucous membranes and are usually caused by failure of the digestive tract to withstand the action of pepsin and hydrochloric acid. This usually occurs because the mucous membranes become thinner, rather than as a result of excess pepsin or hydrochloric acid. A major cause of peptic ulcers is *Helicobacter pylori* (also known as *Campylobacter pylori*) infection [63]. Additional triggers include excess intake of NSAIDs, which results in thinning of the gastric mucosa and large dosages of pharmaceutical glucocorticosteroids. This influences the production of excessive quantities of pepsin, excessive long-term consumption of alcohol (ethanol) and the increased ingestion of the nicotinic acid form of vitamin B3 on an empty stomach releasing high levels of stomach acid. Stress has a significant impact on existing peptic ulcers and heartburn can be frequently experienced. Risk factors for developing a peptic ulcer are being over 40 years of age, cigarette smoking and family or past medical history of ulcer disease.

General references used in this diagnosis: 2, 6–11, 57, 59, 65

PRESCRIBED MEDICATION
- Proton pump inhibitor: drugs that inhibit the production of gastric acid [14]
- Eradication of *Helicobacter pylori* using antiobiotic therapy

Treatment aims
- Reduce inflammation and promote healing of gastric mucosa [16, 17].
- Enhance integrity of gastric mucosa and gastroduodenal mucosal defence [16–18].
- Normalise gastric acid secretion [15, 18].
- Modulate Dan's immune and inflammatory response [16].
- Support Dan's stress response and help reduce his stress levels [16–18].
- Identify and reduce or eliminate contributing factors to Dan's peptic ulcer [15, 18, 32].
- Determine whether Dan has any food allergies and manage accordingly [15, 18].

Lifestyle alterations/considerations
- Encourage Dan to reduce his stress levels [16–18, 25, 26]. He may find relaxation therapies such as meditation, yoga, tai chi or progressive muscle relaxation helpful to manage his stress levels.
- Encourage Dan to make the time to take a regular lunch break and eat his lunch slowly in a quiet and peaceful environment.
- Encourage Dan to find ways of reducing his work-related stress by reviewing his work schedule and workload. He may need to delegate tasks and/or enlist the help of others where necessary.
- Encourage Dan to take time away from work to enjoy other activities.
- Encourage Dan to exercise daily. Regular exercise is strongly associated with reduced stress levels [27, 28].
- Encourage Dan to stop taking aspirin or other non-steroidal anti-inflammatory medications. These are implicated in the development of peptic ulcers [15–18].
- If Dan smokes, he should stop [15–18].
- Dan may find that raising the head of his bed helps to alleviate symptoms during the night while he is in bed [10].

Dietary suggestions
- Food allergies should be tested for and managed appropriately [17, 18]. Milk should be avoided because it can significantly increase stomach-acid production [17, 18, 33].

- Fermented milk products, such as yoghurt containing live cultures of bifidobacteria and lactobacillus, may be helpful [16, 34, 35]; although, if Dan is allergic or intolerant to dairy products he should avoid them [17, 18].
- Encourage Dan to increase consumption of soluble fibre from fruit and vegetables [16–18].
- Encourage Dan to avoid foods that he knows aggravate his symptoms, and also avoid refined sugars [16, 17].
- Encourage Dan to avoid coffee, alcohol and chocolate [15].
- Encourage Dan to avoid spicy foods, spearmint, peppermint, fatty foods, carbonated beverages, orange juice and tomato juice [10].
- Cabbage and other cruciferous vegetables should be included in Dan's diet every day [16– 18]. The juice of half a head of cabbage or eating the cabbage raw may be beneficial during an acute episode [16, 18]. Cabbage can help prevent recurrence of ulcers [16] and has ulcer healing properties [17, 18].
- Encourage Dan to eat bananas every day. Bananas stimulate gastric mucosal cell growth and help maintain the protective layer on the gastric mucosa [17, 18]. Banana is also helpful to relieve acute symptoms of dyspepsia and heartburn [16].
- Ginger tea may reduce symptoms of dyspepsia [16, 18].
- One tablespoon of unpasteurised Manuka honey taken on an empty stomach at bedtime can relieve ulcers [16].
- Encourage Dan to increase his intake of foods rich in vitamin A. Vitamin A helps maintain the integrity of the mucosal barrier and protect gastric mucosa from damage [16, 17, 19, 22].
- Encourage Dan to reduce consumption of fatty foods and saturated fat [15, 16] and increase consumption of foods containing omega-3 fatty acids [16]. Olive oil is a good choice due to its antioxidant properties [16]. Diets high in olive oil are associated with a higher percentage of ulcer healing and reduced ulcerogenesis from NSAIDs [16].
- Encourage Dan to consume garlic and onions every day [18]. Garlic is effective against *Helicobacter pylori* [19]. If Dan's reflux symptoms persist he may find avoiding garlic and onions reduces oesophageal pressure and therefore symptoms of reflux [10].
- Encourage Dan to take lecithin granules daily. The phosphatidylcholine in lecithin is gastroprotective [17, 44].

Physical treatment suggestions
- Dan may find massage therapy very helpful in reducing his stress levels and improve his ability to deal with stress [29, 30].
- A course of acupuncture therapy may be beneficial [31, 32].
- Hydrotherapy would be beneficial, such as dry skin brushing every day followed by a long, relaxing bath [49].
- Try a hot trunk wrap [50].
- Briefly tread in a cold foot bath followed by a hot compress to the abdomen, contrasted with a cold compress at the end [49].
- Taking neutral temperature baths for 30 minutes improves indigestion [49].
- Alternate brief hot and cold sitz baths [49].
- Constitutional hydrotherapy for toning of digestion and stress release [50, 51].

TABLE 3.10 HERBAL TEA

Alternative to coffee

HERB	FORMULA	RATIONALE
Chamomile flowers *Matricaria recutita*	2 parts	Anti-inflammatory [16, 19, 20]; spasmolytic [16, 19, 20]; carminative [16, 19, 20]; antimicrobial [19, 20]; alpha-bisabolol in chamomile promotes tissue granulation and tissue regeneration in ulcers [19, 20, 36]; chamomile can prevent formation of ulcers [19, 36] and reduces healing time [19, 36]; anti-inflammatory action interrupts tissue destruction cycle and provides symptomatic relief [16]
Ginger root powder *Zingiber officinale*	½ part	Anti-nausea [19, 20]; anti-ulcer activity [19, 20]; anti-inflammatory [19, 20]; analgesic [19, 20]; inhibitory effect on *H. pylori* [19, 37]
Lemon balm *Melissa officinalis*	1 part	Anti-inflammatory [19]; analgesic [19]; antispasmodic [19, 21, 23]; antimicrobial [19, 23]; anxiolytic [19, 23]; sedative [19, 21, 23]; beneficial for gastrointestinal conditions associated with nervousness or anxiety [19, 21]
Chickweed *Stellaria media*	2 parts	Demulcent [19, 23]; antiulcer [23]; beneficial in gastric irritation [23]

Infusion: 1 tsp per cup – 1 cup 3–4 times daily

TABLE 3.11 HERBAL POWDER

HERB	FORMULA	RATIONALE
Deglycyrrhizated licorice root powder [15, 18] *Glycyrrhiza glabra*	1 part	Anti-inflammatory [19, 20]; mucoprotective [19, 20]; promotes mucosal repair and reduces symptoms of active ulcers [19, 20]; antimicrobial [19, 20]; anti-*H. pylori* properties [38]; adrenal tonic [20]
Slippery elm bark powder *Ulmus fulva*	1 part	Nutritive demulcent [19, 21]; emollient [19, 21]; traditionally used for inflammatory conditions of the gastrointestinal tract [19, 21] and for dyspepsia [19], gastric reflux [19] and peptic ulcers [19]
Marshmallow root powder *Althea officinalis*	1 part	Demulcent [21, 23]; emollient [21, 23]; vulnerary [21, 23]

One heaped teaspoon mixed to a smooth paste with a little water 3 times daily before meals. Two heaped teaspoons in water can be taken as required to alleviate acute symptoms of heartburn.

TABLE 3.12 **HERBAL FORMULA (1:2 LIQUID EXTRACTS)**		
Made with ethanolic extract herbal liquids (alcohol removed)		
HERB	**FORMULA**	**RATIONALE**
Meadowsweet *Filipendula ulmaria*	70 mL	Anti-inflammatory [19, 23]; analgesic [19, 23]; gastroprotective [19, 23]; normalises stomach acid [16]; promotes healing of stomach ulcers [19, 39]; positive effect on antioxidant status of gastric tissue [40]; traditionally used for dyspepsia, heartburn and hyperacidity [21, 23]
Golden seal *Hydrastis canadensis* (cultivated/plantation source)	40 mL	Antimicrobial [19, 23]; mucous membrane trophorestorative [19, 23]; anti-inflammatory [19, 23]; vulnerary [19, 23]; bitter tonic [19, 23]; traditionally used for dyspepsia and gastritis [41]; beneficial for peptic ulcers [23]; inhibits growth of *H. pylori* [48]
Siberian ginseng *Eleutherococcus senticosus*	30 mL	Adaptogenic [19, 20]; immunomodulator [19, 20]; tonic [19, 20]; beneficial to improve stress response and increase energy levels [19, 20]
Skullcap *Scutellaria lateriflora*	30 mL	Nervine tonic [23]; spasmolytic [23]; mild sedative [21, 23]; traditional indications include nervous tension and anxiety [21, 23]
Rhodiola *Rhodiola rosea*	30 mL	Adaptogenic [42]; tonic [42]; traditionally used to treat fatigue, depression and nervous system disorders [42]; effective in reducing symptoms of generalised anxiety disorder [43]
Dosage:	200 mL	Dose: 10 mL twice daily before meals

TABLE 3.13 **NUTRITIONAL SUPPLEMENTS**	
SUPPLEMENT AND DOSE	**RATIONALE**
Supplement providing a daily dose of approx 2000 mg vitamin C, 500 IU vitamin E, 5000 IU vitamin A, 2000 mg mixed bioflavanoids and 10 mg elemental zinc in divided doses [17, 18]	Vitamins C, E and zinc enhance wound healing and recovery [17, 18, 22, 24]; zinc supplementation reduces the incidence, severity and number of gastric lesions [17, 18]; lower levels of vitamin C have been found in people with peptic ulcers [68]; bioflavanoids have anti-allergic properties [18, 22]; may inhibit *H. pylori* [18] and help prevent ulcer formation [18]; vitamins A [18, 24] and E [18] help maintain integrity of the mucosal barrier
Omega-3 fish oil 3 × 1000 mg capsules twice daily [17, 19]	Anti-inflammatory [17, 19, 22]; protective against peptic ulcer disease [17]
L-glutamine 1500 mg daily in divided doses [18]	Protects gastrointestinal mucosa from damage and promotes repair [19, 45]; indicated for use to prevent and heal peptic ulcers [22, 45]

▶

High-potency practitioner-strength **multivitamin and mineral complex** providing therapeutic doses of B-group vitamins Dosage as recommended by manufacturer	B vitamins are beneficial to support Dan's stress response [19, 22]; a broad-spectrum multivitamin and mineral supplement can help increase levels of essential nutrients and antioxidants which may be deficient due to Dan's diet and lifestyle
High-potency practitioner-strength **probiotic supplement** containing therapeutic levels of human strain *Lactobacillus* and *Bifidobacterium* organisms [46, 47] Dosage as recommended by manufacturer	Probiotic supplementation can inhibit *H. pylori* [46, 47] and in combination with antibiotic therapy may increase its eradication rate [46, 47] and reduce antibiotic side effects [46]; probiotics can stabilise gastric barrier function [46] and decrease mucosal inflammation [46]

References

[1] N.J. Talley, S. O'Connor, Pocket Clinical Examination, third edn, Churchill Livingstone Elsevier, Australia, 2009.

[2] P. Kumar, C. Clark, Clinical Medicine, sixth edn, Elsevier Saunders, London, 2005.

[3] J. Silverman, S. Kurtz, J. Draper, Skills for Communicating with Patients, second edn, Radcliff Publishing, Oxford, 2000.

[4] R. Neighbour, The Inner Consultation: how to develop an effective and intuitive consulting style, Radcliff Publishing, Oxon, 2005.

[5] M. Lloyd, R. Bor, Communication Skills For Medicine, third edn, Churchill Livingstone Elsevier, Edinburgh, 2009.

[6] G. Douglas, F. Nicol, C. Robertson, Macleod's Clinical Examination, twelfth edn, Churchill Livingstone Elsevier, 2009.

[7] J. Jamison, Differential Diagnosis for Primary Care, second edn, Churchill Livingstone Elsevier, London, 2006.

[8] A. Polmear (Ed.), Evidence- Based Diagnosis in Primary Care, Churchill Livingstone Elsevier, 2008, pp. 274–283.

[9] R.M.D. Berkow, A.J.M.D. Fletcher, M.H.M.D. Beers, The Merck Manual, sixteenth edn, Merck Research Laboratories, Rathway, N.J, 1993 (later edition).

[10] R.H. Seller, Differential Diagnosis of Common Complaints, fifth edn, Saunders Elsevier, Philadelphia, 2007.

[11] R.D. Collins, Differential Diagnosis in Primary Care, fourth edn, Lippincott Williams & Wilkins, Philadelphia, 2008.

[12] D. Peters, L. Chaitow, G. Harris, S. Morrison, Integrating Complementary Therapies in Primary Care, London, Churchill Livingstone, 2002.

[13] K.D. Pagna, T.J. Pagna, Mosby's Diagnostic and Laboratory Test reference, third edn, Mosby, USA, 1997 (later edition).

[14] M. Numans, J. Lau, N. de Wit, et al., Short-term treatment with protonpump inhibitors as a test for gastroesophageal reflux disease, Ann Intern Med 140 (2004) 518–527.

[15] S. El-Hashemy, Naturopathic Standards of Primary Care, CCNM Press Inc, Toronto, 2007.

[16] J. Jamison, Clinical Guide to Nutrition & Dietary Supplements in Disease Management, Churchill Livingstone, Edinburgh, 2003.

[17] H. Osiecki, The Physicians Handbook of Clinical Nutrition, seventh edn, Eagle Farm: Bioconcepts, 2000.

[18] J.E. Pizzorno, M.T. Murray, H. Joiner-Bey, The Clinicians Handbook of Natural Medicine, second edn, St Louis, Churchill Livingstone, 2008.

[19] L. Braun, M. Cohen, Herbs & Natural Supplements: An evidence based guide, second edn, Elsevier, Sydney, 2007.

[20] S. Mills, K. Bone, Principles & Practice of Phytotherapy; Modern Herbal Medicine. Edinburgh, Churchill Livingstone, London, 2000.

[21] British Herbal Medicine Association, British Herbal Pharmacopoeia, BHMAA, 1983.

[22] H. Osiecki, The Nutrient Bible, seventh edn, Eagle Farm: BioConcepts Publishing, 2008.

[23] S. Mills, K. Bone, The Essential Guide to Herbal Safety, Churchill Livingstone, St Louis, 2005.

[24] J. Higdon, An Evidence Based Approach to Vitamins and Minerals, Thieme, New York, 2003.

[25] S. Levenstein, Stress and peptic ulcer: life beyond helicobacter, British Medical Journal 316 (1998) 538–541.

[26] S. Levenstein, S. Ackerman, J.K. Kiecolt-Glaser, A. Dubois, Stress and Peptic Ulcer Disease, Journal of the American Medical Association 281 (1) (1999) 10–11.

[27] A.F. Jorm, H. Christensen, K.M. Griffiths, R.A. Parslow, B. Rodgers, K.A. Blewitt, Effectiveness of complementary and self-help treatments for anxiety disorders, Medical Journal of Australia 181 (7) (2004) S29–S46.

[28] A. Byrne, G.D. Byrne, The effect of exercise on depression, anxiety and other mood states: A review, J Psychosom Res 37 (6) (1993) 565–574.

[29] C.A. Moyer, J. Rounds, J.W. Hannum, A Meta-Analysis of Massage Therapy Research, Psychological Bulletin 130 (1) (2004) 3–18.

[30] T. Field, G. Robinson, F. Scafidi, R. Nawrocki, A. Goncalves, Massage therapy reduces anxiety and enhances EEG pattern of alertness and math computations, International Journal of Neuroscience 86 (1996) 197–205.

[31] Y. Li, G. Tougas, S.G. Chiverton, R.H. Hunt, The Effect of Acupuncture on Gastrointestinal Function and Disorders, The American Journal of Gastroenterology 87 (10) (2008) 1372–1381.

[32] T. Takahashi, Acupuncture for functional gastrointestinal disorders, Journal of Gastroenterology 41 (2006) 408–417.

[33] A.F. Ippoliti, V. Maxwell, J.I. Isenberg, The Effect of Various Forms of Milk on Gastric-Acid Secretion, Annals of Internal Medicine 84 (3) (1976) 286–289.

[34] C. Rodriguez, M. Medici, A.V. Rodriguez, F. Mozzi, F. de Valdez, Prevention of chronic gastritis by fermented milks made with exopolysaccharide-producing Streptococcus thermophilus strains, Journal of Dairy Science 92 (2009) 2423–2434.

[35] S. Elmstahl, U. Svenssen, G. Berglund, Fermented milk products are associated to ulcer disease, Results from a cross sectional population study, European Journal of Clinical Nutrition 52 (1998) 668–674.

[36] I. Szelenya, O. Isaac, K. Thiemer, Pharmacological experiments with compounds of chamomile. III. Experimental studies of the ulcerprotective effect of chamomile, Planta Med 35 (3) (1979) 218–227.

[37] A. Nostro, L. Cellini, S. DiBartolomeo, M.A. Cannatelli, E. DiCampli, F. Procopio, R. Grande, et al., Effects of combining extracts (from propolis or Zingiber officinale) with clarithromycin on Helicobacter pylori, Phytotherapy Research 20 (3) (2006) 187–190.

[38] T. Fukai, A. Maruma, K. Kaitou, T. Kanda, S. Terada, T. Nomura, Anti-Helicobacter pylori flavonoids from licorice extract, Life Sciences 71 (2002) 1449–1463.

[39] O.D. Barnaulov, P.P. Denisenko, Anti-ulcer action of a decoction of the flowers of the dropwort, Filipendula ulmaria (L.) Maxim [Article in Russian], Farmakol Toksikol 43 (6) (1980) 700–705.

[40] A. Vasiliauskas, A. Keturkienė, L. Leonavièienė, D. Vaitkienė, Influence of Herb Filipendula ulmaria (L.) Maxim Tincture on Pro-/antioxidant Status in Gastric Tissue with Indomethacin-induced Gastric Ulcer in Rats, Acta Medica Lituanica 11 (1) (2004) 31–36.

[41] Goldenseal (Hydrastis Canadensis), An annotated bibliography, in: M. Predny, J. Chamberlain (Eds.), Gen. Tech. Rep. SRS-88, U.S. Department of Agriculture, Forest Service, Southern Research Station, Asheville, NC, 2005. Available from http//www.sfp.forprod.vt.edu/.

[42] M. Morgan, K. Bone, Rhodiola rosea – Rhodiola, Mediherb Phytotherapist's Perspective 47 (2005) 1–4.

[43] A. Bystritsky, L. Kerwin, J.D. Feusner, A Pilot Study of Rhodiola rosea (Rhodax®) for Generalized Anxiety Disorder (GAD), The J Altern Complement Med 14 (2) (2008) 175–180.

[44] B.S. Dunjic, J. Axelson, A. Ar'Rajab, K. Larsson, S. Bengmark, Gastroprotective capability of exogenous phosphatidylcholine in experimentally induced chronic gastric ulcers in rats, Scandinavian Journal of Gastroenterology 28 (1) (1993) 89–94.

[45] M. Elia, P.G. Lunn, The Use of Glutamine in the Treatment of Gastrointestinal Disorders in Man, Nutrition 13 (7–8) (1997) 743–747.

[46] M. Gotteland, O. Brunser, S. Cruchet, Systematic review: are probiotics useful in controlling gastric colonization by Helicobacter pylori? Alimentary Pharmacology and Therapeutics 23 (8) (2006) 1077–1086.

[47] C. Felley, P. Michetti, Probiotics and Helicobacter pylori, Best Practice & Research Clinical Gastroenterology 17 (5) (2003) 785–791.

[48] G.B. Mahady, S.L. Pendland, A. Stoia, L.R. Chadwick, in: Vitro Susceptibility of Helicobacter pylori to Isoquinoline Alkaloids from Sanguinaria canadensis and Hydrastis canadensis, Phytotherapy Research 17 (2003) 217.

[49] D.D. Buchman, The complete book of water healing, Contemporary Books, McGraw-Hill Companies, New York, 2001.

[50] E. Blake, Philadelphia, in: L. Chaitow, E. Blake, P. Orrock, M. Wallden, P. Sinder, J. Zeff (Eds.), Naturopathic Physical Medicine: Theory and Practice for Manual Therapists and Naturopaths, Churchill Livingstone Elsevier, 2008.

[51] W. Boyle, A. Saine, Lectures in Naturopathic Hydrotherapy, Oregon: Eclectic Medical Publications, 1988.

[52] M. Lin, G. Triadafilopoulos, Belching: dyspepsia or gastroesophageal reflux disease? Am J Gastroenterol 98 (2003) 2139–2145.

[53] M.A. Ahmad, D.C. Metz, Dyspepsia and heartburn, Rheum Dis Clin North Am 25 (1999) 703–718.

[54] O.V. Bazaldua, F.D. Schneider, Evaluation and management of dyspepsia, Am Fam Physician 60 (1999) 1773–1788.

[55] J. Dent, Definitions of reflux disease and its separation from dyspepsia, Gut 50 (Suppl. 4) (2002) 17–20.

[56] M.P. Jones, Evaluation and treatment of dyspepsia, Posgrad Med J 79 (2003) 225–229.

[57] J.E. Richter, Dyspepsia: organic causes and differential characteristics from functional dyspepsia, Scand J Gastroenterol 26 (Suppl. 182) (1991) 11–16.

[58] L.M. Dickerson, D.E. King, Evaluation and management of nonulcer dyspepsia, Am Fam Physician 70 (1) (2004) 107–114.

[59] B.M. Schroeder, Evaluation of epigastric discomfort and management of dyspepsia and GERD, Am Fam Physician 68 (6) (2003) 1215–1216, 1219–1220.

[60] P. Moayyedi, N. Talley, M. Fennerty, et al., Can the clinical history distinguish between organic and functional dyspepsia? JAMA 295 (2006) 1566–1576.

[61] R. Spiller, Anorexia, nausea, vomiting and pain, BMJ 323 (2001) 1354–1357.

[62] A. Ford, M. Qume, P. Moayyedi, et al., Helicobacter pylori 'test and treat' or endoscopy for managing dyspepsia: an individual patient data meta-analysis, Gastroenterology 128 (2005) 1838–1844.

[63] C. Weijnen, M. Numans, N. de Wit, et al., Testing for Helicobacter pylori in dyspeptic patients suspected of peptic ulcer disease in primary care: cross sectional study, BMJ 323 (2001) 71–75.

[64] F. Chan, J. Wu, J. Ching, et al., Effect of Helicobacter pylori eradication on treatment of gastro-oesophageal reflux disease: a double blind, placebo controlled, randomized trial, Gut 53 (2004) 174–179.

[65] M. Heikkinen, P. Pikkarainen, M. Eskelinen, et al., GP's ability to diagnose dyspepsia based only on physical examination and patient history, Scand J Prim Healthcare 18 (2000) 99–104.

[66] J.G. Fox, T.C. Wang, Helicobacter pylori–not a good bug after all, N Engl J Med 345 (2001) 829–831.

[67] P. Hohenberger, S. Gretschel, Gastric Cancer, Lancet 362 (2003) 305–315.

[68] H. O'Connor, C. Schorah, N. Habibzedah, et al., Vitamin C in the human stomach: relation to gastric pH, gastroduodenal disease, and possible sources, Gut 30 (1989) 436–442.

Irritable bowel syndrome

Case history

Adrian Nixon, 45, is a sound engineer who works on theatre productions. Adrian works long hours and loves his work. He is here at the recommendation of a colleague to get an alternative perspective on the digestive problems he is experiencing.

Adrian has experienced episodes of alternating diarrhoea and constipation associated with left-sided lower abdominal pain over the past four years. He can also feel quite bloated at times and suffers from excessive wind.

Adrian had this problem when he was in his early 20s but it seemed to settle down. The return of his symptoms has coincided with his divorce four years ago. Adrian explains that the divorce was very stressful and he believes his emotional turmoil had a lot to do with the problem returning. He would like to explore and address this aspect of his problem.

Adrian explains that his abdominal pain can be quite acute and the only thing that seems to relieve it is when he passes a bowel motion. When he experiences diarrhoea he can pass up to six motions a day, which are quite small and thin. Sometimes the diarrhoea is watery or slimy, but he hasn't noticed any blood or froth. Adrian's digestive problems are not accompanied by a loss of appetite, nausea or vomiting.

When you ask Adrian about his diet he admits it is not very good. He lives on his own and doesn't enjoy cooking. Since his divorce he has eaten mostly takeaway or frozen convenience meals. His favourite foods are Thai and Chinese. Adrian drinks a lot of tea and coffee at work, eats on the run and doesn't think he drinks enough water. Adrian is a social drinker but that happens rarely these days as he has not felt like socialising with friends and colleagues for a while now. He prefers to just go home and says he has never enjoyed drinking alcohol alone.

TABLE 3.14 **COMPLAINT** [1–10]	
Analogy: Skin of the apple	**Complaint:** Define the presenting complaint and symptoms; understand the complaint *Diarrhoea and constipation*
AREAS OF INVESTIGATION AND EXAMPLE QUESTIONS	**CLIENT RESPONSES**
Your practitioner impression	Adrian is open to being helped and is interested in amelioration of symptoms along with understanding underlying cause. Adrian has vitality.
Rating scale *How would you rate the diarrhoea and constipation discomfort out of 10, with 10 being as bad as can be?*	*With acute pain it can feel like a 9 out of 10 and on a daily level it can be 6 out of 10.*

TABLE 3.15 **CONTEXT**	
Analogy: Flesh of the apple	**Context:** Put the presenting complaint into context to understand the disease
AREAS OF INVESTIGATION AND EXAMPLE QUESTIONS	**CLIENT RESPONSES**
Family health history *Is there a family history of similar symptoms to what you have been experiencing?*	*My brother used to complain a lot of digestive concerns before he died in a motorcycle accident 10 years ago.*
Trauma and pre-existing illness *Have you experienced any other illness that may seem unrelated to your current symptoms?*	*I've been tested for haemochromatosis. My mother has this condition passed down from both her parents. I have one gene but have been told I won't develop symptoms.*
Functional disease *Do you experience urgency to pass a watery bowel motion in the morning when you wake? (colon and functional disorder)*	*Sure do, right on time!*
Infection and inflammation *Is your abdominal pain alleviated by lying down or remaining completely still? (inflammation)* *Do you need to get up during the night because you have diarrhoea or pain in your stomach? (organic cause, inflammatory bowel syndrome)*	*No, but it can be helped by passing a bowel motion sometimes.* *No, I never need to get up at night, and only pass diarrhoea during the day.*

TABLE 3.16 **CORE**	
Analogy: Core of the apple with the seed of ill health	**Core:** Holistic assessment to understand the client
AREAS OF INVESTIGATION AND EXAMPLE QUESTIONS	**CLIENT RESPONSES**
Emotional health *Can you remember a time when you felt extremely healthy and happy?*	*I felt great around my 40th birthday. My wife and son were with me and we had a really special day. I remember feeling I had everything I needed to make me happy.*
Education and learning *Do you feel like you have learned anything significant about yourself through the process of your divorce over the past four years?*	*I was surprised at how much sadness and anger I had to deal with and how long it took me to let go. I learned that I've been working through much underlying grief from my brother's death. I have learned that I really miss seeing my son.*

TABLE 3.17 **ADRIAN'S SIGNS AND SYMPTOMS**	
Pulse	70 bpm
Blood pressure	125/75
Temperature	37°C
Respiratory rate	12 resp/min
Body mass index	20
Waist circumference	82 cm
Face	Pale
Urinalysis	No abnormality detected (NAD)

Results of medical investigations

No investigations have been performed at this stage.

TABLE 3.18 **UNLIKELY DIAGNOSTIC CONSIDERATIONS** [1, 3–6, 11]	
CONDITIONS AND CAUSES	**WHY UNLIKELY**
OBSTRUCTION AND FOREIGN BODY	
Kidney stones: hyperoxaluria disorders of uric acid metabolism may develop with inflammatory bowel disease and dehydration	Colic pain usually radiates from the loin to the groin about every 10 minutes; it can be very sharp pain in acute episodes; urinalysis NAD
DEGENERATIVE AND DEFICIENCY	
Peptic/duodenal ulcer: abdominal pain and bloating	Not common to be associated with diarrhoea; usually severe episodes of upper or midgut abdominal pain; usually will not eat due to pain after ingesting food
INFECTION AND INFLAMMATION	
Gastroenteritis: abdominal pain, diarrhoea	Associated with vomiting, nausea and fever; Adrian has no low-grade fever; acute gastritis is usually self-limiting and lasts less than a week; it is possible, however, to develop functional bowel disease after an acute infective episode [62]
Bacterial infection: e.g. *Yersinia enterocolitica, Escherichia coli, Shigella, Staphylococcal enterocolitis,* ileocaecal TB; diarrhoea is the main symptom; may cause ulceration and inflammation; diarrhoea, abdominal pain, bloating [73, 74]	Usually self-limiting and acute in duration between 1 and 10 days depending on bacterial toxin; violent vomiting can be associated; no bloody diarrhoea reported
Viral infection: retrovirus, hepatitis; diarrhoea, tired, nausea, fatigue, weight loss; recently travelled to new environment	No history or signs of jaundice; stools are not pale; no fever, nausea or change in appetite
Parasitic infection: giardia, amoebiasis *Giardia:* symptoms include diarrhoea and abdominal discomfort *Amoebiasis:* symptoms of chronic mild intermittent diarrhoea with abdominal discomfort	Stools become very pale with mucus; loss of appetite or weight loss is not a dominant symptom for Adrian; no nausea, headache or blood or significant mucus in stools

▶

▶

Hepatitis/fatty liver: can be due to family history of haemochromatosis	No jaundice or yellow sclera; usually upper abdominal pain or middle of gut; no loss of appetite or nausea
Cholecystitis: chronic and acute gall bladder inflammation; symptoms can be vague gastrointestinal disturbance; biliary colic that resembles functional bowel disorders	Usually severe right-sided, upper abdominal pain; no fever or nausea associated with symptoms
Causal factor: *H. pylori* infection: abdominal pain, bloating	Pain usually clearly located in middle of the abdomen; usually nausea is associated with stomach bloating; often do not feel like eating
ENDOCRINE/REPRODUCTIVE	
Diabetes: diabetic neuropathy causes chronic diarrhoea, gastric stasis and bacterial overgrowth	Adrian has not reported increased urination or thirst; abdominal pain can be general as well as local to the left side; urinalysis NAD
Addison's disease: weight loss, dehydration, nausea, diarrhoea, abdominal pain	No loss of body hair or skin pigmentation reported; urinalysis NAD

Case analysis

TABLE 3.19 **POSSIBLE DIFFERENTIAL DIAGNOSIS**		
Not ruled out by tests/investigations already done [1, 3–7, 11, 13, 57–59]		
CONDITIONS AND CAUSES	**WHY POSSIBLE**	**WHY UNLIKELY**
ALLERGIES AND IRRITANTS		
Food allergy: typically to cow's milk, egg, soya, peanut, wheat and fish [29, 67]	Diarrhoea, cramping colic	Often presents with swelling of lips and tongue, urticaria skin rash, conjunctivitis, rhinitis, anaphylaxis and difficulty breathing; has not linked symptoms to a particular food yet
Lactose and fructose intolerance [29, 78]	Abdominal pain, bloating, watery and frothy diarrhoea; possible recurrent abdominal pain with onset of lactose ingestion	No nausea; need to investigate how Adrian's diet has changed
CANCER AND HEART DISEASE		
Bowel cancer, polyps, gastrointestinal lymphoma [58]	Usually associated with alternating diarrhoea and constipation; more common in middle-aged men; carcinomas and polyps can cause irritation and hypermotility	Usually presents with blood in the stool; abdominal pain is more often an advanced symptom

▶

Lymphoma: malignant lymphadenopathies may infiltrate the small intestine and cause diarrhoea and malabsorption; increased risk if coeliac disease present	Diarrhoea	No significant weight loss and fatigue recently; usually associated with significant fever and night sweats
OBSTRUCTION AND FOREIGN BODY		
Intestinal obstruction e.g. faecal impaction with overflow	Abdominal pain, constipation, diarrhoea, abdominal distension; can be acute and recurrent abdominal pain	Can cause vomiting; Adrian's abdominal pain is not exclusively worse after eating meals
FUNCTIONAL DISEASE		
Functional abdominal pain syndrome [59]	Abdominal discomfort that can be continuous	Abdominal pain is not exclusively connected with physiological events such as eating or passing a bowel motion
Functional diarrhoea [59]	Chronic diarrhoea and anxiety; no bleeding from the bowel, weight loss or ongoing fatigue; bowel motions are watery and mushy	Usually symptoms are in absence of abdominal pain; Adrian has bowel motions first thing in morning but need to clarify if he also has further passing during the day; defecation not exclusively after eating food for Adrian
Functional constipation: more than 1 in 4 bowel motions are lumpy, hard and need to strain, has feeling of incomplete evacuation or blockage; has fewer than 3 evacuations a week and may need manual help to facilitate bowel motions [59]	Constipation	Adrian has constipation that alternates with diarrhoea and has more than 3 evacuations a week
Functional abdominal bloating [59]	Bloating and visible distension	Functional bloating will not usually be relieved by passing a bowel motion
Irritable bowel syndrome: a combination of functional pain, diarrhoea, constipation and bloating [57, 59]	Diarrhoea, recurrent episodes, symptom-free episodes, stress; abdominal pain on lower left side; usually alternates between constipation and diarrhoea; bowel motions are rarely nocturnal; poor diet	

DEGENERATIVE AND DEFICIENCY		
Ulcerative colitis	Diarrhoea and lower abdominal pain	Usually affects the rectum alone; may spread to the whole colon but rarely affects the ileum; no blood and mucus in stools, which would usually be present; no significant weight loss, fever or fatigue
Diverticular disease: diverticula and diverticulitis	Chronic symptoms include abdominal pain and diarrhoea; usually pain in the left lower abdomen; can experience erratic bowel habits; more common for those eating a low-fibre diet	Usually affects people who are over 50 years of age; usually would present with blood or mucus in stools
Causal factor: **Bile acid malabsorption:** due to conditions such as Crohn's disease, coeliac disease, increased small intestine transit, diabetic diarrhoea, postinfective gastroenteritis [62]	Under-diagnosed cause of chronic diarrhoea; when terminal ileum fails to reabsorb bile salts causes diarrhoea and increases colonic motility	
INFECTION AND INFLAMMATION		
Appendicitis	Abdominal pain, constipation; can be vague symptoms before an acute episode	More common to be right-sided abdominal pain, but can refer to the left side in some cases; usually associated with midgut belly button pain; diarrhoea not as common as a key symptom; no fever, vomiting or loss of appetite
Crohn's disease	Diarrhoea, recurrent episodes of watery bowel and lower abdominal pain	No key symptoms of weight loss, fever, nausea or blood and mucus in stools; Adrian only passes a bowel motion during the day
Small-bowel disease	Chronic bacteria overgrowth due to small-bowel obstruction – diarrhoea, lower abdominal discomfort	Weight loss is not a key symptom
Candidiasis and dysbiosis	Diarrhoea and abdominal distension	Adrian has not been on medication or antibiotics recently; no reports of feeling significant fatigue; abdominal pain is not a key symptom of candidiasis

▶

SUPPLEMENTS AND SIDE EFFECTS MEDICATION/DRUGS		
Supplement or food additive abuse: excess vitamin C or magnesium?	Diarrhoea, abdominal pain	Adrian is not taking any supplements at this time
Drug induced (e.g. *Pseudomembranous colitis*)	Diarrhoea caused by recent antibiotic use (allow overgrowth of fungi), laxatives, antihypertensives, NSAIDs	Not usually associated with episodic abdominal pain; no recent antibiotic use
ENDOCRINE/REPRODUCTIVE		
Pancreatic disorders: chronic pancreatitis, vipoma (endocrine pancreatic tumour), Zollinger-Ellison syndrome [79]	Symptoms of abdominal pain, episodes of diarrhoea, fatty diet; slimy bowel motion	Constipation not usually a symptom; no significant blood or mucus reported in stools; usually upper abdominal pain similar to ulcer or gall bladder colic
Hyperthyroidism	Diarrhoea and anxiety, weight loss; common to present between 20 and 40 years of age	No goitre or eye symptoms presenting as clinical markers; Adrian not experiencing high levels of anxiety now or restlessness, energy levels are moderate
AUTOIMMUNE DISEASE		
Coeliac disease [71]	Abdominal pain, poor diet, diarrhoea	More often upper abdominal pain with bloating
STRESS AND NEUROLOGICAL DISEASE		
Depression [65, 69, 72]	Often presents as physical symptoms such as diarrhoea; spending more time on his own since his divorce 4 years ago	No loss of appetite, still very active at work, no significant fatigue reported
Anxiety [69, 70, 72, 79]	Not as socially active as he used to be, diarrhoea	No reports on lack of sleep, palpitations, tight chest, difficulty breathing, loss of appetite, fast talking
Phobia: intense fear to specific or set of stimuli that are predictable	Has mentioned not socialising as much recently	Adrian is not experiencing symptoms of anxiety that are restricted to a specific event; has not mentioned avoidance of a specific object or event
EATING HABITS AND ENERGY		
Causal factor: **Dehydration**	Chronic diarrhoea, not drinking much water, drinking a lot of tea and coffee; symptoms can be asymptomatic, however, colicky pain in the abdomen may be present that can be dull, constant and intermittent	

TABLE 3.20 **DECISION TABLE FOR REFERRAL** [1, 3–6, 12]		
COMPLAINT	**CONTEXT**	**CORE**
Referral for presenting complaint	Referral for all associated physical, dietary and lifestyle concerns	Referral for contributing emotional, mental, spiritual, metaphysical, lifestyle and constitutional factors
REFERRAL FLAGS	**REFERRAL FLAGS**	**REFERRAL FLAGS**
• Adrian experiences diarrhoea associated with severe abdominal pain • Duration of diarrhoea has been more than 3 months • Adrian may be at risk of dehydration due to diarrhoea	• Possible dehydration due to lack of water	• Isolation
ISSUES OF SIGNIFICANCE	**ISSUES OF SIGNIFICANCE**	**ISSUES OF SIGNIFICANCE**
• Alternating diarrhoea with constipation can be signs of a more benign functional bowel disorder or serious colon cancer	• Excessive consumption of caffeine • Lack of water • Prefers to eat takeaway food rather than cook at home	• Digestive symptoms began when Adrian went through a divorce 4 years ago • Not as socially active since his divorce
REFERRAL DECISION	**REFERRAL DECISION**	**REFERRAL DECISION**
• Immediate referral to medical practitioner to rule out serious organic causes for abdominal discomfort, diarrhoea and constipation [67]	• Adrian needs dietary guidance and cooking/eating/drinking alternatives	• Counselling may help Adrian deal with unresolved issues from his divorce and help him move forward socially

TABLE 3.21 **FURTHER INVESTIGATIONS THAT MAY BE NECESSARY** [1–6, 11, 14]	
TEST/INVESTIGATION	**REASON FOR TEST/INVESTIGATION**
FIRST-LINE INVESTIGATIONS:	
Abdominal examination: guarding, rebound tenderness, palpation, abdnormal pulsations (auscultation)	Monitor bloating and distension for abdominal mass
Full blood count	Low haemoglobin in Crohn's disease, detect anaemia of chronic disease (usually normocytic, normochromic anaemia, and rarely megaloblastic due to B12 deficiency), inflammation, infection or tumour; iron deficiency anaemia; white-blood-cell count raised in appendicitis
ESR (erythrocyte sedimentation rate)/CRP (C-reactive protein)	Inflammation, tumour, infection
Blood electrolytes	Addison's disease, kidney infection, dehydration
Stool test [68]	Detect ova, parasites, bacteria, calprotectin and fat levels, and occult blood; if acidic stools are passed it indicates lactose intolerance

▶

Abdominal x-ray	Appendicitis, intestinal obstruction, ulcerative colitis
Elimination diets	Detect food intolerance
IF NECESSARY:	
Hydrogen breath test	To detect bacterial overgrowth; when bacteria is metabolised by lactose or glucose there is a production of hydrogen; can detect fructose intolerance
Liver function test	Hepatitis, substance abuse
Fasting blood glucose test	Diabetes, Addison's disease, raised in pancreatitis
Antigliadin antibodies	Check if antibodies to gluten are present in blood
Sigmoidoscopy	To test for Crohn's disease
Colonoscopy and biopsy	Rule out bowel cancer, polyps, inflammatory bowel disease, diverticulitis or haemorrhoids
Serum B vitamins and iron	Possible malabsorption and poor diet [16]
Hair tissue mineral analysis	To determine the presence of heavy metals [16] and ascertain tissue mineral status due to malabsorption and poor diet

Confirmed diagnosis

ADRIAN AND IRRITABLE BOWEL SYNDROME

Adrian has come to the clinic for help with a longstanding digestive concern that returned four years ago after he went through a divorce. Adrian has maintained his employment as a sound engineer and really enjoys his work. He has become socially isolated following his divorce and experienced significant emotional turmoil resulting from the failure of his marriage. Adrian does not enjoy cooking and prefers to eat out alone.

Adrian's digestive symptoms required immediate referral to rule out organic and inflammatory causes for the diarrhoea, abdominal pain and constipation. The confirmed diagnosis is a **functional bowel disorder**, which is extremely common and usually has a clinical presentation of left iliac fossa pain in the abdomen relieved by wind or passing a bowel motion.

The condition of **irritable bowel syndrome** (IBS) has a working criteria [57] of symptoms including abdominal discomfort for 12 or more weeks with at least two of the following features [59]:

- pain relieved by passing a bowel motion
- onset of abdominal discomfort associated with change in bowel motion
- more than three abnormal stools a day alternating with fewer than three stools a week
- consistent abnormal stool formation that can appear ribbon-like
- needing to strain when passing a bowel motion
- feeling of urgency with incomplete evacuation of stool
- abdominal bloating.

A more generalised criterion for IBS is that the condition involves abdominal discomfort with changeable bowel motions in the absence of structural or biochemical disorders [57]. However, it is suggested more research is needed to ascertain whether low-grade inflammation may be present for some individuals with IBS [65].

The pain experienced with IBS can be very acute and intense requiring hospitalisation at times. Abdominal bloating is a common symptom and the condition is more prevalent in women than men, often associated with the menstrual cycle. The history of the condition can be longstanding with varying episodes of discomfort.

There can be symptom-free intervals and symptoms are often associated with: increased stress, sexual and emotional abuse and trauma; family history of bowel disease and other social factors; and diet [57, 69, 72].

General references used in this diagnosis: 2, 4, 5, 11, 57–61, 63, 75

PRESCRIBED MEDICATION

• Antidepressants [61]

Adrian has chosen not to take prescribed antidepressant medication until he has tried natural therapies and works through his emotional issues. He has agreed to work collaboratively and be monitored regularly by his GP while trying a more natural approach.

TABLE 3.22 **DECISION TABLE FOR TREATMENT (ONCE DIAGNOSIS IS CONFIRMED)**		
COMPLAINT	**CONTEXT**	**CORE**
Treatment for the presenting complaint and symptoms	Treatment for all associated symptoms	Treatment for mental, emotional, spiritual, constitutional, lifestyle issues and metaphysical considerations
TREATMENT PRIORITY	**TREATMENT PRIORITY**	**TREATMENT PRIORITY**
• Lifestyle recommendations to reduce stress-induced symptoms • Dietary recommendations to avoid potential dietary triggers and increase consumption of foods with a positive effect of bowel function • Physical therapy suggestions to help reduce frequency and severity of symptoms • Herbal tea, tonic or tablets, powder and/or capsules to help reduce frequency and severity of symptoms • Nutritional supplements to help reduce frequency and severity of symptoms	• Lifestyle recommendations to improve general health and wellbeing • Dietary recommendations to improve nutritional status and general health • Dietary recommendations to consume foods with anti-inflammatory properties to reduce potential gastrointestinal inflammation • Supplemental nutrients to improve nutritional status and gastrointestinal health • Herbal tonic and tablets with adaptogenic and tonic action to improve Adrian's vitality and general health	• Lifestyle and physical treatment recommendations to reduce stress • Recommendation for Adrian to attend counselling to deal with his emotional issues • Recommendation for Adrian to become more socially active • Herbal tea, tonic and tablets to support Adrian's nervous system and stress response • Herbal tonic or tablets with antidepressant action **NB:** If Adrian decides to take the prescribed antidepressant medication his herbal tonic or tablets will need to be reformulated to exclude St John's wort

Treatment aims

- Identify and eliminate foods that may be causing or aggravating Adrian's symptoms [15–18, 29].
- Reduce or eliminate symptoms of bloating, flatulence and abdominal pain [15–18].
- Reduce exaggerated gut response to stress [15–18, 26].
- Support Adrian's stress response [16–18].
- Support normal serotonergic signalling and response [16, 17, 24, 25].
- Reduce mucosal inflammation and modulate the inflammatory response in Adrian's gastrointestinal tract [27, 28].
- Support healthy intestinal microflora [15–18, 46].
- Determine whether Adrian has any micronutrient deficiencies; improve his diet and nutritional status [81].
- Help Adrian address his emotional issues.

Lifestyle alterations/considerations

- Encourage Adrian to use stress-management techniques such as meditation, yoga and other relaxation techniques [16–18, 30].
- Encourage Adrian to exercise regularly [17, 32]. Exercise will help to improve Adrian's sense of general wellbeing and reduce stress and depression [31]. Regular physical activity is likely to provide symptom improvement [17, 32].
- Encourage Adrian to cook proper meals for himself. He may find cooking classes are beneficial and may help him to enjoy cooking.
- Encourage Adrian to seek counselling to help him deal with the break-up of his marriage. Psychotherapy [35] and cognitive behavioural therapy [33, 34] are also likely to provide ongoing benefit for his physical symptoms.
- Adrian may find hypnotherapy is beneficial [37].
- Encourage Adrian to get out socially. He may try joining a club or sporting group where he can meet new people and become less isolated. He may even find a new partner.

Dietary suggestions

- Identify and eliminate any foods to which Adrian is allergic or intolerant [15–18, 29, 37]. Food intolerance is a major factor in the pathogenesis of IBS [17, 18, 29, 37]. Commonly implicated foods include barley [15, 17], chocolate [15], citrus fruit [15], coffee [15, 16], corn [15, 17], dairy food [15, 37], eggs [15, 37], garlic [15], nuts [15], oats [15, 17], onions [15], potatoes [15], rye [15, 17], soy [15], tea [15, 16] and wheat [15, 17, 37].
- Encourage Adrian to also eliminate alcohol, refined carbohydrates, sugar, fats and hot spices from his diet [15, 17, 18].
- Encourage Adrian to avoid sugar alternatives such as sorbitol, xylitol or mannitol as these may exacerbate flatulence [15].
- Encourage Adrian to eat a fibre-rich whole-food diet [15–17]. Soluble fibre is particularly beneficial to Adrian [51].
- If Adrian finds legumes and beans aggravate his symptoms, he may find them tolerable if they are soaked in water prior to cooking and the water used to soak them is discarded [15].
- Encourage Adrian to increase his intake of water [15, 16].
- Adrian will benefit from including soluble fibre in his diet [15–18, 51]. Ensure Adrian is not sensitive to cereal grains before recommending cereal fibre [16].
- Adrian could include ginger and turmeric in his diet [16].

Physical treatment suggestions

- Adrian may find acupuncture helpful in managing his symptoms. It may also improve his general wellbeing and stress response [80].
- Massage therapy [36] or aromatherapy massage [38] is likely to help Adrian as part of a stress-management program.
- Hydrotherapy: alternating hot and cold showers to the abdomen and spine [52]. Hot trunk wrap [52]. A hot sitz bath for abdominal pain [53]. A hot apple cider vinegar and water compress on the abdomen [53]. For acute diarrhoea, brief cold sitz baths with apple cider vinegar from a few seconds up to 10 minutes every day for a week, then every second day after symptoms subside [53].
- Constitutional hydrotherapy [52, 54, 55].
- For constipation place a hot compress on the abdomen, cover it in plastic, then place a hot water bottle or heating pad on top for 12 minutes. Follow this with cold mitten friction for 30 seconds. Repeat this process three times [56].
- Take a hot shallow bath or hot foot bath for abdominal bloating and pain [56].
- To tone the abdomen when not experiencing pain, apply a cold, wet compress on the abdominal area, covered by a dry towel with an elastic bandage around the trunk at night for at least three months [53].

TABLE 3.23 **HERBAL FORMULA (1:2 LIQUID EXTRACTS)**		
HERB	**FORMULA**	**RATIONALE**
Damiana *Turnera diffusa*	50 mL	Traditionally used in Western herbal medicine as an antidepressant and anxiolytic [19, 21, 22]; particularly beneficial where there is a sexual factor involved [19]
Skullcap *Scutellaria laterifolia*	40 mL	Nervine tonic [45]; spasmolytic [15, 45]; mild sedative [15, 45]; BHP indication for nervous tension [21]
St John's wort *Hypericum perforatum*	60 mL	Antidepressant [19, 20, 39]; anxiolytic [20, 39]; nervine [19, 20]
Rhodiola *Rhodiola rosea*	50 mL	Adaptogen [42, 44]; tonic [42, 44]; antidepressant [42, 43]; anxiolytic [42–44]
Supply:	200 mL	Dose: 10 mL twice daily

TABLE 3.24 **HERBAL TEA**		
Alternative to tea and coffee		
HERB	**FORMULA**	**RATIONALE**
Chamomile *Matricaria recutita*	3 parts	Antispasmodic [19, 20]; sedative [19, 20]; anti-inflammatory [19, 20]; carminative [20]; traditionally used to treat gastrointestinal conditions such as colic, flatulence, cramping, diarrhoea, restlessness and anxiety [19, 20, 39, 21]
Peppermint *Mentha × piperita*	2 parts	Spasmolytic [19, 20]; carminative [19, 20]; traditionally use therapeutically for digestive disorders such as colic, flatulence, cramping [19, 20]; peppermint oil has been shown to improve symptoms of IBS [19, 39]

▶

Lemon balm *Melissa officinalis*	1 part	Anxiolytic [19, 22] sedative [19, 22]; spasmolytic [19, 22]
Ginger root powder *Zingiber officinalis*	¼ part	Carminative [19, 20]; spasmolytic [19, 20]; traditionally used therapeutically for digestive disorders such as colic, cramping and flatulence [19, 20, 39]
Infusion: 1 tsp per cup, 1 cup three to four times daily		

TABLE 3.25 TABLET ALTERNATIVE TO HERBAL LIQUID: MAY IMPROVE COMPLIANCE

HERB	DOSE PER TABLET	RATIONALE
St John's wort *Hypericum perforatum*	750 mg	See above
Damiana *Turnera diffusa*	675 mg	See above
Schisandra *Schisandra chinensis*	625 mg	Adaptogen [19, 23]; hepatoprotective [19]; nervine tonic [23]
Skullcap *Scutellaria laterifolia*	500 mg	See above
Dose: 2 tablets twice daily		

TABLE 3.26 ADDITIONAL FORMULA TO HERBAL TONIC OR TABLET

HERB	DOSE	RATIONALE
Slippery elm bark powder capsules or powder *Ulmus fulva*	One 500 mg capsule 4 times daily [21, 39] or ½ tsp powder mixed with hot water 3–4 times daily [19]	Nutritive demulcent [19, 21]; bulking agent and prebiotic [40]; traditionally used for diarrhoea and constipation [19, 39]; indicated for use in IBS [19, 39, 40]
Peppermint oil *Mentha × piperita*	One 200 mg enteric coated capsule 3 times daily [41]	See above Enteric-coated peppermint oil improves symptoms of IBS [16–19, 39, 41]

TABLE 3.27 NUTRITIONAL SUPPLEMENTS

SUPPLEMENT AND DOSE	RATIONALE
High-potency practitioner-strength **probiotic supplement** containing *Lactobacillus plantarum* [15–17, 37, 46, 47] and *Lactobacillus GG* [37] Dosage as directed by the manufacturer	Supplementation with specific strains of probiotics may improve symptoms of IBS [15–18, 37, 46, 47]; probiotic supplementation can improve intestinal health [50]

▶ **Prebiotic supplement** containing fructo-oligosaccharides (FOS) [16, 37] Dosage as directed by the manufacturer	Taking a prebiotic together with a probiotic supplement can support growth of the probiotic organisms [48]; supplemental FOS may improve symptoms of IBS [16, 49]
High-potency practitioner-strength **multivitamin and mineral supplement** providing therapeutic doses of essential micronutrients Dosage as directed by the manufacturer	Adrian's diet is poor and lacking in important micronutrients; diarrhoea may have depleted nutrient levels [81]; particularly important if tests show Adrian has specific micronutrient deficiencies

References

[1] G. Douglas, F. Nicol, C. Robertson, Macleod's Clinical Examination, twelfth edn, Churchill Livingstone Elsevier, Edinburgh, 2009.

[2] N.J. Talley, S. O'Connor, Pocket Clinical Examination, third edn, Churchill Livingstone Elsevier, Australia, 2009.

[3] P. Kumar, C. Clark, Clinical Medicine, sixth edn, Elsevier Saunders, London, 2005.

[4] A. Polmear, Evidence- Based Diagnosis in Primary Care, Churchill Livingstone Elsevier, Edinburgh, 2008.

[5] J. Jamison, Differential Diagnosis for Primary Care, second edn, Churchill Livingstone Elsevier, London, 2006.

[6] R.D. Collins, Differential Diagnosis in Primary Care, fourth edn, Lippincott Williams & Wilkins, Philadelphia, 2008.

[7] R.H. Seller, Differential Diagnosis of Common Complaints, fifth edn, Saunders Elsevier, Philadelphia, 2007.

[8] M. Lloyd, R. Bor, Communication Skills For Medicine, third edn, Churchill Livingstone Elsevier, Edinburgh, 2009.

[9] R. Neighbour, The Inner Consultation: how to develop an effective and intuitive consulting style, Radcliff Publishing, Oxon, 2005.

[10] J. Silverman, S. Kurtz, J. Draper, Skills for Communicating with Patients, second edn, Radcliff Publishing, Oxford, 2000.

[11] R. Berkow, A.J. Fletcher, M.H. Beers, The Merck Manual, sixteenth edn, Merck Research Laboratories, Rathway, N.J, 1993 (later edition).

[12] D. Peters, L. Chaitow, G. Harris, S. Morrison, Integrating Complementary Therapies in Primary Care, London, Churchill Livingstone.

[13] L. Chaitow, E. Blake, P. Orrock, M. Wallden, P. Sinder, J. Zeff, Natropathic physical Medicine: Theory and Practice for Manual Therapists and Naturopaths, Churchill Livingstone Elsevier, Philadephia, 2008.

[14] K.D. Pagna, T.J. Pagna, Mosby's Diagnostic and Laboratory Test reference, third edn, Mosby, USA, 1997 (later edition).

[15] J. Jamison, Clinical Guide to Nutrition & Dietary Supplements in Disease Management, Churchill Livingstone, Edinburgh, 2003.

[16] H. Osiecki, The Physicians Handbook of Clinical Nutrition, seventh edn, Eagle Farm: Bioconcepts, 2000.

[17] J.E. Pizzorno, M.T. Murray, H. Joiner-Bey. The Clinicians Handbook of Natural Medicine, second edn, St Louis: Churchill Livingstone

[18] S. El-Hashemy, Naturopathic Standards of Primary Care, CCNM Press Inc, Toronto, 2007.

[19] L. Braun, M. Cohen, Herbs & Natural Supplements: An evidence based guide, 2nd edn, Elsevier, Sydney, 2007.

[20] S. Mills, K. Bone, Principles & Practice of Phytotherapy; Modern Herbal Medicine, Churchill Livingstone, Edinburgh, London, 2000.

[21] British Herbal Medicine Association. British Herbal Pharmacopoeia. BHMAA.

[22] S. Mills, K. Bone, The Essential Guide to Herbal Safety, Churchill Livingstone, St Louis, 2005.

[23] K. Bone, Clinical Applications of Chinese and Ayurvedic Herbs: Monographs for the Western Herbal Practitioners, Warwick. Phytotherapy Press, 1996.

[24] M.D. Coates, C.R. Mahoney, D.R. Linden, J.E. Sampson, J. Chen, H. Blaszyk, M.D. Crowell, et al., Molecular Defects in Mucosal Serotonin Content and Decreased Serotonin Reuptake Transporter in Ulcerative Colitis and Irritable Bowel Syndrome, Gastroenterology 126 (2004) 1657–1664.

[25] G.M. Mawe, M.D. Coates, P.L. Moses, Intestinal Serotonin Signalling In Irritable Bowel Syndrome, Alimentary Pharmacology & Therapeutics 23 (8) (2006) 1067–1076.

[26] S. Fukudo, T. Nomura, M. Hongo, Impact of corticotropin-releasing hormone on gastrointestinal motility and adrenocorticotropic hormone in normal controls and patients with irritable bowel syndrome, Gut 42 (1998) 845–849.

[27] S.M. Collins, T. Piche, P. Rampal, The putative role of inflammation in the irritable bowel syndrome, Gut 49 (2001) 743–745.

[28] G. Barbara, R. DeGiorgio, V. Stanghellini, C. Cremon, R. CorinalAdriani, A role for inflammation in irritable bowel syndrome? Gut 51 (2002) i41–i44.

[29] V. Alun Jones, M. Shorthouse, P. McLaughlan, E. Workman, J.O. Hunter, Food intolerance: a major factor in the pathogenesis of irritable bowel syndrome, Lancet 320 (8303) (1982) 1115–1117.

[30] G. Shaw, E.D. Srivastava, M. Sadlier, P. Swann, J.Y. James, J. Rhodes, Stress management for irritable bowel syndrome: a controlled trial, Digestion 50 (1) (1991) 36–42.

[31] P. Salmon, Effects of physical exercise on anxiety, depression, and sensitivity to stress: A unifying theory, Clinical Psychology Review 21 (1) (2001) 33–61.

[32] M. Lustyk, B. Kathleen, M.E. Jarrett, J.C. Bennett, M.M. Heitkemper, Does a Physically Active Lifestyle Improve Symptoms in Women With Irritable Bowel Syndrome? Gastroenterology Nursing 24 (3) (2001) 129–137.

[33] A.M. Van Dulmen, J.F. Fennis, G. Bleijenberg, Cognitive Behavioural Group Therapy for Irritable Bowel Syndrome: Effects and Long Term Follow Up, Psychosomatic Medicine 58 (1996) 508–514.

[34] P. Boyce, J. Gilchrist, N.J. Talley, D. Rose, Cognitive-behaviour therapy as a treatment for irritable bowel syndrome: a pilot study, Australian and New Zealand Journal of Psychiatry 34 (2) (2000) 300–309.

[35] E. Guthrie, F. Creed, D. Dawson, B. Tomenson, A randomised controlled trial of psychotherapy in patients with refractory irritable bowel syndrome, The British Journal of Psychiatry 163 (1993) 315–321.

[36] T. Field, G. Robinson, F. Scafidi, R. Nawrocki, A. Goncalves, Massage therapy reduces anxiety and enhances EEG pattern of alertness and math computations, International Journal of Neuroscience 86 (1996) 197–205.

[37] J.A. Spanier, C.W. Howden, M.P. Jones, A Systematic Review of Alternative Therapies in the Irritable Bowel Syndrome, Archives of Internal Medicine 163 (2003) 265–274.

[38] J. Edge, A pilot study addressing the effect of aromatherapy massage on mood, anxiety and relaxation in adult mental health, Complementary Therapies in Nursing & Midwifery 9 (2003) 90–97.

[39] E.M. Basch, C.E. Ulbricht, Natural Standard Herb & Supplement Handbook: The Clinical Bottom Line, Elsevier Mosby, St Louis, 2005.

[40] M. Morgan, The numerous healing properties of Slippery Elm, A Phytotherapist's Perspective 42 (2004) 1–2.

[41] H.G. Grigoleit, P. Grigoleit, Peppermint Oil in Irritable Bowel Syndrome, Phytomedicine 12 (8) (2005) 601–606.

[42] M. Morgan, Rhodiola rosea: Rhodiola, A Phytotherapists Perspective 47 (2005) 1–4.

[43] A. Bystritsky, L. Kerwin, J.E. Feusner, A Pilot Study of Rhodiola rosea (Rhodax®) for Generalised Anxiety Disorder (GAD), The J Altern Complement Med 14 (2) (2008) 175–180.

[44] M. Morgan, K. Bone, Herbs to Enhance Energy and Performance, A Phytotherapist's Perspective 124 (2008) 1–3.

[45] R. Awad, J.T. Arnason, V. Trudeau, C. Bergeron, J.W. Budzinski, B.C. Foster, Z. Merali, Phytochemical and biological analysis of Skullcap (Scutellaria laterifolia L.): A medicinal plant with anxiolytic properties, Phytomedicine 10 (8) (2003) 640–649.

[46] E.M.M. Quigley, B. Flourie, Probiotics and irritable bowel syndrome: a rationale for their use and an assessment of the evidence to date, Neurogastroenterology and Motility 19 (3) (2007) 166–172.

[47] Z. Hussain, E.M.M. Quigley, Systematic review: complementary and alternative medicine in the irritable bowel syndrome, Alimentary Pharmacology and Therapeutics 23 (2006) 465–471.

[48] G.T. Macfarlane, J.H. Cummings, Probiotics and prebiotics: can regulating the activities of intestinal bacteria benefit health? British Medical Journal 318 (1999) 999–1003.

[49] M. Olesen, E. Gudmand-Høyer, Efficacy, safety, and tolerability of fructooligosaccharides in the treatment of irritable bowel syndrome, American Journal of Clinical Nutrition 72 (2000) 1570–1575.

[50] P. Maretau, P. Seksik, R. Jian, Probiotics and intestinal health effects: a clinical perspective, British Journal of Nutrition 88 (S1) (2002) S51–S57.

[51] C.J. Bijkerk, N.J. de Wit, J.W. Muris, P.J. Whorwell, J.A. Knotterus, A.W. Hoes, Soluble or insoluble fibre in irritable bowel syndrome in primary care? Randomised placebo controlled trial, British Medical Journal 339 (2009) b3154.

[52] E. Blake, in: L. Chaitow, E. Blake, P. Orrock, M. Wallden, P. Sinder, J. Zeff (Eds.), Naturopathic Physical Medicine: Theory and Practice for Manual Therapists and Naturopaths, Philadelphia, Churchill Livingstone Elsevier, 2008.

[53] D.D. Buchman, The complete book of water healing, Contemporary Books, McGraw-Hill Companies, New York, 2001.

[54] W. Boyle, A. Saine, Lectures in Naturopathic Hydrotherapy, Oregon: Eclectic Medical Publications, 1988.

[55] L.M. Watrous, Constitutional hydrotherapy: from nature cure to advanced naturopathic medicine, Journal of Naturopathic Medicine 7 (2) (1997) 72–79.

[56] M. Sinclair, Modern Hydrotherapy for the Massage Therapist, Lippincott Williams & Williams, Baltimore, 2008.

[57] N. Talley, A. Weaver, A. Zinsmeister, et al., Onset and disappearance of gastrointestinal and functional gastrointestinal disorders, American Journal of Epidemiol 136 (1992) 117–165.

[58] W. Hamilton, A. Round, D. Sharp, et al., Clinical features of colorectal cancer before diagnosis: a population based case-control study, British Journal of Cancer 93 (2005) 399–405.

[59] W. Thompson, G. Longstreth, D. Drossman, et al., Functional bowel disorders and functional abdominal pain, Gut 45 (Supp. II) (1999) 43–47.

[60] M. Camilleri, Management of irritable bowel syndrome, Gastroenterology 120 (2001) 652–668.

[61] M.Z.D. Castle, D.B.A. Silk, G.W. Libby, Review article: the rationale for antidepressant therapy in functional gastrointestinal disorders, Alimentary Pharmacology and Therapeutics 19 (2004) 969–979.

[62] R.C. Spiller, Postinfectious irritable bowel syndrome, Gastroenterology 124 (2003) 1662–1671.

[63] S. Wilson, L. Roberts, et al., Prevalence of irritable bowel syndrome: a community survey, Br J Gen Pract 54 (2004) 495–502.

[64] M.D. Coates, et al., Molecular Defects in Mucosal Serotonin Content and Decreased Serotonin Reuptake Transporter in Ulcerative Colitis and Irritable Bowel Syndrome, Gastroenterology 126 (2004) 1657–1664.

[65] G. Barbara, R. DeGiorgio, V. Stanghellini, C. Cremon, R. CorinalAdriani, A role for inflammation in irritable bowel syndrome? Gut 51 (2002) i41–i44.

[66] M. Heyman, Gut barrier dysfunction in food allergy, European Journal of Gastroenterology and Hepatology 17 (12) (2005) 1270–1285.

[67] N. Talley, When to conduct testing in patients with suspected irritable bowel syndrome, Rev Gastroenterol Discord 3 (Suppl. 3) (2003) S18–S24.

[68] J. Tibble, G. Sightorsson, R. Foster, et al., Use of surrogate markers of inflammation and Rome criteria to distinguish organic from nonorganic intestinal disease, Gastronenterology 123 (2002) 450–460.

[69] W. Whitehead, O. Palsson, K. Jones, Systematic review of the comorbidity of irritable bowel syndrome with other disorders; what are the causes and implications? Gastroentorology 122 (2002) 1140–1156.

[70] M.J. Ford, M.J. Camilleri, R.B. Hanson, Hyperventilation, central autonomic control, and colonic tone in humans, Gut 37 (1995) 499–504.

[71] D. Sanders, M. Carter, D. Hurlstone, et al., Association of adult celiac disease with irritable bowel syndrome: a case–control study in patients fulfilling the ROME II criteria referred to secondary care, Lancet 358 (2001) 1504–1508.

[72] D. Drossman, D. McKee, R. Sandler, et al., Psychosocial factors in the irritable bowel syndrome. A multivariate study of patients and nonpatients with irritable bowel syndrome, Gastroenterology 95 (1988) 701–708.

[73] B. Kass, Traveller's diarrhoea, Australian Family Physician 34 (4) (2005) 243–247.

[74] P.R. Hunter, Drinking water and diarrheal disease due to Escherichia coli, Journal of Water Health 1 (2) (2003) 65–72.

[75] P. Thomas, A. Forbes, J. Green, et al., Guidelines for the investigation of chronic diarrhoea, Gut 52 (Suppl. v) (2003) v1–v15.

[76] A. Shaw, G. Davies, Lactose intolerance problems in diagnosis and treatment, Journal of Clinical Gastroenterol 28 (1999) 208–216.

[77] B. Etemad, D.C. Whitcomb, Chronic Pancreatitis: diagnosis, classification, and new genetic developments, Gastroenterology 120 (2001) 682–707.

[78] Y. Tache, V. Martinez, M. Million, L. Wang, Stress and the gastrointestinal tract III. Stress-related alternations of gut motor function: role of brain corticotropin-releasing factor receptors, American Journal of Physiology. Gastrointestinal and Liver Physiology 280 (2) (2001) G173–G177.

[79] R. Wapnir, Zinc Deficiency, Malnutrition and the Gastrointestinal Tract, The Journal of Nutrition 130 (2000) 1388S–1392S.

[80] T. Takahashi, Acupuncture for functional gastrointestinal disorders, Journal of Gastroenterology 41 (2006) 408–417.

Gallstones (cholecystitis)

Case history

Karin Andersen, 29, has been travelling in Australia for the past six months and is currently working as a nanny for a farming family in order to save some money so she can do more travelling. Before coming to Australia Karin had been working in the family business in Denmark, which she had been doing since she left high school. Last year she decided she needed a radical change in her life and chose to take some time off to travel and see the world.

Karin has been experiencing pain in the upper right quadrant of her abdomen. Initially the pain was quite mild and only occurred intermittently. It would come on quite suddenly and then quickly subside. More recently she noticed the pain gradually building in intensity and becoming very severe and accompanied by a feverish feeling, sometimes taking up to an hour to abate. Karin has not experienced this pain before and has become anxious about what might be causing it. Karin has also been feeling slightly nauseous recently and her appetite has decreased. Additionally, she has noticed a pain in her right shoulder that radiates down her back, which she thought might have been caused by lifting little children. She went to a local GP who diagnosed gallstones with associated episodes of acute cholecystitis. The GP performed several medical investigations and advised Karin that if she develops more gallstones or if the acute attacks of pain become more frequent, she will need to consider having a laparoscopic cholecystectomy to remove her gall bladder. Prior to surgery she would be given intravenous antibiotics and pain relief. Because Karin's symptoms have settled down over the past two days her GP has given her some time to rest without intervention other than oral analgesics.

Karin has come to the clinic at the recommendation of a neighbour and she is seeking an alternative opinion about how her gallstones could be managed. She would also like to learn how to prevent her condition getting any worse or returning in the future.

Karin's menstrual period is regular and she has never suffered from pain or heavy bleeding. She has noticed a change in her bowel motions in the last six months though, which she forgot to tell her doctor. She experiences diarrhoea alternating with constipation and wonders whether her current diet may be contributing to that.

Karin has been consuming a lot more milk, cheese, red meat and bread since she started working as a nanny. This is not the diet she was used to in Denmark. She would like to eat a more balanced diet but is not comfortable talking to her employers about it because it's the way they have always eaten.

When she was in Denmark Karin used to be more physically active, playing sport and cycling with her friends. When Karin first began working as a nanny she lost a lot of weight very quickly but now seems to be putting it back on, which she thinks is because of her new diet!

Karin tells you she sometimes feels homesick, but when she left home her relationship with her parents was very strained and she has not had contact with them for 12 months (although they know where she is staying in Australia). Karin says she had to make a break and begin a life of her own away from the confines of her family. She still feels bitterness towards her parents because they resisted supporting her making her own decisions about her life. Karin is looking forward to more travel and would like to meet other people her own age. She is currently saving money so she can go on an organised tour.

During the consultation Karin reveals that her mother has experienced similar symptoms. Karin did not tell this to her GP in case the doctor insisted she contact her parents to find about her family health history and to tell them about what is happening.

TABLE 3.28 **COMPLAINT** [1–10]	
Analogy: Skin of the apple	**Complaint:** Define the presenting complaint and symptoms; understand the complaint *Abdominal pain*
AREAS OF INVESTIGATION AND EXAMPLE QUESTIONS	**CLIENT RESPONSES**
Onset *When did you first notice the abdominal pain?*	*About 3 months after I started working as a nanny.*
Rating scale *How would you rate the abdominal pain out of 10, with 10 being as bad as can be?*	*When the pain is bad it feels like a 10 out of 10 and then it can subside to a 2.*

TABLE 3.29 **CONTEXT**	
Analogy: Flesh of the apple	**Context:** Put the presenting complaint into context to understand the disease
AREAS OF INVESTIGATION AND EXAMPLE QUESTIONS	**CLIENT RESPONSES**
Obstruction *How does movement affect your abdominal pain?* (obstruction of gall bladder, biliary tree or ureter from stones will be relieved by movement)	*Yes. Sometimes when I have the pain I just need to keep moving, I feel really restless and cannot keep still.*
Recreational drug use *Have you had any significant amounts of alcohol recently?*	*I have not told my host family, but the daughter of the family next door and I like to go out on a weekend and drink a fair bit of beer and spirits and I stay with her overnight. It helps me feel like I'm still on holiday.*

TABLE 3.30 **CORE**	
Analogy: Core of the apple with the seed of ill health	**Core:** Holistic assessment to understand the client
AREAS OF INVESTIGATION AND EXAMPLE QUESTIONS	**CLIENT RESPONSES**
Home life *How are you getting on with the family you are living with in Australia?*	*They are nice people and very accepting of me. They are hard workers though and expect a lot of me. They don't know how much pain I'm in sometimes.*
Action needed to heal *If your parents were here now, what would you want to say to them regarding how you left each other?*	*I wish they took the time to listen to me before judging me.*

TABLE 3.31 **KARIN'S SIGNS AND SYMPTOMS** [1, 3, 5]	
Pulse	88 bpm
Blood pressure	130/80 sitting
Temperature	37.7°C
Respiratory rate	16 resp/min
Body mass index	23
Waist circumference	78.5 cm
Face	Flushed appearance, slight yellow tinge to skin
Eyes	Sclera of eye appears slightly yellow
Urinalysis	Bilirubin detected, dark urine

TABLE 3.32 RESULTS OF MEDICAL INVESTIGATIONS [1–3, 5, 6, 11, 13]

TEST	RESULTS
Abdominal examination: guarding, rebound tenderness, palpation, abnormal pulsations (auscultation)	No sign of appendicitis, pancreatitis, kidney swelling, enlarged liver, bowel obstruction or perforated ulcer; positive Murphy's sign for inflamed gall bladder
Cholecystography: oral ingestion of radio-opaque iodinated dye with x-ray	Lack of all dye passing through bile duct into the gall bladder indicates mild acute cholecystitis
Plain abdominal x-ray	Reveals gallstones, rules out intestinal obstruction, appendicitis
Ultrasound examination	Reveals distension of gall bladder for acute cholecystitis, shows gall bladder wall thickening, distention of gall bladder and presence of biliary sludge
Full blood count	Moderate leucocytosis
ESR/CRP	Inflammation status raised
Cholesterol blood test	Raised
Fasting blood lipid test	High LDL, low HDL
Liver biochemistry blood work	Serum bilirubin, alkaline phosphatase (ALP), γ-glutamyl transpeptidase (γ-GT) and aminotransferase slightly raised
Serum amylase levels	Not elevated
Serum albumin levels	Not elevated
Stool test	No ova, parasites, bacteria and fat, or occult blood; stools not acidic stools, which would indicate lactose intolerance
Electrolyte blood test	All within normal range
Urine microscopic investigation	No urine crystals and red blood cells
Serum assay for β-HCG	Negative
Fasting blood-sugar test	NAD

TABLE 3.33 UNLIKELY DIAGNOSTIC CONSIDERATIONS

Diagnostic considerations that have been ruled out [1, 3, 5–7, 11]

CONDITIONS AND CAUSES	WHY UNLIKELY
FAMILY HEALTH – INHERITED	
Choledochal cyst: due to congenital cystic disease of the bile duct	Symptoms similar to bile duct stones usually present in childhood; has not experienced current symptoms in the past

▶

Caroli's syndrome: rare inherited disease of bile duct and liver; can be associated with gallstones; intermittent abdominal pain and fever with mild jaundice present; family history of symptoms	No dilated intrahepatic ducts detected on ultrasound
CANCER AND HEART DISEASE	
Gall bladder polyp: adenomas most common benign neoplasm of gall bladder; polyps are inflammatory and composed of cholesterol deposits	Ultrasound did not pick up polyp size masses
Primary cancer of the gall bladder: adenocarcinoma; may only be detected at time of cholecystectomy for gallstones; more common in women; gall bladder stones and polyps, and chronic cholecystitis has been associated with gall bladder cancer; symptoms of rapid weight loss and gallstones	Usually occurs from 60 years of age and onwards; CRP did not indicate cancer
Primary cancer of the bile duct: cholangiocarcinoma	Rare cancer; associated with significant jaundice and imaging did not show signs; CRP did not indicate cancer
Hypertension	Blood pressure is in normal range
OBSTRUCTION AND FOREIGN BODY	
Acute cholangitis (inflammation of bile duct) and **bile duct stones:** abdominal pain, biliary colic symptoms	Fever is rare unless biliary sepsis has caused septicaemia; usually has significant jaundice; x-ray and ultrasound did not reveal stones in the common bile duct; serum amylase usually mildly elevated
Bile pigment gallstones: black and brown stones (less common than cholesterol)	No significant haemolytic disease or duct disease
Kidney stones: severe abdominal pain	Abdominal pain usually is lower and radiates to the lower back and groin rather than the upper abdomen and shoulder; no urine crystals and red blood cells
Intestinal obstruction: pain in the abdomen, nausea, decreased appetite and change in bowel motion	Usually nausea, vomiting and constipation as key symptoms; abdominal x-ray and ultrasound did not detect obstruction
Constipation: can cause slow colonic transit time that influences bile salt pool	Abdominal x-ray showed no faecal mass
DEGENERATIVE AND DEFICIENCY	
Perforated peptic ulcer: pain in the abdomen that is radiating, nausea, decreased appetite [41]	Usually vomiting on onset and previous history of ulcer disease; serum amylase levels not raised significantly; ultrasound did not detect any sign of ulcers; the pain of gallstone colic/cholecystitis does not have periodicity like an ulcer

▶

INFECTION AND INFLAMMATION	
Non-calculous cholecystitis: chronic inflammation in the wall of the gall bladder without gallstones	Ultrasound scanning revealed the presence of gallstones; this condition is more common in the elderly and critically ill
Appendicitis: pain in the upper right quadrant of the abdomen that is radiating, nausea, loss of appetite, increased diarrhoea and constipation, change in diet	Abdominal ultrasound did not detect an inflammation of the appendix
Acute gallstone pancreatitis: pain in the abdomen that is radiating, nausea, decreased appetite, change in bowel motions; commonly caused by gallstones that block the pancreatic drainage; often associated with alcoholic binge	Usually associated with significant fever, nausea and vomiting; upper abdominal pain radiates to the lower back rather than the shoulder like gallstone pain; serum amylase levels usually markedly raised; no pancreatic swelling shown in the abdominal examination or ultrasound; no dilated intrahepatic ducts detected on ultrasound
Hepatitis: pain in the upper right quadrant of the abdomen that is radiating, nausea, loss of appetite, increased diarrhoea and constipation, change in diet; serum bilirubin, alkaline phosphatase (ALP), γ-Glutamyl transpeptidase (γ-GT) and aminotransferase slightly raised	Serum albumin levels not elevated; no anaemia or viral markers in full blood count; no liver abnormalities detected on the abdominal ultrasound examination
Crohn's disease: can affect bile salt content in the colon to predispose to cholesterol gallstones; diarrhoea experienced with change of diet; ESR raised indicating inflammation	Usually low haemoglobin in Crohn's disease, did not detect anaemia of chronic disease (usually normocytic, normochromic anaemia, and rarely megablastic due to B12 deficiency); no blood or mucus in stools; abdominal x-ray showed no indication of inflammation in the large intestine or colon
ENDOCRINE/REPRODUCTIVE	
Diabetes: can influence gall bladder motility to predispose to cholesterol gallstones	Urinalysis NAD; fasting blood-sugar NAD
Pregnancy/ectopic or normal: Karin is of child-bearing age and may be sexually active; pain is building in intensity, pain in the abdomen with nausea and loss of appetite	Will have symptoms of missed or delayed menstrual period, vaginal discharge, lower abdominal pain; serum assay for β-HCG test is negative
Ovarian cyst: abdominal pain	Abdominal ultrasound did not detect a cyst on the ovaries; abdominal pain is usually lower and radiates to the lower back rather than the upper abdomen and shoulder
AUTOIMMUNE DISEASE	
Primary sclerosing cholangitis: chronic autoimmune cholestatic liver disease with fibrosis and inflammation of the bile duct; often associated with inflammatory bowel disease; often raised serum alkaline phosphatase	More common in men over 40 years of age; no itching of skin or significant jaundice

TABLE 3.34 **CONFIRMED DIAGNOSIS** [3, 5, 11, 40]	
CONDITION	**RATIONALE**
Acute cholecystitis/gallstone colic (cholesterol gall stones)	Pain in the right upper quadrant that can be mild, subside quickly and then gradually build in intensity; severe upper right abdominal pain develops; feverish feeling and nausea are associated symptoms; pain radiating to the right shoulder is indicative of referred pain from the gall bladder; can be asymptomatic for years; change of diet to include more high-cholesterol foods; episode of rapid weight loss recently; feeling 'bitter' towards family with suppressed anger; can present with family history of gall bladder symptoms
Test results	Positive Murphy's sign for inflamed gall bladder; ultrasound revealed minimal gallstones that have caused pressure on the neck of the gall bladder and cystic duct

Case analysis

TABLE 3.35 **POSSIBLE FURTHER DIFFERENTIAL DIAGNOSIS** [3–7, 11]		
Not ruled out by tests/investigations already done		
CONDITIONS AND CAUSES	**WHY POSSIBLE**	**WHY UNLIKELY**
ALLERGIES AND IRRITANTS		
Lactose intolerance	Abdominal pain, bloating, watery and frothy diarrhoea; possible recurrent abdominal pain with onset of lactose ingestion; Karin's diet has significantly changed since she came to Australia	No nausea; need to understand more how Karin's diet has changed
RECREATIONAL DRUG USE		
Alcohol abuse: γ-GT raised in liver biochemistry	Can be raised even with a small intake of alcohol; binge drinking will exacerbate symptoms of cholecystitis	Can be raised in parallel to ALP in gall bladder disorders; if raised when serum ALP is normal that is more likely to indicate alcohol abuse

▶

FUNCTIONAL DISEASE		
Irritable bowel syndrome	Pain in the abdomen, alternating between diarrhoea and constipation; pain often presents similar to cholecystitis and may have in conjunction	Pain not necessarily relieved by passing a bowel motion
INFLAMMATION		
Chronic cholecystitis: chronic inflammation of the gall bladder giving rise to vague symptoms of indigestion, distension and upper abdominal discomfort; can be similar to functional bowel disease; can be clinically connected to gallstones	Thickening of gall bladder wall detected on ultrasound	Not an isolated condition because connected with gallstones; not clear whether Karin had this before her gallstones developed; has not had current symptoms ever before
AUTOIMMUNE DISEASE		
Coeliac disease	Abdominal pain, poor diet, diarrhoea; more often upper abdominal pain; diet has significantly changed since being in Australia; family history of symptoms	Significant lower abdominal bloating not reported
STRESS AND NEUROLOGICAL		
Causal factor: **Stress**	Being away from home, wanting more finances to go travelling, unresolved issues with parents, significant health concern while being in a foreign country; can exacerbate functional bowel disease	
EATING HABITS AND ENERGY		
Causal factor: **Hypercholesterolaemia:** increased cholesterol	Karin has been eating more red meat, dairy products and bread than she used to	

Working diagnosis

KARIN AND GALLSTONES (CHOLECYSTITIS)

Karin is a woman travelling alone in Australia and is currently working as a nanny to save some money to do more travelling. Karin's plans may need to be revised, however, because she has just been diagnosed with gallstones causing periods of acute cholecystitis (biliary colic). Karin left her home in Denmark in strained circumstances after a bitter argument with her parents and is now resisting contacting them. During the consultation we learn that Karin has not told her doctor about symptoms of alternating diarrhoea and constipation. Karin's mother has had abdominal symptoms and alternating diarrhoea and constipation similar to those Karin is currently experiencing.

GALLSTONES

It is difficult to ascertain the prevalence of gallstones in the general population because they are often asymptomatic (silent) producing no significant physical symptoms for years. However, gallstones do seem to be more common in North America, Scandinavia and South America and young women are likely to report having gallstones more frequently than men. The difference between male and female prevalence is thought to decrease with age. Although gallstones are mostly asymptomatic, they may lodge in the neck of the gall bladder or in the cystic duct giving rise to biliary pain or acute cholecystitis. Gallstones can also move into the common bile duct causing biliary obstruction and producing severe pain and jaundice. It is medically understood that gallstones themselves do not produce colicky pain, indigestion, chronic right abdominal pain or intolerance to fatty foods they are often correlated with. However, if there is a temporary obstruction of the common bile duct by a stone moving from the gall bladder, physical symptoms of gallstone colic/dyspepsia can be experienced. When this occurs symptoms may include feelings of fullness after eating, increased belching, flatulence and abdominal distension, particularly after overindulgence in fatty foods.

Gallstones are classified into those made up of cholesterol (80 per cent of all gallstones) and those made up of bile pigment. Karin has been diagnosed with cholesterol stones. These stones are partly derived from dietary sources, and are also synthesised in the liver, small intestine, skin and adrenals. Cholesterol stones develop in bile when there is an excess of cholesterol relative to bile salts and phospholipids (supersaturated bile). This can occur due to an excess of cholesterol or a decrease in bile salts. Risk factors for cholesterol stones developing include:
• eating foods high in cholesterol
• being female due to increased oestrogen decreasing solubility and excretion of cholesterol
• rapid weight loss or fasting due to an increase in leptin, which can increase cholesterol secretion
• bile salt loss occurring in conditions such as Crohn's disease
• chronic constipation causing a slow colonic transit time and influencing the composition of the bile salt pool in the colon
• gall bladder motility disorders that may occur during pregnancy and diabetes
• obesity
• taking the oral contraceptive pill
• liver disease.

ACUTE CHOLECYSTITIS

About 90 per cent of acute cholecystitis cases result from an obstruction of the neck of the gall bladder by gallstones. This leads to lack of gall bladder emptying, distension and inflammation. Sometimes the inflammation is mild and quickly subsides and the person may only feel a small amount of pain. It is more common for inflammation to become more severe giving rise to an acute rapid onset of pain that is localised to the middle of the abdomen or specifically in the right upper quadrant. It is at this stage that many people realise for the first time they have gallstones. The pain is continuous and increases gradually in intensity and can radiate to the back and the right shoulder. An episode of pain will slowly ease and there will usually be pain-free periods for between 30 and 360 minutes. The person may also feel nauseous, feverish and often will vomit. At this stage mild jaundice may occur.

General references used in this diagnosis: 1, 3, 5, 6, 11, 40

TABLE 3.36 DECISION TABLE FOR TREATMENT PRIOR TO REFERRAL

COMPLAINT	CONTEXT	CORE
Treatment for the presenting complaint and symptoms	Treatment for all associated symptoms	Treatment for mental, emotional, spiritual, constitutional, lifestyle issues and metaphysical considerations
TREATMENT PRIORITY	**TREATMENT PRIORITY**	**TREATMENT PRIORITY**
• Lifestyle recommendations to reduce the incidence of acute episodes • Dietary recommendations to reduce recurrence of attacks • Physical therapy recommendations for symptomatic relief • Herbal tonic to support bile flow and formation and to help reduce further stone formation **NB:** Herbal choleretics and cholagogues are contraindicated in septic cholecystitis where there is a risk of peritonitis; collaborative management of Karin's case with her GP is therefore essential to ensure there are no contraindications to herbal therapy • Herbal tea to help reduce nausea and improve production and flow of bile	• Lifestyle recommendations to help reduce stone formation • Specific dietary recommendations to help reduce and/or prevent formation and enlargement of stones • Dietary recommendations to improve general nutrition and reduce dietary risk factors for stone development • Herbal tonic and tea to support digestive and liver function • Specific nutritional supplements to help reduce and/or prevent formation and enlargement of stones	• Lifestyle recommendations to help reduce stress and anxiety • Recommendation for counselling to help Karin deal with unresolved family conflict • Physical therapy suggestions to help reduce stress and anxiety • Herbal tea with anxiolytic and sedative action

TABLE 3.37 DECISION TABLE FOR REFERRAL [3, 5, 11, 12]

COMPLAINT	CONTEXT	CORE
Referral for presenting complaint	Referral for all associated physical, dietary and lifestyle concerns	Referral for contributing emotional, mental, spiritual, metaphysical, lifestyle and constitutional factors
REFERRAL FLAGS	**REFERRAL FLAGS**	**REFERRAL FLAGS**
• Being far away from home with a potentially serious medical condition • Karin has not communicated with her GP that she is investigating 'alternative' rather than 'complementary' approaches to treating her gallstones	• γ-GT enzyme raised could indicate alcohol abuse	• Karen did not tell her doctor her mother has similar symptoms out of worry that she would be forced to contact her parents

▶

ISSUES OF SIGNIFICANCE	ISSUES OF SIGNIFICANCE	ISSUES OF SIGNIFICANCE
• Potential family history of gall bladder disease with her mother having had similar symptoms	• Possible family history of food allergy with her mother having had similar symptoms • Karin's diet is unbalanced and contributing to the development of gallstones • Karin is not as physically active as she used to be, which may be contributing to the development of gallstones	• Karin has unresolved bitterness and issues with her parents, which may be causing stress and contributing to her current condition • Wanting to keep travelling and meet people her own age
REFERRAL DECISION	**REFERRAL DECISION**	**REFERRAL DECISION**
• Contact with Karin's parents may shed light on family health history and potential severity of gallstone prognosis • Karen needs medical monitoring and collaboration between her CAM therapist and GP regarding treatment for gallstones	• A dietary evaluation is necessary for Karin to assess food allergies/intolerances	• A counsellor and long-distance mediator may help Karin to resolve issues with her parents and help alleviate stress

TABLE 3.38 **FURTHER INVESTIGATIONS THAT MAY BE NECESSARY** [1, 3–6, 11, 13]

TEST/INVESTIGATION	REASON FOR TEST/INVESTIGATION
FIRST-LINE INVESTIGATIONS:	
Hydrogen breath test	To detect bacterial overgrowth; when bacteria is metabolised by lactose or glucose there is a production of hydrogen
Elimination diet	Detect food intolerance
IF NECESSARY:	
Oral tolerance lactose test	Determine lactose metabolism
Antigliadin antibodies	Check if antibodies to gluten are present in blood indicating coeliac disease
p-ANCA (anti-neutrophil cytoplasmic antibody)	Detect primary sclerosing cholangitis
Serum immunoglobulins IgG and IgM	Cirrhosis of the liver, postviral disease and autoimmune disease of the liver
Serum autoantibodies AMA	Primary biliary cirrhosis of the liver
Magnetic resonance cholangiography (MRC)	Delineates fluid volume in bile tree, detect primary sclerosing cholangitis

▶

Sprial CT scanning	Detect bile duct dilatation; can exclude carcinoma as the cause of the bile duct obstruction; define if opaque or cholesterol stones; acute pancreatitis
Endoscopic ultrasound scanning of the bile duct and gall bladder	Identify stones at the distal end of the common bile duct; invasive procedure
Endoscopic retrograde cholangiography (ERC)	Detects primary sclerosing cholangitis
Endoscopy	Peptic ulcer
Sigmoidoscopy	Confirm Crohn's disease and eliminate from differential diagnosis list
Liver histology	Confirms primary sclerosing cholangitis

Confirmed diagnosis

Gallstones (cholecystitis) with hypercholesterol and stress

PRESCRIBED MEDICATION

• Analgesics as required for the pain

TABLE 3.39 DECISION TABLE FOR TREATMENT (ONCE DIAGNOSIS IS CONFIRMED)		
COMPLAINT	CONTEXT	CORE
Treatment for the presenting complaint and symptoms	Treatment for all associated symptoms	Treatment for mental, emotional, spiritual, constitutional, lifestyle issues and metaphysical considerations
TREATMENT PRIORITY	TREATMENT PRIORITY	TREATMENT PRIORITY
• Continue with lifestyle and dietary recommendations to reduce the incidence of acute episodes • Continue with physical therapy recommendations as required for symptomatic relief • Continue with herbal tonic and tea for at least 10 weeks, and then review formulae based on Karin's symptoms	• Continue with lifestyle and dietary recommendations to improve nutrition and reduce risk factors for further stone development • Continue with herbal tonic and tea to support digestive and liver function; review formulae after 10 weeks • Continue with supplemental nutrients to improve general health and digestive function; review supplements after 8–10 weeks	• Continue with lifestyle and physical therapy recommendations to help reduce stress and anxiety • Encourage Karin to continue counselling • Continue with herbal tea; review formula after 10 weeks

Treatment aims

• Prevent bile stasis and supersaturation [14–16].
• Stimulate production and flow of bile [21].

- Increase solubility of bile [15] and solubility of cholesterol in bile [15, 19].
- Prevent further stone formation and enlargement [15].
- Reduce dietary risk factors [15–17] and improve Karin's diet [15, 16].

Lifestyle alterations/considerations

- Encourage Karin to not be encouraged to use gall bladder flushing techniques because stones may lodge and block her bile duct [16, 17].
- Encourage Karin to ensure she protects her skin from excessive exposure to sunlight and avoids sunburn [15].
- Karin would benefit from dealing with her emotional stress [15]. Chronic stress can increase bile retention and inhibit gall bladder emptying [15]. Stress-management techniques would therefore be helpful to her.
- Karin may find counselling helpful to help her deal with the unresolved conflict with her parents [27].
- Karin would benefit from increasing her physical activity. Symptomatic cholelithiasis can be prevented by physical activity [26]. Regular exercise is associated with lower levels of stress and anxiety [29, 30].

Dietary suggestions

- Encourage Karin to drink six to eight glasses of water every day to ensure the water content of the bile is maintained [15].
- Encourage Karin to try to include turmeric in her diet as often as possible [15]. Turmeric is a choleretic [21] and is used traditionally to improve poor digestion [21]. It has also been demonstrated to reduce gallstone size [24].
- Encourage Karin to reduce her consumption of animal protein, refined carbohydrates, sugar, saturated fats and dietary cholesterol [15, 16].
- Encourage Karin to avoid all fried foods [15].
- Encourage Karin to increase consumption of fruit, vegetables and legumes [15, 16].
- Encourage Karin to increase her consumption of foods containing omega-3 fatty acids, particularly from cold-water fish [15].
- Encourage Karin to increase her consumption of soluble fibre [15, 16].
- Determine whether Karin has any food allergies and manage accordingly [15].
- Karin could include buckwheat regularly in her diet [15]. Buckwheat enhances bile acid synthesis, reduces concentration of cholesterol in the gall bladder and decreases gallstone formation [15].
- Karin could consume 1–2 tsp of lecithin granules daily [15, 16]. The phosphatidyl choline in lecithin increases phospholipids in bile, which can improve bile solubility, therefore reducing the risk of stone formation [16].
- Karin may benefit from drinking lemon juice. Lemon juice increases hepatobiliary excretion and therefore may improve digestive function [25].

Physical treatment suggestions

- Acupuncture may relieve Karin's abdominal pain and nausea [22, 23]. It may also help reduce her anxiety and stress [29, 30].
- Karin may find massage helpful to reduce stress and anxiety [31, 32].
- Hydrotherapy: hot trunk wrap [33]. Constitutional hydrotherapy [33–35].
- Hot fomentations (5–10 minutes) with vinegar water alternating with cold (1–5 minutes) mitten frictions to abdomen and lower back [34, 35].

TABLE 3.40 HERBAL FORMULA (1:2 LIQUID EXTRACTS)

HERB	FORMULA	RATIONALE
Fringe tree *Chionanthus virginicus*	40 mL	Choleretic [18, 21]; cholagogue [18, 19, 21]; traditionally used for cholecystitis
Dandelion root *Taraxacum officinale*	40 mL	Choleretic [18, 20]; cholagogue [19]; traditionally used to treat cholecystitis and gall stones [18, 19]
Boldo *Peumus boldo*	20 mL	Cholagogue [18, 19]; liver stimulant [18, 19]; traditionally used to treat gall bladder pain and gallstones [18, 19]; indicated for use in cholelithiasis with pain [19]
Globe artichoke *Cynara scolymus*	40 mL	Choleretic [21, 20]; cholagogue [21, 20]; antiemetic [21]; hepatoprotective [21, 20]
St Mary's thistle *Silybum marianum*	60 mL	Choleretic [21]; hepatoprotective [21, 20]
Supply:	200 mL	Dose: 5 mL 3 times daily

TABLE 3.41 HERBAL TEA

Alternative to tea and coffee

HERB	FORMULA	RATIONALE
Peppermint leaf *Mentha × piperita*	3 parts	Choleretic [20, 21]; antispasmodic [20, 21]; relieves nausea [20, 21]
Chamomile flower *Matricaria recutita*	3 parts	Choleretic [20]; antispasmodic [20, 21]; anti-inflammatory [20, 21]; mild sedative [20, 21]
Ginger root (powdered) *Zingiber officinale*	¼ part	Anti-emetic [20, 21]; anti-nausea [20, 21]; choleretic [20]; anxiolytic [20]; traditionally used to enhance digestion [21]

Infusion: 1 tsp per cup – 1 cup 3–4 times daily

TABLE 3.42 NUTRITIONAL SUPPLEMENTS

SUPPLEMENT AND DOSE	RATIONALE
Omega-3 fish oil 3 × 1000 mg capsules twice daily [16, 38]	Omega-3 oils are essential for the normal formation of bile [15, 16, 38]; supplementation decreases biliary cholesterol saturation in gallstone disease [38] and improves gall bladder dysmotility [39]
Vitamin C 1000 mg twice daily [15, 16, 37]	High-dose vitamin C supplementation may reduce cholesterol stone formation by altering bile acid composition and increasing the time taken for gallstones to develop [16, 37]

▶

Soluble fibre supplement 10 g twice daily [15]	Soluble fibre reduces biliary cholesterol saturation and cholesterol stone formation [16, 36]
Lipotropic supplement providing approx. 1000 mg choline [15, 16], 800 mg l-methionine [15, 16] and 3 g taurine [5, 15, 16] daily	Lipotropic factors are essential for normal liver metabolism of fat and bile flow [15, 16]; taurine increases bile acid pool and prevents gallstone formation [5, 28]

References

[1] G. Douglas, F. Nicol, C. Robertson, Macleod's Clinical Examination, twelfth edn, Churchill Livingstone Elsevier, Edinburgh, 2009.
[2] N.J. Talley, S. O'Connor, Pocket Clinical Examination, third edn, Churchill Livingstone Elsevier, Australia, 2009.
[3] P. Kumar, C. Clark, Clinical Medicine, sixth edn, Elsevier Saunders, London, 2005.
[4] A. Polmear, Evidence-Based Diagnosis in Primary Care, Churchill Livingstone Elsevier, 2008.
[5] J. Jamison, Differential Diagnosis for Primary Care, second edn, Churchill Livingstone Elsevier, London, 2006.
[6] R.D. Collins, Differential Diagnosis in Primary Care, fourth edn, Lippincott Williams & Wilkins, Philadelphia, 2008.
[7] R.H. Seller, Differential Diagnosis of Common Complaints, fifth edn, Saunders Elsevier, Philadelphia, 2007.
[8] M. Lloyd, R. Bor, Communication Skills For Medicine, third edn, Churchill Livingstone Elsevier, Edinburgh, 2009.
[9] R. Neighbour, The Inner Consultation: how to develop an effective and intuitive consulting style, Radcliff Publishing, Oxon, 2005.
[10] J. Silverman, S. Kurtz, J. Draper, Skills for Communicating with Patients, second edn, Radcliff Publishing, Oxford, 2000.
[11] R. Berkow, A.J. Fletcher, M.H. Beers, The Merck Manual, sixteenth edn, Merck Research Laboratories, Rathway, N.J, 1993 (later edition).
[12] D. Peters, L. Chaitow, G. Harris, S. Morrison, Integrating Complementary Therapies in Primary Care, London, Churchill Livingstone, 2002.
[13] K.D. Pagna, T.J. Pagna, Mosby's Diagnostic and Laboratory Test reference, third edn, Mosby, USA, 1997 (later edition).
[14] J. Jamison, Clinical Guide to Nutrition & Dietary Supplements in Disease Management, Churchill Livingstone, Edinburgh, 2003.
[15] J.E. Pizzorno, M.T. Murray, H. Joiner-Bey, The Clinicians Handbook of Natural Medicine, second edn, Churchill Livingstone, St Louis, 2008.
[16] H. Osiecki, The Physicians Handbook of Clinical Nutrition, seventh edn, Eagle Farm: Bioconcepts, 2000.
[17] S. El-Hashemy, Naturopathic Standards of Primary Care, CCNM Press Inc, Toronto, 2007.
[18] S. Mills, K. Bone, The Essential Guide to Herbal Safety, Churchill Livingstone, St Louis, 2005.
[19] British Herbal Medicine Association, British Herbal Pharmacopoeia, BHMAA, 1983.
[20] L. Braun, M. Cohen, Herbs & Natural Supplements: An evidence based guide, second edn, Elsevier, Sydney, 2007.
[21] S. Mills, K. Bone, Principles & Practice of Phytotherapy: Modern Herbal Medicine, Churchill Livingstone, Edinburgh, London, 2000.
[22] D.L. Diehl, Acupuncture for Gastrointestinal and Hepatobiliary Disorders, The J Altern Complement Med 5 (1) (1999) 27–45.
[23] T. Takahashi, Acupuncture for functional gastrointestinal disorders, Journal of Gastroenterology 41 (2006) 408–417.
[24] K. Srinivasan, Spices as influencers of body metabolism: an overview of three decades of research, Food Research International 38 (2005) 77–86.
[25] S.C. Cherng, Y.H. Chen, M.S. Lee, S.P. Yang, W.S. Huang, C.Y. Cheng, Acceleration of hepatobiliary excretion by lemon juice on 99mTc-tetrofosmin cardiac SPECT, Nuclear Medicine Communications 27 (11) (2006) 859–864.
[26] H.P.F. Peters, W.R. DeVries, G.P. Vanberge-Henegouwen, L.M.A. Akkermans, Potential benefits and hazards of physical activity and exercise on the gastrointestinal tract, Gut 48 (2001) 435–439.
[27] T.R. Nielsen, D.S. Carlson, M.J. Lankau, The Supportive Mentor as a Means of Reducing Work–Family Conflict, Journal of Vocational Behavior 59 (2001) 364–381.
[28] J.D. Militante, J.B. Lombardini, Dietary taurine supplementation: hypolipidemic and antiatherogenic effects, Nutrition Research 24 (2004) 787–801.
[29] A.F. Jorm, H. Christensen, K.M. Griffiths, R.A. Parslow, B. Rodgers, K.A. Blewitt, Effectiveness of complementary and self-help treatments for anxiety disorders, Medical Journal of Australia 181 (7) (2004) S29–S46.
[30] A. Byrne, G.D. Byrne, The effect of exercise on depression, anxiety and other mood states: A review, J Psychosom Res 37 (6) (1993) 565–574.
[31] T. Field, G. Robinson, F. Scafidi, R. Nawrocki, A. Goncalves, Massage therapy reduces anxiety and enhances EEG pattern of alertness and math computations, International Journal of Neuroscience 86 (1996) 197–205.
[32] C.A. Moyer, J. Rounds, J.W. Hannum, A Meta-Analysis of Massage Therapy Research, Psychological Bulletin 130 (1) (2004) 3–18.

[33] E. Blake, in: L. Chaitow, E. Blake, P. Orrock, M. Wallden, P. Sinder, J. Zeff (Eds.), Naturopathic Physical Medicine: Theory and Practice for Manual Therapists and Naturopaths, Churchill Livingstone Elsevier, Philadelphia, 2008.

[34] D.D. Buchman, The complete book of water healing, Contemporary Books, McGraw-Hill Companies, New York, 2001.

[35] W. Boyle, A. Saine, Lectures in Naturopathic Hydrotherapy, Oregon: Eclectic Medical Publications, 1988.

[36] W.H. Schwesinger, W.E. Kurtin, C.P. Page, R.M. Stewart, R. Johnson, Soluble Dietary Fiber Protects against Cholesterol Gallstone Formation, American Journal of Surgery 177 (1999) 307–310.

[37] U. Gustafsson, F.H. Wang, M. Axelson, A. Kallner, S. Sahlin, K. Einarsson, The effect of vitamin C in high doses on plasma and biliary lipid composition in patients with cholesterol gallstones: prolongation of the nucleation time, European Journal of Clinical Investigation 27 (5) (2003) 387–391.

[38] F. Berr, J. Holl, D. Jungst, S. Fischer, W.O. Richter, B. Seifferth, et al., Dietary N-3 Polyunsaturated Fatty Acids Decrease Biliary Cholesterol Saturation in Gallstone Disease, Hepatology 16 (1992) 960–967.

[39] I. Jonkers, A. Smelt, M. Ledeboer, M. Hollum, I. Biemond, F. Kuipers, et al., Gall bladder dysmotility: a risk factor for gall stone formation in hypertriglyceridaemia and reversal on triglyceride lowering therapy by bezafibrate and fish oil, Gut 52 (2003) 109–115.

[40] R.H. Dowling, Review: pathogenesis of gallstones, Alimentary Pharmacology and Therapeutics 14 (Suppl. 2) (2000) 39–47.

[41] R.E. Marshall, A. Anggiansah, W.A. Owen, et al., The relationship between acid and bile reflux and symptoms in gastro-oesophageal reflux disease, Gut 40 (2) (1997 Feb) 182–187.

Coeliac disease

Case history

Nine-month-old Sam has been brought to the clinic by his parents, Ally and Rod, for help with a digestive problem. Ally and Rod are exhausted and desperate to get help for Sam, and are hoping a gentle natural treatment will fix Sam's problem. Sam is Ally and Rod's first child and they are feeling anxious and completely out of their depth.

Sam was fully breastfed until the age of five months when he started eating solid foods. Since then Sam has experienced frequent episodes of abdominal bloating and diarrhoea after meals. The bloating appears to be painful as Sam usually screams and lifts his legs to his chest when his abdomen is bloated. Ally and Rod are concerned because Sam appears to be losing weight and is always tired and irritable. Sam also has an itchy rash on his elbows, scalp and buttocks, which is causing him considerable distress and keeping him awake at night. Sam is very clingy and miserable and spends most of his time sleeping face down on Ally's chest, which seems to help relieve his symptoms. Ally and Rod have had a number of suggestions from family and friends as to the cause of Sam's problems including early teething, colic and eczema.

Ally tells you that Sam is always hungry and she tries to give him a broad and balanced diet. He has porridge or Weet-Bix with warm milk for breakfast, and loves pasta and rice with vegetables. Ally has tried giving Sam organic vegetables to see if that helped, but it hasn't made much difference. Sam also eats small amounts of fish and chicken but hasn't had red meat yet. He is still having two feeds of breast milk each day and Ally is concerned that Sam's problems may be caused by something she is eating.

Rod tells you he thinks Sam's problem may be inherited from his side of the family. His mother often complained of stomach pain and was always very thin.

In the past three months Sam has been taken to emergency by Ally and Rod when he has shown signs of intense symptoms of abdominal pain. Each time tests such as abdominal ultrasound, rectal and testicular examination came back clear. They have been advised to seek medical advice for dietary reasons that may be causing Sam's symptoms. Ally and Rod have never been to a natural therapist before but are willing to try anything to help Sam.

TABLE 3.43 **COMPLAINT** [1–5, 40]	
Analogy: Skin of the apple	**Complaint:** Define the presenting complaint and symptoms; understand the complaint *Abdominal bloating and diarrhoea*
AREAS OF INVESTIGATION AND EXAMPLE QUESTIONS	**CLIENT RESPONSES**
Timing (duration, frequency) *How long does the diarrhoea last and how often does it occur?*	*The diarrhoea seems to come a couple of hours after food and a large amount will be passed and then it will settle down until the next feed.*
Account and description *What volume of diarrhoea is Sam passing?*	*I need to change Sam's nappy 3 to 4 times an hour after eating. Then it settles down.*

TABLE 3.44 **CONTEXT**	
Analogy: Flesh of the apple	**Context:** Put the presenting complaint into context to understand the disease
AREAS OF INVESTIGATION AND EXAMPLE QUESTIONS	**CLIENT RESPONSES**
Functional disease *Does Sam cry for more than 3 hours a day, more than 3 days a week and more than 3 weeks in a row?* (commonly infantile colic)	*Sam can cry all day every day for weeks, it seems! That's why we knew something was seriously wrong.*
Degenerative and deficiency *Has Sam experienced a decreased urine output while having diarrhoea?* (dehydration)	*Sometimes after a big episode of diarrhoea he doesn't seem to pass urine as much. I tried giving him fluids again with breast milk, but I think that's causing the problem, so I'm trying to give him more water.*
Eating habits and energy *How soon after eating does Sam appear to have symptoms of abdominal bloating?*	*Sam appears to be in pain and can scream sometimes as early as 15 to 40 minutes after eating or having a breastfeed.*

TABLE 3.45 **CORE**	
Analogy: Core of the apple with the seed of ill health	**Core:** Holistic assessment to understand the client
AREAS OF INVESTIGATION AND EXAMPLE QUESTIONS	**CLIENT RESPONSES**
Emotional health *Describe, if any, a time you both felt relaxed as first-time parents.*	*We're both exhausted and have not felt really elated to be parents since Sam was a few weeks old.*

▶

Home life *How would you describe the family environment at home?*	*Stressful. We are not sleeping well and the cries and screaming from Sam bring us to our knees with worry most of the time.*
Has not been well since *What do you think might be causing Sam's symptoms?*	*We really think it has something to do with either Ally's diet or what we're feeding Sam.*

TABLE 3.46 SAM'S SIGNS AND SYMPTOMS [4,6]

Pulse	100 bpm
Blood pressure	Not taken
Temperature	37.5°C
Respiratory rate	40 resp/min
Physical development	9.3 kg – 50th percentile for an infant of Sam's age
Face	Pale, dark under the eyes
Abdominal examination	Distended abdomen
Skin examination	Red plaques present on elbows, scalp and buttocks; plaques are excoriated from scratching, crusted over in areas; new blister vesicles are present and appear to be spreading
Urinalysis	Not done due to difficulty in obtaining a urine sample

TABLE 3.47 RESULTS OF MEDICAL INVESTIGATIONS [1–5, 7]

TEST/INVESTIGATION	REASON FOR TEST/INVESTIGATION
Abdominal examination: guarding, rebound tenderness, palpation, abnormal pulsations (auscultation)	No palpable mass found; intussusception would present with a palpable lump either rectally or abdominally; appendicitis, constipation mass, enlarged kidney, hernia may also be palpable
Rectal and testicular examination	No mass associated with hernia and intussusception
Abdominal ultrasound	No appendicitis, intussusception, intestinal obstruction found

TABLE 3.48 CONDITIONS THAT HAVE BEEN MEDICALLY INVESTIGATED [1–5]

CONDITIONS AND CAUSES	WHY UNLIKELY
OBSTRUCTION AND FOREIGN BODY	
Intussusception: part of the small intestine slides into another part, like a collapsible telescope; abdominal pain in babies from birth to 1 year; baby will scream and pull its legs to the chest	Cause of sudden and acute severe abdominal pain in children as opposed to recurrent pain; vomiting can be common; red current jelly stool (blood and mucus mixed with stool); will show signs of difficulty breathing; not usual to have significant diarrhoea as an associated symptom; can feel a banana-shaped mass in the upper abdomen

Volvulus (twisted bowel): common in infants, usually congenital intestinal malrotation	Acute abdominal pain; usually associated with vomiting; requires emergency surgery as can cause death quickly; not usual to have significant diarrhoea as an associated symptom
Hernia strangulation	Cause of acute abdominal pain in children as opposed to recurrent pain; not usual to have significant diarrhoea as an associated symptom; often presents with vomiting
Hirschsprung's disease: congenital disorder causing enlarged colon; abdominal pain in babies aged birth to 1 year; causes chronic constipation	Diarrhoea not a prominent symptom; common to show signs of food refusal or vomiting
Intestinal obstruction (constipation): abdominal pain, distended abdomen; can be acute and recurrent	Pain is usually relieved by passing a bowel motion; pain often in right lower quadrant; abdominal pain can be made worse or better by eating meals; abdominal examination and ultrasound will clarify diagnosis
INFECTION AND INFLAMMATION	
Appendicitis: diagnosis may be missed because it is not common in children aged under 5; perforation can cause death without fast surgical intervention [39]	Not common in this age group; usually associated with severe abdominal pain and fever – it is good practice to further investigate this diagnosis

Case analysis

TABLE 3.49 POSSIBLE DIFFERENTIAL DIAGNOSIS		
Not ruled out by tests/investigations already done [1–5, 7, 38, 40, 47]		
CONDITIONS AND CAUSES	WHY POSSIBLE	WHY UNLIKELY
ALLERGIES AND IRRITANTS		
Lactose and fructose intolerance	If diarrhoea and abdominal pain occurs in an in infant less than 1 year old who has been introduced to dairy and friut products, lactose and/or fructose intolerance needs to be considered	Not necessarily associated with skin rash
Causal factor: Food allergy: typically to cow's milk, egg, soya, peanut, wheat and fish [43, 44]	Diarrhoea, cramping colic, skin rash, abdominal pain	Often presents with swelling of lips and tongue, urticarial skin rash, conjunctivitis, rhinitis, anaphylaxis and difficulty breathing
CANCER AND HEART DISEASE		
Lymphoma	May infiltrate the small intestine and cause diarrhoea and malabsorption; increased risk with coeliac disease; weight loss, fatigue	

FUNCTIONAL DISEASE		
Infantile colic [48]	The baby will scream and pull the legs to the chest; abdominal pain, distended abdomen, diarrhoea; can begin when weaning the baby onto solids and during teething	Need to define what pattern of crying and how long the abdominal distension has been present
DEGENERATIVE AND DEFICIENCY		
Causal factor: **Dehydration**	Diarrhoea; colicky pain in the abdomen may be present that can be dull, constant and intermittent	Clarify if there has been a decreased urine output
Pernicious anemia	Diarrhoea, tiredness, irritability, B12 deficiency can be associated with coeliac disease	
Iron deficiency anaemia	Tiredness, lack of iron-rich foods in diet; can be associated with coeliac disease	
Causal factor: **Failure to thrive**	Weight loss, fatigue	
INFECTION AND INFLAMMATION		
Dermatitis herpetiformis	Abdominal pain, skin rash, diarrhoea, came on with introduction of solid foods, associated with coeliac disease	More common to present in early adulthood
Eczema	Rash on extensor surfaces, rash associated with foods; can be aggravated by dairy foods, wheat allergies	Not necessarily associated with diarrhoea
Gastroenteritis: rotavirus, *Salmonella*, *Shigella*	Abdominal pain, diarrhoea; can have transient lactose intolerance	More often acute presentation and not recurrent; check if the abdominal pain is generalised; usually associated with a low-grade fever; severe presentation in infants; check if the peak incidence of diarrhoea occurs in winter (rotavirus in infants)
Parasite infestation: giardia	Causes diarrhoea, weight loss and malnutrition; infants can be susceptible; may persist for weeks and months	Check if other family members have experienced similar symptoms recently and if they have shared water with Sam
Urinary tract infection	Abdominal pain in children	Check if the abdominal pain seems to radiate; urinalysis check; not necessarily associated with diarrhoea; abdominal examination and ultrasound can assist diagnosis

Crohn's diease	Abdominal pain, diarrhoea, symptoms associated with foods, weight loss	Common to have low-grade fever, blood and/or mucous in stools; more common to first present in adolescence
ENDOCRINE/REPRODUCTIVE		
Diabetes	Abdominal pain in children; diarrhoea	Need to explore family history
AUTOIMMUNE DISEASE		
Coeliac disease	Abdominal pain from bloating, weight loss, tiredness, skin rash, diarrhoea; came on when weaned onto solids foods; family history of symptoms	
EATING HABITS AND ENERGY		
Causal factor: Poisoning	Frequent cause of abdominal pain in children	Need to explore if recurrent abdominal symptoms could be due to food or environmental poisoning; usually associated with vomiting

TABLE 3.50 DECISION TABLE FOR REFERRAL		
COMPLAINT	**CONTEXT**	**CORE**
Referral for presenting complaint	Referral for all associated physical, dietary and lifestyle concerns	Referral for contributing emotional, mental, spiritual, metaphysical, lifestyle and constitutional factors
REFERRAL FLAGS	**REFERRAL FLAGS**	**REFERRAL FLAGS**
• Consistent diarrhoea since the introduction of solid food	• Dehydration due to diarrhoea • Chronic diarrhoea is likely to be causing significant nutritional deficiencies, which are affecting Sam's development – failure to thrive • Weight loss since onset of symptoms • Sam is below the expected weight and height percentile for an infant of his age – failure to thrive • Fatigue – failure to thrive • Family history of similar symptoms	• Ally and Rod are exhausted and anxious about Sam's health
ISSUES OF SIGNIFICANCE	**ISSUES OF SIGNIFICANCE**	**ISSUES OF SIGNIFICANCE**
Nil	• Sam is likely to have dysbiosis of intestinal microflora • Skin rash associated with onset of symptoms • Skin rash is interfering with Sam's sleep	• Sam is tired, clingy and often miserable and in pain

REFERRAL DECISION	REFERRAL DECISION	REFERRAL DECISION
• Encourage collaborative healthcare management with GP and natural therapist/dietician	• Dietician/natural therapist for dietary assessment and food elimination [42] • Skin specialist to assess skin rash • Medical investigation for autoimmune food-related disorders such as coeliac disease	• Counselling and support for Ally and Rod

TABLE 3.51 FURTHER INVESTIGATIONS THAT MAY BE NECESSARY [1–7, 40, 42, 47]

TEST/INVESTIGATION	REASON FOR TEST/INVESTIGATION
FIRST-LINE INVESTIGATIONS:	
Abdominal examination: guarding, rebound tenderness, palpation, abnormal pulsations (auscultation)	Monitor bloating and distension for abdominal mass
Breath smell test	Sweet fruity smell in ketoacidosis, generalised abdominal pain – diabetic ketoacidosis
Stool sample	Rule out parasites, occult blood; if acidic stools are passed it indicates lactose intolerance
Urinalysis	Urinary tract infection, diabetes
Skin assessment by a dermatologist	Eczema, dermatitis herpetiformis
Dietary elimination diets for mother and baby – gluten-free diet [41, 42, 46]	Coeliac disease, lactose intolerance, typical food allergies
IF NECESSARY:	
Full blood count	Anaemia, appendicitis, allergic response, lymphoma; determine iron and B12 levels
ESR	Inflammation
Serum IgE [42, 45, 46]	Allergies
Skin-prick test [42]	Food and environmental allergies and intolerances
Antigliadin antibodies	Check if antibodies to gluten are present in blood
Jejunal biopsy	The appearance of the mucosa is a definitive diagnosis for coeliac disease

Working diagnosis

SAM AND COELIAC DISEASE WITH ASSOCIATED DERMATITIS HERPETIFORMIS [1–4, 47]

Sam is a nine-month-old baby who has been brought in by his parents to see a complementary therapist for help with recurrent abdominal bloating, diarrhoea and a skin rash. Sam is an only child and his parents are worried about the distress he is experiencing along with progressive symptoms of fatigue, weight loss and irritability.

Sam was referred for medical assessment and has been diagnosed with coeliac disease with associated dermatitis herpetiformis. Coeliac disease is a condition where the jejunal mucosa in the small intestine is damaged when consuming gluten-containing foods. Gluten is found in the cereals of wheat, barley, rye and oats. A skin disorder called *Dermatitis herpetiformis* can be associated with gluten-sensitive enteropathy.

The mucosa of the small intestine is most affected and the microvilli become flat, causing malabsorption of nutrients in food. Coeliac disease can present at any age and in children it can first present when they are weaned onto solid foods.

Vague symptoms can present including tiredness, diarrhoea, abdominal pain, weight loss, mouth ulcers, muscle weakness and malnutrition, with a greater incidence of autoimmune disorders and inflammatory bowel conditions.

Dermatitis herpetiformis is a condition that produces a rash symmetrically distributed over extensor surfaces of the body. It can occur at any age but is most commonly seen in the second, third and fourth decades. The rash blisters, excoriates and crusts and is very itchy. The vesicles usually burst through scratching and then crust over. Most people with this condition also have a gluten-sensitive enteropathy; however, bowel symptoms may not be as severe as those with coeliac disease.

TABLE 3.52 **DECISION TABLE FOR TREATMENT (ONCE DIAGNOSIS IS CONFIRMED)**		
COMPLAINT	**CONTEXT**	**CORE**
Treatment for the presenting complaint and symptoms	Treatment for all associated symptoms	Treatment for mental, emotional, spiritual, constitutional, lifestyle issues and metaphysical considerations
TREATMENT PRIORITY	**TREATMENT PRIORITY**	**TREATMENT PRIORITY**
• Dietary recommendations to eliminate gluten from both Sam and Ally's diets • Recommendation for Ally to continue breastfeeding Sam • Dietary changes to allow Sam's digestive tract to heal and function normally • Herbal drops or tea and powder to help alleviate acute digestive symptoms and soothe and heal inflamed gastric mucosa • Nutritional supplementation to ensure Sam is receiving essential nutrients until his digestive function has normalised and he is properly absorbing nutrients again • Topical herbal cream to help soothe and heal Sam's rash until dietary measures prevent it recurring	• Dietary recommendations to eliminate all potentially aggravating foods from Sam and Ally's diets until Sam's symptoms have improved • Dietary recommendations and nutritional supplements to ensure Sam develops normally • Nutritional supplements to replace missing nutrients until Sam's digestive tract is working normally again • Nutritional and probiotic supplementation to help restore normal intestinal microflora and facilitate normal digestive function • Herbal drops or tea plus slippery elm bark powder to help soothe and heal Sam's gut, reduce diarrhoea, improve digestive function and nutrient absorption	• As Sam's condition improves, Ally and Rod's anxieties will be alleviated • Educating Ally and Rod about coeliac disease and how it can be managed will help them understand Sam's condition and empower them to manage his condition themselves; this will significantly reduce their fears and anxieties • As Sam's rash is treated his sleep will improve, which will improve his energy and reduce his fatigue and support normal growth and development • Once Sam is sleeping well Ally and Rod will also get sufficient sleep and have the energy to cope better

Treatment aims

- Eliminate all sources of gluten in Sam's diet [8, 9].
- Correct underlying nutritional deficiencies [8, 9].
- Reduce inflammation in the bowel and soothe the gut [9].
- Restore mucosal integrity and normalise gut function [9].
- Correct bowel dysbiosis [9, 10].
- Eliminate dairy products at least until normal structure and function of the digestive tract is restored [8].

Lifestyle alterations/considerations

- Malabsorption of nutrients can result in growth retardation, bone density problems, dental problems and developmental problems [9, 24]. It would be wise for Sam to be referred to a paediatric specialist for appropriate assessment of growth and development [9].
- Ally and Rod need to learn how to manage his condition. Refer them to coeliac support groups, good-quality literature and websites.
- Ally and Rod may be feeling anxious and stressed and may benefit from a holistic natural therapy program to help them manage their stress.

Dietary suggestions

- Gluten-free diet. Exclude wheat, rye, spelt, barley, oats and triticale. Buckwheat and millet should also be excluded as they contain prolamins with a similar antigenicity to alpha-gliadin [8, 9, 24].
- It is important for Ally and Rod to read food labels carefully to avoid accidental or unintended gluten consumption.
- Encourage Sam to stay off dairy products, at least until his condition stabilises [8]. Dairy intolerance could also be a problem [8, 23], so Sam should not be given dairy-based infant formula, milk, cheese, yoghurt and products made with dairy.
- It may be prudent for Ally to follow a gluten- and dairy-free diet while she is breastfeeding [34].
- Ally should continue breastfeeding Sam until he is two [9, 17, 18] and delay re-introducing dairy products into his diet until his condition has stabilised [8, 23].

Physical treatment suggestions

- Hydrotherapy: a daily neutral-temperature oatmeal bath for the skin [30, 31]. Apply a warm apple cider vinegar and water compress on the abdomen for colic [31, 33]. A warm trunk wrap for abdominal pain [32]. Hot-warm wet sock treatment to divert blood from the abdomen to the lower extremities for colic [33].
- Sam may gain some benefit from acupuncture therapy [26]; however, stimulation of acupuncture points without the use of needles may be more acceptable to both Sam and his parents.
- Massage therapy may help relax Sam and improve his sleep and may help alleviate some of his distress and digestive discomfort [34].

TABLE 3.53 HERBAL FORMULA (1:2 LIQUID EXTRACTS)

Made with ethanolic extract herbal liquids (alcohol removed)

HERB	FORMULA	RATIONALE
Golden seal *Hydrastis canadensis* (cultivated/plantation source)	20 mL	Anti-inflammatory [11]; mucous membrane trophorestorative [11]; antimicrobial [12]; vulnerary [13]; traditionally used for digestive disorders [14]
Chamomile *Matricaria recutita*	60 mL	Anti-inflammatory [15, 16, 25]; antispasmodic [15, 16, 25]; mild sedative [15, 16, 25]; specifically indicated for gastrointestinal disturbance with associated nervous irritability in children [14]
Licorice *Glycyrrhiza glabra*	20 mL	Demulcent [14, 15]; mucoprotective [14, 15, 25]; anti-inflammatory [14, 15, 25]
Supply:	100 mL	Dose: 2 mL TDS (based on Sam's weight as a percentage of adult dose)

Slippery elm bark powder (*Ulmus rubra*) ¼ tsp mixed with 100 mL boiling water, then cooled before drinking [14]
Demulcent; emollient; nutritive; indicated for use in diarrhoea [14]

Herbal drops and **slippery elm bark powder** may be mixed into stewed fruit or mashed vegetables

Calendula (*Calendula officinalis*) cream or ointment can be applied 3–4 times daily to Sam's skin to help soothe and heal the rash [14, 25]

TABLE 3.54 HERBAL TEA

Alternative to herbal tonic if Ally prefers giving Sam a tea

HERB	FORMULA	RATIONALE
Chamomile flowers *Matricaria recutita*	2 parts	See above
Lemon balm leaves *Melissa officinalis*	1 part	Anti-inflammatory [25]; carminative [14]; antispasmodic [14, 25]; sedative [14, 25]. indicated for use in flatulent dyspepsia [14]
Licorice root powder *Glycyrrhiza glabra*	1 part	See above

Infusion: ½ tsp per ½ cup consumed during the course of the day

TABLE 3.55 NUTRITIONAL SUPPLEMENTS

SUPPLEMENT AND DOSE	RATIONALE
High-potency practitioner-strength **probiotic supplement** designed for infants containing therapeutic levels of human strain organisms Dose: as directed by the manufacturer for a child of Sam's age and weight	Dysbiosis of intestinal microflora is associated with coeliac disease [19]; supplemental probiotics have a beneficial effect in coeliac disease [19]

▶

High-potency practitioner-strength **children's multivitamin and mineral supplement** providing therapeutic doses of vitamins, particularly B-group vitamins and minerals zinc, magnesium, calcium and potassium [8, 35] Dose: as directed by the manufacturer for an infant of Sam's age/weight	Deficiency of macro- and micronutrients is associated with coeliac disease [8, 18, 20]; zinc deficiency can hinder recovery [8]
Glutamine Dose: calculated as a percentage of the adult dose of 500 mg daily [21] Can be mixed in with probiotic powder	Glutamine facilitates repair of villi [21, 22] and is indicated in conditions causing villi atrophy and irritation of the intestinal wall [21, 22]
Cod liver oil Dose: approx. 2 mL to provide no more than 1500 IU of vitamin A daily [21]	Vitamin A and omega-3 supplement; both these nutrients are necessary for the health of Sam's digestive system [9, 21]
Liquid iron supplement suitable for infants Dose: To provide 6 mg iron daily [36, 37] or as per the manufacturer's instructions for an infant of Sam's weight and age	Iron deficiency anaemia is common in coeliac disease [23] and iron supplementation may be necessary if deficiency is present [27]

References

[1] R.H. Seller, Differential Diagnosis of Common Complaints, fifth edn, Saunders Elsevier, Philadelphia, 2007.

[2] J. Jamison, Differential Diagnosis for Primary Care, second edn, Churchill Livingstone Elsevier, London, 2006.

[3] R. Berkow, A.J. Fletcher, M.H. Beers, The Merck Manual, sixteenth edn, Merck Research Laboratories, Rathway, N.J, 1993 (later edition).

[4] P. Kumar, C. Clark, Clinical Medicine, sixth edn, Elsevier Saunders, London, 2005.

[5] A. Polmear (Ed.), Evidence-Based Diagnosis in Primary Care, Churchill Livingstone Elsevier, 2008.

[6] G. Douglas, F. Nicol, C. Robertson, Macleod's Clinical Examination, twelfth edn, Churchill Livingstone Elsevier, 2009.

[7] R.D. Collins, Differential Diagnosis in Primary Care, fourth edn, Lippincott Williams & Wilkins, Philadelphia, 2008.

[8] J.E. Pizzorno, M.T. Murray, H. Joiner-Bey, The Clinicians Handbook of Natural Medicine, second edn, Churchill Livingstone, St Louis, 2008.

[9] H. Osiecki, The Physicians Handbook of Clinical Nutrition, seventh edn, Eagle Farm: Bioconcepts, 2000.

[10] B. Tjellstrom, L. Stenhammar, L. Hogberg, K. Falth-Magnusson, T. Midtveldt, T. Sundqvist, E. Norin, Gut Microflora Associated Characteristics in Children with Celiac Disease, American Journal of Gastroenterology 100 (2005) 2784–2788.

[11] M. Predny, J. Chamberlain, Goldenseal (Hydrastis Canadensis): An annotated bibliography. 2005. Gen. Tech. Rep. SRS-88. Asheville, NC: U.S. Department of Agriculture, Forest Service, Southern Research Station. Retrieved 20 August 2009 from http//www.sfp.forprod.vt.edu.

[12] F. Scassocchio, M.F. Cometa, L. Tomassini, M. Palmery, Antibacterial activity of Hydrastis canadensis extract and its major isolated alkaloids, Planta Med 67 (6) (2001) 561–564.

[13] S. Mills, K. Bone, The Essential Guide to Herbal Safety, Churchill Livingstone, St Louis, 2005.

[14] British Herbal Medicine Association, British Herbal Pharmacopoeia, BHMAA, 1983.

[15] S. Mills, K. Bone, Principles & Practice of Phytotherapy. Modern Herbal Medicine, Churchill Livingstone, Edinburgh, London, 2000.

[16] D. McKay, J. Blumberg, A review of the bioactivity and potential health benefits of chamomile tea (Matricaria recutita), Phytotherapy Research 20 (7) (2006) 519–530.

[17] A. Ivarsson, O. Hernell, H. Stenlund, L. Ake, Breast-feeding protects against celiac disease, American Journal of Clinical Nutrition 75 (5) (2002) 914–921.

[18] Y. Naveh, A. Lightman, O.A. Zinder, Prospective study of serum zinc concentration in children with celiac disease, The Journal of Pediatrics 102 (5) (1983) 734–736.

[19] K. Lindfors, T. Blomqvist, K. Juuti-Uusitalo, S. Stenman, J. Venalainen, M. Maki, K. Kaukinen, Live probiotic Bifidobacterium lactis bacteria inhibit the toxic effects induced by wheat gliadin in epithelial cell culture, Clinical and Experimental Immunology 152 (3) (2008) 552–558.

[20] N.W. Solomons, I.H. Rosenberg, H.H. Sandstead, Zinc Nutrition in Celiac Sprue, The American Journal of Clinical Nutrition 29 (4) (1976) 371–375.

[21] H. Osiecki, The Nutrient Bible, seventh edn, Eagle Farm: AG Publishing, 2008.

[22] T.R. Zigeler, N. Bazargan, L. Leader, R.G. Martindale, Glutamine and the Gastrointestinal Tract, Current Opinion in Clinical Nutrition and Metabolic Care 3 (5) (2000) 355–362.

[23] D. Schuppan, M.D. Dennis, C.P. Kelly, Celiac Disease: Epidemiology, Pathogenesis, Diagnosis and Nutritional Management, Nutrition in Clinical Care 8 (2) (2005) 54–69.

[24] I.D. Hill, M.H. Dirks, G.S. Liptak, R.B. Colletti, A. Fasano, S. Guandalini, et al., Guideline for the Diagnosis and Treatment of Celiac Disease in Children: Recommendations of the North American Society for Pediatric Gastroenterology, Hepatology and Nutrition, Journal of Pediatric Gastroenterology and Nutrition 40 (1) (2005) 1–19.

[25] L. Braun, M. Cohen., Herbs & Natural Supplements: An evidence based guide, second edn, Elsevier, Sydney, 2007.

[26] H. Ouyang, J.D. Chen, Review article: therapeutic roles of acupuncture in functional gastrointestinal disorders, Alimentary Pharmacology & Therapeutics 20 (2004) 831–841.

[27] B. Annibale, C. Severi, A. Chistolini, G. Antonelli, E. Lahner, et al., Efficacy of Gluten-Free Diet Alone on Recovery From Iron Deficiency Anemia in Adult Celiac Patients, The American Journal Of Gastroenterology 96 (1) (2001) 132–137.

[28] M. Sinclair, Modern Hydrotherapy for the Massage Therapist, Lippincott Williams & Williams, Baltimore, 2008.

[29] D.D. Buchman, The complete book of water healing, Contemporary Books, McGraw-Hill Companies, New York, 2001.

[30] E. Blake, in: L. Chaitow, E. Blake, P. Orrock, M. Wallden, P. Sinder, J. Zeff (Eds.), Naturopathic Physical Medicine: Theory and Practice for Manual Therapists and Naturopaths, Churchill Livingstone Elsevier, Philadelphia, 2008.

[31] W. Boyle, A. Saine, Lectures in Naturopathic Hydrotherapy, Oregon: Eclectic Medical Publications, 1988.

[32] I.R. Chertok, The importance of exclusive breastfeeding in infants at risk for celiac disease, The American Journal of Maternal/Child Nursing 32 (1) (2007) 50–54.

[33] C.C. Tuchtan, V.M. Tuchtan, D. Stelfox, Foundations of Massage, second edn, Elsevier, Marrickville, New South Wales, 2005.

[34] J. Jamison, Clinical Guide to Nutrition & Dietary Supplements in Disease Management, Churchill Livingstone, Edinburgh, 2003.

[35] J. Higdon, An Evidence-Based Approach to Vitamins and Minerals: Health Benefits and Intake Recommendations, Thieme, New York, 2003.

[36] R. Kohli, B.K. Li, Differential diagnosis of recurrent abdominal pain: new considerations, Paediatr Ann 33 (2004) 113–122.

[37] D.J. Humes, J. Simpson, Acute appendicitis, BMJ 333 (2006) 530–534.

[38] A.M. Lake, Chronic abdominal pain in childhood: diagnosis and management, Am Fam Physician 59 (7) (1999) 1823–1830.

[39] J.C. Guarderos, Is it food allergy? Differentiating the causes of adverse reactions to food, Postgrad Med 109 (2001) 125–134.

[40] K. Beyer, S.S. Teuber, Food allergy diagnostics: scientific and unproven procedures, Curr Opin Allergy Clin Immunol 5 (2005) 261–266.

[41] J. Grundy, S. Matthews, B. Bateman, et al., Rising prevalence of allergy to peanut in children: Data from 2 sequential cohorts, J Allergy Clin Immunol 110 (2002) 784–789.

[42] A. Sheikh, S. Walker, Ten-Minute consultation: food allergy, BMJ 325 (2002) 1337.

[43] H.A. Sampson, Improving in-vitro tests for the diagnosis of food hypersensitivity, Curr Opin Allergy Clin Immunol 2 (2002) 27–261.

[44] S. Celik-Bilgili, A. Mehl, A. Verstege, et al., The predicitive value of specific immunoglobulin E levels in serum for the outcome of oral food challenges, Clin Exp Allergy 35 (2005) 268–273.

[45] D.P. Westerberg, J.M. Gill, B. Dave, M.J. DiPrinsio, A. Quisel, A. Foy, New strategies for diagnosis and management of celiac disease, Journal of the American Osteopathic Association 106 (3) (2006) 145–151.

[46] D.M. Roberts, M. Ostapchuk, J.G. O'Brien, Infantile colic, Am Fam Physician 70 (2004) 735–742.

Crohn's disease

Case history

David Feinberg is 30 years old and has come to your clinic seeking help for a digestive complaint, which he confesses has been causing him problems for the past two years. He experiences intermittent episodes of diarrhoea that can last for up to a month, often accompanied by lower abdominal pain on his right side. He originally thought he had a recurring gastrointestinal infection. When he experiences an episode of diarrhoea he thinks he must have had an infection that resolves itself and then returns. He describes the pain as a griping, colicky sensation that tightens and then releases. When he has diarrhoea it causes problems at work because he can have watery bowel motions up to 10 times a day, which are brown and slimy. He usually gets something from the chemist to stop the diarrhoea. He is now realising these symptoms are not normal and is wondering whether he has an unidentified food intolerance or allergy. When the symptoms are particularly bad he experiences nausea, may vomit and even have watery bowel motions during the night. Sometimes he notices blood in his stools when he has diarrhoea, but he hasn't mentioned this to anyone. Privately he is beginning to consider his symptoms may be due to a serious illness, but because this would worry his family enormously, he has not told anyone he is experiencing symptoms and has chosen to avoid seeing a doctor for tests. David has tried to work on the problem himself by eliminating particular foods from his diet, but because of weight loss and fatigue he is concerned about taking out too many foods. He says he is now trying to put on weight by eating fatty foods like burgers and chips, peanut butter sandwiches, pizza, meat pies and sausage rolls. He doesn't drink much water but drinks plenty of tea and coffee during the day to help him keep going and cope with the long hours he has to work. He smokes a pack of cigarettes a day (which his family do not realise) and doesn't think he could give the habit up easily.

David has been working in corporate law since he graduated from university. His employment provides him with a good income and opportunity for advancement. His parents are proud that their son is a lawyer. Recently his mother has been encouraging him to find a nice girl, settle down and have a family since he is now established in his career. He says in his Jewish culture a man of his age should be thinking about getting married, and some of his mother's friends have been trying to match him up with the perfect Jewish woman. David is not against the idea of finding a life partner but is unsettled at the moment. Despite his career success, David wonders whether he will be happy working as a corporate lawyer for the rest of his life. In his first couple of years at university he seriously considered working for Greenpeace and using his career to make a difference to the planet. Once he got his job the dream seemed to fade into the background. He loves and respects his parents and does not want to disappoint them. He believes they will think he is throwing his career away if he leaves his current position to pursue his dream.

TABLE 3.56 **COMPLAINT** [1–10]	
Analogy: Skin of the apple	**Complaint:** Define the presenting complaint and symptoms; understand the complaint. *Diarrhoea and abdominal pain*
AREAS OF INVESTIGATION AND EXAMPLE QUESTIONS	**CLIENT RESPONSES**
Exacerbating factors *Have you noticed anything that makes the symptoms worse?* *Does the diarrhoea prevent you from doing anything in your daily life?*	*I think some foods I'm eating don't help. I notice it's bad after having pasta sauce or some breakfast cereals.* *I need to be really close to the toilet at all times at work. It's difficult when I have a client interview and need to excuse myself often.*
Rating scale *How would you rate the abdominal pain and diarrhoea symptoms out of 10, with 10 being as bad as can be?*	*The pain can be 8 out of 10 and the diarrhoea is really causing me grief now so I will say 7 most days.*

TABLE 3.57 **CONTEXT**	
Analogy: Flesh of the apple	**Context:** Put the presenting complaint into context to understand the disease
AREAS OF INVESTIGATION AND EXAMPLE QUESTIONS	CLIENT RESPONSES
Obstruction and foreign body *Is there any undigested food present when you are forced to vomit?* (obstruction near stomach or peptic condition)	*No. It's just acid and fluid, it seems.*
Functional disease *Do you pass a bowel motion at a certain time of day or in a certain environment more often?*	*No. I can pass a motion any time of day or night and anywhere if I need to go.*

TABLE 3.58 **CORE**	
Analogy: Core of the apple with the seed of ill health	**Core:** Holistic assessment to understand the client
AREAS OF INVESTIGATION AND EXAMPLE QUESTIONS	CLIENT RESPONSES
Stress release *It sounds like you've been under stress with your job and family expectations. How do you let off steam?*	*I love sailing and could work on a boat for long periods of time with no problem.*
Has not been well since *What was happening in your life when you first began experiencing diarrhoea?*	*I think the first time my family began to focus on my need to get married I began to feel stressed. To tell you the truth I am not sure I want to get married ... to a woman anyway!*

TABLE 3.59 **DAVID'S SIGNS AND SYMPTOMS** [4, 7]	
Pulse	86 bpm
Blood pressure	115/70
Temperature	37.3°C
Respiratory rate	12 resp/min
Body mass index	22
Waist circumference	84.2 cm
Face	Dark under the eyes and tired looking
Eyes	Bloodshot eyes, pale conjunctiva and conjunctival rim
Mouth	Three small ulcers
Abdominal inspection	Mildly tender in the lower right quadrant
Urinalysis	NAD

Results of medical investigations

No investigations have been carried out yet.

TABLE 3.60 **UNLIKELY DIAGNOSTIC CONSIDERATIONS [1, 4–12, 74]**	
CONDITIONS AND CAUSES	**WHY UNLIKELY**
CANCER AND HEART DISEASE	
Hypertension	Blood pressure is in normal range
OBSTRUCTION AND FOREIGN BODY	
Kidney stones: hyperoxaluria; disorders of uric acid metabolism may develop in Crohn's disease, especially with fistulisation into the urinary tract; can cause symptoms of diarrhoea; may develop due to dehydration	Colicky pain usually radiates from the loin to the groin and occurs every 10 minutes; pain can be very sharp in acute episodes; urinalysis NAD
FUNCTIONAL DISEASE	
Functional diarrhoea: chronic diarrhoea, anxiety and uncertainty about bowel function	Usually symptoms are not accompanied by abdominal pain; bowel motions are watery and occur first thing in morning with no more passing during the day; defecation may only occur after eating food; usually there is no bleeding, weight loss or ongoing fatigue
INFECTION AND INFLAMMATION	
Ischaemic colitis: abdominal pain, blood from the rectum can be accompanied by diarrhoea, the abdomen can be tender	Usually occurs in older age groups; underlying cardiovascular disease may be present; onset is usually sudden
Bacterial infection: e.g. *Yersinia enterocolitica*, *Escherichia coli*, *Shigella*, *Staphylococcal enterocolitis*, ileocaecal TB; diarrhoea is the main symptom; may cause ulceration and inflammation, bloody diarrhoea and nausea [72, 73]	Usually self-limiting and acute in duration between 1 and 10 days depending on bacterial toxin; violent vomiting can be associated
Fungal infection: histoplasmosis; weight loss	David did not report having mild influenza symptoms or a cough recently
ENDOCRINE/REPRODUCTIVE	
Diabetes: diabetic neuropathy causes chronic diarrhoea, gastric stasis and bacterial overgrowth	David has not reported increased urination or thirst; urinalysis NAD
Addison's disease: weight loss, dehydration, nausea, diarrhoea, abdominal pain	No loss of body hair or skin pigmentation reported; urinalysis NAD

Case analysis

TABLE 3.61 **POSSIBLE DIFFERENTIAL DIAGNOSIS**		
Not ruled out by tests/investigations already done [1, 4–12, 74]		
CONDITIONS AND CAUSES	**WHY POSSIBLE**	**WHY UNLIKELY**
ALLERGIES AND IRRITANTS		
Lactose intolerance	Diarrhoea, abdominal pain	Fever not usually associated
CANCER AND HEART DISEASE		
Bowel cancer, polyps, gastrointestinal lymphoma [71, 75]	Chronic diarrhoea, blood in stools; carcinomas and polyps can cause irritation, hypermotility	Usually associated with alternating diarrhoea and constipation; more common in middle-aged men
TRAUMA AND PRE-EXISTING ILLNESS		
Causal factor: **Congenital lesions** of the colon	Symptoms of chronic diarrhoea	
OBSTRUCTION AND FOREIGN BODY		
Small-bowel disease	Chronic bacteria overgrowth due to small-bowel obstruction; diarrhoea, abdominal discomfort, weight loss	
Intestinal obstruction e.g. faecal impaction with overflow	Can cause vomiting, constipation, diarrhoea, abdominal distension and pain	
Causal factor: **Anal fissures, haemorroids, anal skin tags**	Bloody stools, diarrhoea, secondary to inflammatory bowel disease	
DEGENERATIVE AND DEFICIENCY		
Causal factor: **Bile acid malabsorption:** due to conditions such as Crohn's disease, coeliac disease, increased small intestine transit, diabetic diarrhoea, postinfective gastroenteritis	Under-diagnosed cause of chronic diarrhoea; when terminal ileum fails to reabsorb bile salts causes diarrhoea and increases colonic motility	
Anaemia: of chronic disease	Fatigue, weight loss, pale conjunctiva, pale face, diarrhoea and blood in stools indicating inflammatory condition	

▶

INFECTION AND INFLAMMATION		
Crohn's disease: inflammatory bowel disease [71]	Diarrhoea, weight loss, recurrent episodes of watery bowel motions during day and night, abdominal pain, low-grade fever and nausea; abdominal pain occasionally felt on the right lower abdomen due to a right iliac mass; inflammation is deep and patchy; lesions can be from mouth to anus	
Ulcerative colitis [71]	Diarrhoea, weight loss, fever, fatigue	Inflammation is usually mucosal and continuous [1] usually affects the rectum alone; may spread to the whole colon but rarely affects the ileum
Diverticular disease: diverticula and diverticulitis	Chronic symptoms include abdominal pain and diarrhoea; can experience erratic bowel habits; more common for those eating a low-fibre diet	Usually affects people over 50 years of age; the pain is usually experienced in the left lower abdomen
Appendicitis	Right-sided abdominal pain, diarrhoea	More likely to have abdominal pain in midgut region
Cholecystitis: chronic and acute gall bladder inflammation	Symptoms can be a vague gastrointestinal disturbance; biliary colic, right abdominal pain	More likely to be moderately severe pain of sudden onset referred to above the belly button in the abdomen rather than lower
Parasitic infection: giardia, amoebiasis [73]	*Giardia:* symptoms include diarrhoea, nausea, abdominal discomfort, steatorrhoea, malabsorption *Amoebiasis:* symptoms of chronic mild intermittent diarrhoea with abdominal discomfort, bloody diarrhoea and mucus, headache, nausea	Stools usually become very pale with mucus in parasitic infections; usually loss of appetite is a predominant symptom
Viral infection: retrovirus, hepatitis	Diarrhoea, tired, nausea, fatigue, weight loss	No history or signs of jaundice and stools not pale
Fatty liver	Common in Crohn's disease [4]; diarrhoea, nausea, anorexia	
Perianal/ischiorectal abscesses/anal fistula	Abdominal pain, fever, generalised wasting; common with inflammatory bowel disease	

SUPPLEMENTS AND SIDE EFFECTS MEDICATION AND DRUGS		
Causal factor: **Medicine/drug induced**: (e.g. *Pseudomembranous colitis*)	Diarrhoea caused by recent antibiotic use (causing overgrowth of fungi), laxatives, antihypertensives, NSAIDs	
Causal factor: **Supplement or food additive abuse:** excess vitamin C or magnesium, dandelion root coffee	Diarrhoea, weight loss	
ENDOCRINE/REPRODUCTIVE		
Hyperthyroidism	Diarrhoea and anxiety, weight loss; common to present between the ages of 20 and 40	No goitre or eye symptoms presenting as clinical markers
Pancreatic disorders: chronic pancreatitis, vipoma (endocrine pancreatic tumour), Zollinger-Ellison syndrome [76]	Symptoms of abdominal pain, episodes of pain, steatorrhoea, fatty diet	
AUTOIMMUNE DISEASE		
Coeliac disease	Diarrhoea, abdominal pain, weight loss, nausea, anaemia, inflammatory condition until diet changed	Fever not usually associated
STRESS AND NEUROLOGICAL DISEASE		
Causal factor: **Anxiety**	Functional causes of diarrhoea	
Causal factor: **Stress**	Diarrhoea, anxiety, feeling of pressure and responsibility for family concerns, confusion about career development; stress can exacerbate Crohn's disease via the hypothalamic-pituitary-adrenal axis and sympathetic-adrenal-medullary axis, which modulate gut barrier function and secretory absorption [24] and the autonomic and enteric nervous systems, which influences gut inflammation [25, 26]	
EATING HABITS AND ENERGY		
Causal factor: **Dehyration**	Chronic diarrhoea, not drinking much water, drinking a lot of tea and coffee, smoking a pack of cigarettes a day; symptoms can be asymptomatic – colicky pain in the abdomen may be present and be dull, constant and intermittent	

TABLE 3.62 DECISION TABLE FOR REFERRAL [4–9, 11]

COMPLAINT	CONTEXT	CORE
Referral for presenting complaint	Referral for all associated physical, dietary and lifestyle concerns	Referral for contributing emotional, mental, spiritual, metaphysical, lifestyle and constitutional factors
REFERRAL FLAGS	**REFERRAL FLAGS**	**REFERRAL FLAGS**
• Blood in watery stools • Duration of diarrhoea has been more than 3 months [74] • Diarrhoea lasting up to 4 weeks • Can have watery diarrhoea up to 10 times a day • Bowel motions can disturb sleep • David has not seen a doctor about his symptoms although they have worsened over 2 years	• Nausea and vomiting accompanying diarrhoea • Dehydration • Unexplained weight loss and fatigue • Lower abdominal pain in the right side • Smoking a pack of cigarettes a day	• Stress from family pressures • David believes he may have a serious illness
ISSUES OF SIGNIFICANCE	**ISSUES OF SIGNIFICANCE**	**ISSUES OF SIGNIFICANCE**
Nil	• Eating fatty foods to gain weight when digestion is not stable • Not drinking sufficient water	• Does not want to disappoint his family • David has not told anyone about his ongoing digestive symptoms • Would like a career change • David's family would like him to get married
REFERRAL DECISION	**REFERRAL DECISION**	**REFERRAL DECISION**
• To a GP for further medical investigation [75]	• To a GP for a medical investigation • Dietary assessment	• Counselling

TABLE 3.63 FURTHER INVESTIGATIONS THAT MAY BE NECESSARY [1, 4–12, 14–16, 74]

TEST/INVESTIGATION	REASON FOR TEST/INVESTIGATION
FIRST-LINE INVESTIGATIONS:	
Full blood count	Low haemoglobin in Crohn's disease, detect anaemia of chronic disease (usually normocytic, normochromic anaemia, and rarely megaloblastic due to B12 deficiency), inflammation, infection or tumour; check for viral or fungal causes to symptoms; anaemia in Addison's disease
ESR/CRP	Raised in Crohn's – inflammation
Blood electrolytes	Addison's disease, dehydration
Saccharomyces cerevisiae antibody	Present in Crohn's and not in ulcerative colitis
p-ANCA antibody test	Present in ulcerative colitis and not in Crohn's

►

SeHCAT test	Bile acid malabsorption
Serum gastrin	Gastrinoma
Stool test	Detect ova, parasites, bacteria and fat levels, and occult blood
Liver function test	Eliminate hepatitis; sometimes in Crohn's disease liver biochemistry can present as abnormal; check for fatty liver
IF NECESSARY:	
Abdominal x-ray	Appendicitis, intestinal obstruction, ulcerative colitis
Sigmoidoscopy	Confirm Crohn's disease and eliminate differential diagnosis list
Small-bowel follow through	Confirm diagnosis of Crohn's disease and eliminate small-bowel tumour, obstruction, adhesions, anatomic anomalies or perforation
Cortisol serum test/ACTH stimulation test/ serum aldosterone/adrenal antibodies	Addison's disease
Fasting blood glucose test	Raised in pancreatic cancer, pancreatitis, diabetes, Addison's disease
CT scan of pancreas	Eliminate chronic pancreatitis

Confirmed diagnosis

DAVID AND CROHN'S DISEASE

David is a young man who has been experiencing chronic gastrointestinal symptoms at a time of his life when he is busy with his career and unsure of his future direction regarding career and marriage. David feels great responsibility towards his family and feels under pressure to please them through making the right life decisions. Consequently he is experiencing some stress and anxiety about this situation.

David has been diagnosed with Crohn's disease, a condition more common in Western culture and possibly even more common in the Jewish community. It is difficult to distinguish between Crohn's disease and ulcerative colitis as both conditions have a familial characteristic and increased risk among the smoking population. Many immunological abnormalities and possible infectious agents have been identified as factors influencing the pathogenesis of inflammatory bowel disease. Crohn's disease is a chronic inflammatory condition that can affect the whole gastrointestinal tract (GIT) but seems to commonly affect the lower bowel [71]. A right lower quadrant mass may be present in the abdomen that is tender on physical examination. The condition may affect one small area of the gut or several sections at the one time and clinical features depend on what part of the bowel is affected. Crohn's disease can occur at any age but more commonly occurs between the ages of 30 and 40, and both men and women seem equally affected. Symptoms include diarrhoea, blood and mucus in watery stools, abdominal pain and weight loss and may be accompanied by fatigue, anorexia, low-grade fever, nausea and vomiting. Further complications such as anaemia, conjunctivitis, mouth ulcers, arthralgia, dehydration, kidney stone formation, fatty liver and inflammatory back pain may also be experienced. Crohn's disease can be asymptomatic for periods of time, or acute and chronically recurrent episodes may develop.

General references used in this diagnosis: 1, 4, 6, 7–14

PRESCRIBED MEDICATION

- Antibiotics
- Mesalazine

TABLE 3.64 **DECISION TABLE FOR TREATMENT (ONCE DIAGNOSIS IS CONFIRMED)**		
COMPLAINT	**CONTEXT**	**CORE**
Treatment for the presenting complaint and symptoms	Treatment for all associated symptoms	Treatment for mental, emotional, spiritual, constitutional, lifestyle issues and metaphysical considerations
TREATMENT PRIORITY	**TREATMENT PRIORITY**	**TREATMENT PRIORITY**
• Lifestyle recommendations to reduce the severity and frequency of episodes • Physical therapy suggestions to reduce the severity and frequency of symptoms • Dietary recommendations to eliminate aggravating or triggering foods and increase consumption of foods that have a beneficial effect on digestive function • Specific dietary recommendations to consume foods with anti-inflammatory, gut healing and normalising action on digestive function • Herbal tonic or tea, tablets and powders with anti-inflammatory, antimicrobial, carminative, demulcent and mucous membrane trophorestorative action to help reduce symptom severity • Supplemental nutrients to help reduce inflammation, promote healing of the gut and improve GIT microflora balance **NB:** It is essential David's case is managed collaboratively with his GP to ensure his condition is properly monitored and to minimise the changes of negative interactions between complementary and conventional treatments; David's herbal and nutritional supplements should be taken at least two hours from prescribed medication to ensure optimal absorption of both complementary and conventional medications [27].	• Lifestyle recommendations to improve David's general health and wellbeing • Physical therapy suggestions to promote health and normal immune system and gastrointestinal function • Dietary recommendations to improve nutritional status, general health and vitality, support immune system balance and maintain normal GIT function • Specific dietary recommendations and supplements to improve absorption of nutrients • Herbal tonic or tea, tablets and powders to support immune system balance and enhance GIT function • Supplemental nutrients to correct deficiencies; testing can be done after 6 weeks, and then again every 8–12 weeks to monitor vitamin A and zinc levels; dosages can be adjusted according to test results	• Stress-management recommendations • Physical therapy recommendations to help improve David's stress response • Counselling

Treatment aims

- Reduce inflammation in the gastrointestinal tract [13, 17]. Soothe and heal inflamed gut mucosa [13, 17] and improve nutrition to the epithelial lining [17].
- Balance David's immune system [17, 18, 43].
- Reduce levels of pathogenic microflora in the bowel, and support healthy bowel flora [13, 19, 20, 43].
- Dietary modification to maximise David's nutritional status [13] and to identify and eliminate dietary antigens and other trigger foods that may be contributing to gut inflammation [12, 13, 17, 21, 43].
- Reduce small intestinal permeability and the resultant 'leaky gut' [13, 17, 43].
- Support healthy gut mucosa and healthy gut function [13, 17, 22, 43].
- Correct nutritional deficiencies that have resulted from malabsorption [12, 13, 17, 23, 43].
- Reduce oxidative stress [17, 43].
- Support David's nervous system and stress response [13, 24, 43].

Lifestyle alterations/considerations

- Encourage David to quit smoking. Smoking is implicated in the development of Crohn's disease, its degree of severity and rate of relapse after surgery [4, 8, 9, 43, 55].
- David will benefit from managing his stress levels [13, 43, 56]. Mind–body stress-management techniques such as meditation, yoga or tai-chi may be helpful [64].
- Encourage David to exercise each day. Exercise is strongly associated with decreased levels of stress, anxiety and depression [59, 61].
- David may find counselling helpful in dealing with the pressure he feels his family is placing on him [13, 43, 56].

Physical treatment suggestions

- A course of acupuncture may be helpful. Acupuncture may be beneficial in mild to moderately active Crohn's disease [57]. Acupuncture can also help reduce David's anxiety levels and improve his stress response [59, 60].
- David may find massage therapy helpful to reduce stress and anxiety [62, 63].
- Hydrotherapy: alternating hot (three minutes) and cold (one minute) showers to the abdomen and spine [67]. Hot trunk wrap [67]. A hot sitz bath for abdominal pain [68]. A hot apple cider vinegar and water compress on the abdomen followed by cold mitten friction for 30 seconds (repeat three times once a day) [68, 69]. For acute diarrhoea, brief cold sitz baths with apple cider vinegar from a few seconds up to 10 minutes every day for a week, then every second day after symptoms subside [68].
- Constitutional hydrotherapy [70].

Dietary suggestions

- David's diet should be nutrient and antioxidant dense and contain minimal levels of aggravating foods and non-food substances [13, 17].
- David should eliminate all likely allergens: wheat, corn, dairy products and yeast [12, 13, 17, 43]. Sensitivities to dietary antigens may contribute to inflammation [21]. Elimination of foods known to cause symptom exacerbation can prolong disease remission [42].
- David should eliminate all dietary sources of carrageenan [12, 13, 43]. Carrageenan is a stabiliser used in foods such as ice-cream, cottage cheese, milkshakes, desserts, sauces, milk chocolate, pâtés, processed meats and beer and is implicated in the development of intestinal inflammation [41].

- Encourage David to avoid all sugar and refined carbohydrates and increase consumption of complex carbohydrates and fibre [12, 17].
- Encourage David to increase dietary consumption of omega-3 fatty acids [13, 17, 43].
- Encourage David to include plenty of ginger and turmeric in his diet. They are both potent anti-inflammatories [35, 40].
- Drinking cabbage juice may help heal David's gut as it contains substance 'U', which has ulcer-healing properties [43, 44].
- Encourage David to increase his intake of filtered water [43] and reduce his consumption of tea and coffee [43].

TABLE 3.65 HERBAL FORMULA (1:2 LIQUID EXTRACTS)

HERB	FORMULA	RATIONALE
Rhemannia *Rhemannia glutinosa*	60 mL	Anti-inflammatory [27, 34]; immunomodulator [27]; adrenal tonic [34]; beneficial in inflammatory disorders involving the immune system [27]
Turmeric *Curcuma longa*	70 mL	Anti-inflammatory [28, 35, 39]; antioxidant [28, 35, 39]; immunomodulator [39]; antimicrobial [28, 35, 39]; carminative [28, 35]; curcumin inhibits several of the cytokines and genes involved in the pathogenesis of Crohn's disease [23]
Golden seal *Hydrastis canadensis* (cultivated/plantation source)	30 mL	Anti-inflammatory [32, 34, 39]; mucous membrane trophorestorative [32, 34]; antimicrobial [32, 33, 34, 39]; antidiarrhoeal [39]; bitter digestive tonic [34, 39]; vulnerary [34]; traditionally used for digestive disorders and colitis [34, 31]
Chamomile *Matricaria recutita*	40 mL	Anti-inflammatory [28, 29, 39]; antispasmodic [28, 29, 39]; antimicrobial [28, 29, 39]; antiulcer [39]; antioxidant [39]; mild sedative [28, 30, 39]; traditionally used for flatulent dyspepsia, nervous diarrhoea, restlessness and anxiety [31]
Supply:	200 mL	Dose: 5 mL 3–4 times daily

It may be prudent to start David off with a smaller dose, e.g. 2 mL two or 3 times daily. If any of the constituents of the formula cause irritation or discomfort, it will be minimised by the smaller dose. Gradually increase the dose to the maximum level over a period of 2 weeks. In the clinical experience of the authors, some clients with inflammatory bowel disease can react when started at higher doses of herbs but tolerate them when taken at lower doses which are gradually increased over time.

Ginkgo (*Ginkgo biloba*)
1 mL of standardised extract three to four times daily or 6–10 g daily of dried leaf in divided doses
Reduces PAF activity [28, 36]; antioxidant [28, 36, 39]; tissue perfusion enhancer [28, 36, 39]; circulatory stimulant [28, 36, 39]
Ginkgo may cause mild gastrointestinal complaints in some individuals [34], therefore commence David on the lowest dose and gradually increase the dose and monitor for any adverse reactions. Review the use of ginkgo after 3 months [34].

▶

Boswellia (*Boswellia serrata*)
Tablet or powder equivalent to 4 g of dried resin daily in divided doses [37]
Anti-inflammatory [34]; boswellic acids are specific nonredox inhibitors of leukotriene synthesis and specifically inhibit the 5-lipoxygenase product LTB4, which has been implicated in Crohn's disease [38]; boswellia is an effective therapy for Crohn's disease [37]

Slippery elm bark powder (*Ulmus rubra*)
1 heaped teaspoon twice daily [39]
Nutritive demulcent [31, 39], soothes irritated and inflamed tissue [23, 31, 39]; antioxidant [39]; prebiotic [23, 39]; indicated for use in Crohn's disease [23, 31, 39]
May be combined with probiotics, glutamine and glucosamine to reduce the number of individual supplements and improve compliance

---

TABLE 3.66 HERBAL TEA

Alternative to herbal liquid tonic if David prefers a tea

HERB	FORMULA	RATIONALE
Chamomile flowers *Matricaria recutita*	2 parts	See above
Golden seal root *Hydrastis canadensis* (cultivated/plantation source)	1 part	See above
Wild yam root *Dioscorea villosa*	1 part	Spasmolytic [39]; anti-inflammatory [39]; traditionally used for intestinal colic [31]
Marshmallow root *Althea officinalis*	1 part	Demulcent; emollient; BHP indication for enteritis [31]
Ginger root *Zingiber officinale*	½ part	Anti-inflammatory [28, 40, 39]; carminative [28, 39]; spasmolytic [28, 39]; antiemetic [28, 39]; antiulcer activity [39]; digestive stimulant [28, 39]; traditionally used for colic and flatulent dyspepsia [31]; combines well with wild yam root for intestinal colic [31]

Decoction: 1 cup 3 times daily

TABLE 3.67 NUTRITIONAL SUPPLEMENTS

SUPPLEMENT AND DOSE	RATIONALE
Omega-3 fish oil 3 × 1000 mg capsules 3 × daily [39, 58]	Anti-inflammatory [17, 39, 58]; inhibits leukotrienes, thromboxanes and TNF alpha [45] and is indicated for use in inflammatory bowel disease [39, 45, 58]
High-potency practitioner-strength **probiotic supplement** containing therapeutic levels of human-strain lactobacillus and bifidus organisms [13, 43] and *Saccharomyces boulardii* [43] 1 capsule twice daily with meals [49]	Inhibits pathogenic bacteria via growth suppression or epithelial binding [46]; improves epithelial and mucosal barrier function [47]; alters immuno-regulation via stimulation of secretory IgA or reduction in TNF alpha [47, 48]; clinical trial showed higher remission rates in Crohn's patients taking 1 g *Saccharomyces boulardii* daily [50]

▶

► **Zinc supplement** [12, 17] containing 75 mg elemental zinc daily [51]; 2 mg of copper should be included if zinc supplement is taken for more than a month [17] Review dose after one month	Zinc deficiency is common in Crohn's disease [13, 17]; daily supplementation of 75 mg zinc daily reduces intestinal permeability in Crohn's patients [51]
Vitamin A 20,000 IU daily [58]	Low levels of vitamin A are found in Crohn's patients [23]
Vitamin E 500 IU daily [58]	Low levels of vitamin E are found in Crohn's patients [23]
High-potency practitioner-strength **multivitamin, mineral and antioxidant supplement** providing therapeutic doses of B-group vitamins [13, 43] Liquid form is likely to be absorbed more readily than tablet form	Helps reduce free radical damage and ensure adequate levels of essential nutrients [12, 13, 17, 23, 43]
Glucosamine sulphate 6 g daily in divided doses [52]	Glucosamine supplementation can reduce the severity of inflammatory bowel disease [52]
Glutamine 500 mg 3 times daily [12] Glutamine may be combined with slippery elm bark powder, glucosamine and probiotic supplement to reduce the amount of individual supplements and improve compliance	Glutamine facilitates repair of villi [65, 66] and is indicated in conditions causing villi atrophy and irritation of the intestinal wall [65, 66]
Quercetin 1200 mg daily before meals, in divided doses [58]	Anti-inflammatory [39, 53]; antioxidant [39]; immunomodulator [39]; gastroprotective [39]; inhibits platelet-activating factor (PAF) [53]
Digestive enzyme tablets or capsules Taken with meals Dose: as per manufacturer's instruction	To help enhance upper digestive function and improve nutrient absorption [43, 54]

References

[1] N.J. Talley, S. O'Connor, Pocket Clinical Examination, third edn, Churchill Livingstone Elsevier, Australia, 2009.

[2] J. Silverman, S. Kurtz, J. Draper, Skills for Communicating with Patients, second edn, Radcliff Publishing, Oxford, 2000.

[3] R. Neighbour, The Inner Consultation; how to develop an effective and intuitive consulting style, Radcliff Publishing, Oxon, 2005.

[4] P. Kumar, C. Clark, Clinical Medicine, sixth edn, Elsevier Saunders, London, 2005.

[5] D. Peters, L. Chaitow, G. Harris, S. Morrison, Integrating Complementary Therapies in Primary Care, Churchill Livingstone, London, 2002.

[6] R.D. Collins, Differential Diagnosis in Primary Care, fourth edn, Lippincott Williams & Wilkins, Philadelphia, 2008.

[7] R.H. Seller, Differential Diagnosis of Common Complaints, fifth edn, Saunders Elsevier, Philadelphia, 2007.

[8] A. Polmear, Evidence-Based Diagnosis in Primary Care, Churchill Livingstone Elsevier, 2008.

[9] J. Jamison, Differential Diagnosis for Primary Care, second edn, Churchill Livingstone Elsevier, London, 2006.

[10] M. Lloyd, R. Bor, Communication Skills For Medicine, third edn, Churchill Livingstone Elsevier, Edinburgh, 2009.

[11] R. Berkow, A.J. Fletcher, M.H. Beers, The Merck Manual, sixteenth edn, Merck Research Laboratories, Rathway, N.J, 1993 (later edition).

[12] S.E. El-hashemy, Naturopathic Standards of Primary Care, CCNM Press, Toronto, 2008.

[13] J.E. Pizzorno, M.T. Murray, H. Joiner-Bey, The Clinicians Handbook of Natural Medicine, Missouri. second edn, Churchhill and Livingstone Elsevier, 2008.

[14] G. Douglas, F. Nicol, C. Robertson, Macleod's Clinical Examination, twelfth edn, Churchill Livingstone Elsevier, 2009.

[15] K.D. Pagna, T.J. Pagna, Mosby's Diagnostic and Laboratory Test reference, third edn, Mosby, USA, 1997 (later edition).

[16] H.M. Seidal, J.W. Ball, J.E. Dains, G.W. Benedict, Mosby's Guide To Physical examination, third edn, Mosby, U.S.A, 1995 (later edition).

[17] J. Jamison, Clinical Guide to Nutrition & Dietary Supplements in Disease Management, Churchill Livingstone, Edinburgh, 2003.

[18] T.T. Macdonald, G. Monteleone, S.L.F. Pender, Recent developments in the Immunology of Inflammatory Bowel Disease, Scandinavian Journal of Immunology 51 (1) (2000) 2–9.

[19] N.S. Ambrose, M. Johnson, D.W. Burdon, M.R.B. Keighley, Incidence of pathogenic bacteria from mesenteric lymph nodes and ileal serosa during Crohn's disease surgery, British Journal of Surgery 71 (8) (2005) 623–625.

[20] F. Shanahan, Probiotics and inflammatory bowel disease: Is there a scientific rationale? Inflammatory Bowel Diseases 6 (2) (2007) 107–115.

[21] J. Van Den Bogaerde, M.A. Kamm, S. Knight, Immune sensitization to food, yeast and bacteria in Crohn's disease, Alimentary Pharmacology & Therapeutics 15 (10) (2001) 1647–1653.

[22] P.R. Gibson, Increased Gut Permeability in Crohn's disease: is TNF the link? GUT 53 (2004) 1724–1725.

[23] K. Head, J. Jurenka, Inflammatory bowel disease part II: Crohn's disease—pathophysiology and conventional and alternative treatment options, Alternative Medicine Review (4) (2004) 9.

[24] S.M. Collins, Stress and the gastrointestinal tract IV. Modulation of intestinal inflammation by stress: basic mechanisms and clinical relevance, Am J Physiol Gastrointest Liver Physiol 280 (2001) G315–G318.

[25] Y. Kawahito, H. Sano, M. Kawata, K. Yuri, S. Mukai, Y. Yamamura, et al., Local secretion of corticotropin-releasing hormone by enterochromaffin cells in human colon, Gastroenterology 106 (1994) 859–865.

[26] Y. Tache, M.H. Perdue, Role of peripheral CRF signalling pathways in stress-related alterations of gut motility and mucosal function, Neurogastroenterology and Motility 16 (1) (2004) 137–142.

[27] K. Bone, Clinical Applications of Chinese and Ayurvedic Herbs: Monographs for the Western Herbal Practitioners, Warwick. Phytotherapy Press, 1996.

[28] S. Mills, K. Bone, Principles & Practice of Phytotherapy: Modern Herbal Medicine, Churchill Livingstone, Edinburgh, London, 2000.

[29] D. McKay, J. Blumberg, A review of the bioactivity and potential health benefits of chamomile tea (Matricaria recutita), Phytotherapy Research 20 (7) (2006) 519–530.

[30] G. Beaubrun, G. Gray, A review of herbal medicines for psychiatric disorders, Psychiatric Services 51 (2000) 1130–1134.

[31] British Herbal Medicine Association, British Herbal Pharmacopoeia, BHMAA, 1983.

[32] Goldenseal (Hydrastis canadensis), An annotated bibliography, in: M. Predny (Ed.), Chamerlain J. Gen. Tech. Rep. SRS-88, U.S. Department of Agriculture, Forest Service, Southern Research Station, Asheville, NC, 2005. Available from http//www.sfp.forprod.vt.edu/.

[33] F. Scassocchio, M.F. Cometa, L. Tomassini, M. Palmery, Antibacterial activity of Hydrastis canadensis extract and its major isolated alkaloids, Planta Med 67 (6) (2001) 561–564.

[34] S. Mills, K. Bone, The Essential Guide to Herbal Safety, Churchill Livingstone, St Louis, 2005.

[35] I. Chattopadhyay, K. Biswas, U. Bandyopadhyay, R.J. Bannerjee, Turmeric, Curcumin: Biological, Actions and Medicinal Applications, Current Science (1) (2004) 87.

[36] K.F. Chung, G. Dent, M. McCusker, P. Guinot, C.P. Page, P.J. Barnes, Effect of a ginkgolide mixture (BN 2063) in antagonising skin and platelet responses to platelet activating factor in man, Lancet 1 (8527) (1987) 248–251.

[37] H. Gerhardt, F. Seifert, P. Buvari, H. Vogelsang, R. Repges, Therapy of active Crohn disease with Boswellia serrata extract H 15, Z Gastroenterol 39 (2001) 11–17. [Article in German].

[38] H.P. Ammon, T. Mack, G.B. Singh, H. Safayhi, Inhibition of leukotriene B4 formation in rat peritoneal neutrophils by an ethanolic extract of the gum resin exudate of Boswellia serrata, Planta Med 57 (1991) 203–207.

[39] L. Braun, M. Cohen, Herbs & Natural Supplements: An evidence based guide, second edn, Elsevier, Sydney, 2007.

[40] R. Grzanna, L. Lindmark, C.G. Frondoza, Ginger—An Herbal Medicinal Product with Broad Anti-Inflammatory Actions, Journal of Medicinal Food 8 (2) (2005) 125–132.

[41] S. Bhattacharyya, A. Borthakur, P.K. Dudeja, J. Tobacman, Carrageenan Induces Cell Cycle arrest in Human Intestinal Epithelial Cells in Vitro, The Journal of Nutrition 138 (2008) 469–475.

[42] T.S. King, J.T. Woolner, J.O. Hunter, The dietary management of Crohn's disease, Alimentary Pharmacology & Therapeutics 11 (1) (1997) 17–31.

[43] H. Osiecki, The Physicians Handbook of Clinical Nutrition, seventh edn, Eagle Farm: Bioconcepts, 2006.

[44] G. Cheney, Rapid Healing of Peptic Ulcers in Patients receiving fresh cabbage juice, Calif Med 70 (1) (1949) 10–15.

[45] A. Beluzzi, C. Brignola, M. Campieri, A. Pera, S. Boschi, M. Miglio, Effect of an enteric-coated fish-oil preparation on relapses in Crohn's disease, N Engl J Med 334 (1996) 1557–1560.

[46] F. Yang, D. Brent-Polk, Probiotic Bacterium Prevents Cytokine-induced Apoptosis in Intestinal Epithelial Cells, The Journal of Biological Chemistry 277 (52) (2002) 50959–50965.

[47] A.F. Mattar, D.H. Teitelbaum, R.A. Drongowski, et al., Probiotics up-regulate MUC-2 mucin gene expression in a Caco-2 cell culture model, Pediatric Surgery International 18 (2002) 586–590.

[48] M. Malin, H. Suomalainen, M. Saxelin, E. Isolauri, Promotion of IgA immune response in patients with Crohn's disease by oral bacteriotherapy with Lactobacillus GG, Ann Nutr Metab 40 (1996) 137–145.

[49] Shanahan F. (2007). Probiotics and inflammatory bowel disease: Is there a scientific rationale?

[50] M. Guslandi, G. Mezzi, M. Sorghi, P.A. Testoni, Saccharomyces boulardii in maintenance treatment of Crohn's disease, Dig Dis Sci 45 (2000) 1462–1464.

[51] G.C. Sturniolo, V. Di Leo, A. Ferronato, A. D'Odorico, R. D'Incà, Zinc Supplementation Tightens 'Leaky Gut' in Crohn's Disease, Inflammatory Bowel Diseases 7 (2) (2001) 94–98.

[52] S. Salvatore, R. Heuschkel, S. Tomlin, et al., A pilot study of N-acetylglucosamine, a nutritional substrate for glycosaminoglycan synthesis, in paediatric chronic inflammatory bowel disease, Aliment Pharmacol Ther 14 (2000) 1567–1579.

[53] P. Ruiz, A. Braune, G. Hölzlwimmer, L. Quintanilla-Fend, and D. Haller, Quercetin Inhibits TNF-Induced NF-KB Transcription Factor Recruitment to Proinflammatory Gene Promoters in Murine Intestinal Epithelial Cells. The Journal of Nutrition 137 (2007) 1208–1215.

[54] L. Gullo, Indication for pancreatic enzyme treatment in non-pancreatic digestive diseases, Digestion 54 (Suppl. 2) (1993) 43–47.

[55] E. Lindberg, G. Jarnerot, B. Huitfeldt, Smoking in Crohn's disease: effect on localisation and clinical course, Gut 33 (1992) 779–782.

[56] S. Collins, Stress and the gastrointestinal tract IV. Modulation of intestinal inflammation by stress: basic mechanisms and clinical relevance, Am J Physiol Gastrointest Liver Physiol 280 (2001) G315–G318.

[57] S. Joos, B. Brinkhaus, C. Maluche, N. Maupai, R. Kohnen, N. Kraehmer, E.G. Hahn, D. Schuppan, Acupuncture and moxibustion in the treatment of active Crohn's disease: a randomized controlled Study, Digestion 69 (3) (2004) 131–139, Epub 2004 Apr 26.

[58] J. Higdon, An Evidence-Based Approach to Vitamins and Minerals: Health Benefits and Intake Recommendations, Thieme, New York, 2003.

[59] A.F. Jorm, H. Christensen, K.M. Griffiths, R.A. Parslow, B. Rodgers, K.A. Blewitt, Effectiveness of complementary and self-help treatments for anxiety disorders, Medical Journal of Australia 181 (7) (2004) S29–S46.

[60] D.W. Spence, L. Kayumov, A. Chen, A. Lowe, U. Jain, M.A. Katzman, et al., Acupuncture increases nocturnal melatonin secretion and reduces insomnia and anxiety: A preliminary report, Journal of Neuropsychiatry and Clinical Neurosciences 16 (1) (2004) 19–28.

[61] A. Byrne, G.D. Byrne, The effect of exercise on depression, anxiety and other mood states: A review, J Psychosom Res. 37 (6) (1993) 565–574.

[62] T. Field, G. Robinson, F. Scafidi, R. Nawrocki, A. Goncalves, Massage therapy reduces anxiety and enhances EEG pattern of alertness and math computations, International Journal of Neuroscience 86 (1996) 197–205.

[63] C.A. Moyer, J. Rounds, J.W. Hannum, A Meta-Analysis of Massage Therapy Research, Psychological Bullettin 130 (1) (2004) 3–18.

[64] S. Cotton, Y. Humenay Roberts, J. Tsevat, M.T. Britto, P. Succop, et al., Mind-body complementary alternative medicine use and quality of life in adolescents with inflammatory bowel disease, Inflammatory Bowel Diseases, 2009. August 24. DOI 10.1002/ibd.21045.

[65] H. Osiecki, The Nutrient Bible, seventh edn, Eagle Farm: AG Publishing, 2008.

[66] T.R. Zigeler, N. Bazargan, L. Leader, R.G. Martindale, Glutamine and the Gastrointestinal Tract, Current Opinion in Clinical Nutrition and Metabolic Care 3 (5) (2000) 355–362.

[67] E. Blake, in: L. Chaitow, E. Blake, P. Orrock, M. Wallden, P. Sinder, J. Zeff, (Eds.), Naturopathic Physical Medicine, Theory and Practice for Manual Therapists and Naturopaths, Churchill Livingstone Elsevier, Philadelphia, 2008.

[68] D.D. Buchman, The complete book of water healing, Contemporary Books, McGraw-Hill Companies, New York, 2001.

[69] M. Sinclair, Modern Hydrotherapy for the Massage Therapist, Lippincott Williams & Williams, Baltimore, 2008.

[70] W. Boyle, A. Saine, Lectures in Naturopathic Hydrotherapy, Oregon: Eclectic Medical Publications, 1988.

[71] W. Hamilton, A. Round, D. Sharp, et al., Clinical features of colorectal cancer before diagnosis: a population based case-control study, British Journal of Cancer 93 (2005) 399–405.

[72] P.R. Gibson, J. Iser, Inflammatory bowel disease, Australian Family Physician 34 (4) (2005) 233–237.

[73] B. Kass, Traveller's diarrhoea, Australian Family Physician 34 (4) (2005) 243–247.

[74] P.R. Hunter, Drinking water and diarrheal disease due to Escherichia coli, Journal of Water Health 1 (2) (2003) 65–72.

[75] P. Thomas, A. Forbes, J. Green, et al., Guidelines for the investigation of chronic diarrhoea, Gut 52 (Suppl. v) (2003) v1–v15.

[76] W. Hamilton, A. Round, D. Sharp, et al., Clinical features of colorectal cancer before diagnosis: a population based case-control study, British Journal of Cancer 93 (2005) 399–405.

[77] B. Etemad, D.C. Whitcomb, Chronic Pancreatitis: diagnosis, classification, and new genetic developments, Gastroenterology 120 (2001) 682–707.

Lactose intolerance

Case history

Nine-year-old Yoshimi Koboyashi is an only child and she and her parents recently moved to Australia from Japan. Yoshimi's father has a two-year contract, which will keep the family in Australia for at least that time. If the family decide they like Australia, they may stay longer. Yoshimi has been in her new school for four months and finds it difficult to keep up with the language and cultural differences at times, and still hasn't found a special friend. Yoshimi's mother tells you Yoshimi is very shy, which is obvious to you as she looks at the floor most of the time and when you ask her questions she keeps her eyes averted and appears very uncomfortable. Yoshimi's mother goes on to tell you that Yoshimi can speak English quite well, but she chooses to communicate in Japanese wherever possible. Yoshimi is missing her grandparents and her parents have heard her calling out for them in her sleep.

Yoshimi's mother brought her to the clinic today because for the past three months Yoshimi has been experiencing stomach pain associated with frothy and watery diarrhoea. Yoshimi is complaining of nausea with bloating in her stomach and her parents have noticed she seems to be losing weight. Sometimes when she has the stomach pain she refuses to eat. Her mother is not sure whether these symptoms are occurring because she is homesick or because of the change in Yoshimi's diet since they moved to Australia. For the first two months in Australia, the family stayed with friends. They ate much more wheat, sugar, meat and dairy foods than they ate in Japan. In Japan Yoshimi rarely had cheese, milk or yoghurt and ate rice more often than pasta or bread. Yoshimi's mother explains that she and her husband did not feel it was polite to refuse the food offered by their friends who wanted to give them a taste of real Aussie cuisine and culture.

In Japan Yoshimi's family had a natural therapist who took care of their healthcare needs, so her parents have brought her to the clinic before seeing a doctor. They are interested to know how Yoshimi can be helped and if it is necessary for her to see a doctor, or to ask for a recommendation for a doctor who is willing to work with natural therapies.

TABLE 3.68 COMPLAINT [1–4, 12, 39]	
Analogy: Skin of the apple	**Complaint:** Define the presenting complaint and symptoms; understand the complaint *Chronic diarrhoea and stomach pain*
AREAS OF INVESTIGATION AND EXAMPLE QUESTIONS	**CLIENT RESPONSES**
Relieving factors *Can you tell me what makes the pain go away or get better?*	*Holding my tummy and lying down with a hot water bottle helps.*
Location and radiation *Can you point to where you feel the stomach pain?*	Yoshimi shows you that the pain can radiate over the entire stomach area.
Account and description *Does the stomach pain feel like butterflies or like a needle in your stomach?*	*It can feel more like a balloon is in my tummy!*

TABLE 3.69 **CONTEXT**	
Analogy: Flesh of the apple	**Context:** Put the presenting complaint into context to understand the disease
AREAS OF INVESTIGATION AND EXAMPLE QUESTIONS	CLIENT RESPONSES
Allergies and irritants *Did the stomach pain and diarrhoea get worse over a few weeks after eating different sorts of foods in Australia?* (more likely to be food intolerance) *Did the stomach pain and diarrhoea begin as soon as you ate different foods when you first arrived in Australia?* (more likely to be allergy)	*I didn't have the pain at first, it took a little while and then it would not go away.*
Infection and inflammation *Did the stomach pain begin with diarrhoea, nausea and vomiting?* (gastroenteritis)	*I did feel sick in my tummy but didn't throw up.*
Eating habits and energy *Do you not want to eat because you get the stomach pain after eating or are you just not feeling hungry?*	*I'm scared of the pain, but I do get hungry.*

TABLE 3.70 **CORE**	
Analogy: Core of the apple with the seed of ill health	**Core:** Holistic assessment to understand the client
AREAS OF INVESTIGATION AND EXAMPLE QUESTIONS	CLIENT RESPONSES
Home life *How do you feel about living in Australia now?*	*It is okay I guess...*
Action needed to heal *Is there anything you can think of that would make it easier for you to live in Australia now?*	*A puppy!*

TABLE 3.71 **YOSHIMI'S SIGNS AND SYMPTOMS** [5–7]	
Pulse	90 bpm
Blood pressure	130/80
Temperature	37°C (ear temp)
Respiratory rate	16 resp/min
Body mass index	Not applicable for a 9-year-old child. Yoshimi's weight is 31 kg, which puts her at around the 40th percentile for a child of her age
Face	Pale and tired looking; dark under the eyes
Urinalysis	No abnormality detected (NAD)

Results of medical investigations

No investigations have been carried out yet.

TABLE 3.72 **UNLIKELY DIAGNOSTIC CONSIDERATIONS** [1, 2, 7, 35]	
CONDITIONS AND CAUSES	**WHY UNLIKELY**
INFECTION AND INFLAMMATION	
Gastroenteritis: abdominal pain, diarrhoea, nausea and vomiting; most common cause of acute abdominal pain in this age group; can have transient lactose intolerance	Associated with vomiting, fever; check if generalised cramping abdominal pain; no low-grade fever; acute gastritis usually self-limiting and lasts less than a week
Bacterial infection: e.g. *Yersinia enterocolitica*, *Escherichia coli*, *Shigella*, *Staphylococcal enterocolitis*, ileocaecal TB; diarrhoea is the main symptom; may cause ulceration and inflammation; diarrhoea, abdominal pain, bloating, travelled recently	Usually self-limiting and acute in duration between 1 and 10 days depending on bacterial toxin; violent vomiting can be associated; no bloody diarrhoea reported
Viral infection: retrovirus, hepatitis; diarrhoea, tired, nausea, fatigue, weight loss; recently travelled to new environment	No history or signs of jaundice; check if stools are pale; no fever
Urinary tract infection: abdominal pain in children	Urinalysis NAD; not necessarily associated with diarrhoea
Mesenteric adenitis: inflamed swollen lymph glands in the abdomen; temporary abdominal pain in children; can experience nausea and diarrhoea	No recent fever/common cold reported prior to the abdominal pain developing; check if the abdominal guarding is only when Yoshimi experiences pain; no fever; not necessarily associated with diarrhoea
ENDOCRINE/REPRODUCTIVE	
Diabetes: diabetic neuropathy causes chronic diarrhoea, gastric stasis and bacterial overgrowth; abdominal pain in children	Has not reported increased urination or thirst; check if the abdominal pain is generalised rather than local; urinalysis NAD

Case analysis

TABLE 3.73 **POSSIBLE DIFFERENTIAL DIAGNOSIS**		
Not ruled out by tests/investigations already done [1, 2, 5–10, 35, 37, 43]		
CONDITIONS AND CAUSES	**WHY POSSIBLE**	**WHY UNLIKELY**
ALLERGIES AND IRRITANTS		
Lactose intolerance	Abdominal pain, bloating, nausea, watery and frothy diarrhoea, change in diet; recurrent abdominal pain with onset of lactose ingestion	

▶

Fructose intolerance	Abdominal pain, bloating, diarrhoea	Need to determine which fruit Yoshimi is eating and how much
Food allergy: typically to cow's milk, egg, soya, peanut, wheat and fish [45, 46]	Diarrhoea, cramping colic	Often presents with swelling of lips and tongue, urticaria skin rash, conjunctivitis, rhinitis, anaphylaxis and difficulty breathing
OBSTRUCTION AND FOREIGN BODY		
Small-bowel disease	Chronic bacterial overgrowth due to small-bowel obstruction; diarrhoea, abdominal discomfort, weight loss	
Intestinal obstruction e.g. faecal impaction with overflow	Diarrhoea, abdominal pain, constipation, diarrhoea, abdominal distension and pain; can be acute and recurrent abdominal pain	Can cause vomiting; check if recurrent cramping pain worse after eating meals
FUNCTIONAL DISEASE		
Irritable bowel syndrome [36, 37]	Diarrhoea, stress, abdominal pain and bloating	Usually alternates between constipation and diarrhoea; bowel motions are rarely nocturnal; check if the abdominal pain is relieved by passing a bowel motion
Functional diarrhoea [37]	Common for children in times of stress; usually weight loss or ongoing fatigue	Usually no abdominal pain associated; bowel motions are watery and first thing in morning with no more passing during the day; bowel motions may only occur after eating food
Functional abdominal pain [37]	Common in children at times of moving, travel, school pressures	Usually symptoms of abdominal pain are central and not radiating (need to clarify); usually not associated with recurrent diarrhoea; often has multiple symptoms of headache and pain in the arms and legs
Nonspecific abdominal pain (NSAP) [37]	Abdominal pain in children; presents with no increased pulse, fever; urinalysis clear	Check if similar abdominal pain and episodes are relieved within 24 hours (common to NSAP); check if full blood count and stool test all clear; not necessarily associated with diarrhoea
DEGENERATIVE AND DEFICIENCY		
Peptic ulcer [39]	Can develop in children experiencing stress, abdominal pain; refusing to eat	Usually can point to where the abdominal pain is

Causal factor: **Dehydration**	Diarrhoea; colicky pain in the abdomen may be present that can be dull, constant and intermittent	
Anaemia	Weight loss, diarrhoea, not sleeping well; fatigue, weight loss, pale; can be associated with malabsorption disorder of the gut	
Causal factor: **Bile acid malabsorption:** due to conditions such as Crohn's disease, coeliac disease, increased small intestine transit, diabetic diarrhoea, postinfective gastroenteritis	Under-diagnosed cause of chronic diarrhoea; when terminal ileum fails to reabsorb bile salts causes diarrhoea and increases colonic motility	
INFECTION AND INFLAMMATION		
Appendicitis [38]	Diarrhoea, abdominal pain, nausea; common in this age group with peak incidence between 10 and 15 years; pain can come on gradually and mimic mild colic pain in young children; refuses food; pain not always present in right iliac area in children if the appendix is not located in the right side of the abdomen; poor appetite	Acute abdominal pain that often presents with vomiting and doubling over in pain; pain is gradual in onset with a cramping feeling (need to clarify); check if abdominal guarding is present all the time, even when not experiencing pain; check if the local rebound pain is in the right lower quadrant of the abdomen; not usual to have significant diarrhoea as an associated symptom; no fever or raised pulse rate
Inflammatory bowel disease: Crohn's disease	Diarrhoea, abdominal pain, change in diet; diarrhoea has persisted more than one month	Usually associated with low-grade fever, significant blood or mucus in stools; more common to present at adolescence
Chronic gastritis	Abdominal pain, bloating, nausea, diarrhoea; symptoms made worse by eating	Check if pain is located in the middle of the abdomen
Causal factor: **Helicobacter pylori**	Abdominal pain, nausea, bloating; recurrent abdominal pain in children; refusing to eat	Check if pain is clearly located in the middle of the abdomen

Parasite infection: giardia, amoebiasis	Loss of appetite *Giardia:* symptoms include diarrhoea, nausea, abdominal discomfort, malabsorption *Amoebiasis:* symptoms of chronic mild intermittent diarrhoea with abdominal discomfort, nausea	Stools become very pale with mucus; no bloody diarrhoea and mucus; no headache
SUPPLEMENTS AND SIDE EFFECTS MEDICATION AND DRUGS		
Causal factor: **Supplement or food additive abuse:** excess vitamin C or magnesium?	Diarrhoea, weight loss	
ENDOCRINE/REPRODUCTIVE		
Pancreatic disease: rare in children but can develop due to mumps, steroid therapy, obstruction of common bile duct	Lactose intolerance, diarrhoea, nausea, abdominal pain	Usually associated with vomiting, low-grade fever, abdominal pain radiating to the back
AUTOIMMUNE DISEASE		
Coeliac disease	Diarrhoea, pain in the abdomen, change in diet; can be associated with lactose intolerance; having more wheat and dairy	
STRESS AND NEUROLOGICAL DISEASE		
Depression	Often presents as physical symptoms in children such as loss of appetite, diarrhoea, fatigue; recently moved to Australia and missing family and home in Japan	
Abdominal migraine [40]	Can develop in children as recurrent abdominal pain; associated symptoms can be nausea, diarrhoea and pale complexion	Pain is often localised in the middle of the abdomen; need to investigate a family history of migraine
EATING HABITS AND ENERGY		
Poisoning: food, lead	Abdominal pain in children, diarrhoea	Can be diffuse pain associated with constipation (lead poisoning)

TABLE 3.74 **DECISION TABLE FOR REFERRAL** [1, 2, 7, 8, 11]		
COMPLAINT	**CONTEXT**	**CORE**
Referral for presenting complaint	Referral for all associated physical, dietary and lifestyle concerns	Referral for contributing emotional, mental, spiritual, metaphysical, lifestyle and constitutional factors
REFERRAL FLAGS	**REFERRAL FLAGS**	**REFERRAL FLAGS**
• Dehydration risk from diarrhoea and refusing to eat • Duration of diarrhoea has been 3 months	• Weight loss • Malabsorption	• Yoshimi is feeling overwhelmed with life • Yoshimi's loneliness and social isolation • Yoshimi is feeling grief for leaving Japan
ISSUES OF SIGNIFICANCE	**ISSUES OF SIGNIFICANCE**	**ISSUES OF SIGNIFICANCE**
Nil	Nil	• Missing her grandparents • Choosing to speak Japanese rather than English
REFERRAL DECISION	**REFERRAL DECISION**	**REFERRAL DECISION**
• Yoshimi needs a medical doctor to investigate organic causes for abdominal pain and diarrhoea that could develop into emergency symptoms	• For weight check and monitoring	• Yoshimi/parents may like to speak with a family counsellor if her emotional symptoms persist

TABLE 3.75 **FURTHER INVESTIGATIONS THAT MAY BE NECESSARY** [1, 2, 5–10, 26, 35, 39, 41, 43, 44]	
TEST/INVESTIGATION	**REASON FOR TEST/INVESTIGATION**
FIRST-LINE INVESTIGATIONS:	
Abdominal examination: guarding, rebound tenderness, palpation, abnormal pulsations (auscultation)	Appendicitis
Kidney flank test	Pyelonephritis
Urinalysis	Urinary tract infection; blood in the urine may indicate kidney stones, kidney infection or appendicitis
Hydrogen breath test	To detect bacterial overgrowth; when bacteria is metabolised by lactose or glucose there is a production of hydrogen; if there is lactose in the small intestine that has not been broken down there will be an early rise in breath hydrogen; this is a safe and non-invasive test to perform for children; can detect fructose intolerance

▶

Stool test	If acidic stools are passed it indicates lactose intolerance; parasites, viral, bacteria, occult blood can be detected in stools
Elimination diets [42, 44]	Detect food intolerance
Skin-prick test [44]	Food and environmental allergies and intolerances
IF NECESSARY:	
Oral tolerance lactose test	Determine lactose metabolism
Full blood count	Anaemia, inflammation, infection or tumour; white blood cell count raised in appendicitis/not raised in mesenteric adenitis
ESR/CRP	Inflammation, tumour or infection
Differential white blood cell count IgE (eosinophils antibody blood test)	Definitive diagnosis for allergic triggers, appendicitis
Antigliadin antibodies	Check if antibodies to gluten are present in blood indicating coeliac disease
Blood-sugar test	Diabetes
Abdominal x-ray	Appendicitis, intestinal obstruction or abnormality
Small-bowel follow through and jejunal biopsy	Detect low lactase enzyme activity
CT scan of pancreas/abdomen	Eliminate pancreatitis, pancreatic cancer causing low lactase activity

Confirmed diagnosis

YOSHIMI AND LACTOSE INTOLERANCE

Yoshimi is a nine-year-old girl who recently moved with her family to Australia from Japan after her father took up a job opportunity abroad. Yoshimi has not coped well with the move and is choosing not to speak English although she is able to. Major life changes, such as going to a new school, living in a new culture and moving to a new country, have left Yoshimi feeling overwhelmed. During their integration into Australia her family stayed with an Australian family who introduced them to a typical Australian diet consisting of more dairy, wheat, meat and sugar than Yoshimi was used to in Japan. Coinciding with this dietary change, Yoshimi has developed stomach pain and diarrhoea that has continued for more than three months. After referring Yoshimi to a medical doctor, she has been diagnosed with **lactose intolerance**, a condition of lactose enzyme deficiency.

The pancreatic enzyme lactase splits lactose into glucose and galactose. When there is a deficiency of lactase the unsplit disaccharides remain in the lumen and cause fluid retention and diarrhoea. Bacterial fermentation of the sugar in the colon leads to acidic stools. Because the pancreatic enzymes are located in the brush border of mucosal cells in the small intestine, secondary related conditions, such as coeliac disease, may develop. Lactase deficiency is relatively normal in adults and particularly affects people of Asian origin. When diarrhoea occurs in children who have been recently introduced to diary foods, lactose intolerance should be considered.

General references used in this diagnosis: 7, 10, 35, 37, 43

TABLE 3.76 **DECISION TABLE FOR TREATMENT**		
COMPLAINT	**CONTEXT**	**CORE**
Treatment for the presenting complaint and symptoms	Treatment for all associated symptoms	Treatment for mental, emotional, spiritual, constitutional, lifestyle issues and metaphysical considerations
TREATMENT PRIORITY	**TREATMENT PRIORITY**	**TREATMENT PRIORITY**
• Dietary recommendation to eliminate lactose • Herbal powder, tonic or tea to help reduce gastrointestinal inflammation heal and restore gut function • Nutritional supplements to heal gastrointestinal mucosa and normalise gastrointestinal microflora	• Educating Yoshimi's parents about managing lactose intolerance and providing information about dairy food alternatives • Supplemental nutrients to increase levels of essential nutrients; particularly important until Yoshimi's GIT has returned to optimal function and she is correctly absorbing dietary nutrients • Herbal formula and nutritional therapy heal and restore gut function to improve absorption of nutrients • Dietary recommendations to optimise dietary intake of essential nutrients • Lactase supplement to help improve Yoshimi's tolerance to lactose; beneficial in situations where it may be difficult to completely avoid lactose	• Herbal tea or tonic with nervine and sedative action to help reduce Yoshimi's anxiety and stress • Helping Yoshimi to make connections with other Japanese children by encouraging her parents to get involved with other expatriate Japanese families • Suggesting Yoshimi join a sporting club or community group • Encouraging Yoshimi's parents to bring her grandparents to Australia for a visit

Treatment aims

• Soothe inflamed digestive mucosa and heal gut wall [13].
• Remove all lactose from Yoshimi's diet, providing specific guidelines to Yoshimi's parents regarding which foods to avoid.
• Treat intestinal dysbiosis and possible leaky gut syndrome resulting from lactose intolerance [14, 15].

- Address Yoshimi's emotional issues.
- Identify and correct nutritional deficiencies [14, 15].
- In the longer term, improve Yoshimi's tolerance to lactose so she can occasionally consume it. This is important for her to feel normal and part of activities such as children's parties and other activities.

Lifestyle alterations/considerations

- Encourage Yoshimi's parents to get involved with community groups where Yoshimi can meet children from other expatriate Japanese families. Helping Yoshimi make friends will make her happier.
- Yoshimi may benefit from joining a local sporting club or organisation such as Scouts Australia where she may make new friends.
- Provide Yoshimi's parents with detailed information regarding lactose intolerance and direct them to books and websites where they can find useful information regarding lactose-free products and recipes.
- Yoshimi may benefit from a visit by her grandparents.

Dietary suggestions

- Eliminate all sources of lactose from Yoshimi's diet: milk, cheese, yoghurt, ice-cream, custard, sherbet and foods containing them. Depending on the severity of the condition, she may not tolerate foods with dairy products cooked into them such as some lollies, cakes (and icing), biscuits, processed meats, dessert mixes, sauces and gravies, some soups, drink mixes and even salad dressings.
- Yoshimi may tolerate lactose-free milk.
- Yoshimi's parents need detailed information on hidden sources of lactose and need to read labels and avoid foods with milk, milk solids, skim milk powder, cream, buttermilk, malted milk, whey lactose, curds and margarine.
- Soy milk and rice milk are an alternative to milk. Custards and ice-cream made with soy milk are an alternative to ones made with milk.
- Ensure Yoshimi gets important nutrients contained in dairy products such as calcium from other sources [15].
- Encourage Yoshimi to eat a whole-food diet high in fresh fruit and vegetables and low in refined carbohydrates. Yoshimi's diet should be more like the diet she used to eat in Japan.
- Encourage Yoshimi to drink sufficient water, particularly when she has diarrhoea, to help prevent dehydration [13].

Physical treatment suggestions

- Hydrotherapy: consitutional hydrotherapy [31, 32]. A hot shallow bath or hot foot bath for bloating [30]. Alternating hot/cold showers to the abdomen and spine [33]. Hot trunk wrap [33]. A hot sitz bath for abdominal pain [30]. A hot apple cider vinegar and water compress on the abdomen [30]. To tone the abdomen, apply a cold-wet compress on the abdomen, covered by a dry towel with an elastic bandage around the trunk at night for at least three months [30]. For acute diarrhoea, brief cold sitz baths with apple cider vinegar from a few seconds up to 10 minutes every day for a week, then every second day after symptoms subside [30].
- Yoshimi may find massage helpful to reduce her anxiety and improve her general health and wellbeing [29].

TABLE 3.77 HERBAL FORMULA (1:2 LIQUID EXTRACTS)

Made with ethanolic extract herbal liquids (alcohol removed)

HERB	FORMULA	RATIONALE
Witch hazel leaf *Hamamalis virginiana*	30 mL	Anti-inflammatory [19, 20]; astringent [16, 19, 20]; traditionally used for diarrhoea [16, 20]
Chamomile *Matricaria recutita*	70 mL	Anti-inflammatory [20, 21]; antispasmodic [20, 21]; antimicrobial [20, 21]; mild sedative [20, 22]; traditionally used for flatulent dyspepsia, nervous diarrhoea, restlessness and anxiety [19]
Fennel *Foeniculum vulgare*	70 mL	Carminative, anti-inflammatory; indicated for flatulent colic in children [19]
Peppermint *Mentha × piperita*	30 mL	Spasmolytic, carminative, cholagogue, antimicrobial, sedative [20]; BHP indication for flatulent digestive pains [19]; helpful to improve taste in herbal formulas for children
Supply:	200 mL	Dose: 2½ mL three times daily

Slippery elm bark powder (*Ulmus rubra*) 1 tsp twice daily, mixed with boiling water and then cooled before drinking [23]
Demulcent [19, 23]; emollient [19, 23]; nutritive [19, 23]; indicated for use in diarrhoea [19, 23]

TABLE 3.78 HERBAL TEA

Alternative to herbal liquid if there are compliance problems with a liquid tonic

HERB	FORMULA	RATIONALE
Chamomile flowers *Matricaria recutita*	2 parts	See above
Lemon balm leaves *Melissa officinalis*	1 part	Anti-inflammatory [23]; anxiolytic [23]; carminative [19]; antispasmodic [19, 23]; sedative [19, 23]; indicated for use in flatulent dyspepsia [19]
Peppermint *Mentha × piperita*	1 part	See above
Fennel *Foeniculum vulgare*	2 parts	See above

Infusion: 1 tsp per cup, half a cup 3 times daily

TABLE 3.79 NUTRITIONAL SUPPLEMENTS

SUPPLEMENT AND DOSE	RATIONALE
High-potency practitioner-strength **probiotic supplement** suitable for children containing therapeutic levels of human strain lactobacillus and bifidus organisms Dose: Child's dose as directed by the manufacturer for a child of Yoshimi's weight and age	To correct dysbiosis resulting from lactose intolerance [24]; probiotic supplementation can reduce symptoms of lactose intolerance [25]

►

High-potency practitioner-strength children's **multivitamin and mineral supplement** providing therapeutic doses of B-group vitamins Dose: As directed by the manufacturer for a child of Yoshimi's weight and age	Diarrhoea can result in reduced absorption of essential nutrients [15]
Calcium supplement Dose: Up to 1000 mg daily depending on Yoshimi's dietary calcium intake [27]	Calcium supplement may be necessary depending on Yoshimi's intake of calcium from other sources [13]
Glutamine Dose: 500 mg twice daily [23]	To assist with gut repair [23]; leaky gut syndrome may result from lactose intolerance [15]
Lactase supplement as required when Yoshimi occasionally consumes lactose-containing foods Dose: As directed by the manufacturer for a child of Yoshimi's weight and age	Supplemental lactase enzyme can help break down lactase; this may help improve Yoshimi's lactose tolerance [28]

References

[1] R.H. Seller, Differential Diagnosis of Common Complaints, fifth edn, Saunders Elsevier, Philadelphia, 2007.

[2] J. Jamison, Differential Diagnosis for Primary Care, second edn, Churchill Livingstone Elsevier, London, 2006 pp. 315, 394, 414, 460, 541–542, 574, 630–631.

[3] M. Lloyd, R. Bor, Communication Skills For Medicine, third edn, Churchill Livingstone Elsevier, Edinburgh, 2009.

[4] R. Neighbour, The Inner Consultation; how to develop an effective and intuitive consulting style, Radcliff Publishing, Oxon, 2005.

[5] G. Douglas, F. Nicol, C. Robertson, Macleod's Clinical Examination, twelfth edn, Churchill Livingstone Elsevier, Edinburgh, 2009.

[6] N.J. Talley, S. O'Connor, Pocket Clinical Examination, third edn, Churchill Livingstone Elsevier, Australia, 2009.

[7] P. Kumar, C. Clark, Clinical Medicine, sixth edn, Elsevier Saunders, London, 2005 pp. 640–643, 651, 663.

[8] A. Polmear (Ed.), Evidence-Based Diagnosis in Primary Care, Churchill Livingstone Elsevier, 2008, pp. 92–100.

[9] R.D. Collins, Differential Diagnosis in Primary Care, fourth edn, Lippincott Williams & Wilkins, Philadelphia, 2008 pp. 332, 360, 439–444.

[10] R. Berkow, A.J. Fletcher, M.H. Beers, The Merck Manual, sixteenth edn, Merck Research Laboratories, Rathway, N.J, 1993 (later edition).

[11] D. Peters, L. Chaitow, G. Harris, S. Morrison, Integrating Complementary Therapies in Primary Care, Churchill Livingstone, London, 2002.

[12] J. Silverman, S. Kurtz, J. Draper, Skills for Communicating with Patients, second edn, Radcliff Publishing, Oxford, 2000.

[13] M.B. Heyman, Lactose Intolerance in Infants, Children, and Adolescents, Pediatrics 118 (3) (2006) 1279–1286.

[14] H. Osiecki, The Physicians Handbook of Clinical Nutrition, seventh ed., Eagle Farm: Bioconcepts, 2000.

[15] J. Walker-Smith, J. Barnard, Z. Bhutta, J. Heubi, Z. Reeves, J. Schmitz, Chronic Diarrhea and Malabsorption (Including Short Gut Syndrome): Working Group Report of the First World Congress of Pediatric Gastroenterology, Hepatology and Nutrition, Journal of Pediatric Gastroenterology and Nutrition 35 (2002) S98–S105.

[16] D. Hoffman, The New Holistic Herbal, Element Books Ltd, Shaftesbury, Dorset, 1990.

[17] F. Scassocchio, M.F. Cometa, L. Tomassini, M. Palmery, Antibacterial activity of Hydrastis canadensis extract and its major isolated alkaloids, Planta Med 67 (6) (2001) 561–564.

[18] S. Mills, K. Bone, The Essential Guide to Herbal Safety, Churchill Livingstone, St Louis, 2005.

[19] British Herbal Medicine Association, British Herbal Pharmacopoeia, BHMA, 1983.

[20] S. Mills, K. Bone, Principles & Practice of Phytotherapy: Modern Herbal Medicine, Churchill Livingstone, Edinburgh, London, 2000.

[21] D. McKay, J. Blumberg, A review of the bioactivity and potential health benefits of chamomile tea (Matricaria recutita), Phytotherapy Research 20 (7) (2006) 519–553.

[22] G. Beaubrun, G. Gray, A review of herbal medicines for psychiatric disorders, Psychiatric Services 51 (2000) 1130–1134.

[23] L. Braun, M. Cohen, Herbs & Natural Supplements: An evidence based guide, second edn, Elsevier, Sydney, 2007.

[24] M. deVrese, A. Stegelman, B. Richter, S. Fensleau, C. Laue, J. Schrezenmeir, Probiotics – compensation for lactose insufficiency, American Journal of Clinical Nutrition 73 (2001) 421–429.

[25] L. Kipp-Hoolihan, Prophylactic and therapeutic uses of probiotics: a review, Journal of the American Dietetic Association 101 (2) (2001) 229–238.

[26] S.A. Bock, Diagnostic evaluation, Paediatrics 111 (2003) 1638–1644.

[27] J. Higdon, An Evidence Based Approach to Vitamins and Minerals, Thieme, New York, 2003.

[28] M.S. Medow, K.D. Thek, L.J. Newman, S. Berezin, M.S. Glassman, S.M. Schwarz, Beta-galactosidase tablets in the treatment of lactose intolerance in pediatrics, American Journal of Diseases in Children 144 (11) (1990) 1261–1264.

[29] S. Beider, C.A. Moyer, Randomized Controlled Trials of Pediatric Massage: A Review, ECAM 4 (1) (2007) 23–34.

[30] D.D. Buchman, The complete book of water healing, Contemporary Books, McGraw-Hill Companies, New York, 2001.

[31] W. Boyle, A. Saine, Lectures in Naturopathic Hydrotherapy, Oregon: Eclectic Medical Publications, 1988.

[32] L.M. Watrous, Constitutional hydrotherapy: from nature cure to advanced naturopathic medicine, Journal of Naturopathic Medicine 7 (2), 1997.

[33] E. Blake, in: L. Chaitow, E. Blake, P. Orrock, M. Wallden, P. Sinder, J. Zeff, Natropathic Physical Medicine (Eds.), Theory and Practice for Manual Therapists and Naturopaths, Philadelphia, Churchill Livingstone Elsevier, 2008.

[34] P.R. Hunter, Drinking water and diarrheal disease due to Escherichia coli, Journal of Water Health 1 (2) (2003) 65–72.

[35] P. Thomas, A. Forbes, J. Green, et al., Guidelines for the investigation of chronic diarrhoea, Gut 52 (Suppl. v) (2003) v1–v15.

[36] A. Shaw, G. Davies, Lactose intolerance problems in diagnosis and treatment, Journal of Clinical Gastroenterol 28 (1999) 208–216.

[37] R. Kohli, B.K. Li, Differential diagnosis of recurrent abdominal pain: new considerations, Paediatr Ann 33 (2004) 113–122.

[38] D.J. Humes, J. Simpson, Acute appendicitis, BMJ 333 (2006) 530–534.

[39] A.M. Lake, Chronic abdominal pain in childhood: diagnosis and management, Am Fam Physician 59 (7) (1999) 1823–1830.

[40] G. Russell, I. Abu-Arafeh, D.N. Symon, Abdominal migraine: evidence for existence and treatment options, Paediatr Drugs 4 (2002) 1–8.

[41] P.J. Strouse, Imaging the child with abdominal pain, Singapore Med J 44 (2003) 312–322.

[42] J.C. Guarderos, Is it food allergy? Differentiating the causes of adverse reactions to food, Postgrad Med 109 (2001) 125–134.

[43] D.L. Swagerty, A.D. Walling, R.M. Klein, Lactose intolerance, Am Fam Physician 65 (2002) 1845–1856.

[44] K. Beyer, S.S. Teuber, Food allergy diagnostics: scientific and unproven procedures, Curr Opin Allergy Clin Immunol 5 (2005) 261–266.

[45] J. Grundy, S. Matthews, B. Bateman, et al., Rising prevalence of allergy to peanut in children: Data from 2 sequential cohorts, J Allergy Clin Immunol 110 (2002) 784–789.

[46] A. Sheikh, S. Walker, Ten-Minute consultation: food allergy, BMJ 325 (2002) 1337.

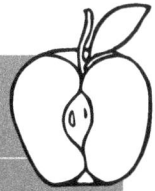

CHAPTER 4

Endocrine system

Hypothyroidism

Case history

Suzanne Beaumont is 32 years old. She has come to the clinic at the recommendation of her friend. Suzanne is here primarily for help with weight loss. During your consultation you discover Suzanne is experiencing significant fatigue despite sleeping at least 10 hours every night and is feeling more depressed than she has ever felt before.

Suzanne tells you she is experiencing worsening constipation, her hair and skin have become very dry and, in recent months, has been having problems with facial hair growth and a recurrence of facial acne (she had some problems with acne in her teen years, but that was nearly 15 years ago). Suzanne explains that she is embarrassed about her weight and is beginning to feel isolated from her friends and family because her physical appearance makes her reluctant to go out in public.

Suzanne is also experiencing aches and pains in her body. She doesn't exercise very much, and is too embarrassed to go to the gym or go walking because of her appearance. She is currently unemployed and, apart from having to go shopping, she rarely leaves the house.

Suzanne has hopes of having children one day; however, she is not currently in a relationship and says she doesn't really think anyone would be interested in her at the moment anyway. Her parents want her to find a husband and settle down to having children soon so they can enjoy having grandchildren before they are too old. Suzanne has had irregular periods for the past couple of years and she never knows when they will come but they are at least three months apart. When she does get her period the blood flow is extremely heavy and that is another reason she does not like to go out much after a few months without having had a period in case she is caught out. She is thankful she does not experience any period pain these days.

Suzanne can't understand why she has put on so much weight over the past three years when her appetite has decreased and she doesn't seem to enjoy food the way she used to. Apart from concerns about her appearance, she would really like to feel well and energetic again.

Suzanne has not been to a doctor in years and doesn't know if we can help her but says it feels good to finally talk about her problems with someone.

TABLE 4.1 **COMPLAINT**	
Analogy: Skin of the apple	**Complaint:** Define the presenting complaint and symptoms; understand the complaint *Overweight and fatigue*
AREAS OF INVESTIGATION AND EXAMPLE QUESTIONS	**CLIENT RESPONSES**
Onset *How long have you had problems with your weight?* *How long have you been feeling fatigue?*	*I've always been large, but in recent years it's just gotten worse and worse.* *It's gotten worse the more weight I put on.*
Understanding the cause (client) *What do you think has been causing the significant increase in weight?*	*I don't know, but something is really wrong, I think. Even my periods are going wrong.*
Your practitioner impression Suzanne is obviously obese. Your first impression of her is someone who lacks confidence and is quite unsure of herself.	

TABLE 4.2 **CONTEXT**	
Analogy: Flesh of the apple	**Context:** Put the presenting complaint into context to understand the disease.
AREAS OF INVESTIGATION AND EXAMPLE QUESTIONS	**CLIENT RESPONSES**
Family health *Has anyone else in your family experienced similar problems?*	*My mum is pretty big, but not as big as I am. Her sister is a lot like me, she's really big.*
Supplements and side effects of medication *Are you taking any supplements or medications from the doctor?*	*I went to the chemist and got a multivitamin and I also bought some weight-loss tablets, but they haven't helped my energy or my weight.*
Endocrine/reproductive *Did your irregular period cycle come on suddenly or begin to slow down gradually?*	*I used to be more regular and then it began to slow down and chop and change. Now I get confused about when it's going to come.*
Stress and neurological *Do you feel stressed at the moment?*	*Yes. I feel so bad about putting on this weight and I know I don't do enough exercise, but I feel so tired all of the time.*

▶

Eating habits and energy *Describe your diet.*	Suzanne's description of her diet indicates it is quite healthy, containing good amounts of whole foods, fresh fruit and vegetables. She insists her portion sizes are normal and on further questioning her description of her portion sizes indicates she is not eating excessive amounts at mealtimes.

TABLE 4.3 **CORE**	
Analogy: Core of the apple with the seed of ill health	**Core:** Holistic assessment to understand the client
AREAS OF INVESTIGATION AND EXAMPLE QUESTIONS	**CLIENT RESPONSES**
Support systems *Do you have a good support system?*	*I have my parents and some friends.*
Emotional health *Do you think you are depressed?*	*I think I am.*
Stress release *How do you manage your stress?*	*I don't know, I just usually read or watch TV.*
Family and friends *Do you spend much time with family or friends?*	*I see my parents at least once a week. I haven't seen my friends much recently since I feel really embarrassed whenever I go out with them. They're always nice to me, but I just feel they think I should try harder.*
Action needed to heal *What do you think you need to do to get better?*	*I really don't know, I've tried dieting and exercising but it didn't really work. I'm hoping you can help me.*
Long-term goals *What are your long-term goals?*	*To get slimmer and fitter and to get my energy back. I want to get a job and am thinking of retraining and doing something different.*

TABLE 4.4 **SUZANNE'S SIGNS AND SYMPTOMS** [2, 6–8]	
Pulse	55 bpm
Blood pressure	140/85
Temperature	35.8°C
Respiratory rate	14 resp/min
Body mass index	35 (obese)
Waist circumference	97 cm
Face	Pale, slight facial hair, puffy eyes, thin eyebrows, dry hair
Neck	Enlarged non-nodular thyroid gland
Nails	Inspection of nails – dry cuticles and surrounding skin
Urinalysis	No abnormality detected (NAD)
General observations	Deep voice, dry skin, slow movements and speech

Results of medical investigations

Suzanne has not had any medical investigations.

TABLE 4.5 **UNLIKELY DIAGNOSTIC CONSIDERATIONS** [2, 7–11]	
CONDITIONS AND CAUSES	**WHY UNLIKELY**
INFECTION AND INFLAMMATION	
Chronic salpingo-oophoritis: irregular cycle; can be minimal or excessive menstrual bleed	Usually congestive dysmenorrhoea is the predominant symptom; associated with purulent discharge, fever, period pain and abdominal pain
Postpartum thyroiditis: transient hypothyroid after pregnancy	No pregnancies that we know of
ENDOCRINE/REPRODUCTIVE	
Diabetes: anovulatory cycles	Urinalysis NAD
Primary dysmenorrhoea: lower abdominal pain, can get worse with menstrual cycle	Period pain usually begins at menarche and is often associated with no pelvic abnormality, nausea vomiting, headache and dizziness
Secondary dysmenorrhoea: acquired due to pathology; period pain begins several years after menarche and due to a pelvic abnormality	No menstrual pain
Endometriosis: irregular periods	No significant pelvic pain or pain on menstrual bleed reported; no bleeding from the bowel; usually brown discharge with associated abdominal and pelvic pain
Premenstrual syndrome: pain in the abdomen before menses	Will experience premenstrual mood changes, feel teary, bloated and swollen 1–12 days before her period; experiences a dull pelvic ache, abdominal bloating

▶

Ovarian cyst: irregular periods	Ovarian cysts almost never cause heavy menstrual bleeding
Ovulatory bleed: have a bleed mid-cycle as well as regular menses and ovulation has occurred	Feel emotional, premenstrual symptoms such as ovulation pain (mittelschmerz) and mood changes; usually spotting or light bleed at time of ovulation, regular cycle; check basal body temperature as it will be biphasic and fluctuate indicating ovulation has occurred

Case analysis

TABLE 4.6 POSSIBLE DIFFERENTIAL DIAGNOSIS

NOT RULED OUT BY TESTS/INVESTIGATIONS ALREADY DONE [2, 7–11, 56–58]

CONDITIONS AND CAUSES	WHY POSSIBLE	WHY UNLIKELY
FAMILY HEALTH		
Familial or idiopathic hirsutism: excess hair growth would not be typically androgenic	Excess hair appearing on hormonal influenced areas of the body where hair will grow, such as the face	Check if family history of excess hair growth for females
ALLERGIES AND IRRITANTS		
Food intolerance/allergy	Fatigue, depression; skin and hair changes; constipation	Need to gain more insight into Suzanne's diet and associated symptoms
CANCER AND HEART DISEASE		
Thyroid cancer	Deep voice, thyroid swelling	Will have signs of pain in neck or throat, difficulty swallowing, nodule or lump around laryngeal prominence, trouble breathing, difficulty speaking, hoarse throat; thyroid gland will have a single firm nodule that has developed rapidly
Ovarian, uterine cancer	Heavy irregular bleeding	No vaginal discharge reported
Adult onset and congenital adrenal hyperplasia/adrenal tumour: can cause primary and secondary amenorrhoea anovulatory cycles	Usually presents with severe acne and hirsutism; can present with anovulatory irregular menstrual bleeding	Check if there was rapid development of symptoms and how severe symptoms of virilisation are; usually will be severe and can include symptoms such as frontal balding, enlarged clitoris

TRAUMA AND PRE-EXISTING ILLNESS		
Congenital – dyshormonogenesis: genetic defects in synthesis of thyroid hormone – primary cause	Goitre and hypothyroid symptoms	Rare condition; may have associated deafness; need to investigate for family history of thyroid disease; will present with childhood symptoms such as dwarfism, mental retardation, pot belly, delayed bone age
OBSTRUCTION AND FOREIGN BODY		
Intestinal obstruction (bowel cancer, adhesions, hernias, faecal impaction with overflow)	Abdominal constipation	No vomiting, abdominal pain and distension
FUNCTIONAL DISEASE		
Thyroid benign nodules: follicular adenomas, cysts, focal thyroiditis	Deep voice, thyroid swelling, hypothyroid symptoms	Nodules develop rapidly
Fibromyalgia: pain in axial skeleton with tender points that has lasted more than 3 months	Tiredness, aches and pains more common in women; can be worse from being in cold weather; depression	Will often present with irritable bowel symptoms, difficulty sleeping; normal laboratory results; rule out organic reasons for symptoms
Obstructive sleep apnoea	Fatigue during the day; more common when overweight or obese; does not usually complain of 'sleepiness' but fatigue generally	Need to define if Suzanne does not feel well rested in the morning and if she snores during the night; can be made worse by alcohol consumption prior to sleeping
Obesity	BMI 35; lack of exercise; usually general distribution of weight gain	Goitre visible; usually no other abnormal health features other than being overweight; appetite is usually increased; oedema present (unusual); need to define if Suzanne has a family history of obesity; need to define if Suzanne's weight gain has been gradual with increased caloric intake and/or with eating more sugar
Chronic fatigue syndrome: fatigue for at least 6 months that has no physical, psychoses, bipolar affective disorder, eating disorder or organic brain disease	Severe disabling fatigue affects both mental and physical functioning for at least 6 months; sleeping more, depression, feelings of guilt, social withdrawal, crying spells; muscular aches and pains	Goitre indicates a physical reason for fatigue; need to define if Suzanne's fatigue improves as the day progresses

Functional constipation	Constipation, lack of exercise, stress	Need to check if more than 1 in 4 bowel motions is lumpy and hard, and causes strain, a feeling of incomplete evacuation or blockage; need to check if manual help is needed to facilitate a bowel motion passing; does she have fewer than 3 evacuations in a week?
DEGENERATIVE AND DEFICIENCY		
Iodine deficiency: iodine required for thyroid hormone synthesis – primary cause	Goitre and hypothyroid or euthyroid	In mountainous areas of Alps, Himalayas, South America, Central Africa; thyroid gland can have multiple nodules
Pernicious anaemia: lack of B12 absorption due to immune destruction of intrinsic factor in atrophic gastritis and loss of stomach parietal cells	Fatigue, slow movements, cognitive impairment, can present with hypothyroidism	Usually low blood pressure and rapid heart rate, shortness of breath, swollen red tongue, diarrhoea, can also present with hyperthyroidism
Anaemia: iron deficiency, pernicious anaemia, due to heavy menstrual bleeding	Fatigue, depression	Usually signs of shortness of breath, palpitations, increased heart rate
INFECTION AND INFLAMMATION		
Post-subacute thyroiditis: primary cause	Goitre and hypothyroid symptoms	Would be a transient condition of infective origin rather than the symptoms gradually building up over time; soft tender, sometimes painful goitre
Riedel's thyroiditis: fibrous tissue infiltrates and replaces the thyroid gland	Goitre hypothyroid symptoms; more common in women	Very hard goitre; rare form of thyroid disease
Osteoarthritis	Pain in many joints and more common in women	Usually develops in older age groups; presents with signs of limited range of movement, bony swellings and instability of joints; not necessarily associated with severe fatigue; need to check family history as it can be congenital and begin at an early age
Postviral infection	Depression, fatigue	Need to rule out if Suzanne has had viral symptoms prior to feeling fatigued and depressed

SUPPLEMENTS AND SIDE EFFECTS OF MEDICATION		
Drugs: lithium, antithyroid medication, cytokines	Cause hypothyroid symptoms	Need to check medication history
ENDOCRINE/REPRODUCTIVE		
Hypothalamic-pituituary disease: tumour, hypopituitarism is secondary cause of hypothyroidism	Goitre; symptoms of hypothyroid such as irregular periods, depression, weight gain, slow pulse, constipation, low body temperature	Blood tests will rule out secondary causes of hypothyroidism
Hypothyroidism: cause of secondary amenorrhoea due to hyperprolactinaemia and endocrine disorder; anovulatory cycles	Goitre, weight gain, fatigue, depression, irregular periods, heavy menses, constipation, increased facial hair (hirsutism), puffy eyes, deep voice, dry hair, low body temperature, slow pulse, muscle aches, slow movements, change in appetite	
Subclinical hypothyroidism [59, 60]	Weight gain, fatigue, depression, irregular periods, heavy menses, constipation, change in appetite	Need to check if serum TSH levels are above limit and T3 and T4 levels present as normal; could indicate clinical hypothyroidism may develop
Pregnancy	Irregular periods; missed periods; most common cause of secondary amenorrhoea; can present with vaginal discharge and pelvic/abdominal pain	Suzanne claims she is not sexually active at the moment and has no partner; pregnancy can present with fever; will have signs of breast tenderness and may have morning sickness
Uterine fibroids and polyps: fibroids form due to excess oestrogen and can cause symptoms of heavy bleeding, uterine enlargement	Usually causes menorrhagia (blood loss of 80 mL per day and lasting more than 7 days)	Often maintains normal cycle unless submucosal or nearly extruded
Polycystic ovarian syndrome (PCOS): extremely common cause of secondary amenorrhoea; anovulatory cycles	Irregular menstrual cycles, acne, increased facial hair (hirsutism), weight gain; irregular periods came on slowly	Can occur with androgenic alopecia (thinning of hair on the head such as men have); may not be associated with heavy menstrual bleeding

▶

Cushing's syndrome: cause amenorrhoea, irregular menstrual cycles	Irregular menstrual cycles, increased facial hair, depression, weight gain, higher scale blood pressure	There was not a rapid development of symptoms; no moon-shaped face or frontal balding; urinalysis NAD and indicating no glucose intolerance or diabetes that can be associated with Cushing's syndrome
Dysfunctional uterine bleeding (DUB): endometrial hyperplasia, PCOS, from taking exogenous oestrogen; endocrine dysfunction; (not associated with inflammation, tumour or pregnancy) anovulatory hormone-related bleeding is most common	Usually causes bleeding with unpredictable volume and frequency; often accompanied by menorrhagia (heavy bleed with regular cycle) but interval between periods is shorter to make the cycle appear irregular	No use of exogenous oestrogen reported
Anovulatory bleeding: have irregular bleed that appears menstrual although no ovulation has occurred; can be associated with both short and long cycles	Irregular cycle; no significant premenstrual symptoms reported to show evidence of regular association with menses cycle; bleed is painless and unexpected; blood volume can be excessive but irregular; physical findings will often include hirsutism, acne	Check basal body temperature; if anovulatory it will not fluctuate (monophasic)
Oestrogen-withdrawal bleeding: causes intermenstrual bleeding; occurs when the endometrium proliferates and becomes unstable when oestrogen drops below threshold; can happen outside of the secretory phase or in the absence of progesterone	Common cause of irregular periods in reproductive years, especially if ovulation has not occurred; menstrual bleeding is prolonged and profuse when it does occur; bleed is painless	
Progesterone-withdrawal bleeding: only occurs when there is an oestrogen-primed endometrium; can occur when oestrogen therapy continued and progesterone stopped; also when progesterone is administered to test endogenous oestrogen	Irregular menstrual bleed; often present in conditions such as amenorrhoea	

▶

Oestrogen-breakthrough bleeding – 1st type: when oestrogen levels are low but constant causing sections of endometrium to degenerate	Intermenstrual bleed	Need to investigate if experience any spotting of blood
Oestrogen-breakthrough bleeding – 2nd type: oestrogen levels are well above threshold causing endometrium to become hyperplastic and outgrow blood-borne hormone supply	Causes degeneration of endometrium with prolonged and irregular bleeding	More common in oestrogen-based tumours
AUTOIMMUNE DISEASE		
Atrophic thyroiditis: (autoimmune) most common cause of primary hypothyroidism; will cause atrophy and fibrosis of the thyroid gland	Goitre; may be intermittent and recover; symptoms of hypothyroidism; common in women	Check for the presence of antithyroid antibodies and pernicious anaemia; thyroid gland will be enlarged, sometimes painful and soft swelling
Hashimoto's thyroiditis: [58] important to rule out an autoimmune cause of primary hypothyroidism	Goitre; common in women	More often presents in late middle age
Rheumatoid arthritis	Muscle aches and pain; common in women, fatigue due to anaemia of chronic disease	Check if family history of rheumatoid arthritis
Systemic lupus erythematosus	Generalised aches and pains, skin changes, more common in women, increased fatigue	See if there is a butterfly rash on Suzanne's face
STRESS AND NEUROLOGICAL DISEASE		
Depression: important differential diagnosis to rule out before exploring other possibilities of mental or organic causes for fatigue symptoms		
Primary origins Primary depression and endogenous depression are associated conditions that are regarded as primary disorders, i.e. that do not occur secondarily to other medical or psychiatric disorders; these terms refer to depression that is caused by internal chemical and biological factors rather than external stressors		

▶

Type 1 – major (clinical) depression	Has at least five symptoms of depression every day for more than 2 weeks, which causes considerable incapacity with daily activities; people often describe symptoms in physical terms; depressed daily, loss of interest in daily activities, change of appetite, weight gain, increased fatigue, slower movements, feelings of worthlessness	Need to define if Suzanne feels worse in the morning and has a sense of apprehension; visible goitre indicates the feelings of depression come from a secondary origin
Dysthymia: mild depressive illness	Could be experiencing 'double depression' if Suzanne has had intermittent periods of depression in the past; symptoms include tiredness, lack of interest in life and low mood	Lasts intermittently for 2 years or more; need to determine if Suzanne has had a tendency to have episodes of feeling low prior to the onset of her physical changes
Secondary origins Reactive depression and associated conditions that occur after or in response to a pre-existing medical or psychiatric disorder; brought on by external life experiences		
Seasonal affective disorder: secondary to the winter months	Symptoms include increased sleep, tiredness, change in appetite, weight gain	Need to determine if Suzanne has experienced episodes of depression during the winter months in the past; usually appetite increases
Psychological **Functional fatigue** (depression)	Tiredness that has lasted several months	Need to determine if Suzanne's fatigue improves as the day progresses; determine if her fatigue began after a specific life event or only when her physical symptoms began
EATING HABITS AND ENERGY		
Causal factor: **Diet high in brassica and cassava foods:** when in excess can cause hypothyroid symptoms	Symptoms of underactive thyroid	Need to ask if Suzanne regularly eats broccoli, spinach, cabbage, cauliflower, brussels sprouts, kale, collard greens, pak choi and tapioca is in Suzanne's diet
Causal factor: **Lack of exercise**	Weight gain, fatigue, depression	

TABLE 4.7 **DECISION TABLE FOR REFERRAL** [2, 7–12]		
COMPLAINT	**CONTEXT**	**CORE**
Referral for presenting complaint	Referral for all associated physical, dietary and lifestyle concerns	Referral for contributing emotional, mental, spiritual, metaphysical, lifestyle and constitutional factors
REFERRAL FLAGS	**REFERRAL FLAGS**	**REFERRAL FLAGS**
• BMI over 30 indicating obesity • Weight gain associated with goitre	• A menstruating woman of any age can bleed from pregnancy complications • Irregular bleeding in menstrual cycle for years • Change in volume of menstrual bleed • Hirsutism associated with menstrual change and other virilising symptoms such as acne • Weight gain with decreased appetite • Pattern of premenstrual symptoms have stopped, indicating lack of ovulation	• Social isolation • Significant depression • Symptoms have worsened without Suzanne seeking medical help
ISSUES OF SIGNIFICANCE	**ISSUES OF SIGNIFICANCE**	**ISSUES OF SIGNIFICANCE**
• Lack of exercise	• Puffy eyes, dry hair and skin • Significant fatigue although sleeping well at night • Worsening constipation	• Embarrassed about weight and hirsutism • Unemployed • Would like to have children and a husband • Family pressure regarding marriage
REFERRAL	**REFERRAL**	**REFERRAL**
• Signs and symptoms warrant further investigations for a definitive diagnosis of hypothyroidism [56, 57]; we have a duty of care to Suzanne to encourage her to be informed regarding possible treatment using thyroxine medication [58, 60] • Dietary assessment	• Medical assessment on associated menstrual, metabolic and virilising symptoms	• Mental health assessment and counselling • Career advice

TABLE 4.8 **FURTHER INVESTIGATIONS THAT MAY BE NECESSARY** [2, 6–11, 13, 57, 60]	
TEST/INVESTIGATION	**REASON FOR TEST/INVESTIGATION**
FIRST-LINE INVESTIGATIONS:	
Pelvic, vaginal, abdominal examination	Check for bulging uterus, ovaries can be palpable in PCOS, abdominal rebound tenderness, overactive bowel sounds, genital deformities, signs of trauma
Musculoskeletal examination	Back strain, trauma, deformities, inflammation
Human chorionic gonadotropin (HCG) **blood test/radioimmunoassay** (RIA)	Pregnancy, ectopic pregnancy
Full blood count	Check for signs of infection, virus or allergic reaction; rule out anaemia
Thyroid function test **Thyroid stimulating hormone** (TSH) **Thyroid hormones** (T4, T3 synthesised in the thyroid gland)	*TSH:* High in primary and subclinical hypothyroidism; normal or low in secondary hypothyroidism (hypothalamic-pituitary cause) *T4:* Low in primary and secondary hypothyroidism; normal reading in subclinical hypothyroidism *T3:* Low in primary and secondary hypothyroidism; normal reading in subclinical hypothyroidism
'Free' T4: available for tissue action	Measures only the unbound active T4 hormone; will be low in hypothyroid
Thyroxine-binding globulin (TBG) – binds T4 and T3 in plasma	Will be increased in hypothyroidism
Thyroid antibody: blood test thyroid perioxidase antibody, antithyroglobulin antibody	Autoimmune causes of hypothyroidism
Serum cholesterol	Can be raised in hypothyroidism
ESR/CRP	Inflammation such as in systemic lupus erythematosus (SLE) and rheumatoid arthritis
Progesterone level	Test 7 days before menstruation due to see if ovulation has occurred; low serum progesterone level in anovulatory cycles
Oestradiol	*Normal:* PCOS, weight loss, excess exercise *Raised:* pregnancy, ovarian tumour, testicular tumour, adrenal tumour *Low:* PCOS, polycystic ovarian disease, ovarian failure, anorexia nervosa, weight loss, excess exercise, hypothyroidism, Cushing's syndrome, adrenal hyperplasia, menopause, Turner's syndrome, failing pregnancy, fetal death

▶

FSH (follicle-stimulating hormone)	*Normal:* PCOS, pregnancy, anorexia, weight loss, excess exercise *Raised:* ovarian failure, menopause *Low:* polycystic ovarian disease, anorexia, weight loss, excess exercise, hypothyroidism, Cushing's syndrome, adrenal tumour/hyperplasia
LH (luteinising hormone) due to pulsatile action of this hormone it may not be accurately measured on one random sample	*Normal:* pregnancy, anorexia, weight loss, excess exercise *Raised*: PCOS, polycystic ovarian disease, ovarian failure, menopause *Low:* anorexia, weight loss, excess exercise, hypothyroidism, Cushing's syndrome, adrenal tumour/hyperplasia
PRL (prolactin) commonly raised in secondary amenorrhoea	*Normal:* ovarian failure, anorexia, weight loss, excess exercise, adrenal tumour/hyperplasia *Raised*: PCOS (mildly), hypothyroidism, Cushing's syndrome, pregnancy, amenorrhoea *Low:* pituitary destruction from tumour
Testosterone	*Normal:* ovarian failure, anorexia, weight loss, excess exercise, hypothyroidism, pregnancy *Raised*: PCOS, Cushing's syndrome, adrenal tumour/hyperplasia, testicular tumour, ovarian tumour *Low:* corticosteriod use
SHBG (sex hormone-binding globulin)	Low SHBG would indicate the presence of elevated levels of free androgens
Fasting blood glucose test	Raised levels can indicate diabetes mellitus, Cushing's syndrome
Cervical smear	To detect cervical cancer
HOME TESTS:	
Basal body temperature	Normally drops 24–36 hours after menses commences; with endometriosis there is often a delay in basal body temperature to the second or third day of menses; a decrease indicates preovulation and an increase of 5 degrees occurs after ovulation Monitors thyroid function; low temperature readings consistently over a period of days can indicate subclinical or clinical hypothyroidism
Ovulation prediction kits	Designed to detect an increase in urinary luteinising hormone (LH) excretion 24–36 hrs prior to ovulation
Diet dairy	Assess caloric intake and possible food sensitivities

▶

IF NECESSARY:	
Serum aspartate transferase	Will be increased from muscle and liver in hypothyroid
Serum creatine kinase levels	Increased with associated myopathy in hypothyroidism
Sodium levels	Low due to increase in ADH and slow free water clearance
Thyrotropin releasing hormone (TRH)	TRH is released in the hypothalamus to stimulate release of TSH from pituitary; determine hypothalamic-pituitary disease
Anti-nuclear antibody	Autoimmune disorders, SLE, rheumatoid arthritis
RH factor	Rheumatoid arthritis
Epstein-Barr virus blood test	Postviral symptoms, may show that Suzanne has had this virus in the past without realising it
Abdominal and pelvic x-ray/ultrasound	Most accurate diagnosis of PCOS, ovarian mass, ovarian cyst or tumour, retroverted uterus, tubo-ovarian abscesses, fibroids, trauma; intestinal obstruction
Brain scan CT/MRI	Pituitary tumour
Back x-ray CT scan and MRI	Degenerative disc disease, disc prolapse, *Ankylosing spondylitis*, Paget's disease, osteoporosis

Confirmed diagnosis

SUZANNE AND HYPOTHYROIDISM

Suzanne is a 32-year-old woman who has come to the clinic asking for help with weight loss – she has now reached a BMI of 35. Additionally Suzanne is experiencing significant fatigue despite sleeping long hours at night, has worsening constipation, a lack of appetite and is depressed. She has also been experiencing irregular and heavy periods, has developed facial hair growth and acne, dry skin and hair and suffers from generalised aches and pains in her body. On the whole Suzanne is feeling very low about herself and this is not made any better by her family being disappointed that she does not yet have a husband and children. Suzanne is currently unemployed and does not leave her home often. She is not exercising because she is too embarrassed to do so outside of her home and is not motivated on her own.

On physical examination it became evident that Suzanne has a visible goitre, deep voice, puffy eyes, slow movements and speech, low body temperature and pulse rate and high blood pressure. Suzanne required immediate referral for a medical and mental health assessment. A medical diagnosis of **hypothyroidism** was confirmed, which explains the range of symptoms she has been experiencing.

Hypothyroidism is an ailment characterised by under-activity of the thyroid gland (i.e. insufficient production of thyroid hormones). The most 'observable' sign of hypothyroidism is a goitre and low basal temperature in the morning. Other symptoms include fatigue, weight gain, memory and mental impairment, dry skin, cold intolerance, decreased concentration, constipation, depression, loss of hair, coarse hair, muscle and joint pain, goitre, hyperlipidaemia, irregular periods, infertility, hoarseness, yellow skin, lowered body temperature, drooping swollen eyes, reduced or excessive sweating, brittle nails, diminished sex drive and slow healing.

Hypothyroidism occurs most frequently in women over the age of 40 (however, men and teenagers may also have hypothyroidism). It is possible for a woman or man to have symptoms of subclinical hypothyroidism for many years before developing a clinical manifestation of the disease. Approximately 50 per cent of people with hypothyroidism are unaware they have the condition [56]. Although clients with this disorder can be asymptomatic, some clients have subtle findings including alteration in lipid metabolism as well as abnormalities in cardiac, gastrointestinal, neuropsychotic and reproductive functions [57].

General references used in this diagnosis: 2, 7, 8, 10, 11, 56–58

PRESCRIBED MEDICATION

• Thyroxine

TABLE 4.9 **DECISION TABLE FOR TREATMENT**		
COMPLAINT	**CONTEXT**	**CORE**
Treatment for the presenting complaint and symptoms	Treatment for all associated symptoms	Treatment for mental, emotional, spiritual, constitutional, lifestyle issues and metaphysical considerations
TREATMENT PRIORITY	**TREATMENT PRIORITY**	**TREATMENT PRIORITY**
• Improve thyroid function and endogenous production of thyroid hormones via recommendations to increase dietary intake of nutrients essential for thyroid hormone production • Improve thyroid function and endogenous production of thyroid hormones via physical therapy suggestions and recommendation to increase exercise • Improve thyroid function and endogenous production of thyroid hormones by identifying and addressing chemical or heavy metal exposure, which may affect thyroid function	• Dietary and supplement recommendations to assist with weight loss • Recommendation for Suzanne to increase physical activity to assist with weight loss, improve metabolic rate and improve general health • Herbal tea to assist with weight loss • Increasing antioxidant intake to enhance general health and protect against damage from oxidative stress through diet, herbal tea and nutritional supplements • Dietary and nutritional supplementation recommendations to assist with balancing reproductive hormones	• Recommendation to increase physical activity to assist with stress and depression • Herbal liquid or tablets with anxiolytic and adaptogenic properties • Recommendations to improve dietary intake of essential fatty acids and essential nutrients to help improve depression • Recommendation for counselling or cognitive behavioural therapy to help improve Suzanne's body image and general emotional health

▶

▶

• Improve thyroid function and endogenous production of thyroid hormones by reducing or avoiding exposure to dietary and environmental substances that may adversely affect thyroid function, e.g. avoiding fluoride, caffeine and goitrogens • Improve thyroid function and endogenous production of thyroid hormones via nutritional supplement suggestions • Improve thyroid function and endogenous production of thyroid hormones via herbal tincture or tablets **NB:** Collaborative management of Suzanne's case is essential to ensure potential interactions between prescribed thyroxine and herbal and nutritional supplements are managed appropriately; it may be possible to reduce the dose of thyroxine as the dietary, lifestyle, herbal and supplement treatments improve Suzanne's thyroid function		

Treatment aims

- Improve thyroid function and increase endogenous production of T4 [14, 15].
- Optimise nutritional status and ensure adequate dietary intake of nutrients required for hormone production and conversion of T4 to T3 [14, 15, 32].
- Identify and address any environmental chemical or heavy metal exposure, which may be implicated in the development and/or progression of Suzanne's condition [15, 35].
- Identify and correct any nutritional deficiencies that may be contributing to Suzanne's condition [14, 15, 32].
- Improve Suzanne's nutritional and antioxidant status. This is essential for both normal thyroid function [14, 15, 31, 32], to reduce oxidative stress associated with hypothyroidism [14, 31, 32] and to help manage symptoms of depression [14, 15].
- Improve Suzanne's reproductive hormone balance [14].
- Improve Suzanne's associated symptoms of dry skin, hair and nails, excessive fatigue, musculoskeletal pain and psychological symptoms [2, 8, 14].
- Assist Suzanne with weight loss.

- Improve Suzanne's physical activity levels [14, 15].
- Support Suzanne's cardiovascular health and manage hyperhomocysteinaemia, hyperlipidaemia and insulin resistance if present [14, 32, 33].
- Support Suzanne's emotional health.

Lifestyle alterations/considerations

- Encourage Suzanne to exercise daily. Exercise stimulates thyroid hormone secretion and increases tissue sensitivity to the thyroid hormone [14, 15, 22, 23]. Exercise also helps improve depression and anxiety [47].
- Encourage Suzanne not to eat a very low calorie diet in an effort to lose weight. It can reduce metabolic rate as the body seeks to conserve energy [14, 24].
- Suzanne may benefit from a course of cognitive behavioural therapy [25, 28]. Improving thyroid function is likely to improve response to psychological treatment [26, 27].

Dietary suggestions

- Encourage Suzanne to avoid or significantly reduce consumption of foods containing goitrogens and thiocanates (cabbage, cauliflower, brussels sprouts, soy fibre, apples, walnuts, almonds) [14, 15]. If Suzanne chooses to eat goitrogenic foods they should be cooked to reduce levels of goitrogens [15, 29, 30].
- If Suzanne eats soy-based foods it is important to ensure her iodine intake is adequate to ensure thyroid function is not affected [17, 38].
- Encourage Suzanne to increase consumption of foods containing iodine, selenium, copper, iron, zinc, B-group vitamins and tyrosine, which are essential nutrients for thyroid function [14, 15].
- Encourage Suzanne to eat whole organic foods [14] and increase consumption of antioxidant-rich foods [14, 15, 31].
- Encourage Suzanne to increase her dietary intake of essential fatty acids, particularly omega-3 and -6 fatty acids and decrease consumption of saturated fats [15, 34]. Omega-3 fatty acids are essential to reduce or treat depression [48].
- Suzanne's weight-loss program should incorporate a higher protein and lower carbohydrate intake and include adequate levels of essential fatty acids [36, 37] that comprise low GI/GL foods. This is likely to assist Suzanne with weight loss [46].
- Suzanne would benefit from incorporating turmeric into her diet for its antioxidant, anti-inflammatory and liver function enhancing properties [14, 17, 18].
- Suzanne should reduce consumption of caffeinated beverages [15, 40].

Physical treatment suggestions

- Cold hydrotherapy can stimulate thyroid function [14, 55].
- Cold sitz baths to prevent heavy menstrual bleeding [50]. Place an ice pack on the inside of the thighs to stop heavy bleeding [50].
- Whole body cold mitten friction for circulation and depression [51].
- Constitutional hydrotherapy [50, 52, 53].
- For constipation place a hot compress on the abdomen, then cover in plastic with a hot water bottle/heating pad on top for 12 minutes, followed by cold mitten friction for 30 seconds (repeat process three times) [54].
- Alternating hot and cold showers to improve immune function and decrease fatigue [51, 53].

- Arm, wrist, ankle cold shower affusions for fatigue [50, 53, 54].
- Neutral baths (note: whole body heat treatments contraindicated) [54].
- Exercise therapy program incorporating resistance training to support metabolic function and weight loss [14, 15, 22, 23, 49].

TABLE 4.10 **HERBAL TEA**		
Alternative to tea and coffee		
HERB	**FORMULA**	**RATIONALE**
Green tea *Camellia sinensis* Decaffeinated [40]	4 parts	Thermogenic [17, 39]; antioxidant [17]; may be beneficial to aid weight loss [17, 39]
Ginger root powder *Zingiber officinale*	½ part	Anti-inflammatory [17, 18]; antioxidant [17]
Bitter orange peel *Citrus aurantium*	3 parts	Antioxidant [17]; may be beneficial to aid weight loss [17]
Infusion: 1 tsp per cup – 3–4 cups daily		

TABLE 4.11 **HERBAL FORMULA (1:2 LIQUID EXTRACTS)**		
HERB	**FORMULA**	**RATIONALE**
Withania *Withania somnifera*	70 mL	Adaptogen [17, 18]; tonic [18]; anti-inflammatory [17, 18, 19]; stimulates thyroid activity [17, 41]; enhances serum T4 concentration [17, 41]
Brahmi *Bacopa moniera*	65 mL	Adaptogen [17]; nervine tonic [19]; increases T4 concentration [17, 42]
Bladderwrack *Fucus vesiculosus*	50 mL	Thyroid stimulating [20]; aids with weight loss [20]; contains iodine [20]
Korean ginseng *Panax ginseng*	15 mL	Adaptogenic [17, 18]; tonic [17, 18]; antioxidant [17]
Supply:	200 mL	Dose: 10 mL twice daily
Suzanne's thyroid hormone levels should be monitored regularly due to the potential for interaction with thyroxine [17]		

TABLE 4.12 TABLET ALTERNATIVE TO HERBAL LIQUID: MAY IMPROVE COMPLIANCE

HERB	DOSE PER TABLET	RATIONALE
Bladderwrack *Fucus vesiculosus*	440 mg	See above
Brahmi *Bacopa moniera*	1000 mg	See above
Withania *Withania somnifera*	250 mg	See above

Dose: 1 tablet 3 times daily. Suzanne's thyroid hormone levels should be monitored regularly due to the potential for interaction with thyroxine [17]

TABLE 4.13 NUTRITIONAL SUPPLEMENTS

SUPPLEMENT AND DOSE	RATIONALE
Iodine 250 mcg daily [16, 17, 21, 43] If Suzanne choose not to take the herbal liquid or tablets that contain bladderwrack Suzanne's thyroid hormone levels should be monitored regularly due to the potential for interaction with thyroxine [17]	Essential for the manufacture of T4 and T3 [16, 17, 21] and for normal thyroid function [43]; combines with tyrosine to form thyroid hormones [16]; deficiency may be associated with decreased plasma levels of T4 and T3 [21] and hypothyroidism [16, 21, 43]; supplementation of 250 mcg takes into account recommendations to increase dietary intake of iodine [14, 15] and to ensure Suzanne does not exceed the upper prescribing limit for iodine [16, 17, 21, 43]
Zinc citrate 50 mg elemental zinc daily [16, 21]	Necessary for normal thyroid function [44]; antioxidant [16, 17, 21, 43]; required for normal function of the reproductive system and reproductive hormones [17, 43]
Selenium 200 mcg daily [16, 17, 21, 43] 2 mg daily of copper to be included if zinc supplement taken for more than a month [16]	Required for thyroid hormone synthesis [21]; facilitates conversion of T3 to T4 [16, 17, 43]; regulates thyroid hormones [17, 43, 44]; antioxidant [16, 17, 21, 43]; necessary for normal function of reproductive hormones [21]; reduces heavy metal toxicity [17, 21]
Vitamin C 1000 mg twice daily [16, 17, 21, 43]	Required for thyroid hormone synthesis [14, 17]; antioxidant [16, 17, 21, 43]
High-potency practitioner-strength **multivitamin and antioxidant supplement** providing therapeutic doses of B-group vitamins [16, 17, 21, 45]	There is an increased need for antioxidant intake in hypothyroidism [14, 31, 32]; thyroid hormone insufficiency increases the need for vitamin B2 [17]; deficiency of B-group vitamins adversely effects mitochondrial energy production [45]; vitamin B6 is essential for reproductive hormone synthesis [16, 17, 21, 43]; inadequate nutritional status is implicated in depression [14, 15]

▶

Tyrosine 1500 mg daily in divided doses [17, 21] Suzanne's thyroid hormone levels should be monitored regularly due to the potential for interaction with thyroxine [17]	Thyroid hormone precursor [17, 21]; combines with iodine to form thyroid hormones [16]; low levels of tyrosine can be associated with hypothyroidism [17, 21]; supplementation may be beneficial to improve stress adaptation [17, 21]; improve energy levels [17] and aid with weight loss [17]

References

[1] N.J. Talley, S. O'Connor, Pocket Clinical Examination, third edn, Churchill Livingstone Elsevier, Australia, 2009.

[2] P. Kumar, C. Clark, Clinical Medicine, sixth edn, Elsevier Saunders, London, 2005.

[3] J. Silverman, S. Kurtz, J. Draper, Skills for Communicating with Patients, second edn, Radcliff Publishing, Oxford, 2000.

[4] R. Neighbour, The Inner Consultation: how to develop an effective and intuitive consulting style, Radcliff Publishing, Oxon, 2005.

[5] M. Lloyd, R. Bor, Communication Skills For Medicine, third edn, Churchill Livingstone Elsevier, Edinburgh, 2009.

[6] G. Douglas, F. Nicol, C. Robertson, Macleod's Clinical Examination, twelveth edn, Churchill Livingstone Elsevier, 2009.

[7] J. Jamison, Differential Diagnosis for Primary Care, second edn, Churchill Livingstone Elsevier, London, 2006.

[8] A. Polmear (Ed.), Evidence-Based Diagnosis in Primary Care, Churchill Livingstone Elsevier, 2008, pp. 274–283.

[9] R.D. Collins, Differential Diagnosis in Primary Care, fourth edn, Lippincott Williams & Wilkins, Philadelphia, 2008.

[10] R.H. Seller, Differential Diagnosis of Common Complaints, 5th edn, Saunders Elsevier, Philadelphia, 2007.

[11] R.M.D. Berkow, A.J.M.D. Fletcher, M.H.M.D. Beers, The Merck Manual, sixteenth edn, Merck Research Laboratories, Rathway, N.J, 1993 (later edition).

[12] D. Peters, L. Chaitow, G. Harris, S. Morrison, Integrating Complementary Therapies in Primary Care. London: Churchill Livingstone.

[13] K.D. Pagna, T.J. Pagna, Mosby's Diagnostic and Laboratory Test reference, third edn, Mosby, USA, 1997 (later edition).

[14] J.E. Pizzorno, M.T. Murray, H. Joiner-Bey, The Clinicians Handbook of Natural Medicine, second edn, Churchill Livingstone, St Louis, 2008.

[15] H. Osiecki, The Physicians Handbook of Clinical Nutrition, seventh edn, Eagle Farm: Bioconcepts, 2000.

[16] J. Jamison, Clinical Guide to Nutrition & Dietary Supplements in Disease Management, Churchill Livingstone, Edinburgh, 2003.

[17] L. Braun, M. Cohen, Herbs & Natural Supplements: An evidence based guide, second edn, Elsevier, Sydney, 2007.

[18] S. Mills, K. Bone, Principles & Practice of Phytotherapy: Modern Herbal Medicine, Churchill Livingstone, Edinburgh: London, 2000.

[19] K. Bone, Clinical Applications of Chinese and Ayurvedic Herbs: Monographs for the Western Herbal Practitioners, Warwick. Phytotherapy Press, 1996.

[20] S. Mills, K. Bone, The Essential Guide to Herbal Safety, Churchill Livingstone, St Louis, 2005.

[21] H. Osiecki, The Nutrient Bible, seven edn, Eagle Farm: BioConcepts Publishing, 2008.

[22] M.J. Gawel, D.M. Park, J. Alaghband-Zadeh, F.C. Rose, Exercise and hormonal secretion, Postgraduate Medical Journal 55 (1979) 373–376.

[23] R.G. McMurray, A.G. Hackney, Interactions of Metabolic Hormones, Adipose Tissue and Exercise, Sports Medicine 35 (5) (2005) 393–412.

[24] D.L. Elliot, L. Goldberg, K.S. Kuehl, W.M. Bennett, Sustained depression of the resting metabolic rate after massive weight loss, The American Journal of Clinical Nutrition 49 (1989) 93–96.

[25] J.C. Rosen, P. Orosan, J. Reiter, Cognitive behavior therapy for negative body image in obese women, Behaviour Therapy 26 (1) (1995) 25–42.

[26] R. Joffe, Z. Segal, W. Singer, Change in thyroid hormone levels following response to cognitive therapy for major depression, American Journal of Psychiatry 153 (3) (1996) 411–413.

[27] M. Gitlin, L.L. Altshuler, M.A. Frye, R. Suri, E.L. Huynm, L. Fairbanks, M. Bauer, et al., Peripheral thyroid hormones and response to selective serotonin reuptake inhibitors, The Journal of Psychiatry and Neuroscience 29 (5) (2004) 383–386.

[28] T.A. Wadden, G.D. Foster, Behavioural Treatment of Obesity, Medical Clinics of North America 84 (2) (2000) 441–461, vii.

[29] E. Ciska, H. Kozlowska, The effect of cooking on the glucosinolates content in white cabbage, European Food Research and Technology 212 (5) (2001) 582–587.

[30] M. McMillan, E.A. Spinks, G.R. Fenwick, Preliminary Observations on the Effect of Dietary Brussels Sprouts on Thyroid Function, Human & Experimental Toxicology 5 (1) (1986) 15–19.

[31] U. Resch, G. Helsel, F. Tatzber, H. Sinzinger, Antioxidant Status in Thyroid Dysfunction, Clinical Chemistry and Laboratory Medicine 40 (11) (2002) 1132–1134.

[32] M.S. Morris, A.G. Bostom, P.F. Jacques, J. Selhub, I.H. Rosenberg, Hyperhomocysteinemia and hypercholesterolemia associated with hypothyroidism in the third US National Health and Nutrition Examination Survey, Atherosclerosis 155 (1) (2001) 195–200.

[33] A.R. Cappola, P.W. Ladenson, Hypothyroidism and Atherosclerosis, The Journal of Clinical Endocrinology & Metabolism 88 (6) (2003) 2438–2444.

[34] G. Krey, O. Braissant, F. L'Horeset, E. Kalkhoven, M. Perroud, M.G. Parker, W. Wahli, Fatty Acids, Eicosanoids, and Hypolipidemic Agents Identified as Ligands of Peroxisome Proliferator-Activated Receptors by Coactivator-Dependent Receptor Ligand Assay, Molecular Endocrinology 11 (6) (1997) 779–791.

[35] N. Osius, W. Karmaus, H. Kruse, J. Witten, Exposure to Polychlorinated Biphenyls and Levels of Thyroid Hormones in Children, Environmental Health Perspectives 107 (10) (1999) 843–849.

[36] J.S. Volek, M.J. Sharman, A.L. Gomez, D.A. Judelson, M.R. Rubin, G. Watson, B. Sokmen, et al. Comparison of energy-restricted very low-carbohydrate and low-fat diets on weight loss and body composition in overweight men and women,

[37] D.K. Laymen, R.A. Boileau, D.J. Erickson, J.E. Painter, H. Shiue, C. Sather, D.D. Christou, A Reduced Ratio of Dietary Carbohydrate to Protein Improves Body Composition and Blood Lipid Profiles during Weight Loss in Adult Women, The Journal of Nutrition 133 (2) (2003) 411–417.

[38] M. Messina, G. Redmond, Effects of soy protein and soybean isoflavones on thyroid function in healthy adults and hypothyroid patients: a review of the relevant literature, Thyroid 16 (3) (2006) 249–258.

[39] A.G. Dulloo, J. Seydoux, L. Girardier, P. Chantre, J. Vandermander, Green tea and thermogenesis: interactions between catechin-polyphenols, caffeine and sympathetic activity, International Journal of Obesity Related Metabolic Disorders 24 (2) (2000) 252–258.

[40] E. Spindel, M. Arnold, B. Cusack, R.J. Wurtman, Effects of caffeine on anterior pituitary and thyroid function in the rat, Journal of Pharmacology and Experimental Therapeutics 214 (1980) 58–62.

[41] S. Panda, A. Kar, Changes in thyroid hormone concentrations after administration of ashwagandha root extract to adult male mice, Journal of Pharmacy and Pharmacology 50 (9) (1998) 1065–1068.

[42] A. Kar, S. Panda, S. Bharti, Relative efficacy of three medicinal plant extracts in the alteration of thyroid hormone concentrations in male mice, Journal of Ethnopharmacology 81 (2) (2002) 281–285.

[43] J. Higdon, An Evidence Based Approach to Vitamins and Minerals, Thieme, New York, 2003.

[44] J.R. Arthur, J.G. Beckett, Thyroid Function, British Medical Bulletin 55 (3) (1999) 658–668.

[45] F. Depeint, W.R. Bruce, N. Shangari, R. Mheta, P.J. O'Brien, Mitochondrial function and toxicity: Role of the B vitamin family on mitochondrial energy metabolism, Chemico-Biological Interactions 163 (2006) 94–112.

[46] M.A. Pereira, J. Swain, A.B. Goldfine, N. Rifai, D.S. Ludwig, Effects of a Low–Glycemic Load Diet on Resting Energy Expenditure and Heart Disease Risk Factors During Weight Loss, Journal of the American Medical Association 292 (20) (2004) 2482–2490.

[47] P. Salmon, Effects of physical exercise on anxiety, depression, and sensitivity to stress: A unifying theory, Clinical Psychology Review 21 (1) (2001) 33–61.

[48] B.M. Ross, J. Seguin, L.E. Sieswerda, Omega-3 fatty acids as treatments for mental illness: Which disorder and which fatty acid? Lipids in Health and Disease 6 (2007) 21.

[49] R.W. Bryner, I.H. Ullrich, J. Sauers, D. Donley, G. Hornsby, M. Kolar, R. Yeater, Effects of Resistance vs. Aerobic Training Combined With an 800 Calorie Liquid Diet on Lean Body Mass and Resting Metabolic Rate, Journal of the American College of Nutrition 18 (1) (1999) 115–121.

[50] W. Boyle, A. Saine, Lectures in Naturopathic Hydrotherapy, Oregon: Eclectic Medical Publications, 1988.

[51] D.D. Buchman, The complete book of water healing, Contemporary Books, McGraw-Hill Companies, New York, 2001.

[52] E. Blake, in: L. Chaitow, E. Blake, P. Orrock, P. Wallden, P. Sinder, J. Zeff (Eds.), Naturopathic Physical Medicine: Theory and Practice for Manual Therapists and Naturopaths, Philadelphia, Churchill Livingstone Elsevier, 2008.

[53] L. Chaitow, Hydrotherapy, water therapy for health and beauty, Element, Dorset, 1999.

[54] M. Sinclair, Modern Hydrotherapy for the Massage Therapist, Lippincott Williams & Williams, Baltimore, 2008.

[55] F. De Lorenzo, M. Mukherjeem, Z. Kadziolaz, R. Sherwood, V.V. Kakkar, Central cooling effects in patients with hypercholesterolaemia, Clinical Science 95 (1998) 213–217.

[56] R. Indra, S. Patil, R. Joshi, et al., Accuracy of physical examination in the diagnosis of hypothyroidism: a cross-sectional, double-blind study, J Postgrad Med 50 (2004) 7–10.

[57] C.M. Dayan, Interpretation of thyroid function tests, Lancet 357 (2001) 619–624.

[58] C. Roberts, P. Ladenson, Hypothyroidism. Lancet 363 (2004) 793–803.

[59] M. Surks, E. Ortiz, G. Daniels, et al., Subclinical thyroid disease: scientific review and guidelines for diagnosis and management, JAMA 291 (2004) 228–238.

[60] J. Guirguis-Blake, C.M. Hales, Screening for thyroid disease, American Family Physician 71 (7) (2005) 1369–1370.

Diabetes mellitus: type 2

Case history

Anita Bloom is a 58-year-old medical secretary who has come to the clinic for help with a personal health problem she is finding very embarrassing. Anita has chosen to come to the clinic because she is too shy about talking to her boss, who is also her GP. She would prefer to deal with this problem without having to consult any of the doctors at work. She feels it is just too personal to talk about with people she works with.

The symptom causing Anita the most embarrassment is an itchy bottom. She has taken worming tablets and has tried a number of creams from the pharmacy. Sometimes she notices blood on the toilet paper after passing a bowel motion but experiences no discomfort or pain when passing a motion. When you ask her about her bowel habits, Anita tells you she has regular bowel motions and hasn't noticed any abdominal bloating, wind or pain. She has not noticed whether any food or drink makes her symptoms better or worse.

Anita tells you she feels there is something just 'not right' in her body recently. She feels 'sluggish' and has been gaining weight over the past six months. She is aware that she has been eating far too many lollies and biscuits recently. Because they are being sold from a stand on the reception desk at work it is just too tempting for her to resist.

Anita tells you she has been waking several times a night to urinate, and thinks this is why she is feeling so tired. Some days she feels so exhausted that she just drags herself through the day and collapses in a chair when she gets home.

Anita is more thirsty recently and has been drinking more tea and coffee. Her appetite has also increased. Anita enjoys a wide range of foods, she enjoys cooking and particularly likes red wine, cheese, fish and fresh salads. She tells you she is a sociable person who enjoys spending time with friends and usually laughs a lot. She often has friends and colleagues over for dinner parties, where she enjoys serving her own home-grown organic vegetables. Anita has been living alone for the past 10 years, a situation she is more than happy with.

Anita went through menopause about nine years ago and didn't experience any problems. Up until recently she has felt very well. Anita has not been exercising much recently because her muscles ache and she feels weak. She is also concerned that her eyesight isn't as good as it used to be. She hasn't gone to the optometrist for an eye check because she is afraid they will find something wrong with her eyes. Anita loves reading and needlework, and is concerned that eye problems will stop her from being able to do these favourite pastimes.

TABLE 4.14 **COMPLAINT**	
Analogy: Skin of the apple	**Complaint:** Define the presenting complaint and symptoms; understand the complaint *Itchy bottom* *Feeling 'something is not right'*
AREAS OF INVESTIGATION AND EXAMPLE QUESTIONS	**CLIENT RESPONSES**
Onset *When did you start noticing your bottom was itchy?* *When did you start feeling something wasn't right?*	*It started about 6 or 8 months ago, and comes and goes.* *I suppose I haven't been feeling completely myself for about 18 months.*

▶

▶

Understanding the cause (client) *What do you think might be causing your problem?*	*I really don't know. I thought it might be 'intestinal worms' but it wasn't.*
Exacerbating factors *Have you noticed if anything makes it worse?*	*Not really.*
Relieving factors *Have you noticed if anything makes it better?*	*Anti-fungal creams help, but it keeps coming back.*
Your practitioner impression Anita is quite overweight and appears slightly anxious.	

TABLE 4.15 **CONTEXT**	
Analogy: Flesh of the apple	**Context:** Put the presenting complaint into context to understand the disease
AREAS OF INVESTIGATION AND EXAMPLE QUESTIONS	**CLIENT RESPONSES**
Family health *What is your family health history?*	*My father passed away from bowel cancer, but he had been a smoker most of his life. My mum is still with us; she has diabetes. My sister and brothers are fairly healthy although one has arthritis.*
Allergies and irritants *Is the itching worse after being in contact with particular soaps, bath oils, bubble baths, perfume or lubricants?*	*I don't think so.*
Recreational drug use *How much alcohol would you usually have per week?* *Do you take any recreational drugs?*	*Probably about 3 or 4 glasses a week, perhaps more when I'm socialising.* *No.*
Degenerative and deficiency *Did you experience a sudden onset of blurred vision in both eyes?* (changes in blood-sugar levels)	*Yes, sometimes my vision is blurry when I feel a bit faint … and yes, it will be in both eyes.*
Supplements and side effects of medications *Are you taking any supplements or medications?*	*Just a multivitamin, which I thought might help improve my energy levels.*

▶

Stress and neurological disease *Did the increased need to pass urine develop after menopause?* (stress incontinence connected with oestrogen deficiency)	*I didn't have any of these symptoms initially after going through menopause, they just seemed to creep up on me.*
Eating habits and energy *Can you tell me about your diet?*	Anita's diet appears to be quite healthy, with plenty of fresh whole foods, although she snacks on sugary biscuits and lollies and has been drinking more tea and coffee recently.

TABLE 4.16 **CORE**	
Analogy: Core of the apple with the seed of ill health	**Core:** Holistic assessment to understand the client
AREAS OF INVESTIGATION AND EXAMPLE QUESTIONS	**CLIENT RESPONSES**
Daily activities *Tell me about your daily routine.*	*I usually get up around 6.30 and have breakfast. I get to work by 8 and get home around 5.30. I try to walk in the mornings, but recently I've felt too tired. Dinner is around 7.30 and I'm usually in bed by 10 or 10.30.*
Occupation *Do you enjoy your work?*	*I love my work; the doctors and other staff at the medical centre are all great. It's just that I feel this problem is too personal to share with work colleagues.*
Family and friends *What about your family and friends?*	*I have a wonderful daughter and son-in-law. They have a little boy and another on the way. I really love spending time with them all. I have great friends and we often go out on the weekends or they come to my house and I cook for all of us.*
Action needed to heal *How are you hoping I can help you?*	*I was hoping you might know what was wrong with me and what I could do about it. I suppose I need to stop eating all the biscuits and lollies and exercise more. If I had more energy I think I would get back to walking every morning.*

TABLE 4.17 **ANITA'S SIGNS AND SYMPTOMS** [1–3]	
Pulse	70 bpm
Blood pressure	140/88
Temperature	36.9°C
Respiratory rate	16 resp/min
Body mass index	32
Waist circumference	109 cm
Face	Slightly flushed
Urinalysis	Glucose detected, low pH (acidic), increased specific gravity; no protein or ketones

Results of medical investigations

No medical tests have been carried out.

TABLE 4.18 **UNLIKELY DIAGNOSTIC CONSIDERATIONS** [4–8]	
CONDITIONS AND CAUSES	**WHY UNLIKELY**
CANCER AND HEART DISEASE	
Congestive heart failure: weight gain (need to determine if weight gain is due to fluid increase)	No protein in urine, no hypertension, extreme tachycardia, shortness of breath; changes in weight due to fluid usually occur suddenly
Systemic hypertension	Anita's blood pressure is within normal range but in the 'high' normal end of the scale
OBSTRUCTION AND FOREIGN BODY	
Renal calculi – **hypercalcaemia**	Most common causes are hyperparathyroidism, vitamin D ingestion and sarcoidosis
Renal calculi – **hypercalciuria**	Most common metabolic abnormality detected in calcium stone-formers; causes can be due to excess dietary intake of calcium, excess resorption of calcium from the skeleton in prolonged immobilisation, idiopathic reasons where there is an increased absorption of calcium from the gut; these conditions would usually present with alkaline urine (high pH)
FUNCTIONAL DISEASE	
Primary renal diseases	Medullary sponge kidney, renal tubular acidoses
Female urethral syndrome: irritative bladder symptoms in the absence of urologic findings; pain in the urethra; can be a component of interstitial cystitis; usually does not present with blood in the urine; urinalysis usually detects no bacteria; fever is usually not present	Will experience pain on urination, increased frequency, pelvic pain, associated with sexual activity; onset of symptoms over 2–7 days; level of urinary urgency not noted yet in Anita's history; female urethral syndrome does not necessarily have nocturia as a symptom

►

Paget's disease	Rapid bone remodelling causing calcium excess
DEGENERATIVE AND DEFICIENCY	
Osteoporosis	Lower back pain, rapid bone remodelling causing calcium excess
Osteomalacia	Buffering of H^+ by Ca^{2+} in bone resulting in depletion of calcium from bone; excess calcium excretion can develop
INFECTION AND INFLAMMATION	
Interstitial cystitis: painful bladder syndrome; middle aged, marked frequency, nocturia	No significant recurrent pain on urination and pelvic pain reported
Glomerulonephritis (advanced kidney infection): common in diabetes due to diabetic nephropathy	Would show protein in the urine and possible macrocytic blood; low specific gravity, and would present often with high blood pressure and high fever
SUPPLEMENTS AND SIDE EFFECTS OF MEDICATION	
Causal factor: **Lithium intake**	Lithium can cause hypercalcaemia
Causal factor: **Vitamin D intoxication**	Can cause excess calcium levels due to producing excess bone resorption
ENDOCRINE/REPRODUCTIVE	
Primary parahyperthyroidism	Caused by single or multiple adenomas or by hyperplasia of the parathyroid gland, or compensatory response due to renal failure or vitamin D deficiency
Hyperthyroidism	Excess calcium

Case analysis

TABLE 4.19 POSSIBLE DIFFERENTIAL DIAGNOSIS

NOT RULED OUT BY TESTS/INVESTIGATIONS ALREADY DONE [2, 4–8]

CONDITIONS AND CAUSES	WHY POSSIBLE	WHY UNLIKELY
FAMILY HEALTH		
Rare genetic causes of type 2 diabetes: insulin receptor mutations, maternally inherited diabetes and deafness, Wolfram syndrome, severe obesity and diabetes, disorders of intracellular insulin signalling	Weight gain, insulin resistance, glucose in urine, visual disturbances	No skin pigmentation, no deafness, usually occurs in younger age group; no significant mental deficiencies are evident

ALLERGIES AND IRRITANTS		
Food intolerance/allergy	Fatigue, potential recent dietary change with eating more sugar since feeling low; may be eating foods she did not previously; itchy skin [50]	Need to gain more insight into Anita's previous and current diet and associated symptoms
CANCER AND HEART DISEASE		
Acromegaly/pituitary tumour	Glucose in urine; can develop diabetes; visual disturbance, tiredness, weight gain, increased urination, muscle weakness	No significant change in the size of the hands and feet or change in appearance mentioned; no goitre, excess sweating, headaches, deeper voice; no increase in body and facial hair, oedema
Bowel cancer/polyps	Blood on toilet paper	Need to determine if itching is associated with a lump or discharge
Pancreatic cancer/ insulinomas	Sugar cravings, visual disturbances and weakness; can have recurrent hypoglycaemia for a long time before diagnosis	Need to determine whether Anita is experiencing double vision, sweating, palpitations, loss of concentration or seizures; symptoms are worse with fasting or exercise
Transient ischaemic attack [51]	Visual disturbance	Need to establish if blurred vision or double vision comes and goes and is associated with dizziness
Carotid atherosclerosis	Acute and painless loss of vision; more common in older age group	No hypertension or prior myocardial infarction; need to test blood lipids
High 'normal' blood pressure [52]	Leading to hypertension; risk factor for diabetes, cardiovascular and kidney conditions	Need to test several times to see if get the reading remains constant
TRAUMA AND PRE-EXISTING ILLNESS		
Seasonal affective disorder	Secondary to the winter months; symptoms include tiredness, increased appetite, weight gain	Need to determine whether Anita has experienced episodes of depression during winter months in the past
OBSTRUCTION AND FOREIGN BODY		
Renal calculi: primary hyperoxaluria, hyperuricaemia and hyperuriosuria, and cystinuria	Acidic urine, increased urination, increased thirst; increased risk of developing if Anita has diabetes	Back pain has not been reported as a predominant symptom; normal appetite

FUNCTIONAL DISEASE		
Fibromyalgia	Tiredness, aching and weakness in body; more common in women	Need more specific information regarding the multiple sites of muscle pain
Ophthalmic migraine	Visual disturbances, prodromal migraine symptoms without developing the migraine headache	
Obesity [46, 52]	Anita's BMI is 32 and waist circumference is 109 cm; increased caloric intake, eating more sugar, increased appetite and lack of exercise; usually general distribution of weight gain can cause increased fatigue	Usually no other health features other than being overweight; need to determine whether there is any family history of obesity; need to determine whether Anita's weight gain has been gradual and if there is any oedema present (which is unusual for obesity without a cardiovascular condition)
Eye conditions of older adults: cataracts, glaucoma, senile macular degeneration, drug side effects, dry eyes [47, 48]	Visual changes	Need to establish if Anita experiences significant visual blurring; are the visual changes unilateral or happening in both eyes; is the visual disturbance constant or does it come and go; does Anita have visual field loss or see halos around objects
Obstructive sleep apnoea	Feels tired; often occurs in those who are overweight; can be made worse with drinking alcohol prior to sleeping; does not usually complain of 'sleepiness' but rather fatigue generally	Need to determine if Anita does not feel not well rested in the morning and if she snores during the night
Nocturnal polyuria syndrome	Nocturia and increased volume of urine; common in older people from conditions such as diabetes, heart disease and from certain medications	
Anal fissures **Haemorrhoids** **Anal skin tags**	Blood on toilet paper; itchy rectum	Need to determine whether stools with blood may be secondary to inflammatory bowel disease; need to determine if the itching is associated with a discharge or if pain is experienced on passing a bowel motion

INFECTION AND INFLAMMATION		
Chronic pancreatitis	Glucose in urine, diabetes can be a complication of chronic pancreatitis	No jaundice, abdominal pain or mucus in stools
Ischaemic colitis	Blood from rectum; usually occurs in older people; may have underlying cardiovascular disease (CVD)	Abdominal pain; usually presents suddenly
Candidiasis (moniliasis, *Candida albicans*)	Itchy bottom, having sweet cravings; common in diabetes	Need to determine if Anita experiences external pain or irritation on urination and whether there is vaginal discharge; more likely if she has taken antibiotics or other medication recently
Recurrent cystitis (lower urinary tract infection/ bladder infection)	Increased urination at night; common due to diabetic neuropathy and bladder dysfunction; acidic urine can indicate infection/ bacteria	These symptoms not present at this stage: painful passing of urine, blood in urine, smelly urine, exacerbated by sexual intercourse, high temperature; symptoms develop quickly; recurrent same symptoms; urinalysis nitrates, leukocytes (pyuria), blood, foul odour to urine; pain on urination with pus (pyuria) in urine is diagnostic for cystitis
Parasites/infestations: scabies, lice, pinworms	Itchiness in rectum; no associated discharge	Need to determine if itching is worse at night and associated with a rash and excoriation (scabies, lice) or if it is worse in morning (pinworm)

SUPPLEMENTS AND SIDE EFFECTS OF MEDICATION		
Medication/recreational drug reaction	Can get symptoms of thrush, increased weight due to increased appetite; increased fatigue and sugar cravings; visual changes; contribute to dysbiosis of the bowel to cause fungal overgrowth	Need to determine if Anita has recently taken antibiotics (resulting in overgrowth of fungi), laxatives, antihypertensives, NSAIDs, steroids, antihypertensives, antidepressants, lithium or oestrogens; need to establish if weight gain has a basis of fluid retention; psychotropic drugs can cause an increase in craving for carbohydrates; propranolol may cause weight gain due to hypoglycaemia; quitting smoking can increase weight gain; increased alcohol intake causes increased caloric intake and risk of weight gain due to fluid increase, liver and heart conditions; anticholinergic, antihypertensive and psychotropic agents cause blurred vision and defects in accommodation of the vision; chronic corticosteroid use can cause cataract formation and visual blurring; antihistamines decrease tear production and cause hot, dry eyes; chocolate and red wine can provoke migraine visual prodromal symptoms; hormone replacement therapy (HRT) can cause dry eyes
ENDOCRINE/REPRODUCTIVE		
Asymptomatic diabetes/ renal glycosuria: inherited low renal threshold for glucose	Glucose in urine	Requires further investigation to identify causes for glucose detected in urine; usually no other symptoms of ill-health present
Diabetes mellitus: non-insulin dependent diabetes (NIDDM) [52]	Glucose in urine, weight gain, sugar craving, increased thirst, frequent urination during the evening, eyesight worsening, pruritis ani, fatigue, muscle weakness; Anita is in the common age group for NIDDM to develop	Need to determine if Anita's muscle weakness is proximal (upper arms, shoulders, legs) or distal (fingers and feet) and there is clawing of the toes; need to determine whether she is experiencing numbness and tingling in the toes and fingers (common in diabetes)

Cushing's syndrome	Glucose in urine, weight gain, muscle weakness; could have diabetes	Usually accompanied by increased body and facial hair, hypertension, moon-shaped face, 'buffalo hump', acne, oedema; Anita has not reported pain on urination
Hypothyroidism	Fatigue, weight gain, aches and feeling weak; itchy skin [50]	Usually associated with a decrease in appetite, dry and coarse skin and hair, loss of eyebrows, low hoarse voice, goitre, puffy skin and face; need to establish if Anita is intolerant to cold weather; no significant constipation reported
Diabetic eye conditions: refractive errors, diabetic retinopathy, oculomotor palsies (rare) [47, 49]	Increased urination, increased thirst, nocturia, eyesight worsening	Need to determine whether Anita experiences impaired night vision, visual field loss with blurred vision; need to determine if Anita's visual changes were sudden and occurred in both eyes
Impaired glucose tolerance (IGT) [52, 53, 56]	Risk factor for future development of diabetes; weight gain and lack of exercise	Do not develop eye complications as is the case with diabetes; can be due to liver disease or taking certain medications; can be pre-diabetic state where there is a mild impairment to glucose metabolism
Impaired fasting glucose (IFG) [53]	Risk factor for future development of diabetes and CVD	
STRESS AND NEUROLOGICAL DISEASE		
Type 2 – minor depression	Anita would need to show 2–4 symptoms of depression that have lasted 2 weeks; can be mild or moderate depression; significant change in appetite nearly every day with weight gain; fatigue or loss of energy nearly every day; may eat excessively when feeling depressed and celebrate with people with good food and alcohol to alleviate depression	Need to establish if Anita is as happy living on her own as she expresses; are there underlying fears, concerns or sadness she experiences that may affect her appetite?

| **Neurologic disease:** multiple sclerosis (MS), spinal cord injury, cauda equina syndrome, brain tumour | Visual disturbances; symptoms of lower urinary tract symptoms; more common in women; increased urination, nocturia; weakness or tingling in lower limbs | Usually advanced stages of MS; no significant trauma or injury mentioned in health history so far; need to define if the visual disturbance comes and goes; visual disturbance prior to MS is usually unilateral and caused by optic neuritis; need to establish if Anita has double vision; need to establish if Anita has central vision defects (brain tumour and aneurysm) |

TABLE 4.20 DECISION TABLE FOR REFERRAL [4–8,11,12]

COMPLAINT	CONTEXT	CORE
Referral for presenting complaint	Referral for all associated physical, dietary and lifestyle concerns	Referral for contributing emotional, mental, spiritual, metaphysical, lifestyle and constitutional factors
REFERRAL FLAGS	**REFERRAL FLAGS**	**REFERRAL FLAGS**
• Glucose detected in urinalysis • Anita is experiencing a persistent increase in passing urine	• Blood when passing stools • Blood pressure on the high side of the normal scale • Acidic urine can indicate urinary tract infections or renal stones, which can be very problematic for diabetes • BMI is on the obese scale • Dehydration • Visual changes • Pruritis ani, which may be related to intestinal dysbiosis resulting from hyperglycaemia or from haemorrhoids	• Unwillingness to seek medical assistance due to embarrassment • Fear of losing her eyesight preventing Anita from seeking assistance from an optometrist or ophthalmologist
ISSUES OF SIGNIFICANCE	**ISSUES OF SIGNIFICANCE**	**ISSUES OF SIGNIFICANCE**
Nil	• Extreme fatigue and muscle aches • Increased consumption of sugar • Increased consumption of tea and coffee	• Lives alone

REFERRAL	REFERRAL	REFERRAL
• Referral for medical assessment and management	• Refer for medical opinion re: blood from rectum • Blood pressure needs to be monitored • Dietary assessment • Musculoskeletal assessment • Referral to optometrist [45, 49]	• Referral to optometrist and ophthalmologist • Referral to a new GP (who is not known to Anita) for further medical investigations or counselling

TABLE 4.21 **FURTHER INVESTIGATIONS THAT MAY BE NECESSARY** [1–8]	
TEST/INVESTIGATION	**REASON FOR TEST/INVESTIGATION**
FIRST-LINE INVESTIGATIONS:	
Random blood glucose test [54, 55]	< 5.3 mmol/L diabetes unlikely; if between 5.3 and 11.1 further investigation with fasting blood glucose is necessary
Fasting blood glucose test [54, 55]	Can differentiate between diabetes, impaired fasting glycaemia (IFG) and impaired glucose tolerance (IGT); raised levels can indicate diabetes mellitus, Cushing's disease, acromegaly, pancreatic cancer, pancreatitis, drug therapy or acute stress response; decreased levels can indicate hypothyroidism, hypopituitarism, Addison's disease, liver disease
Full blood count	Anaemia, inflammation, infection, tumour
Blood lipids	Carotid atherosclerosis, cardiovascular risk, blood cholesterol
CRP (C-reactive protein) [56], **ESR**	Infection, cancer, inflammation, temporal arteritis
Kidney function: urea, creatinine and electrolytes, sodium, potassium, chloride, bicarbonate, blood test	Signals muscle breakdown and tissue damage and gives an indicator for renal excretory function as urea and blood creatinine is excreted entirely by the kidneys; this will show in renal abnormalities and diabetes; impaired renal function can cause hypertension

TEST/INVESTIGATION	REASON FOR TEST/INVESTIGATION
Eye tests: visual	Looking through a pinhole will improve vision if caused by a refractive error and shows that retinal function is good; if double vision is improved by holding one eye, it may be due to paralysis or a weakness of the extraocular muscles of the eye (causes can be neuropathy, MS, thyroid disease, diabetes, trauma, tumour or aneurysm); if increasing illumination improves the vision then a cataract is suspected; if dimming the lights or looking beside the object improves vision then macular degeneration is probable; early changes in diabetic neuropathy include microaneurysms/haemorrhages in the eye, changes in the blood-retinal barrier, capillary closure, neuronal and glial cell changes in the retina [45, 49]
Snellen chart	Visual acuity
Relative afferent pupillary defect (RAPD): the client looks into distance while a light is shone in one eye, causing a papillary constriction in that eye and should cause simultaneous constriction in the pupil of the adjacent eye; the light is quickly moved in front of the other pupil to constrict the eye further; if the pupil dilates instead, RAPD is present	RAPD is present in optic nerve disease, chronic glaucoma and retinal damage; absent in macular degeneration and cataracts; no eye inflammation or RAPD (cataracts, vitreous opacities, macular degeneration); if there is white eye and RAPD (chronic glaucoma)
Funduscopic examination	Senile macular degeneration, diabetic retinopathy
Stool test	Occult blood, parasites
Rectal examination	Haemorrhoids
IF NECESSARY:	
Endoscopy	Rule out rectal carcinoma, polyps, haemorrhoids
Blood cortisol levels	Cushing's syndrome
Thyroid function test	*Hypothyroidism:* TSH, T4, T3 *TSH:* high *T4:* low in hypothyroidism
Growth hormone levels	Acromegaly, pituitary tumour
Liver function test	Alcohol abuse, cirrhosis, hepatitis
Sleep centre: polysomnogram	Sleep apnoea
Musculoskeletal asssesment	Fibromyalgia
MRI: brain scan	Brain tumour

Confirmed diagnosis

ANITA AND DIABETES MELLITUS (NON-INSULIN DEPENDENT) AND HAEMORRHOIDS

Anita is a 58-year-old woman who has developed myriad symptoms. Anita has been experiencing symptoms of pruritus ani (itchy bottom), feeling sluggish, weight gain, increased sugar cravings, nocturia, blood on the toilet paper after passing a bowel motion, increased appetite and thirst, general fatigue and weakness in her body. Anita works as a medical secretary and is embarrassed to share her health concerns with the doctors she works for. In her personal life, Anita enjoys living on her own and having time to socialise with friends where she can entertain and cook meals at home. Another passion of Anita's is reading books in her spare time. She is currently very concerned about deteriorating eyesight and she is experiencing anxiety about having the cause professionally diagnosed in case she receives a negative prognosis.

Anita has developed several symptoms that are common in non-insulin dependent diabetes mellitus (NIDDM) such as: increased appetite; unexplained fatigue and weakness; pruritus ani and/or vulvovaginitis; and blurred vision [49, 50, 52]. The condition is a secondary form of diabetes where insulin resistance develops over time and may present as subclinical for several years before diagnosis is made. The incidence increases with age and obesity, lack of exercise and can be accelerated by stress, pregnancy and drug treatments. NIDDM is a condition of impaired insulin response to glucose concentration. Complications of type 2 diabetes extend to hypertension, obesity, decreased HDL blood lipids, diabetic neuropathy, retinopathy and nephropathy [47–49]. Both insulin resistance and insulin secretory failure are involved in type 2 diabetes. This will develop over time when a person cannot secrete enough insulin to overcome the dysfunction with insulin uptake. Whether type 2 diabetes is likely to develop is considered to be influenced significantly by genetics; however, when the condition develops it is more commonly due to lifestyle circumstances.

Haemorrhoids are a secondary complication of diabetes that can cause rectal bleeding and itchinesss. Often the person with haemorrhoids will notice red blood on the toilet paper and perhaps blood around the outside of the stools. Haemorrhoids are the most common cause of rectal bleeding.

General references used in this diagnosis: 2, 4–9, 57

PRESCRIBED MEDICATION

• Oral hypoglycaemic medication

TABLE 4.22 DECISION TABLE FOR TREATMENT (ONCE DIAGNOSIS IS CONFIRMED)		
COMPLAINT	**CONTEXT**	**CORE**
Treatment for the presenting complaint and symptoms	Treatment for all associated symptoms	Treatment for mental, emotional, spiritual, constitutional, lifestyle issues and metaphysical considerations

TREATMENT PRIORITY	TREATMENT PRIORITY	TREATMENT PRIORITY
• Lifestyle recommendations to improve glucose control and insulin sensitivity and self-monitoring of blood glucose to assist with glucose control • Dietary recommendations to reduce blood glucose levels, reduce insulin resistance and improve glucose control • Herbal tonic, tea and nutritional supplements to reduce blood glucose levels, reduce insulin resistance and improve glucose control • Herbal and nutritional therapy to improve vascular integrity, microcirculation and retinal health **NB:** Collaborative management of Anita's case is essential to ensure her condition is properly monitored and to ensure any potential interactions between herbal or nutritional treatments and prescribed medication are managed	• Lifestyle recommendations to enhance health and wellbeing and reduce risk factors for CVD and other diabetic complications • Dietary recommendations to increase dietary intake of antioxidants and essential nutrients to enhance health and wellbeing and reduce risk factors for CVD and other diabetic complications • Dietary recommendations and nutritional supplements to improve vascular integrity and support eye health • Dietary recommendations to support normal intestinal microflora and assists with managing haemorrhoids	• Recommendation that Anita finds a medical practitioner from another practice to help reduce her embarrassment • Recommend Anita immediately seeks assistance from an ophthalmologist • To increase foods containing bioflavanoids and anthocyanins to support eye health

Treatment aims

• Bring Anita's blood glucose levels as close as possible to normal range [13, 14].
• Help Anita to lose weight to bring her back into a normal BMI range [13–15] and increase skeletal muscle mass to improve glycaemic control [15].
• Prevent progression of the disease and protect Anita from long-term complications [13, 14].
• Institute dietary measures to keep Anita's blood glucose within normal range [14, 15].
• Improve insulin function and sensitivity [13, 14, 21].
• Aim for optimal nutritional status [15, 21] and prevent nutritional and oxidative stress [14, 21].
• Institute lifestyle practices that will improve Anita's overall health and fitness, improve insulin sensitivity, maintain a healthy weight and prevent progression and long-term complications of diabetes [15].
• Identify and manage any other conditions or existing complications (e.g. haemorrhoids).

Lifestyle alterations/considerations

- Anita would benefit from a weight-loss program to help her achieve her ideal body weight [13–15].
- Encourage Anita to exercise daily [13, 14, 16]. Exercise improves glycaemic control and insulin resistance [16]. Her exercise regimen should involve both strength training and aerobic exercise [16] and the aim of the program should be to reduce body fat and improve skeletal muscle mass and strength, improving glycaemic control [16].
- Encourage Anita to seek assistance from an ophthalmologist as soon as possible.
- Encourage Anita to self-monitor her blood glucose levels to help her improve blood glucose control [27].
- Suggest Anita removes the lollies and biscuits from her work area [14, 21].

Dietary suggestions

- Encourage Anita to have a low GI/GL diet [13, 15, 21]. She should focus on eating foods with a GI of less then 55 [13] and fibre-rich whole foods such as apples, grapefruit, legumes, onions and garlic, dense grainy breads and wholegrain cereals such as whole oats [13, 14, 21]. This is similar to a Mediterranean-style diet, which can postpone the need for oral hypoglycaemic medication in newly diagnosed type 2 diabetics [30].
- Eliminate simple sugars, processed and concentrated carbohydrates [14, 21].
- Increase consumption of fibre, particularly soluble fibre to at least 40 g daily [13, 15, 21]. Soluble fibre can reduce postprandial glucose, lower cholesterol, enhance glycaemic control and reduce insulin [14, 15]. Good sources of soluble fibre include vegetables, oats, wholegrain rice and legumes [13, 14]. Dietary fibre is also beneficial in the management of haemorrhoids [13] and inulin and FOS in dietary fibre from vegetables and fruit positively influences gastrointestinal microbial ecology [25].
- Reduce consumption of saturated fat [13, 14] and increase consumption of omega-3-rich foods and monounsaturated fats [13, 15, 21].
- Encourage Anita to eat antioxidant-rich foods containing B-group vitamins and vitamins C and E [13, 15, 21].
- Encourage Anita to eat low-GI bioflavonoid and anthocyanin-rich foods such as blueberries, strawberries, raspberries, blackberries, citrus fruit and onions [13, 15, 21]. Bioflavanoids and anthocyanins have antioxidant and anti-inflammatory properties [13, 15, 17, 22] and are beneficial to prevent and treat diabetic retinopathy [15, 17, 22]. Anthocyanins from blueberries also enhance microcirculation and improve visual function [17, 13]. Flavonoids and anthocyanins are also beneficial in the management of haemorrhoids [17, 22, 13].
- Encourage Anita to consume foods rich in the minerals zinc, chromium, potassium, magnesium and vanadium, which are essential for blood-sugar balance [13, 15, 21].
- 50–100 mL bitter melon juice containing 100 g fruit per 100 mL can reduce fasting and postprandial glucose levels [17].
- Including cinnamon regularly in the diet can help lower postprandial glucose response [24, 44].
- Encourage Anita to reduce the amount of tea and coffee she is consuming; she should drink water instead. Tea and coffee can inhibit absorption of essential nutrients, especially when consumed with or close to meals [26].

Physical treatment suggestions

- Anita may benefit from massage therapy. Some studies have demonstrated massage may have a positive effect on blood glucose levels and be helpful with diabetic retinopathy [28].
- Hydrotherapy: neutral sitz baths for pruritus ani [39]. Full body cold mitten friction to stimulate circulation [39]. Alternating warm/cool contrast foot baths (*note: hot or icy cold applications contraindicated due to peripheral neuropathy in diabetes*) [40]. A hot apple cider vinegar and water compress on the abdomen for bloating [41]. Alternating warm and cool compress on the eyes to strengthen and tone [40, 41]. Constitutional hydrotherapy for fatigue [42]. Increase energy by running the arms, wrists and ankles under cool water [40, 41]. A short, cool head shower for fatigue [40].
- Acupuncture may be beneficial to Anita because it may help improve symptoms associated with diabetic neuropathy [29].

TABLE 4.23 **HERBAL FORMULA (1:2 LIQUID EXTRACTS)**		
Made with ethanolic extract herbal liquids (alcohol removed)		
HERB	**FORMULA**	**RATIONALE**
Gymnema *Gymnema sylvestre*	100 mL	Hypoglycaemic [17, 18]; antidiabetic [17, 18]; hypocholesterolaemic [17, 18]; improves glucose control [15, 17]; suppresses sweet taste perception [15, 17] and aids fat loss [17]; may assist in the development of a higher muscle to fat ratio [18]
Fenugreek seed *Trigonella foenum-graecum*	60 mL	Hypoglycaemic [17, 19]; hypocholesterolaemic [17, 19]; improves glucose tolerance [15, 17]; improves insulin resistance [17] and improves insulin sensitivity [15, 17]
Ginkgo *Ginkgo biloba*	40 mL	Antioxidant [17, 20]; increases blood flow, tissue oxygenation and tissue nutrition [20]; increases ocular and cerebral blood flow [17, 20]; helpful to assist with prevention of vascular, neurological and ophthalmologic complications [17, 20]; indicated for the treatment of haemorrhoids [17, 13]
Supply:	200 mL	Dose: 5 mL 3 times daily
Bilberry (*Vaccinium myrtillius*): vasoprotective [17, 20]; antioxidant [17, 20]; hypoglycaemic [17]; indicated for peripheral vascular disorders [20]; beneficial in a range of ophthalmic conditions [17, 20] and can be used to help prevent and treat diabetic retinopathy [14, 17, 20]; beneficial for haemorrhoids [17, 13] **Dose:** 20–50 g of fresh fruit daily or extract in tablet or capsule containing 150 mg anthocyanins daily [17]		

TABLE 4.24 **HERBAL TEA**		
Alternative to black tea and coffee		
HERB	**FORMULA**	**RATIONALE**
Green tea leaves *Camellia sinensis*	2 parts	Antioxidant [17, 32, 34]; has an antidiabetic effect [17, 35, 36]; reduces oxidative stress in diabetes [36]; protects against CVD [17, 32, 34]; thermogenic [17, 32, 33]; may be beneficial to aid weight loss [17, 33]
Phyllanthus *Phyllanthus amarus*	2 parts	Hypoglycaemic [18, 37]; antioxidant [37]; indicated for use in type 2 diabetes [18, 37]
Cinnamon bark powder *Cinnamomum cassia*	½ part	Antioxidant [17]; glucose-lowering effect [17, 44]; improves glucose control and lipid levels in type 2 diabetes [38]; antifungal [17, 31]

Infusion: 1 tsp per cup – 1 cup 3–4 times daily
NB: In order to ensure optimal absorption of nutritional supplements, Anita should not take supplements with or within 2 hours of drinking her tea formula [17]

TABLE 4.25 **NUTRITIONAL SUPPLEMENTS**	
SUPPLEMENT AND DOSE	**RATIONALE**
Alpha-lipoic acid 600 µg daily in divided doses [13, 22]	Antioxidant [15, 21, 22]; decreases oxidative stress [21, 22]; improves insulin sensitivity [15, 21, 22]; enhances glucose transport [21, 22]; used for treatment of diabetic neuropathy [13, 15, 21, 22]
Chromium 200 µg daily [13, 21, 22]	Enhances the effects of insulin [22, 23]; reduces skeletal muscle insulin resistance [13, 21]; improves glucose control [13, 22, 23]
Magnesium 400 mg elemental magnesium daily	Magnesium deficiency aggravates insulin resistance [13, 17, 23]; supplemental magnesium improves glucose tolerance [23], metabolism [15, 23] and insulin sensitivity [17, 22, 23]
High-potency practitioner-strength **vitamin, mineral and antioxidant supplement** providing therapeutic doses of essential micronutrients [15, 21]	To increase Anita's essential nutrient and antioxidant levels and to reduce oxidative stress [14, 15, 21]; supplemental multivitamins can reduce the incidence of infection and enhance quality of life in diabetes [43]

▶

▶

Omega-3 fish oil 1000 mg 3 times daily [15, 17, 21]	Anti-inflammatory [13, 17, 22]; lowers triglycerides [17, 22]; lowers LDL [17, 22]; supplementation reduces triglyceride levels in type 2 diabetes [13, 17]
Vitamin E 500 IU daily [15, 21, 17]	Lipid antioxidant [13, 23, 17]; reduces oxidative stress in diabetics [23, 17]; supplementation can help reduce vascular complications [13, 21]; improves retinal blood flow [15, 21]; improves insulin action [13, 21]; decreases diabetic retinopathy [15, 21]; improves kidney function [15]; decreases C-reactive protein [13, 15]

References

[1] K.D. Pagna, T.J. Pagna, Mosby's Diagnostic and Laboratory Test reference, third edn, Mosby, USA, 1997 (later edition).

[2] G. Douglas, F. Nicol, C. Robertson, Macleod's Clinical Examination, twelveth edn, Churchill Livingstone Elsevier, 2009.

[3] N.J. Talley, S. O'Connor, Pocket Clinical Examination, third edn, Churchill Livingstone Elsevier, Australia, 2009.

[4] P. Kumar, C. Clark, Clinical Medicine, sixth edn, Elsevier Saunders, London, 2005.

[5] J. Jamison, Differential Diagnosis for Primary Care, second edn, Churchill Livingstone Elsevier, London, 2006.

[6] A. Polmear (Ed.), Evidence-Based Diagnosis in Primary Care, Churchill Livingstone Elsevier, 2008.

[7] R.D. Collins, Differential Diagnosis in Primary Care, fourth edn, Lippincott Williams & Wilkins, Philadelphia, 2008.

[8] R.H. Seller, Differential Diagnosis of Common Complaints, fifth edn, Saunders Elsevier, Philadelphia, 2007.

[9] J. Silverman, S. Kurtz, J. Draper, Skills for Communicating with Patients, second edn, Radcliff Publishing, Oxford, 2000.

[10] R. Neighbour, The Inner Consultation; how to develop an effective and intuitive consulting style, Radcliff Publishing, Oxon, 2005.

[11] M. Lloyd, R. Bor, Communication Skills For Medicine, third edn, Churchill Livingstone Elsevier, Edinburgh, 2009.

12. D. Peters, L. Chaitow, G. Harris, S. Morrison, Integrating Complementary Therapies in Primary Care, Churchill Livingstone, London, 2002.

[13] J. Jamison, Clinical Guide to Nutrition & Dietary Supplements in Disease Management, Churchill Livingstone, Edinburgh, 2003.

[14] S. El-Hashemy, Naturopathic Standards of Primary Care, CCNM Press Inc, Toronto, 2007.

[15] J.E. Pizzorno, M.T. Murray, H. Joiner-Bey, The Clinicians Handbook of Natural Medicine, second edn, Churchill Livingstone, St Louis, 2008.

[16] A. Maiorana, G. O'Driscoll, C. Goodman, R. Taylor, D. Green, Combined aerobic and resistance exercise improves glycemic control and fitness in type 2 diabetes, Diabetes Research and Clinical Practice 56 (2002) 115–123.

[17] L. Braun, M. Cohen, Herbs & Natural Supplements: An evidence based guide, second edn, Elsevier, Sydney, 2007.

[18] K. Bone, Clinical Applications of Chinese and Ayurvedic Herbs: Monographs for the Western Herbal Practitioners, Phytotherapy Press, Warwick, 1996.

[19] S. Mills, K. Bone, The Essential Guide to Herbal Safety, Churchill Livingstone, St Louis, 2005.

[20] S. Mills, K. Bone, Principles & Practice of Phytotherapy; Modern Herbal Medicine, Churchill Livingstone, Edinburgh: London, 2000.

[21] H. Osiecki, The Physicians Handbook of Clinical Nutrition, seventh edn, Eagle Farm: Bioconcepts: 2000.

[22] H. Osiecki, The Nutrient Bible, seventh edn, Eagle Farm: BioConcepts Publishing, 2008.

[23] J. Higdon, An Evidence Based Approach to Vitamins and Minerals, Thieme, New York, 2003.

[24] J. Hlebowicz, G. Darwiche, O. Björgell, L.O. Almér, Effect of cinnamon on postprandial blood glucose, gastric emptying, and satiety in healthy subjects, American Journal of Clinical Nutrition 85 (6) (2007) 1552–1556.

[25] M. Blaut, Relationship of probiotics and food to intestinal microflora, European Journal of Nutrition 41 (S1) (2002) 11–16.

[26] R.F. Hurrelli, M. Reddy, J.D. Cook, Inhibition of non-haem iron absorption in man by polyphenolic-containing beverages, British Journal of Nutrition 81 (1999) 289–295.

[27] A.J. Karter, L.M. Ackerson, J.A. Darbinian, R.B. D'Agostino, A. Ferrara, J. Liu, J.V. Selby, Self-monitoring of Blood Glucose Levels and Glycemic Control: the Northern California Kaiser Permanente Diabetes Registry, The American Journal of Medicine 111 (1) (2001) 1–9.

[28] J. Ezzo, T. Donner, D. Nickols, M. Cox, Is Massage Useful in the Management of Diabetes? A Systematic Review, Diabetes Spectrum 14 (4) (2001) 218–224.

[29] B.B. Abuaisha, J.B. Costanzi, A.J.M. Boulton, Acupuncture for the treatment of chronic painful peripheral diabetic neuropathy: a long-term study, Diabetes Research and Clinical Practice 39 (1998) 115–121.

[30] K. Esposito, M.I. Maiorino, M. Ciotola, et al., Effects of a Mediterranean-style diet on the need for antihyperglycemic drug therapy in patients with newly diagnosed type 2 diabetes, Annals of Internal Medicine 151 (2009) 306–314.

[31] British Herbal Medicine Association, British Herbal Pharmacopoeia, BHMAA, , 1983.

[32] M. Morgan, Green Tea for Good Health and Longevity, A Phytotherapist's Perspective 88 (2005) 1–7.

[33] A.G. Dulloo, J. Seydoux, L. Girardier, P. Chantre, J. Vandermander, Green tea and thermogenesis: interactions between catechin-polyphenols, caffeine and sympathetic activity, International Journal of Obesity Related Metabolic Disorders 24 (2) (2000) 252–258.

[34] K. Bone, M. Morgan, Green Tea and Garlic as Cardiovascular Life Extension Strategies, Townsend Letter for Doctors and Patients 269 (2005) 51–56.

[35] H. Tsuneki, M. Ishizuka, M. Terasawa, J.B. Wu, T. Sasaoka, I. Kimura, Effect of green tea on blood glucose levels and serum proteomic patterns in diabetic (db/db) mice and on glucose metabolism in healthy humans, BMC Pharmacology 4 (2004) 18.

[36] M.C. Sabu, K. Smitha, K. Ramadasan, Anti-diabetic activity of green tea polyphenols and their role in reducing oxidative stress in experimental diabetes, Journal of Ethnopharmacology 83 (2002) 109–166.

[37] J. Shabeer, R.S. Srivastava, S.K. Singh, Antidiabetic and antioxidant effect of various fractions of Phyllanthus simplex in alloxan diabetic rats, Journal of Ethnopharmacology 124 (1) (2009) 34–38.

[38] A. Khan, M. Safdar, M.M.A. Khan, K.N. Khattak, R.A. Anderson, Cinnamon Improves Glucose and Lipids of People With Type 2 Diabetes, Diabetes Care 26 (2003) 3215–3218.

[39] W. Boyle, A. Saine, Lectures in Naturopathic Hydrotherapy, Oregon: Eclectic Medical Publications, 1988.

[40] M. Sinclair, Modern Hydrotherapy for the Massage Therapist, Lippincott Williams & Williams, Baltimore, 2008.

[41] D.D. Buchman, The complete book of water healing, Contemporary Books, McGraw-Hill Companies, New York, 2001.

[42] L. Chaitow, Hydrotherapy, water therapy for health and beauty, Element, Dorset, 1999.

[43] T.A. Barringer, J.K. Kirk, A.C. Santaniello, K.L. Foley, R. Michielutte, Effect of a Multivitamin and Mineral Supplement on Infection and Quality of Life: A Randomized, Double-Blind, Placebo-Controlled Trial, Annals of Internal Medicine 138 (2003) 365–371.

[44] P. Crawford, Effectiveness of cinnamon for lowering hemoglobin A1C in patients with type 2 diabetes: a randomized, controlled trial, J Am Board Fam Med 22 (5) (2009) 507–512.

[45] J. Cunha-Vaz, R. Bernardes, Nonproliferative retinopathy in diabetes type 2. Initial stages and characterization of phenotypes, Prog Retin Eye Res 24 (3) (2005) 355–377.

[46] A.J. Stunkard, K.C. Allison, Two forms of disordered eating in obesity: binge eating and night eating, Int J Obes 27 (2003) 1–112.

[47] C. Hodge, D. Ng, Dry eyes, menopause, and hormone therapy, Austral Fam Physician 35 (2004) 931–932.

[48] D.A. Quillen, Common causes of vision loss in the elderly, Am Fam Physician 60 (1999) 99–108.

[49] R.N. Frank, Diabetic retinopathy, N Engl J Med 350 (2004) 48–58.

[50] S. Moses, Pruritus, Am Fam Physician 68 (6) (2003) 1135–1142.

[51] N.J. Solenski, Transient ischemic attacks: Part I. Diagnosis and evaluation, Am Fam Physician 69 (7) (2004) 1665–1674.

[52] R.J. Sanchez-Torres, H. Delgado-Osorio, The metabolic syndrome and its cardiovascular manifestations, Boletin-Asociacion Medica de Puerto Rico 97 (4) (2005) 271–280.

[53] S. Raos, P. Disraeli, T. McGregor, Impaired glucose tolerance and impaired fasting glucose, Am Fam Physician 69 (2004) 1961–1968.

[54] S. Anand, F. Razak, V. Vuksan, et al., Diagnostic strategies to detect glucose intolerance in a multiethnic population, Diabetes Care 26 (2003) 290–296.

[55] J. Lawrence, P. Bennet, A. Young, A. Robinson, Screening for diabetes in general practice: cross sectional population study, BMJ 323 (2001) 548–551.

[56] S.M. Haffner, Insulin resistance, inflammation and the prediabetic state, American Journal of Cardiology 92 (suppl) (2003) 18J–26J.

[57] R. Tayor, Causation of type 2 diabetes, N Engl J Med 350 (2004) 639–641.

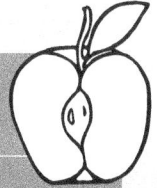

CHAPTER 5

Reproductive system

Polycystic ovarian syndrome

Case history

Gia Galati has come to the clinic for help with hormonal problems. Gia is 24 and is in her final few months of studies for a teaching degree. Gia's symptoms have become more pronounced in the past 12 months and she would really like to get her hormones sorted out.

Gia's cycles have become irregular, and she sometimes misses a period for four to five months. The last menstrual bleed she had was quite heavy but not painful. Between bleeds she notices a white vaginal discharge, which is sometimes quite copious. When Gia did have a regular menstrual cycle she would experience fluctuating emotions 7–10 days before her bleed and find herself more anxious and depressed than usual. Now she does not experience mood swings, which she thinks is great but is not like her. She can feel abdominal pain and a lower backache just before her period starts that she thinks may be due to constipation, something she has been having increasing problems within the past months. She can go for up to three days without passing a bowel motion and she experiences increasing levels of abdominal discomfort and sometimes even pain before finally passing a motion.

Gia has also noticed her skin is breaking out more often and she is becoming worried about having acne at 24. She had mild acne in her early teenage years. Gia is also perplexed about increasing amounts of facial hair on her upper lip and jawline, along with excess hair on her chest, under her armpits, thighs and down the midline of her abdomen. Gia is concerned about the amount of hair and has been waxing frequently to keep it from showing. The facial hair seems to be slowly getting worse and is becoming quite embarrassing. She tells you she does not come from a family of particularly hairy women and is wondering what is going on!

Gia is focused on her studies at the moment and concedes that her diet isn't particularly good. She is drinking a lot of coffee, cola and energy drinks to help her keep going and tends to eat things at odd hours, preferring instant noodles and bowls of cereal and milk, which are quick and easy to prepare so she can spend more time at the computer doing her assignments. She is also eating lots of chocolate at the moment and notices she is craving sugar and carbohydrates. She has put on about 8 kg in the past seven months and thinks it may be to do with her diet and lack of exercise, and is concerned about weight gain. She would like your help with advice to lose the excess weight.

Gia also tells you she has a new boyfriend who she is very happy with. He is very understanding about her need to spend the next few months focused on finishing her studies, but she still manages to spend at least three or four evenings per week with him.

Gia would like to try something more natural before resorting to taking the oral contraceptive pill for birth control and regulating her periods. Additionally, Gia would love some help to reduce stress and anxiety as she completes her studies.

TABLE 5.1 **COMPLAINT**	
Analogy: Skin of the apple	**Complaint:** Define the presenting complaint and symptoms; understand the complaint *Menstrual problems*
AREAS OF INVESTIGATION AND EXAMPLE QUESTIONS	**CLIENT RESPONSES**
Onset *When did you notice your periods starting to become irregular? When did you notice you were getting excessive hair growth?*	*Probably about 18 months or 2 years ago. It has gotten worse recently though. The facial hair began a year ago.*
Understanding the cause (client) *Do you have any ideas about what might have caused these changes?*	*Well, I think it might have something to do with stress and my diet since it seemed to coincide with increased stress and me eating more junk food.*
Examination and inspection Gia appears overweight and slight facial hair and acne is noticeable.	

TABLE 5.2 **CONTEXT**	
Analogy: Flesh of the apple	**Context:** Put the presenting complaint into context to understand the disease
AREAS OF INVESTIGATION AND EXAMPLE QUESTIONS	**CLIENT RESPONSES**
Family health *Has anyone in your family had these problems?*	*Not that I can think of.*
Recreational drug use *How much alcohol would you consume a week?*	*Maybe 6 to 8 glasses a week, mostly on the weekend.*
Functional disease *Do you strain to pass at least 1 in 4 bowel motions and are then left feeling like the evacuation is incomplete or that there's an obstruction?* (functional constipation)	*Yes. I seem to have to strain often to pass a bowel motion. But it does feel complete when I pass a bowel motion.*

►

▶

Infection and inflammation *Have you used any vaginal sprays, douches or had several bubble baths recently?* (chemical vaginitis, vulvovaginitis)	*No, I have not indulged enough in that kind of thing!*
Supplements and side effects of medication *Are you taking any supplements or medications?*	*Just a multivitamin. I thought I should take something since my diet is not good at the moment.*
Endocrine/reproductive *Tell me about your menstrual cycle.*	Gia explains that her periods have become irregular and she is never really sure when it is going to come, when Gia develops a backache or stomachache she realises her period is probably going to come in a couple of days.
Stress and neurological disease *How are you managing your stress at the moment?*	*Mostly with chocolate! My boyfriend is really great, he's a great de-stressor.*
Eating habits and energy *Tell me about your diet and energy levels.*	Gia describes a diet that is high in refined carbohydrates, sugar and caffeine. She does have some whole foods and vegetables but not as much as she knows she should have. She says she finds her energy levels fluctuate, but she finds coffee or cola drinks help with that.

TABLE 5.3 **CORE**	
Analogy: Core of the apple with the seed of ill health	**Core:** Holistic assessment to understand the client
AREAS OF INVESTIGATION AND EXAMPLE QUESTIONS	**CLIENT RESPONSES**
Daily activities *Describe your daily routine.*	*When I get up I have a coffee and cereal and then I either go to uni or I study at home. I try to go out for a jog or swim, but haven't really done much recently. My boyfriend comes over in the evenings 3–4 times a week and I spend all weekend with him if I don't have to work on an assignment.*

▶

Family and friends *What about family and friends?*	*I haven't seen much of anyone in the last few months. I try and catch up with my family every 3 or 4 weeks, and talk to mum and dad on the phone a couple of times a week. My friends are understanding and I try to catch up with them on the weekends if I can.*
Action needed to heal *How do you hope I can help you?*	*I thought you might be able to tell me how to improve my diet and lifestyle. Maybe you have some tablets that could help too.*
Long-term goals *What are your long-term goals?*	*Finish uni and have a holiday! Then get a job teaching. Maybe in four or five years if things go well we might try for a baby. I'd like to get my hormones sorted out before we try for one.*

TABLE 5.4 **GIA'S SIGNS AND SYMPTOMS** [2, 6]	
Pulse	88 bpm
Blood pressure	120/75
Temperature	36.8°C
Respiratory rate	16 resp/min
Body mass index	28
Waist circumference	82 cm
Face	Slight facial hair, acne
Urinalysis	No abnormality detected (NAD)

Results of medical investigations

No medical tests have been carried out.

TABLE 5.5 **UNLIKELY DIAGNOSTIC CONSIDERATIONS** [2, 7–10]	
CONDITIONS AND CAUSES	**WHY UNLIKELY**
FAMILY HEALTH	
Familial or idiopathic hirsutism	Excess hair growth would not be typically androgenic, appearing on hormonally influenced areas of the body where hair will grow, such as the face, armpits, abdomen, chest and thighs; no known family history of excess hair growth
OBSTRUCTION AND FOREIGN BODY	
Polycystic renal disease: lower abdominal and back discomfort	Urinalysis is clear, no high blood pressure

INFECTION AND INFLAMMATION	
Chronic salpingo-oophoritis: irregular cycle; can be minimal or excessive menstrual bleed	Usually congestive dysmenorrhoea is the predominant symptom; associated with purulent discharge, fever, period pain and abdominal pain
Cystitis	Urinalysis NAD
ENDOCRINE/REPRODUCTIVE	
Diabetes: anovulatory cycles	Urinalysis NAD
Primary dysmenorrhoea: lower abdominal pain, can get worse with menstrual cycle	Period pain usually starts when menses first begins and is often associated with no pelvic abnormality, nausea, vomiting, headache or dizziness
Secondary dysmenorrhoea: acquired due to pathology; period pain begins several years after menarche and due to a pelvic abnormality	Menstrual bleed is presenting as painless
Twisted uterine fibroids and polyps: twisted fibroids can cause symptoms of severe dysmenorrhoea, heavy bleeding, back pain and sometimes vaginal discharge	Usually maintains normal cycle unless submucosal or nearly extruded; causes uterine enlargement; usually causes menorrhagia (blood loss of 80 mL per day and lasting more than 7 days); fibroids form due to excess oestrogen
Premenstrual syndrome: pain in the abdomen before menses	Experiences premenstrual mood changes, feels teary, bloated and swollen 1–12 days before period; experiences a dull pelvic ache, abdominal bloating
Ovulatory bleed: have bleed mid-cycle as well as regular menses and ovulation has occurred	Feels emotional, premenstrual symptoms such as ovulation pain (mittelschmerz) and mood changes; usually spotting or light bleed at time of ovulation, regular cycle; check basal body temperature because it will be biphasic and fluctuate, indicating ovulation has occurred

Case analysis

TABLE 5.6 **POSSIBLE DIFFERENTIAL DIAGNOSIS**		
Not ruled out by tests/investigations already done [2, 7–11, 59, 60]		
CONDITION AND CAUSES	WHY POSSIBLE	WHY UNLIKELY
CANCER AND HEART DISEASE		
Ovarian, pituitary or adrenal tumour	Will affect androgen levels, produce symptoms of irregular cycles, lower abdominal pain, acne, increased facial hair, depression, weight gain	No changes in smell or taste; no headaches mentioned indicating a brain tumour

Uterine cancer	Vaginal discharge	Usually brown discharge
Cervical cancer	Vaginal discharge, sexually active	Need to ask if the pain/blood is experienced on intercourse and the date of the last pap smear; vaginal discharge can contain blood
Adult-onset and congenital adrenal hyperplasia/adrenal tumour: can cause primary and secondary amenorrhoea; anovulatory cycles	Usually presents with severe acne and hirsutism; can present with anovulatory irregular menstrual bleeding	Check if rapid development of symptoms and how severe virilisation symptoms are; accompanied by severe virilisation such as frontal balding and enlarged clitoris
TRAUMA AND PRE-EXISTING ILLNESS		
Congenital disorders (spina bifida, scoliosis, spondylolisthesis)	Lower back pain	Back pain only mentioned prior to menstrual period
Trauma (strains, sprains, tear, herniated disc, fracture, disc prolapse)	Lower back pain	
OBSTRUCTION AND FOREIGN BODY		
Intestinal obstruction (bowel cancer, adhesions, hernias, faecal impaction with overflow)	Abdominal distension and pain constipation	No vomiting, abdominal pain associated with menstrual cycle
FUNCTIONAL DISEASE		
Functional constipation	Has 3 or fewer evacuations a week; not drinking enough water, high caffeine intake, not enough fruit, vegetables in diet, lack of exercise, stress	Need to check if more than 1 in 4 bowel motions is lumpy and hard, and causes strain, a feeling of incomplete evacuation or blockage; need to check if manual help is needed to facilitate a bowel motion passing
Faulty posture	Possible if sitting for long periods of time studying	
INFECTION AND INFLAMMATION		
Appendicitis/Meckel's diverticulum	Intermittent lower abdominal pain, constipation; common age group	If pain becomes acute it could be a possible diagnosis
Pelvic inflammatory disorder: abdominal pain, could be from a sexually transmitted disease	Purulent vaginal discharge, sexually active, abdominal pain; irregular periods, lower backache	Unsure whether vaginal discharge is offensive, and unclear at this stage if there is pelvic pain; no fever; need to clarify if there is any pain on sexual intercourse; physical exam will indicate whether pain on motion during physical examination

Acute and chronic cervicitis: *Chlamydia trachomatis*, *Neisseria gonorrhoea*, herpes simplex virus	Vaginal discharge can be produced by cervicitis without vaginal infection; can be profuse discharge with lumbosacral backache	Need to define if the pain is experienced on intercourse associated with purulent discharge; physical exam will indicate whether pain on motion during physical examination
Chlamydia: can be asymptomatic and cause pelvic inflammatory disorder	Sexually active with new boyfriend; vaginal itching not a common symptom	Need to establish if mucopurulent cervicitis is occurring; increased frequency of urination not reported; a physical exam will indicate whether pain motion during physical examination; vaginal discharge usually yellow in colour
Gonorrhoea	Vaginal discharge and abdominal discomfort vaginal discharge can be produced by gonorrhoea without vaginal infection; sexually active with new boyfriend; vaginal itching not a common symptom	Need to define if has had any recent rectal infections, pain on walking or climbing stairs; physical exam will indicate whether pain on motion during physical examination; vaginal discharge usually yellow in colour
Candidiasis (vaginal discharge, sexually active, would be detected when doing a pap smear)	Vaginal discharge, sweet cravings; constipation; *Candida* is common cause of vaginal discharge in adult women	Need to establish if Gia experiences external pain on urination and whether vaginal discharge has strong odour; vaginal discharge can be curdy (most common in yeast infections), recurrent and chronic episodes; symptom of vulvovaginal itching (most common in *Candida* infection); physical exam may indicate vulval inflammation
Inflammatory bowel disease	Abdominal and back pain prior to passing a bowel motion	No blood or mucus or episodes of diarrhoea reported; need to clarify if the abdominal pain is relieved when passing a bowel motion
Inflammatory lower back pain (fibromyositis, osteomyelitis, spinal, tubo-ovarian or rectal abscess, myelitis, endometriosis, cystitis, ankylosing spondylitis)	Lower back pain	Still need to be investigated

Trichomoniasis: a flagellated protozoon that causes vaginitis and urethritis, predominantly sexually transmitted; trichomonal vaginitis often associated with gonococcal or bacteroides cervicitis	Common cause of vaginal discharge in adult women; sexually active; common in women of child-bearing age	Usually severe local irritation and itching in vagina; vaginal discharge is usually frothy, profuse, white-greyish green, smelly discharge; increased frequency of urination not reported; can produce vaginitis with coexisting urethritis that causes pain on urination
Bacterial vaginosis: increase in aerobic bacteria (*Gardnerella vaginalis*) and decrease in lactobacilli	Vaginal discharge; common cause of vaginal discharge in adult women; common during reproductive years; itching not a prominent symptom; usually no symptoms of vaginal inflammation	Need to establish if vaginal discharge is offensive watery grey-white discharge, changes normal flora of the vagina; discharge is homogeneous; no increased frequency of urination reported
ENDOCRINE/REPRODUCTIVE		
Ectopic pregnancy	Irregular periods; can present with no pain (rare) and can leak over several days slowly; may be missed; common cause of secondary amenorrhoea, purulent vaginal discharge	Usually associated with severe and acute abdominal pain, abdominal fullness, increased desire to urinate; may have signs of fever and dull headaches
Pregnancy [65]	Irregular periods; missed periods; most common cause of secondary amenorrhoea; can present with vaginal discharge and pelvic/abdominal pain	Can present with fever; may have signs of breast tenderness and may have morning sickness
Ovarian disease: premature menopause often due to autoimmune disease	Menses beginning to change; can present with symptoms of menopause and irregular periods	No hot flushes
Polycystic ovarian syndrome (PCOS): extremely common cause of secondary amenorrhoea; anovulatory cycles [59, 60]	Irregular menstrual cycles, lower abdominal pain, hormonal acne, increased facial and body hair (hirsutism), sugar cravings, weight gain	Check if symptom development has been slow and steady; may have thinning of hair on the head (like men do) called androgenic alopecia
Hypothyroidism: cause of secondary amenorrhoea due to hyperprolactinaemia and endocrine disorder; anovulatory cycles	Weight gain, irregular periods, constipation, increased facial and body hair (hirsutism), weight gain, constipation	No skin and hair changes mentioned; no significant fatigue, temperature intolerance or visible goitre noted; no significant depression mentioned

Cushing's syndrome: causes amenorrhoea, irregular menstrual cycles	Irregular menstrual cycles, increased facial hair, weight gain	Check if symptom development has been rapid; no moon-shaped face, frontal balding or hypertension and oedema; no significant depression mentioned; urinalysis NAD and no indication of glucose intolerance or diabetes which can be associated with Cushing's syndrome
Adenomyosis: benign invasion of endometrium (inner layer of uterus) into myometrium (thick muscle layer of uterus); can be associated with endometriosis, pregnancy, abortions, caesarean sections, tubal surgery	Heavy bleeding common	Common complaint that often does not cause symptoms; more often occurs between the ages of 30 and 50; can cause painful periods due to excess oestrogen
Endometriosis	Irregular periods; lower back and abdominal pain prior to menstrual bleed; can have symptoms of vaginal discharge	No significant pelvic pain or pain on menstrual bleed reported; no bleeding from the bowel; usually brown discharge with associated abdominal and pelvic pain
Dysfunctional uterine bleeding (DUB): endometrial hyperplasia, PCOS, from taking exogenous oestrogen; endocrine dysfunction not associated with inflammation, tumour or pregnancy; anovulatory hormone related bleeding is most common	Usually causes unpredictable frequency and amount of bleeding; menorrhagia (heavy bleed with regular cycle) common but interval between periods is usually shorter	No use of exogenous oestrogen reported
Anovulatory bleeding: irregular bleeding that appears to be menstrual although no ovulation has occurred; can be associated with both short and long cycles [63]	Irregular cycle; no significant premenstrual symptoms reported to show evidence of regular association with menses cycle; bleed is painless; blood volume can be excessive but irregular; physical findings will often include hirsutism, acne, and indicate PCOS	Check if bleed is unexpected; check basal body temperature, if anovulatory it will not fluctuate (monophasic)

Oestrogen-withdrawal bleeding: causes intermenstrual bleeding; occurs when the endometrium proliferates and becomes unstable when oestrogen drops below threshold; can happen outside of the secretory phase or in the absence of progesterone	Common cause of irregular periods in reproductive years, especially if ovulation has not occurred; menstrual bleeding is prolonged and profuse when does occur	Need to investigate if Gia experiences pain when bleeding as this is not usually present with oestrogen withdrawal [64]
Progesterone-withdrawal bleeding: only occurs when there is an oestrogen-primed endometrium; can occur when oestrogen therapy continued and progesterone stopped; also when progesterone is administered to test endogenous oestrogen	Irregular menstrual bleed often present in conditions such as PCOS	
Oestrogen-breakthrough bleeding – 1st type: when oestrogen levels are low but constant causing sections of endometrium to degenerate	Intermenstrual bleed; common when have PCOS	Need to investigate if she experiences any spotting of blood [64]
Oestrogen-breakthrough bleeding – 2nd type: oestrogen levels are well above threshold causing endometrium to become hyperplastic and outgrow blood-borne hormone supply	Causes degeneration of endometrium with prolonged and irregular bleeding	More common in oestrogen-based tumours
Ovarian cyst	Lower abdominal pain, irregular periods	Ovarian cysts almost never cause heavy menstrual bleeding
Physiologic leukorrhoea: must be in absence of yeast infection, *Trichomonas*	Vaginal discharge; discharge usually thick, greyish white, no odour but profuse; usually no itching associated	More common in girls beginning their menarche
AUTOIMMUNE DISEASE		
Rheumatoid spondylitis	Lower back pain; can be early signs of rheumatoid arthritis	Need further investigation
STRESS AND NEUROLOGICAL DISEASE		
Causal factor: **Stress**	Constipation, dietary changes, increased sugar cravings, lack of exercise	

New sexual relationship	Vaginal discharge, pregnancy, irregular periods	Check if using contraception
EATING HABITS AND ENERGY		
Causal factor: **Diet:** Eating more chocolate, carbohydrates, lack of water, excess caffeine	Insulin resistance connection with symptoms of PCOS, constipation, increase stress	Need to clarify dietary changes and duration of changes
Causal factor: **Lack of exercise**	Affect insulin resistance, PCOS, weight gain, stress, lower back ache	

TABLE 5.7 DECISION TABLE FOR REFERRAL [2, 7–10, 13]

COMPLAINT	CONTEXT	CORE
Referral for presenting complaint	Referral for all associated physical, dietary and lifestyle concerns	Referral for contributing emotional, mental, spiritual, metaphysical, lifestyle and constitutional factors
REFERRAL FLAGS	**REFERRAL FLAGS**	**REFERRAL FLAGS**
• Hirsutism associated with menstrual change and other virilising symptoms such as acne	• A menstruating woman of any age can bleed from pregnancy complications • Irregular bleeding in menstrual cycle • Change in volume of menstrual bleed • Purulent vaginal discharge • Abdominal and lower back discomfort prior to menstrual bleed	• Stress building up due to studies
ISSUES OF SIGNIFICANCE	**ISSUES OF SIGNIFICANCE**	**ISSUES OF SIGNIFICANCE**
Nil	• Pattern of premenstrual symptoms have stopped indicating lack of ovulation • Bowel motion less than three times a week • Increased weight gain and acne with associated menstrual changes • Excess caffeine foods • Lack of exercise • New boyfriend and sexual relations	• New relationship may have potential to effect Gia's studies • Excess body waxing due to hirsutism

REFERRAL	REFERRAL	REFERRAL
• Medical investigation to rule out serious endocrine causes of hirsutism and symptoms of virilisation	• Medical investigations for change in menstrual cycle, abdominal and lower back discomfort • Musculoskeletal assessment for lower back pain • Test for sexually transmitted diseases • Education about contraception options • Dietary assistance to balance food intake	• Massage for relaxation • Student counsellor for time management issues

TABLE 5.8 FURTHER INVESTIGATIONS THAT MAY BE NECESSARY [1, 2, 6–12, 65]	
TEST/INVESTIGATION	**REASON FOR TEST/INVESTIGATION**
FIRST-LINE INVESTIGATIONS:	
Examine genitalia and note secondary sex characteristics	May indicate functional or endocrine disorder
Pelvic, vaginal, abdominal examination	Check for bulging uterus, ovaries can be palpable in PCOS, abdominal rebound tenderness, overactive bowel sounds, genital deformities, signs of trauma
Musculoskeletal examination	Back strain, trauma, deformities, inflammation
Human chorionic gonadotropin (HCG) **blood test/radioimmunoassay** (RIA)	Pregnancy, ectopic pregnancy
Vaginal smear	Evaluation of cervical mucus will indicate if ovarian oestrogen is being produced
Cervical smear	Detect cervical cancer
CA-125 serum marker	Ovarian cancer, endometriosis, pelvic inflammatory disease
Chlamydia cervical culture **Cervical gonorrhoea culture**	Sexually transmitted diseases
Full blood count	Rule out infection, tumour, inflammation, anaemia
Blood lipids	Increased possible risk for cardiovascular disease connected with PCOS [26–29]

Progesterone level	Test 7 days before menstruation to determine if ovulation has occurred; low serum progesterone level in anovulatory cycles
Oestradiol	*Normal:* PCOS, weight loss, excess exercise *Raised:* pregnancy, ovarian tumour, testicular tumour, adrenal tumour *Low:* PCOS, polycystic ovarian disease, ovarian failure, anorexia nervosa, weight loss, excess exercise, hypothyroidism, Cushing's syndrome, adrenal hyperplasia, menopause, Turner's syndrome, failing pregnancy, fetal death
Oestrone	Elevated in PCOS due to peripheral conversion
FSH (follicle-stimulating hormone)	*Normal:* PCOS, pregnancy, anorexia, weight loss, excess exercise *Raised:* ovarian failure, menopause *Low:* polycystic ovarian disease, anorexia, weight loss, excess exercise, hypothyroidism, Cushing's syndrome, adrenal tumour/hyperplasia
LH (luteinising hormone): due to pulsatile action of this hormone it may not be accurately measured on one random sample	*Normal:* pregnancy, anorexia, weight loss, excess exercise *Raised:* PCOS, polycystic ovarian disease, ovarian failure, menopause *Low:* anorexia, weight loss, excess exercise, hypothyroidism, Cushing's syndrome, adrenal tumour/hyperplasia
PRL (prolactin): common in secondary amenorrhoea to be raised	*Normal:* ovarian failure, anorexia, weight loss, excess exercise, adrenal tumour/ hyperplasia *Raised:* PCOS (mildly), hypothyroidism, Cushing's syndrome, pregnancy, amenorrhoea *Low:* pituitary destruction from tumour
Testosterone	*Normal:* ovarian failure, anorexia, weight loss, excess exercise, hypothyroidism, pregnancy *Raised:* PCOS, Cushing's syndrome, adrenal tumour/hyperplasia, testicular tumour, ovarian tumour *Low:* corticosteriod use
SHBG (sex hormone-binding globulin)	Low SHBG would indicate the presence of elevated levels of free androgens
Thyroid function test TSH, T4, T3	TSH (thyroid-stimulating hormone) increased in hypothyroidism
Fasting blood glucose test	Raised levels can indicate diabetes mellitus, Cushing's syndrome

HOME TESTS:	
Basal body temperature	Normally drops 24–36 hours after menses begins; with endometriosis there is often a delay in basal body temperature to the second or third day of menses; a decrease indicates preovulation and an increase of 5 degrees occurs after ovulation; monitors thyroid function
Ovulation prediction kits	Detects increase in urinary luteinising hormone (LH) excretion 24–36 hours prior to ovulation
IF NECESSARY:	
Progesterone withdrawal test	To determine if oestrogen is being produced in the body
17-hydroxyprogesterone	Elevated in congenital adrenal hyperplasia (classic early onset) and after stimulation tests can reveal late onset
Androgens: androstenedione and dehydroepiandrosterone sulphate	Elevated in PCOS and significantly so in congenital adrenal hyperplasia and virilising tumours; androstenedione is a precursor to cortisol, aldosterone, testosterone and oestrogen; will indicate possible adrenal tumour, ovarian tumour or Cushing's syndrome
Serum cortisol blood test	Will determine Cushing's syndrome possible adrenal tumour and stress levels
Abdominal and pelvic x-ray/ultrasound	Most accurate diagnosis of PCOS, ovarian mass, ovarian cyst or tumour, retroverted uterus, tubo-ovarian abscesses, fibroids, trauma; intestinal obstruction
Laparoscopy and biopsy/culdoscopy	Primary diagnostic technique for endometriosis by visualising the lesions
Endometrial, vaginal and cervical biopsies	Detect cancer; during luteal phase (10–12 days after ovulation) to determine inadequate luteal phase production or action of progesterone
Transvaginal ultrasonography	To determine cause of excess and random menstrual bleeding (menometrorrhagia) such as dysfunctional uterine bleeding or cancer
Brain scan CT/MRI	Pituitary tumour
Back x-ray, CT scan and MRI	Degenerative disc disease, disc prolapse, ankylosing spondylitis, Paget's disease, osteoporosis

Confirmed diagnosis

GIA AND POLYCYSTIC OVARIAN SYNDROME WITH ANOVULATORY MENSTRUAL CYCLE AND PHYSIOLOGIC LEUKORRHOEA

Gia is 24 years of age and has come to the clinic for help with a series of symptoms associated with an irregular menstrual cycle. Gia is most concerned about acne, increasing facial and body hair, a vaginal discharge and a change to premenstrual symptoms. Gia is coming to the end of her studies to be a teacher and admits her current lifestyle includes a lot of computer work, lack of exercise, quick meals and consuming more chocolate, cola and energy drinks to get through. She has been craving sugar and has gained weight in the past seven months. Gia has a new boyfriend and enjoys seeing him up to four evenings a week. She is looking for alternative approaches to the oral contraceptive pill for helping her menstrual symptoms.

Gia was referred for a series of medical investigations and has been diagnosed with **polycystic ovarian syndrome**. Gia has classic symptoms of amenorrhoea, lower abdominal pain, backache, hormonal acne, sugar cravings, weight gain and increased facial and body hair (hirsutism). Multiple cysts develop on the ovaries causing increased production of androgens. Due to low levels of follicle-stimulating hormone, excess androgens are converted to testosterone rather than oestrogen. PCOS is a metabolic condition commonly associated with insulin resistance and glucose intolerance. Due to increased levels of insulin there is a decrease in SHBG, which binds increasing free androgens. A propensity to gain weight and develop obesity will make the underlying androgen increase and insulin resistance worse.

Amenorrhoea and oligomenorrhoea associated with symptoms of virilisation, such as acne and hirsutism, develop slowly and steadily shortly after menarche for many young women. Symptoms of PCOS can begin to become very uncomfortable in the second and third decade, affecting fertility and can influence the development of hypertension, hyperlipidaemia and cardiovascular disease. It is believed that a majority of women who do not ovulate regularly have polycystic ovarian syndrome.

General references used in this diagnosis: 2, 7, 9–11, 59, 60, 62

PRESCRIBED MEDICATION

• Oral contraceptive pill [61]

Gia wants to try natural therapies to correct her hormonal balance at this stage. In view of the recommendation to take the oral contraceptive pill, it is important to work collaboratively with Gia's doctor to ensure her condition is monitored. Her treatment program should be reviewed in eight weeks and then again four to six weeks later. If no change has occurred after 12–16 weeks Gia should be encouraged to consider other treatment options.

TABLE 5.9 **DECISION TABLE FOR TREATMENT (ONCE DIAGNOSIS IS CONFIRMED)**		
COMPLAINT	CONTEXT	CORE
Treatment for the presenting complaint and symptoms	Treatment for all associated symptoms	Treatment for mental, emotional, spiritual, constitutional, lifestyle issues and metaphysical considerations

▶

TREATMENT PRIORITY	TREATMENT PRIORITY	TREATMENT PRIORITY
• Dietary recommendations to support hormonal balance and improve glycaemic control, which is essential in managing PCOS • Lifestyle recommendations to improve glycaemic control and control PCOS symptoms • Physical treatment suggestions to help improve hormonal balance • Herbal tonic or tablets to support ovarian function and hormonal balance • Herbal tea to support hormonal balance and glycaemic control • Supplemental nutrients to improve glycaemic control **NB:** Blood pressure and serum potassium should be monitored while Gia is taking the herbal tonic or tablets due to licorice content; dandelion leaf has been added to the herbal tonic and tea to reduce the risk of hypokalaemia and hypertension [14, 19, 20]; dietary recommendation to reduce sodium intake and increase potassium intake while taking herbal tonic or tablets [14, 19, 20] • Review use of chaste tree if menstrual irregularity worsens [14] • Ensure Gia is using appropriate contraception while taking the herbal tonic or tablets due to pregnancy contraindications for schisandra [23, 24] and thuja [23] • If Gia decides to try the oral contraceptive pill, a review of her herbal medicine will be required to ensure there are no negative drug/herb interactions	• Dietary recommendations to improve nutrition, general health and to reduce the risk of type 2 diabetes and cardiovascular disease • Supplemental nutrients to improve nutrient and antioxidant status, as well as to support cardiovascular health • Recommendation for Gia to lose weight to improve general health and reduce the risk of type 2 diabetes and cardiovascular disease	• Lifestyle recommendations to help reduce Gia's stress levels • Herbal tonic and tea containing nervine and adaptogenic herbs to help support Gina's stress response • Supplemental multivitamin to help support Gia's stress response

Treatment aims

- Normalise hormonal balance [14, 27] and restore normal menstrual cycle [14, 27, 48].
- Reduce and manage symptoms of elevated androgens [14, 27, 48].
- Support Gia's ovarian function [14, 48] and maintain her fertility for the future [14, 26, 27].
- Help Gia lose weight and ensure she stays within normal BMI [26, 27, 48].
- Support Gia's stress response [26, 30].
- Improve Gia's diet and lifestyle [26, 27, 50].
- Improve insulin sensitivity [14, 26, 27, 50] and prevent potential progression to type 2 diabetes [15, 26, 27, 48].
- Support Gia's antioxidant status [28] and cardiovascular health [26–29, 48, 58].

Lifestyle alterations/considerations

- Gia will benefit from regular exercise to help reduce her stress levels [32, 33] and improve her symptoms [26, 50]. Exercise should include both strength training and aerobic exercise [31], which will help reduce body fat and improve skeletal muscle mass and strength. This in turn will improve glucose control [26, 31].
- Gia will benefit from a weight-reduction program to bring her back into normal BMI range [26, 27, 50] but should avoid crash dieting and short-term weight loss [26].
- Gia may find relaxation therapies such as meditation, yoga, tai chi or autogenic (self-relaxation) training helpful to reduce her stress levels [26, 33].
- If Gia is a smoker she should quit [26].

Dietary suggestions

- Encourage Gia to follow a low GI and GL diet to improve glucose control [14–18, 35, 36] and improve her skin [34]. Dietary measures are essential for the management of polycystic ovarian syndrome [14, 26, 29, 35, 50].
- Encourage Gia to reduce consumption of saturated [14, 26, 35, 50] and *trans* fats [26] and increase consumption of monounsaturated fats [35, 36] and omega-3 fatty acid-rich foods. Omega-3 oils confer a range of benefits for general and reproductive health in women [38] and can improve glucose metabolism [37, 38].
- Encourage Gia to increase consumption of fibre from low GI sources [14, 26, 35, 36]. Soluble fibre can reduce postprandial glucose response and improve glycaemic control [16, 17, 36].
- Gia's diet should be high in antioxidant-rich foods such as low GI whole grains, fruit, vegetables and legumes [14, 16–18, 26, 28].
- Encourage Gia to consume phyto-oestrogen-containing foods [14]. Lignans can increase levels of SHBG and reduce the biological activity of androgens [14, 41]; they also have a positive effect on ovulation and hormonal balance [14, 39].
- Gia should reduce or eliminate alcohol consumption [26] and significantly reduce her intake of caffeine [26].
- Encourage Gia to eat foods high in B-group vitamins, zinc, chromium, potassium, magnesium and vanadium. These are essential minerals for blood glucose regulation [14, 16–18].
- Encourage Gia to reduce her sodium intake and increase potassium intake while she is taking the herbal tonic or tablets [14, 19, 20].
- Encourage Gia to regularly include cinnamon in her diet to help with glucose control [40].

Physical treatment suggestions

- Gia is likely to benefit from a course of electro-acupuncture [41, 42]. Repeated electro-acupuncture can induce regular ovulation and reduce androgen levels in women with PCOS [41] and positively alter ovarian neuroendrocrine status [42].
- Gia may find massage therapy beneficial in helping reduce her stress levels [43, 44].
- Hydrotherapy: hot sitz baths or full baths are indicated for supressed menses [52, 53]. Taking a shallow cold sitz bath and placing the feet in a hot foot bath simultaneously eases pelvic congestion [52]. Alternatively have hot foot bath with a cold compress on the sacrum (if the feet are warm there is no need to heat the pelvic area – the cold will push blood back into the pelvic organs while the feet keep the core body temperature warm) [57].
- For acute period pain spray the pelvic area with a hot hand shower for two minutes, then alternate and spray with cold water for one minute (repeat three times) [54]. Place a hot compress/fomentation on the back during menstrual pain [54]. Apply a warm castor oil pack on the abdomen/pelvic area for menstrual cramps and constipation [54].
- For constipation place a hot compress on the abdomen, then cover in plastic with a hot water bottle/heating pad on top for 12 minutes, followed by cold mitten friction for 30 seconds (repeat process three times) [54].
- Weekly contrasting treatments between menses with a hot fomentation on the back and abdomen for 15 minutes, followed by 30-second cold mitten friction. Next, apply heat to the pelvic area and back for another 15 minutes, repeat the cold mitten friction with client in the side lying position (repeat alternating procedure three times) then follow with an abdominal massage [54].
- Constitutional hydrotherapy: lumbar wrap [53, 55].
- Use a facial steam treatment to clean the skin, followed by an oatmeal face pack [56]. Finish with a cold shower on the face [52].

TABLE 5.10 **HERBAL FORMULA (1:2 LIQUID EXTRACTS)**		
HERB	**FORMULA**	**RATIONALE**
Paeonia *Paeonia lactiflora*	60 mL	Inhibits testosterone synthesis [14, 24]; enhances aromatase enzymes thereby promoting conversion of oestradiol from testosterone [14]; normalises ovarian function [14]; skeletal muscle relaxant [24]; combined with licorice, paeonia exerts a beneficial effect in PCOS [14, 19, 20, 24, 47] by improving LH:FSH ratio [14, 19, 24], reducing testosterone levels [14, 19, 20, 24, 47] and improving oestradiol to testosterone ratio [14, 24, 47]

▶

Licorice *Glycyrrhiza glabra*	30 mL	Oestrogenic properties [14, 19]; adrenal tonic [19, 20]; antioxidant [19, 20]; beneficial in stress [19, 20]; mild laxative [19, 20]; beneficial in PCOS when combined with paeonia [14, 19, 20, 24, 47] – see above
Dandelion leaf *Taraxacum officinale*	40 mL	Diuretic [14, 20]; liver tonic [20]; rich source of potassium [14, 20]; beneficial to reduce the risk of hypokalaemia and hypertension from long-term use of licorice in herbal tonic or tablets [14]
Black cohosh *Cimicifuga racemosa*	20 mL	Reduces LH secretion [19, 20]; indicated for use in ovarian dysfunction [21] and PCOS [20]
Schisandra *Schisandra chinensis*	50 mL	Antioxidant [19, 23]; nervine tonic [23, 24]; adaptogenic [19, 23, 24]; hepatoprotective [19, 24]; improves mental, physical and sensory performance [24]; to support liver function [24, 48]
Supply:	200 mL	Dose: 5 mL 3 times daily

Chaste tree (*Vitex agnus castus*) 1000 mg tablet once daily
Beneficial for the treatment of latent hyperprolactinaemia [19, 20] and corpus luteum insufficiency [19, 20, 45]; beneficial in PMS [19, 20]; some women may experience a worsening of menstrual irregularity with chaste tree, so its use should be reviewed if this occurs with Gia [14]

TABLE 5.11 **HERBAL TEA**		
Alternative to herbal liquid if Gia prefers a tea		
HERB	**FORMULA**	**RATIONALE**
Paeonia root *Paeonia lactiflora*	2 parts	See above
Licorice root *Glycyrrhiza glabra*	1 part	See above
Black cohosh root *Cimicifuga racemosa*	1 part	See above

Hops *Humulus lupulus*	1 part	Mild sedative [23, 45]; oestrogenic action [19, 46]; anti-androgenic action [45, 46]; beneficial where stress and nervous tension accompanies PCOS [14]
Cinnamon bark powder *Cinnamomum cassia*	½ part	Antioxidant [19]; hypoglycaemic [40]; enhances insulin sensitivity [19]; traditionally used for female reproductive disorders [19]
Dandelion leaf *Taraxacum officinale*	1 part	See above
Infusion: 1 tsp per cup – 3–4 cups daily		

TABLE 5.12 **TABLET ALTERNATIVE TO HERBAL LIQUID: MAY IMPROVE COMPLIANCE**		
HERB	**DOSE PER TABLET**	**RATIONALE**
Paeonia *Paeonia lactiflora*	852 mg	See above
Licorice *Glycyrrhiza glabra*	847 mg	See above
Black cohosh *Cimicifuga racemosa*	300 mg	See above
Thuja *Thuja occidentalis*	250 mg	Traditionally used to support glandular function and to treat abnormal growths [49]
Dose: 2 tablets twice daily		

TABLE 5.13 **NUTRITIONAL SUPPLEMENTS**	
SUPPLEMENT AND DOSE	**RATIONALE**
High-potency practitioner-strength **multivitamin, mineral and antioxidant supplement** providing therapeutic levels of B-group vitamins Dosage as per manufacturer's instructions	To ensure adequate levels of essential nutrient and antioxidants given Gia's current poor dietary intake; to reduce oxidative stress [28]; B-group vitamins are required for glucose metabolism [22, 19]; increased need for B-group vitamins during times of excessive stress [22, 19]; to support Gia's cardiovascular health [28, 51]; PCOS is associated with increased risk of cardiovascular disease [28, 58]

Supplement providing a daily dose of 200 µg **chromium** [16, 22] and 400 mg elemental **magnesium** [22]	Chromium enhances the effects of insulin [22, 25]; reduces skeletal muscle insulin resistance [16]; improves glucose control [16, 22, 25]; magnesium deficiency aggravates insulin resistance [16, 19, 25]; supplemental magnesium improves glucose tolerance [25] and insulin sensitivity [19, 22, 25]
Omega-3 fish oil 3000 mg daily [19]	Beneficial to improve Gia's reproductive health [38] and to improve glucose metabolism [37, 38]

References

[1] N.J. Talley, S. O'Connor, Pocket Clinical Examination, third edn, Churchill Livingstone Elsevier, Australia, 2009.

[2] P. Kumar, C. Clark, Clinical Medicine, sixth edn, Elsevier Saunders, London, 2005.

[3] J. Silverman, S. Kurtz, J. Draper, Skills for Communicating with Patients, second edn, Radcliff Publishing, Oxford, 2000.

[4] R. Neighbour, The Inner Consultation: how to develop an effective and intuitive consulting style, Radcliff Publishing, Oxon, 2005.

[5] M. Lloyd, R. Bor, Communication Skills For Medicine, third edn, Churchill Livingstone Elsevier, Edinburgh, 2009.

[6] G. Douglas, F. Nicol, C. Robertson, Macleod's Clinical Examination, twelth edn, Churchill Livingstone Elsevier, 2009.

[7] J. Jamison, Differential Diagnosis for Primary Care, second edn, Churchill Livingstone Elsevier, London, 2006.

[8] A. Polmear (Ed.), Evidence-Based Diagnosis in Primary Care, Churchill Livingstone Elsevier, 2008, pp. 274–283.

[9] R.D. Collins, Differential Diagnosis in Primary Care, fourth edn, Lippincott Williams & Wilkins, Philadelphia, 2008.

[10] R.H. Seller, Differential Diagnosis of Common Complaints, fifth edn, Saunders Elsevier, Philadelphia, 2007.

[11] R.M.D Berkow, A.J.M.D Fletcher, M.H.M.D Beers, The Merck Manual, sixteenth edn, Merck Research Laboratories, Rathway, N.J, 1993 (later edition).

[12] K.D. Pagna, T.J. Pagna, Mosby's Diagnostic and Laboratory Test reference, third edn, Mosby, USA, 1997 (later edition).

[13] D. Peters, L. Chaitow, G. Harris, S. Morrison, Integrating Complementary Therapies in Primary Care. London: Churchill Livingstone, London, 2002.

[14] R. Trickey, Women, Hormones & The Menstrual Cycle, second edn, Allen & Unwin, Sydney, 2003.

[15] S. El-Hashemy, Naturopathic Standards of Primary Care, CCNM Press Inc, Toronto, 2007.

[16] J. Jamison, Clinical Guide to Nutrition & Dietary Supplements in Disease Management, Churchill Livingstone, Edinburgh, 2003.

[17] H. Osiecki, The Physicians Handbook of Clinical Nutrition, seventh edn, Eagle Farm: Bioconcepts, 2000.

[18] J.E. Pizzorno, M.T. Murray, H. Joiner-Bey, The Clinicians Handbook of Natural Medicine, second edn, St Louis, Churchill Livingstone, 2008.

[19] L. Braun, M. Cohen, Herbs & Natural Supplements: An evidence based guide, second edn, Elsevier, Sydney, 2007.

[20] S. Mills, K. Bone, Principles & Practice of Phytotherapy; Modern Herbal Medicine, Churchill Livingstone, Edinburgh: London, 2000.

[21] British Herbal Medicine Association, British Herbal Pharmacopoeia, BHMAA, 1983.

[22] H. Osiecki, The Nutrient Bible, seventh edn, Eagle Farm: BioConcepts Publishing, 2008.

[23] S. Mills, K. Bone, The Essential Guide to Herbal Safety, Churchill Livingstone, St Louis, 2005.

[24] K. Bone, Clinical Applications of Chinese and Ayurvedic Herbs: Monographs for the Western Herbal Practitioners, Phytotherapy Press, Warwick, 1996.

[25] J. Higdon, An Evidence Based Approach to Vitamins and Minerals, Thieme, New York, 2003.

[26] R.J. Norman, M.J. Davies, J. Lord, L.J. Moran, The role of lifestyle modification in polycystic ovary syndrome, Trends in Endocrinology & Metabolism 13 (6) (2002) 251–257.

[27] D.A. Ehrmann, Polycystic Ovary Syndrome, N Engl J Med 352 (2005) 1223–1236.

[28] V. Fencki, S. Fencki, M. Yilmazer, M. Serteser, Decreased total antioxidant status and increased oxidative stress in women with polycystic ovary syndrome may contribute to the risk of cardiovascular disease, Fertility and Sterility 80 (1) (2003) 123–127.

[29] C.J. Glueck, R. Papanna, P. Wang, N. Goldenberg, L. Sieve-Smith, Incidence and Treatment of Metabolic Syndrome in Newly Referred Women With Confirmed Polycystic Ovarian Syndrome, Metabolism 52 (7) (2003) 908–915.

[30] M. Greiner, A. Paredes, V. Araya, H.E. Lara, Role of Stress and Sympathetic Innervation in the Development of Polycystic Ovary Syndrome, Endocrine 28 (3) (2005) 319–324.

[31] A. Maiorana, G. O'Driscoll, C. Goodman, R. Taylor, D. Green, Combined aerobic and resistance exercise improves glycemic control and fitness in type 2 diabetes, Diabetes Research and Clinical Practice 56 (2002) 115–123.

[32] A. Byrne, G.D. Byrne, The effect of exercise on depression, anxiety and other mood states: A review, J Psychosom Res 37 (6) (1993) 565–574.

[33] A.F. Jorm, H. Christensen, K.M. Griffiths, R.A. Parslow, B. Rodgers, K.A. Blewitt, Effectiveness of complementary and self-help treatments for anxiety disorders, Medical Journal of Australia 181 (7) (2004) S29–S46.

[34] R. Smith, N.J. Mann, A. Braue, H. Makelainen, G.A. Varigos, The effect of a high-protein, low glycaemic load diet versus a conventional, high glycaemic load diet on biochemical parameters associated with acne vulgaris: A randomized, investigator-masked, controlled trial, Journal of the American Academy of Dermatology 57 (2007) 247–256.

[35] K. Marsh, J. Brand-Miller, The optimal diet for women with polycystic ovary syndrome?, British Journal of Nutrition 94 (2005) 154–165.

[36] Z. Hofman, J.D.E. van Drunen, C. de Later, H. Kuipers, The effect of different nutritional feeds on the postprandial glucose response in healthy volunteers and patients with type II diabetes, European Journal of Clinical Nutrition 58 (2004) 1553–1556.

[37] J. Luo, S.W. Rizkalla, J. Boillot, C. Alamowitch, H. Chaib, F. Bruzzo, Desplanque, et al., Dietary (n-3) Polyunsaturated Fatty Acids Improve Adipocyte Insulin Action and Glucose Metabolism in Insulin-Resistant Rats: Relation to Membrane Fatty Acids, The Journal of Nutrition 126 (1996) 1951–1958.

[38] J.M. Bourre, Dietary omega-3 fatty acids for women, Biomedicine & Pharmacotherapy vol. 61 (2007) 105–112.

[39] W.R. Phipps, M.C. Martini, J.W. Lampe, J.L. Slavin, M.S. Kurzer, Effect of flax seed ingestion on the menstrual cycle, Journal of Clinical Endocrinology & Metabolism 77 (1993) 1215–1219.

[40] J. Hlebowicz, G. Darwiche, O. Björgell, L.O. Almér, Effect of cinnamon on postprandial blood glucose, gastric emptying, and satiety in healthy subjects, American Journal of Clinical Nutrition 85 (6) (2007) 1552–1556.

[41] E. Stener-Victorin, U. Waldenstrom, U. Tagnfors, T. Lundeberg, G. Lindstedt, P.O. Janson, Effects of electro-acupuncture on anovulation in women with polycystic ovary syndrome, Acta Obstetrica et Gynecologica Scandinavica 79 (3) (2000) 180–188.

[42] E. Stener-Victorin, T. Lundeberg, U. Waldenstrom, I. Bileviciute-Ljungar, P.O. Janson, Effects of electro-acupuncture on corticotropin-releasing factor in rats with experimentally-induced polycystic ovaries, Neuropeptides 35 (5&6) (2001) 227–231.

[43] C.A. Moyer, J. Rounds, J.W. Hannum, A Meta-Analysis of Massage Therapy Research, Psychological Bulletin 130 (1) (2004) 3–18.

[44] T. Field, G. Robinson, F. Scafidi, R. Nawrocki, A. Goncalves, Massage therapy reduces anxiety and enhances EEG pattern of alertness and math computations, International Journal of Neuroscience 86 (1996) 197–205.

[45] R.F. Weiss, Weiss's Herbal Medicine, sixth edn, Thieme, Stuttgart, 2001.

[46] P. Zanoli, M. Zavatti, Pharmacognostic and pharmacological profile of Humulus lupulus L, Journal of Ethnopharmacology 116 (2008) 383–396.

[47] K. Takahashi, M. Kitao, Effect of TJ-68 (shakuyaku-kanzo-to) on polycystic ovarian disease, International Journal of Fertility and Menopausal Studies 39 (2) (1994) 69–76.

[48] S. Bulloch, Herbal Treatment of PCOS, Modern Phytotherapist 8 (2) (2004) 13–21.

[49] M. Morgan, Herbal Treatment of Polycystic Ovary Syndrome: Focus on Hyperandrogenism & Anovulation, A Phytotherapist's Perspective 49 (2005) 1–2.

[50] H. Farshchi, A. Rane, A. Love, R.L. Kennedy, Diet and nutrition in polycystic ovary syndrome (PCOS): pointers for nutritional management, Journal of Obstetrics and Gynaecology 27 (8) (2007) 762–763.

[51] C.D. Morris, S. Carson, Routine Vitamin Supplementation To Prevent Cardiovascular Disease: A Summary of the Evidence for the U.S. Preventive Services Task Force, Annals of Internal Medicine 139 (2003) 56–70.

[52] D.D. Buchman, The complete book of water healing, Contemporary Books, McGraw-Hill Companies, New York, 2001.

[53] W. Boyle, A. Saine, Lectures in Naturopathic Hydrotherapy, Oregon: Eclectic Medical Publications, 1988.

[54] M. Sinclair, Modern Hydrotherapy for the Massage Therapist, Lippincott Williams & Williams, Baltimore, 2008.

[55] E. Blake, in: L. Chaitow, E. Blake, P. Orrock, M. Wallden, P. Sinder, J. Zeff (Eds.), Naturopathic Physical Medicine: Theory and Practice for Manual Therapists and Naturopaths, Churchill Livingstone Elsevier, Philadelphia, 2008.

[56] L. Chaitow, Hydrotherapy, water therapy for health and beauty, Element, Dorset, 1999.

[57] G.M. Schleinkofer, Lectures on Hydrotherapy according to S.Kneipp, Sebastian Kneipp School, Bad Worishofen, Germany, July 2008.

[58] F. Orio, S. Palomba, L. Spinelli, T. Cascella, L. Tauchmanova, F. Zullo, et al., The Cardiovascular Risk of Young Women with Polycystic Ovary Syndrome: An Observational, Analytical, Prospective Case-Control Study, The Journal of Clinical Endocrinology & Metabolism 89 (8) (2004) 3696–3701.

[59] D.A. Ehrmann, Polycystic ovary syndrome, N Engl J Med 352 (2005) 1223–1236.

[60] D.H. Abbott, D.A. Dumesic, S. Franks, Developmental origin of polycystic ovarian syndrome – a hypothesis, Journal of Endocrinology 174 (2002) 1–5.

[61] D.B. Petitti, Combination estrogen-progestin oral contraceptives, N Engl J Med 349 (2003) 1443–1450.

[62] R.J. Chang, S.E. Katz, Diagnosis of polycystic ovarian syndrome, Endocrinol Metab Clin North Am 28 (1999) 397–408.

[63] D.T. Baird, Amenorrhoea, Lancet 350 (1997) 275–279.

[64] N. O'Flynn, N. Britten, Diagnosing menstrual disorders: a qualitative study of the approach of primary care professionals, Br J Gen Pract 54 (2004) 353–358.

[65] R.B. Kiningham, B.S. Apgar, T.L. Schwenk, Evaluation of amenorrhoea, Am Fam Physican 53 (1996) 1185–1194.

Endometriosis

Case history

Cathy Hall is 29 years old and has come to the clinic for natural help with her hormonal problems. She recently saw her doctor who advised her to take the oral contraceptive pill, but Cathy doesn't think there is any point in taking it because she is not currently sexually active. Cathy explains that her parents always used natural therapies for the family's health when she was growing up and she would like to continue to use natural therapies, partly in their memory but also because she has had positive outcomes with natural therapies in the past. Her parents were killed in a motor vehicle accident nearly four years ago. Her aunt (her father's much younger sister) is only seven years older than Cathy and is happily married with three children. Cathy and her aunt are more like sisters than aunt and niece, and Cathy tells you since her parents died she considers her aunt to be her closest family member. Cathy spends a lot of time at her aunt's house because she feels welcome and at home there.

Cathy's main complaint is irregular and painful periods. She has had problems with irregular periods for the past five years, which has worsened in recent years. This concerns her because she never used to have problems with her cycle. Cathy tells you she knows when her period is coming because she experiences back pain two to three days before her period starts, which increases in intensity the day before her period and also during the bleed. Last month Cathy's aunt took her to the family GP when Cathy was experiencing the premenstrual pain. The doctor did a pelvic and abdominal examination and ordered blood tests. The blood tests showed there was no anaemia, infection or inflammation and the doctor diagnosed her with endometriosis and prescribed the oral contraceptive pill along with ibuprofen. Cathy didn't think to tell her doctor she sometimes has mid-cycle pain and was too embarrassed to tell him that sometimes she notices blood coming from her rectum during her period. Cathy describes the pain as dull and constant, which sometimes becomes severe. She also tells you that her digestion is 'out of balance', with alternating episodes of constipation and diarrhoea. During her period her bowel motions tend to be watery. Premenstrually she feels bloated, teary and generally awful. Cathy has not been sexually active for over four years and is beginning to lose hope that she will ever meet the right person, particularly because she doesn't feel like socialising much these days due to her health problems.

Cathy works as a night shift cleaner and is on her feet for the whole shift. When she has her period she finds it very difficult to manage at work, and she is concerned that she may lose her job soon because she has called in sick so often in the past few months. She knows her shift team leader is getting fed up with the amount of time she is taking off and the pressure it puts on other team members, which she feels really bad about.

Cathy tells you she had considered becoming a nurse when she was much younger, and cleaning was only meant to be a short-term job for a few years to help her save up money so she could study. Eleven years later she is still there and beginning to wonder whether she will ever study. Cathy explains that her father was a member of Australia's 'stolen generation' of Aboriginal children and, in the years just prior to his death, he reconnected with the remote community he originally came from. When she talked about becoming a remote area nurse and working in his community, it made her dad very happy and proud. She confesses she sometimes wonders whether the desire to work as a remote area nurse is really her dream or her father's dream for her.

TABLE 5.14 **COMPLAINT**	
Analogy: Skin of the apple	**Complaint:** Define the presenting complaint and symptoms; understand the complaint *Menstrual pain*
AREAS OF INVESTIGATION AND EXAMPLE QUESTIONS	**CLIENT RESPONSES**
Onset	Menstrual problems started 5 years ago and are worsening
Timing	Pain occurs prior to her period and during her menstrual bleed
Exacerbating factors *Have you noticed anything that makes your symptoms worse?*	*If I'm standing up for a lot of time and doing hard physical work.*
Relieving factors *Have you noticed anything that makes your symptoms better?*	*Ibuprofen, rest and heat packs.*
Location and duration *Can you tell me where you experience the pain and how long it lasts?*	*Lower back before my period and then in my lower abdomen and down into my legs during my period. It starts to get better in the last couple of days of my period.*
Rating scale *Can you rate your pain on a scale of 10, with 1 being no pain and 10 being the worst pain you have ever had?*	*Before my period, the back pain is probably a 5 or 6 and sometimes during my period it gets to an 8.*

TABLE 5.15 **CONTEXT**	
Analogy: Flesh of the apple	**Context:** Put the presenting complaint into context to understand the disease
AREAS OF INVESTIGATION AND EXAMPLE QUESTIONS	**CLIENT RESPONSES**
Family health *Does anyone else in your family have similar problems?*	*I don't think so.*

▶

Trauma and pre-existing illness *Have you ever had trauma to your abdominal or pelvic area?*	*No.*
Recreational drug use *Do you ever take recreational drugs?*	*Not for years.*
Surgery and hospitalisation *Have you ever had surgery or been in hospital?*	*No.*
Occupational toxins and hazards *What kind of cleaning chemicals do you use at work?*	*A few. I always wear gloves and sometimes a mask if it smells really bad. I haven't really asked my boss much about the chemicals we use.*
Infection and inflammation *Have you noticed your bowel motions floating in the toilet bowl with mucus?* (inflammation, pancreatic disorder)	*Not that I've noticed, sometimes they seem to float more.*
Stress and neurological disease *Do you experience more diarrhoea in times of emotional stress?* (nervous diarrhoea with no presence of blood or mucus in stool)	*Yes, I'm scared I might lose my job because I've taken so much time off work. Maybe that would be a good thing because it would make me go back to study.*
Eating habits and energy *Tell me about your daily diet and energy levels.*	Cathy's diet consists of significant amounts of refined carbohydrates, animal protein and smaller amounts of whole grains, fruit and vegetables. She doesn't eat fish often and knows she should drink more water. She has about three cups of coffee a day, and more when she is working. She says her energy levels are good most of the month but not good during her period.

TABLE 5.16 **CORE**	
Analogy: Core of the apple with the seed of ill health	**Core:** Holistic assessment to understand the client
AREAS OF INVESTIGATION AND EXAMPLE QUESTIONS	**CLIENT RESPONSES**
Support systems *Apart from your aunt, who would you go to for support?*	*My older brothers, and my mother's family.*

▶

Emotional health *How do you feel you are emotionally at the moment?*	I'm better than I was a few years ago, but I still get really sad sometimes when I think of my children (if I ever have any) not having grandparents.
Stress release *When you feel stressed what do you do?*	Sometimes I go for a swim or a bike ride and sometimes I talk to my aunt, we're really close.
Family and friends *Tell me more about your other family.*	I am very close to my brothers but neither lives close. I have some friends from work I go out with sometimes and I still keep in touch with a couple of friends from school.
Education and learning *What do you understand about your menstrual problems and what might be causing them?*	I don't really understand it. Maybe if I studied nursing I would understand it better. I think maybe there is something to do with stress since it got much worse after my parents passed away.
Long-term goals *Do you have any long-term goals?*	I don't know, maybe I'm a bit confused about my life and what I'm supposed to be doing. I think I want to study nursing, but maybe I'm only thinking that because I know it would make dad happy and I don't want to be a cleaner for the rest of my life. I think I'd like to have a family like my aunt, but there isn't anyone special in my life right now and sometimes I think there never will be.
Has not been well since *How do you feel your parent's death has impacted your health?*	I think the stress has made my periods worse since the pain got really bad after their accident. I think I struggle with depression sometimes too because of it.

TABLE 5.17 **CATHY'S SIGNS AND SYMPTOMS**	
Pulse	90 bpm
Blood pressure	100/70
Temperature	36.8°C
Respiratory rate	14 resp/min
Body mass index	20
Waist circumference	71 cm
Face	Pale
Urinalysis	No abnormality detected (NAD)

TABLE 5.18 RESULTS OF MEDICAL INVESTIGATIONS [1–4, 7, 10, 11]	
TEST	RESULT
Pelvic and abdominal examination	Tender on palpation
Urinalysis	NAD
Human chorionic gonadotropin (HCG) to test pregnancy, ectopic pregnancy	Negative
Full blood count	NAD
ESR	Raised
Progesterone level	Test 7 days before menstruation revealed ovulation *Result:* low reading
Oestradiol	*Raised:* pregnancy, ovarian tumour, testicular tumour, adrenal tumour, endometriosis [45] ***Ruled out:*** *Normal result:* PCOS, weight loss, excess exercise *Low:* PCOS, polycystic ovarian disease, ovarian failure, anorexia nervosa, weight loss, excess exercise, hypothyroidism, Cushing's syndrome, adrenal hyperplasia, menopause, Turner's syndrome, failing pregnancy, fetal death
FSH (follicle-stimulating hormone)	*Normal result:* PCOS, pregnancy, anorexia, weight loss, excess exercise, endometriosis ***Ruled out:*** *Raised:* ovarian failure, menopause *Low:* polycystic ovarian disease, anorexia, weight loss, excess exercise, hypothyroidism, Cushing's syndrome, adrenal tumour/hyperplasia
LH (luteinising hormone): due to pulsatile action of this hormone it may not be accurately measured on one random sample	*Normal result:* pregnancy, anorexia, weight loss, excess exercise, endometriosis ***Ruled out:*** *Raised:* PCOS, polycystic ovarian disease, Ovarian failure, menopause *Low:* anorexia, weight loss, excess exercise, hypothyroidism, Cushing's syndrome, adrenal tumour/hyperplasia
PRL (prolactin): common in secondary amenorrhoea to be raised	*Normal result:* ovarian failure, anorexia, weight loss, excess exercise, adrenal tumour/ hyperplasia, endometriosis ***Ruled out:*** *Raised:* PCOS (mildly), hypothyroidism, Cushing's syndrome, pregnancy, amenorrhoea *Low:* pituitary destruction from tumour
Testosterone	*Normal:* ovarian failure, anorexia, weight loss, excess exercise, hypothyroidism, pregnancy, endometriosis ***Ruled out:*** *Raised:* PCOS, Cushing's syndrome, adrenal tumour/hyperplasia, ovarian tumour *Low:* corticosteriod use

▶

SHBG (sex hormone-binding globulin)	*Normal result:* low SHBG would indicate the presence of elevated levels of free androgens
CA-125 serum marker	*Raised:* can indicate ovarian cancer, endometriosis, pelvic inflammatory disease
Abdominal and pelvic x-ray/ultrasound [61]	Revealed no acute cholecystitis, aortic aneurysm, acute appendicitis, PCOS, ovarian mass, ovarian cyst or tumour, retroverted uterus, tubo-ovarian abscesses, fibroids, trauma
Laparoscopy and biopsy/culdoscopy	Positive for endometriosis lesions
Cervical pap smear	Regular check for cervical cancer

TABLE 5.19 UNLIKELY DIAGNOSTIC CONSIDERATIONS [1–5, 7, 9, 55]

CONDITIONS AND CAUSES	WHY UNLIKELY
CANCER AND HEART DISEASE	
Ovarian, pituitary or adrenal tumour: will affect androgen levels, produce symptoms of irregular cycles, lower abdominal pain [59]	Full blood count NAD; no changes in smell or taste, headaches mentioned indicating a brain tumour; no significant increased facial hair, depression, weight gain
Abdominal aneurysm **Phlebitis of iliac veins and inferior vena cava:** deep pain in lumbosacral region; can cause acute pain if likely to rupture; steady pain; pain on standing, aching in the groin; history of taking the OCP could be risk factor	Usually indicated in older age groups; unknown if Cathy has previously taken the OCP; abdominal ultrasound clear
Neoplasm: spinal cord, lumbar, Hodgkin's lymphoma, metastatic carcinoma, myeloma, haematoma	Full blood count NAD; no history of primary cancer
OBSTRUCTION AND FOREIGN BODY	
Intestinal obstruction (bowel cancer, adhesions, hernias): abdominal distension and pain	Abdominal ultrasound showed no obstructions; no vomiting or weight change
DEGENERATIVE AND DEFICIENCY	
Anaemia	Full blood count NAD
INFECTION AND INFLAMMATION	
Inflammatory bowel disease: Crohn's disease, diverticulitis, ischaemic colitis, regional ileitis, amoebic colitis, autoimmune granulomatous colitis; ESR raised	No sign of anaemia of chronic disease; abdominal ultrasound did not reveal signs of bowel inflammation
Pelvic inflammatory disorder: abdominal pain, could be from a sexually transmitted disease; causes abdominal pain; irregular periods, lower backache; ESR raised	Purulent vaginal discharge, need to be sexually active; physical exam revealed no motion of cervix

▶

Appendicitis/Meckel's diverticulum: intermittent lower abdominal pain, constipation; common age group	Abdominal ultrasound showed no signs of inflammation at appendix
Cystitis: abdominal pain, ESR raised	Urinalysis NAD
ENDOCRINE/REPRODUCTIVE	
Diabetes: anovulatory cycles	Urinalysis NAD
Hypothyroidism: cause of secondary amenorrhoea due to hyperprolactinaemia and endocrine disorder; anovulatory cycles sadness, fatigue, constipation	Thyroid function tests revealed no abnormality; no weight gain, increased facial and body hair (hirsutism), weight gain; no skin and hair changes mentioned; no significant temperature intolerance or visible goitre noted
Pregnancy: irregular periods; missed periods; most common cause of secondary amenorrhoea; can present with vaginal discharge and pelvic/abdominal pain [59]	Negative HCG blood test; can present with fever; may have signs of breast tenderness and may have morning sickness
Ectopic pregnancy: irregular periods; can present with no pain (rare) and can leak over several days slowly; may be missed; common cause of secondary amenorrhoea; usually associated with severe and acute abdominal pain, abdominal fullness, increased desire to urinate; may have signs of fever and dull headaches	Negative HCG blood test
Primary dysmenorrhoea: period pain and watery stools with menstrual bleed [53, 58]	Period pain usually begins with menarche and is often associated with no pelvic abnormality, nausea vomiting, headache and dizziness
Twisted uterine fibroids and polyps: twisted fibroids can cause symptoms of severe dysmenorrhoea, heavy bleeding, back pain and sometimes vaginal discharge	Usually maintains normal cycle unless submucosal or nearly extruded; causes uterine enlargement; usually causes menorrhagia (blood loss of 80 mL per day and lasting more than 7 days); fibroids form due to excess oestrogen; unless twisted, fibroids do not usually present with pain
Anovulatory bleeding: irregular bleeding that appears to be menstrual although no ovulation has occurred; can be associated with both short and long cycles; blood volume can be excessive but irregular [51]	Usually no significant premenstrual symptoms reported to show evidence of regular association with menses cycle; bleed is painless; physical findings will often include hirsutism, acne, and indicate PCOS; hormonal tests revealed ovulation is occurring
Polycystic ovarian syndrome (PCOS): extremely common cause of secondary amenorrhoea; anovulatory cycles; irregular menstrual cycles, lower abdominal pain	No signs of significant hormonal acne, increased facial and body hair (hirsutism), sugar cravings, weight gain; hormonal levels did not show raised androgens

▶

▶

Ovarian disease: premature menopause often due to autoimmune disease; menses beginning to change; can present with symptoms of menopause and irregular periods	No hot flushes; blood tests did not reveal hormone levels as menopausal
Adenomyosis (benign invasion of endometrium into myometrium)	Common complaint that often does not cause symptoms; more often in late reproductive years; heavy bleeding common
Retroverted uterus (congenital): pelvic pain	Abdominal ultrasound showed uterus not retroverted

TABLE 5.20 CONFIRMED DIAGNOSIS [1–4]	
CONDITION	RATIONALE
Secondary dysmenorrhea (acquired due to a pathology)	Period pain begins several years after menarche and is due to a pelvic abnormality
Endometriosis	Irregular periods, severe episodes of pain before and during menstrual bleed, bleeding from the bowel, lower back pain; pain on passing a bowel motion; period pain becomes worse with every cycle; pelvic and lower back pain
Test results	Laparoscopy revealed endometrial lesions; ESR blood test raised; raised oestradiol levels; low progesterone reading

Case analysis

TABLE 5.21 POSSIBLE FURTHER DIFFERENTIAL DIAGNOSIS [1–4, 6, 9, 55]		
Not ruled out by tests/investigations already done		
CONDITIONS AND CAUSES	WHY POSSIBLE	WHY UNLIKELY
TRAUMA AND PRE-EXISTING ILLNESS		
Causal factor: Trauma: recent curettage, foreign body insertion, sexual abuse, aggressive masturbation	Pelvic and lower back pain; rectal bleeding	No history of pregnancy or sexual abuse revealed at this stage
Causal factor: Trauma: strains, sprains, tear, herniated disc, fracture, disc prolapse	Work strain and lower back pain; standing for long periods of time at work	

▶

▶

Congenital disorders: spina bifida, scoliosis, spondylolisthesis	Lower back pain	
FUNCTIONAL DISEASE		
Irritable bowel syndrome	Symptoms fluctuate between constipation and diarrhoea; bloating, abdominal distension and pain	Pain not necessarily relieved by passing a bowel motion
Causal factor: Faulty posture	Strain and standing for long periods of time at work	
Haemorrhoids	Rectal bleeding	Unsure whether the bleeding is mixed in the stools or from the rectum
Colon polyps	Bleeding, changes in bowel habit, pain in passing a stool	Unsure of the colour of blood and stools
Anal fissures	Painful bowel motions, rectal bleeding; lower back pain	Unsure whether Cathy's bleeding is mixed in the stools or from the rectum
DEGENERATIVE AND DEFICIENCY		
Degenerative and deficiency diseases: osteomalacia, osteoporosis, osteoarthritis, lumbar spondylosis [56]	Lower back pain, physical strain at work; lumbar spondylosis can be symptomless or cause progressive spinal pain and stiffening; ESR blood reading raised	No diagnosed risk factors such as inflammatory bowel disease, vitamin D deficiency; no known familial tendency for osteoarthritis or osteoporosis at this stage
INFECTION AND INFLAMMATION		
Inflammatory lower back pain: fibromyositis, osteomyelitis, spinal, tubo-ovarian or rectal abscess, myelitis, ankylosing spondylitis	Lower back pain; ESR raised	Requires further investigation
ENDOCRINE/REPRODUCTIVE		
Infertility	May be a secondary issue from endometriosis due to distortion of pelvic cavity, impaired ovum pick up and tubal transport mechanisms, increased incidence of luteal phase dysfunction, trapped oocyte, increased peritoneal prostaglandin production and/or increased peritoneal macrophage activity	No history of attempting to become pregnant; unknown at this time

▶

Premenstrual syndrome	Feels teary, bloated and swollen 1–12 days before period; experiences a dull pelvic ache, abdominal bloating	Symptoms not necessarily ameliorated after menses begins
Ovulatory bleed: check basal body temperature – will be biphasic and fluctuate, indicating ovulation has occurred	Feels emotional, premenstrual symptoms such as ovulation pain (mittelschmerz) and mood changes	Has a bleed mid-cycle as well as regular menses and ovulation has occurred; usually spotting or a light bleed at the time of ovulation, regular cycle
Dsyfunctional uterine bleeding (DUB): [60] endometrial hyperplasia, PCOS, from taking exogenous oestrogen; endocrine dysfunction not associated with inflammation, tumour or pregnancy	Usually causes unpredictable frequency and amount of bleeding	No use of exogenous oestrogen reported; menorrhagia (heavy bleed with regular cycle) is common but the interval between periods is usually shorter
AUTOIMMUNE DISEASE		
Coeliac disease	Fluctuation between constipation and diarrhoea, feels bloated; abdominal pain	No indication symptoms become worse with diet
STRESS AND NEUROLOGICAL DISEASE		
Psychogenic back pain	Cathy is not happy with her employment	
Depression	Lack of social support, unhappy in employment, not confident she could have a relationship	
Posttraumatic stress disorder	Parents' sudden death 4 years ago changed her life significantly; stress can contribute to premenstrual symptoms [54, 57]	
Anxiety	Cathy spends most of her time with her aunt; lack of social network; Cathy is worried about how her health is affecting her employment	
Low self-esteem	Cathy does not believe she will meet the right person to have a relationship with	

Working diagnosis

CATHY AND ENDOMETRIOSIS

Cathy is a young woman showing signs of low self-esteem and depression after the death of her parents four years ago. Cathy has experienced worsening reproductive symptoms that suggest endometriosis. This is a benign disease where functioning endometrial tissue is present in sites outside of the uterine cavity. Endometriosis is usually confined to the surfaces of intra-abdominal organs, most commonly the ovaries, posterior broad ligament, posterior cul-de-sac and the uterosacral ligaments. Less commonly it can be found in the small and large bowel, ureters, bladder, vagina, surgical scars and pleural cavity. A retrograde flow of menstrual tissue through the fallopian tubes may cause intra-abdominal endometriosis and lymphatic and circulatory systems may contribute to endometriosis reaching more distant areas in the body. It often develops for women aged 25–45 years who are menstruating and there may be family inheritance pattern and/or late child-bearing. Clinical symptoms that develop include secondary dysmenorrhoea, irregular periods and infertility. Symptoms of endometriosis can range from being asymptomatic to incapacitating pain that can occur after several years of pain-free periods. If endometrial lesions are in the large bowel or bladder symptoms can worsen at the time of menses to include pain on passing a bowel motion, rectal bleeding, abdominal bloating or pain on urination. Bleeding from the endometrial tissue is believed to set up an inflammatory process that causes adhesion formation.

General references used in this diagnosis: 1–4, 45

TABLE 5.22 **DECISION TABLE FOR TREATMENT PRIOR TO REFERRAL**		
COMPLAINT	**CONTEXT**	**CORE**
Treatment for the presenting complaint and symptoms	Treatment for all associated symptoms	Treatment for mental, emotional, spiritual, constitutional, lifestyle issues and metaphysical considerations
TREATMENT PRIORITY	**TREATMENT PRIORITY**	**TREATMENT PRIORITY**
• Acute herbal tea or tonic to be taken during the menstrual bleed. • Lifestyle and self-care practices to help manage acute pain • Physical therapy recommendations to help manage acute pain	• Dietary recommendations to improve general health, hormonal balance and to reduce inflammation • Lifestyle and self-care practices to improve health and wellbeing and help improve reproductive health	• Lifestyle recommendations to address underlying emotional/psychological issues • Physical therapy suggestions to support Cathy's stress response and emotional health

TABLE 5.23 **DECISION TABLE FOR REFERRAL [1–5, 8, 9]**		
COMPLAINT	**CONTEXT**	**CORE**
Referral for presenting complaint	Referral for all associated physical, dietary and lifestyle concerns	Referral for contributing emotional, mental, spiritual, metaphysical, lifestyle and constitutional factors

▶

REFERRAL FLAGS	REFERRAL FLAGS	REFERRAL FLAGS
• Blood from the rectum during menstruation	• Experiences back pain before her period	• Cathy does not believe she can have an intimate relationship
ISSUES OF SIGNIFICANCE	**ISSUES OF SIGNIFICANCE**	**ISSUES OF SIGNIFICANCE**
• Cathy did not feel comfortable to let her GP know about the rectal bleeding	• Back pain is significant enough to be affecting her employment responsibilities • Digestion is not optimal and Cathy experiences both constipation and diarrhoea episodes	• Cathy has concerns about her job security • Spending more time at her aunt's house than her own home
REFERRAL	**REFERRAL**	**REFERRAL**
• Referral to a GP for another opinion on the bleeding	• Suggest musculoskeletal assessment • Suggest digestive assessment	• Suggest Cathy seeks counselling to deal with underlying anxiety and emotional problems

TABLE 5.24 FURTHER INVESTIGATIONS THAT MAY BE NECESSARY [1–4, 7, 10, 11, 56]

TEST/INVESTIGATION	REASON FOR TEST/INVESTIGATION
FIRST-LINE INVESTIGATIONS:	
Musculoskeletal assessment	Deformity, joint movement/pain or swelling, muscle wasting or weakness, gait abnormalities, structure of spine and movement, general posture
Neurological assessment	Assess speech, language, facial expression, neck stiffness, orientation, memory, judgement and reasoning, cranial nerves, motor function (reflexes and tone), coordination, sensory function of skin, joints and temperature feeling, general observation of mood and behaviour
Stool test	Rule out parasitic infections and occult blood that suggests possible diagnosis of diverticulosis, ulcers, polyps, inflammatory bowel disease, and GI tumour, haemorrhoids, *H. pylori*; if acidic stools are passed it indicates lactose intolerance
Basal body temperature	Normally drops 24–36 hours after menses begins; with endometriosis there is often a delay in basal body temperature to the second or third day of menses [3]
IF NECESSARY:	
Sigmoidoscopy	Haemorrhoids, polyps, anal fissures, irritable bowel syndrome, Crohn's disease
Back x-ray, CT scan and MRI	Degenerative disc disease, disc prolapse, ankylosing spondylitis, Paget's disease, osteoporosis
Serum alkaline phosphatase, plasma calcium, serum phosphate, serum 25-hydroxyvitamin D3	Osteomalacia, Paget's disease

Confirmed diagnosis

Cathy has endometriosis with premenstrual syndrome.

PRESCRIBED MEDICATION

• Oral contraceptive pill [52]

Cathy has chosen not to take the OCP at this stage, preferring to try natural therapies first. It is imperative that Cathy's case is managed collaboratively with her GP to ensure appropriate and effective monitoring and treatment of her condition.

TABLE 5.25 DECISION TABLE FOR TREATMENT (ONCE DIAGNOSIS IS CONFIRMED)		
COMPLAINT	**CONTEXT**	**CORE**
Treatment for the presenting complaint and symptoms	Treatment for all associated symptoms	Treatment for mental, emotional, spiritual, constitutional, lifestyle issues and metaphysical considerations
TREATMENT PRIORITY	**TREATMENT PRIORITY**	**TREATMENT PRIORITY**
• Continue with lifestyle and self-care practices for acute pain management as necessary • Continue with physical therapy recommendations for acute pain management as necessary • Continue with acute herbal tea or tonic as required during the menstrual bleed; acute formula reviewed after three months • Continue with dietary recommendations to improve reproductive health and hormonal balance and to reduce inflammation • Continue with nutritional supplements to reduce inflammation and regulate hormone balance; to be reviewed after 3 months **NB:** Cathy's vitamin and mineral levels should be monitored to ensure her levels stay within normal range; supplementation dosage can be reviewed if necessary	• Continue with lifestyle and self-care practices to improve general health and wellbeing and reproductive system health • Continue with dietary recommendations to improve general health, nutrition, hormonal balance and manage food allergies or intolerances (if present) • Continue with physical therapy suggestions to improve general health, enhance detoxification and improve hormonal balance and reproductive health • Herbal tonic or tea with hormonal balancing, detoxification, anti-inflammatory, immunomodulatory and spasmolytic action; to be reviewed after three months; dong quai in Cathy's herbal tonic is contraindicated in heavy menstrual bleeding so her menstrual bleeding should be monitored to ensure there are no problems; reformulate tonic if necessary and review formula after four months of treatment • Nutritional supplements to modulate the immune response, improve digestive health and hepatic detoxification; to be reviewed after 3 months	• Recommendation for counselling to help Cathy deal with her grief and anxieties • Multivitamin support for general health and nervous system support • Regular exercise, massage, acupuncture, meditation and visualisation exercises • Self-care help to increase relaxation and cleansing

Treatment aims

- Relieve pain [13].
- Reduce inflammation at the site of the endometriosis [13, 15].
- Stop further growth of endometriosis, and prevent new growth in other areas [13].
- Normalise Cathy's immune response and identify and manage allergies [9, 50].
- Balance hormones: normalise oestrogen levels [14], enhance clearance of oestroen via liver and bowel [15, 9].
- Improve uterine tone and function; initiate orderly uterine contractions, encourage expulsive uterine action and reduce excessive/abnormal uterine spasm [15].
- Rectify prostaglandin imbalance [15].
- Maintain or restore fertility [15].
- Support Cathy's nervous system, emotional health and stress response.
- Identify and manage any environmental exposure/toxicity that may be contributing to Cathy's endometriosis [33, 34].

Lifestyle alterations/considerations

- Encourage Cathy to take up regular exercise [15].
- Functional breathing exercises [46].
- Cathy may benefit from counselling to deal with the grief associated with the loss of her parents and to work through issues surrounding her desire to study nursing.
- Cathy should avoid using tampons. There is a link between the long-term use of tampons and endometriosis [33].
- Encourage Cathy to minimise her exposure to environmental toxins and xeno-oestrogens, which have been implicated in the development of a variety of hormonal imbalances and reproductive problems [33, 34].
- Skin brushing to encourage circulation and detoxification [40].
- Suggest Cathy uses stress-management techniques such as meditation and visualisation exercises [15].
- Encourage wider social support and group activities that interest Cathy [15].

Dietary suggestions

- Reduce consumption of sugar, dairy foods and red meat [9].
- Increase consumption of soluble fibre [9] and omega-3 essential fatty acids [9, 15].
- Eliminate or significantly reduce consumption of caffeine [25] and alcohol [26].
- Increase consumption of indole-3 carbinole-containing foods (cruciferous vegetables), which help modify oestrogen metabolism [9, 24, 49] and foods that enhance phase 2 liver function to support oestrogen clearance [9, 15]. Adding turmeric to food can help increase bile secretion and decrease inflammation [9, 17, 19].
- Increase consumption of phytoestrogen-rich foods and lignans, which can competitively inhibit endogenous oestrogen and help improve hormonal balance [9, 47, 48].
- Consider a withdrawal challenge followed by an elimination/rotation diet for Cathy. Women with endometriosis have a higher incidence of allergies [27].
- Encourage Cathy to eat a whole-food diet containing plenty of antioxidant-rich foods [28, 29].

Physical treatment suggestions

- Cathy may benefit from a course of acupuncture to assist with hormonal balance and stress management [35].

- Hydrotherapy: for acute period pain spray the pelvis area with a hot hand shower for two minutes, then alternate and spray with cold water for one minute (repeat three times) [40]. Apply a hot compress/fomentation on the back during menstrual pain [40]. Place a warm castor oil pack on the abdomen/pelvic area for menstrual cramps and abdominal discomfort [40].
- A hot foot bath will stimulate menstrual bleed [42].
- Hot sitz baths will ease pain and stimulate menstrual bleed [42, 43].
- Between periods, apply weekly contrasting treatments with a hot fomentation on the back and abdomen for 15 minutes, followed by 30-second cold mitten friction. Next, apply heat to the pelvic area and back for another 15 minutes, repeat cold mitten friction with the client in the side lying position (repeat alternating procedure three times) then follow with an abdominal massage [40].
- Constitutional hydrotherapy: lumbar wrap [41, 44].

HERBAL FORMULA (1:2 LIQUID EXTRACTS)

Given the complex aetiology of, and symptom management required for, this condition, it is likely to be necessary to provide Cathy with two different formulas. One to be taken during her period to assist with symptom relief, and the other to be taken the rest of the month to balance hormones and address underlying causes.

TABLE 5.26 **HERBAL TONIC TO BE TAKEN DURING THE MONTH**		
HERB	**FORMULA**	**RATIONALE**
Dong quai *Angelica sinensis*	40 mL	Anti-inflammatory [15, 16]; regulates uterine function [15, 16]; traditionally used for dysmenorrhoea [17, 18]; contraindicated if there is a tendency to excessive bleeding or heavy menstrual bleeding [18]
Paeony *Paeonia lactiflora*	55 mL	Antispasmodic [15, 18]; anti-inflammatory [15, 18]; traditionally used for dysmenorrhoea [15, 18]
Calendula *Calendula officinalis*	20 mL	Spasmolytic [20]; anti-inflammatory [19, 20]; emmenagogue [20]; antioxidant [19]; immunomodulator [19]
Schisandra *Schisandra chinensis*	45 mL	Nervine [18]; tonic [18]; adaptogenic [18, 19]; liver tonic [18, 19]; antioxidant [19]; anti-inflammatory [19]; used for improving liver function and improve the detoxifying capacity of the liver [18]; improves mental, physical and sensory performance [18]; indicated for use in hormonal disorders related to oestrogen excess [15]
Ginger *Zingiber officinale*	10 mL	Anti-inflammatory [17, 19]; antioxidant [19]; immunomodulator [19]; anxiolytic [19]; circulatory stimulant [17]; traditionally used for dysmenorrhoea [17, 19]

▶

▶

Rosemary *Rosemarinus officinalis*	30 mL	Hepatoprotective [19]; anti-inflammatory [19]; antioxidant [19, 36]; increases oestrogen metabolism [19, 22]; circulatory stimulant [36]
Supply:	200 mL	Dose: 5 mL 3 times daily

Chaste tree (*Vitex agnus castus*) 1000 mg daily (2 mL of 1:2 liquid extract or as a tablet) Enhances development of corpus luteum and can correct relative progesterone deficiency [17], and in conditions such as endometriosis where oestrogen imbalance is involved [23]

TABLE 5.27 **'ACUTE' HERBAL FORMULA TO BE TAKEN DURING THE BLEED**		
HERB	**FORMULA**	**RATIONALE**
Cramp bark *Viburnum opulus*	30 mL	Spasmolytic [15]; mild sedative [21]
Corydalis *Corydalis ambigua*	60 mL	Analgesic [18]; sedative [18]; used for organ pain, blood stasis and dysmenorrhoea [18]
Pasque flower *Pulsatilla vulgaris*	10 mL	Spasmolytic [20, 37]; analgesic [20, 37]; sedative; traditionally used for inflammation or painful conditions of the female reproductive tract [20, 37]
Supply:	100 mL	Dose: 5 mL 3–5 times daily as required during menstrual period

TABLE 5.28 **HERBAL TEAS**		
Alternative to liquid herbal tonic if Cathy prefers a tea Daily formula		
HERB	**FORMULA**	**RATIONALE**
Calendula flowers *Calendula officinalis*	½ part	See above
Black cohosh root *Cimicifuga racemosa*	1 part	Uterine tonic [17, 20]; antispasmodic [17, 20]; traditionally used for dysmenorrhoea [17, 20]
False unicorn root *Chamaelirium luteum* (cultivated/plantation source)	1 part	Uterine tonic [20, 36]; oestrogen modulating [20, 36]; traditionally used for dysmenorrhoea [20, 36]
Chaste tree berries *Vitex agnus castus*	1 part	See above
Ginger root *Zingiber officinale*	½ part	See above
Decoction: 1 cup 3 times daily		

TABLE 5.29 **HERBAL TEA**

'Acute' herbal formula to be taken during the bleed; alternative to liquid herbal tonic if Cathy prefers a tea

HERB	FORMULA	RATIONALE
Cramp bark *Viburnum opulus*	1 part	See above
Pasque flower *Pulsatilla vulgaris*	1 part	See above
Wild yam root *Dioscorea villosa*	1 part	Spasmolytic [19, 20]; anti-inflammatory [19, 20]; autonomic nervous system relaxant [19]; indicated for dysmenorrhoea and uterine pain [19, 20]

Decoction: 1 cup four times daily during menstrual bleed as required

TABLE 5.30 **NUTRITIONAL SUPPLEMENTS**

Omega-3 fish oil 3 × 1000 mg capsule twice daily [38]	Anti-inflammatory [19, 30, 38, 39]; suppress production of pro-inflammatory cytokines [19]; regulates inflammatory prostaglandin formation [38, 39]; regulates prostaglandin imbalance [30]; indicated for use in dysmenorrhoea [19]
High-potency practitioner-strength **women's multivitamin, mineral and antioxidant** supplement containing therapeutic doses of B-group vitamins, beta carotene and selenium [9, 15] Daily dose as recommended by manufacturer	Women with endometriosis have lower antioxidant levels [28]
Vitamin E 500–800 IU daily [15, 19, 39]	Reduces adhesion formation [31]; aids removal of debris in pelvic fluid via white cells [32]; regulates oestrogen ratio [8]
Vitamin C 6000 mg daily in divided doses [9, 38]	Antioxidant [19, 38, 39]; increases cellular immunity and decreases capillary wall fragility [9, 19, 38]; high doses of vitamin C may help reduce pain [38]
Supplement providing approx 1000 mg **choline bitartrate** and 1000 mg of **dl-Methionine** or **cysteine** 3 times daily [9] May be necessary to support detoxification if tests provide evidence of exposure to toxic chemicals or heavy metals	Lipotrophics; supports liver detoxification functions and aids with removal of oestrogen metabolites and environmental toxins [9, 38, 39]

References

[1] P. Kumar, C. Clark, Clinical Medicine, sixth edn, Elsevier Saunders, London, 2005.

[2] R.D. Collins, Differential Diagnosis in Primary Care, fourth edn, Lippincott Williams & Wilkins, Philadelphia, 2008.

[3] R.H. Seller, Differential Diagnosis of Common Complaints, fifth edn, Saunders Elsevier, Philadelphia, 2007.

[4] R.M.D. Berkow, A.J.M.D. Fletcher, M.H.M.D. Beers, The Merck Manual, sixteenth edn, Merck Research Laboratories, Rathway, N.J, 1993 (later edition).

[5] S.E. Shemy, Naturopathic Standards of Primary Care, CCNM Press, 2008.

[6] N.J. Talley, S. O'Connor, Pocket Clinical Examination, third edn, Churchill Livingstone Elsevier, Australia, 2009.

[7] J. Silverman, S. Kurtz, J. Draper, Skills for Communicating with Patients, second edn, Radcliff Publishing, Oxford, 2000.

[8] D. Peters, L. Chaitow, G. Harris, S. Morrison, Integrating Complementary Therapies in Primary Care, Churchill Livingstone, London, 2002.

[9] J.E. Pizzorno, M.T. Murray, H. Joiner-Bey, The Clinicians Handbook of Natural Medicine, Missouri. second edn, Churchill Livingstone Elsevier, 2008.

[10] H.M. Seidal, J.W. Ball, J.E. Dains, G.W. Benedict, Mosby's Guide To Physical examination, third edn, Mosby, U.S.A, 1995 (later edition).

[11] K.D. Pagna, T.J. Pagna, Mosby's Diagnostic and Laboratory Test reference, third edn, Mosby, USA, 1997 (later edition).

[12] C.A. Winkel, Evaluation and Management of Women with Endometriosis, Obstetrics and Gynecology 102 (2) (2003) 397–408.

[13] S.E. Bulun, B. Gurates, Z. Fang, M. Tamura, S. Sebastian, J. Zhou, et al., Mechanisms of excessive estrogen formation in endometriosis, Journal of Reproductive Immunology 55 (1) (2002) 21–33.

[14] R. Trickey, Women, Hormones & The Menstrual Cycle, second edn, Allen & Unwin, Sydney, 2003.

[15] S.R. Wang, Z.Q. Guo, J.Z. Liao, in: R. Trickey (Ed.), Women, Hormones & The Menstrual Cycle, second edn, Allen & Unwin, Sydney, 2003.

[16] S. Mills, K. Bone, Principles & Practice of Phytotherapy: Modern Herbal Medicine, Churchill Livingstone, Edinburgh, London, 2000.

[17] K. Bone, Clinical Applications of Chinese and Ayurvedic Herbs: Monographs for the Western Herbal Practitioners, Phytotherapy Press, Warwick, 1996.

[18] L. Braun, M. Cohen, Herbs & Natural Supplements: An evidence based guide, second edn, Elsevier, Sydney, 2007.

[19] British Herbal Medicine Association, British Herbal Pharmacopoeia, BHMA, Surrey, 1983.

[20] J.A. Nicholson, T.D. Darby, C.H. Jarboe, Viopudial, a hypotensive and smooth muscle antispasmodic from Viburnum opulus, Proc Soc Exp Biol Med 140 (2) (1972) 457–461.

[21] B.T. Zhu, D.P. Loder, M.X. Cai, C.T. Ho, M.T. Huang , A.H. Conney, Dietary administration of an extract from rosemary leaves enhances the liver microsomal metabolism of endogenous estrogens and decreases their uterotropic action in CD-1 mice, Carcinogenesis 19 (1998) 1821–1827.

[22] K. Bone, Vitex Agnus Castus; scientific studies and clinical applications, Mediherb Professional Review 42 (1994) 1–3.

[23] R.S. Lord, B. Bongiovanni, J.A. Bralley, Estrogen Metabolism and the Diet-Cancer Connection: Rationale for Assessing the Ratio of Urinary Hydroxylated Estrogen Metabolites, Alternative Medicine Review 7 (2) (2002) 112–129.

[24] F. Grodstein, M.B. Goldman, L. Ryan, D.W. Cramer, Relation of female infertility to consumption of caffeinated beverages, Am J Epidemiol 137 (12) (1993) 1353–1360.

[25] M.M. Perper, L.J. Breitkopf, R. Breitstein, R.P. Cody, P. Manowitz, MAST scores, alcohol consumption and gynaecological symptoms in endometriosis patient, Alcohol Clin Exp Res 17 (2) (1993) 272–278.

[26] L. Barclay, Endometriosis linked to autoimmune, other chronic diseases, Human Reproduction 17 (10) (2002) 2715–2724.

[27] F. Verit, O. Erel, N. Celik, Serum paraoxonase-1 activity in women with endometriosis and its relationship with the stage of the disease, Human Reproduction 23 (1) (2008) 100–104.

[28] C.A. Hernandez Guerrero, L. Bujalil Montenegro, J. de la Jara Diaz, J. Mier Cabrera, P. Bouchan Valencia, Endometriosis and deficient intake of antioxidant molecules related to peripheral and peritoneal oxidative stress, Ginecol Obstet Mex 74 (1) (2006) 20–28.

[29] A.P. Simopoulos, Omega-3 Fatty Acids in Inflammation and Autoimmune Diseases, Journal of The American College of Nutrition 21 (6) (2002) 495–505.

[30] F. Kalfarentzos, J. Spiliotis, L. Kaklamanis, J. Tsolakis, J. Androulakis, Prevention of peritoneal adhesion formation in mice by vitamin E, Journal of the Royal College of Surgeons Edinburgh 32 (5) (1987) 288–290.

[31] R.P. Tengerty, Vitamin E in immune response and disease resistance, Annals of the New York Academy of Science 570 (1989) 335–344.

[32] L.S. Birnbaum, A.M. Cummings, Dioxins and Endometriosis: a plausible hypothesis, Environmental Health Perspectives 110 (1) (2002) 15–21.

[33] S.E. Rier, The potential role of exposure to environmental toxicants in the pathophysiology of endometriosis, Annals of the New York Academy of Sciences 955 (2002) 201–212.

[34] E. Highfield, C. Kerr, M. Laufer, R. Schnyer, P. Thomas, P.M. Wayne, Adolescent Endometriosis-Related Pelvic Pain Treated with Acupuncture: Two case reports, J Altern Complement Med 12 (3) (2006) 317–322.

[35] S. Mills, K. Bone, The Essential Guide to Herbal Safety, Elsevier Churchill Livingstone, St Louis, 2005.

[36] R.F. Weiss, Weiss's Herbal Medicine Classic Edition, Thieme, Stuttgart, 2001.

[37] J. Jamison, Clinical Guide to Nutrition & Dietary Supplements in Disease Management, Churchill Livingstone, Edinburgh, 2003.

[38] H. Osiecki, The Nutrient Bible, seventh edn, Eagle Farm: BioConcepts Publishing, 2008.

[39] M. Sinclair, Modern Hydrotherapy for the Massage Therapist, Lippincott Williams & Williams, Baltimore, 2008.

[40] W. Boyle, A. Saine, Lectures in Naturopathic Hydrotherapy, Oregon: Eclectic Medical Publications, 1988.

[41] D.D. Buchman, The complete book of water healing, Contemporary Books, McGraw-Hill Companies, New York, 2001.

[42] L. Chaitow, Hydrotherapy, water therapy for health and beauty, Element, Dorset, 1999.

[43] E. Blake, in: L. Chaitow, E. Blake, P. Orrock, M. Wallden, P. Sinder, J. Zeff (Eds.), Naturopathic Physical Medicine: Theory and Practice for Manual Therapists and Naturopaths, Churchill Livingstone Elsevier, Philadelphia, 2008.

[44] S.E. Bulun, Endometriosis, The N Engl J Med 360 (2009) 268–279.

[45] L. Chaitow, E. Blake, P. Orrock, M. Wallden, P. Sinder, J. Zeff, Naturopathic Physical Medicine: Theory and Practice for Manual Therapists and Naturopaths, Philadelphia, Churchill Livingstone Elsevier, 2008.

[46] K.D. Setchell, Phytoestrogens: the biochemistry, physiology, and implications for human health of soy isoflavones, American Journal of Clinical Nutrition 68 (1998) 1333S–1346S.

[47] M.E. Martin, M. Haourigui, C. Pelissero, C. Benassayag, E. Nunez, Interactions between phytoestrogens and sex steroid binding protein, Life Sciences 58 (5) (1996) 429–436.

[48] S. Fan, Q. Meng, K. Auborn, T. Carter, E. Rosen, BRCA1 and BRCA2 as molecular targets for phytochemicals indole-3-carbinol and genistein in breast and prostate cancer cells, British Journal of Cancer 94 (2006) 407–426.

[49] N. Sinaii, S. Clearly, M. Ballweg, L. Nieman, P. Stratton, High rates of autoimmune and endocrine disorders, fibromyalgia, chronic fatigue syndrome and atopic diseases among women with endometriosis: a survey analysis, Human Reproduction 17 (10) (2002) 2715–2724.

[50] D.T. Baird, Amenorrhoea, Lancet 350 (1997) 275–279.

[51] D.B. Petitti, Combination estrogen-progestin oral contraceptives, N Engl J Med 349 (2003) 1443–1450.

[52] L. French, Dysmenorrhea, Am Fam Physician 71 (2005) 285–291.

[53] L.E. Ross, M. Steiner, A biopsychosocial approach to premenstrual dysphoric disorder, Psychiatr Clin North Am 26 (2003) 529–546.

[54] P.A. Baines, G.M. Allen, Pelvic pain and menstrual related illnesses, Emerg Med Clin North Am 19 (2001) 763–780.

[55] J.A. Kanis, Diagnosis of osteoporosis and assessment of fracture risk, Lancet 359 (2002) 1929–1936.

[56] M. Steiner, Premenstrual syndromes, Annu Rev Med 48 (1997) 447–455.

[57] A.S. Coco, Primary dysmenorrhea, Am Fam Physician 60 (1999) 489–496.

[58] J.R. Albers, S.K. Hull, R.M. Wesley, Abnormal uterine bleeding, Am Fam Physician 69 (8) (2004) 1915–1926.

[59] E. Farrell, Dysfunctional Uterine Bleeding, Aust Fam Physician 33 (11) (2004) 906–908.

[60] M.G. Dodson, Use of transvaginal ultrasound in diagnosing the etiology of menometrorrhagia, J Reprod Med 39 (1994) 362–372.

Menopause

Case history

Maggie Lefevre, 49, has come to the clinic with symptoms of fatigue and hot flushes. Maggie has been experiencing increasing fatigue over the past 12 months and flushes for the past three months. During the day the flushes don't particularly bother her, although she gets a bit sweaty and uncomfortable in bed at night, which is disturbing her sleep.

Maggie and her husband Rene live on a small property where they grow organic produce for the restaurant market. Maggie tells you she met Rene while she was travelling in Europe 27 years ago and they married 25 years ago. For many years they travelled the world and enjoyed a nomadic lifestyle and finally settled down in Australia 13 years ago to grow vegetables and start a family. Unfortunately they weren't able to have a baby. Maggie realises now they probably left it too late to start a family when she was 36 and sometimes wishes they had settled down earlier, although Rene wasn't ready to stop travelling before then even though she was ready to settle down in her early 30s. Maggie does have regrets about this, which are intensifying now that she realises her time for having children has passed.

Maggie's cycle has been changing in the past few years. For as long as she can remember her period lasted for around six days and she had a very regular 28-day cycle. Since she turned 47 her cycle has become irregular and usually only lasts 25–26 days. Her bleed has also changed and she gets a couple of days of spotting before her bleed and when it does start it is heavy for about 36 hours and has clots in it; the bleed then tapers off very quickly and is usually all over by the third or fourth day. Maggie is also noticing vaginal dryness and now needs to use lubricants during intercourse.

When asked about her menstrual and reproductive history, Maggie tells you she has no history of menstrual problems although she had an abortion at the age of 22 when she first met Rene. She has been thinking a lot about missed opportunities recently.

Maggie is also noticing changes to her body; her breasts are starting to sag and her skin is getting dryer and she has put on about 2 kg in the past three years even though she doesn't think her diet or lifestyle have changed. Maggie confesses she is a little concerned about losing her youthful looks. Rene is 10 years older than her but is still very vital and good looking. Maggie quickly adds that Rene has given her no reason to be concerned about this but she is aware he comes into contact with a lot of beautiful younger women in the course of his business. She also feels she is more emotional than she used to be.

Maggie feels her diet is very good. Rene worked as a chef for many years and they mostly eat the organic food they grow on their farm. She drinks wine occasionally and has never smoked.

Maggie has been to her doctor who did some blood tests and told her she is perimenopausal. Although she is still ovulating, her hormone levels are dropping. Maggie's doctor referred her to your clinic when she told him she would prefer natural therapies for her symptoms. Maggie feels natural therapies are more in keeping with her lifestyle as an organic farmer.

TABLE 5.31 **COMPLAINT**	
Analogy: Skin of the apple	**Complaint:** Define the presenting complaint and symptoms; understand the complaint. *Hot flushes* *Fatigue*
AREAS OF INVESTIGATION AND EXAMPLE QUESTIONS	**CLIENT RESPONSES**
Onset *When did you first begin to experience the flushes and fatigue?*	*The flushes have been happening for about 3 months and I've been feeling tired for about 12 months.*
Timing *When and how often do you experience the flushes?* *When do you feel fatigue?*	*I feel the flushes during the day, but they don't particularly bother me. They're more of a problem at night because they are disturbing my sleep.* *I'm feeling tired generally, but since the flushes started it's really hard to get out of bed in the morning because I don't feel refreshed.*

▶

▶

Exacerbating factors *Is there anything that makes your symptoms worse?*	*If the weather is warm I notice the flushes more, and it is always worse at night. I'm tired all the time, but I guess it's probably worse in the morning until I have a coffee.*
Relieving factors *Is there anything that makes your symptoms better?*	*Not really. I suppose if I could get better sleep at night I might not feel so tired in the morning.*

TABLE 5.32 **CONTEXT**	
Analogy: Flesh of the apple	**Context:** Put the presenting complaint into context to understand the disease
AREAS OF INVESTIGATION AND EXAMPLE QUESTIONS	**CLIENT RESPONSES**
Surgery and hospitalisation *Have you every had surgery or been in hospital?*	*I had a pregnancy termination when I was 22. Rene and I had just met and when I found out I was pregnant we both felt we weren't ready to have a child.*
Supplements and side effects of medication *Do you take any supplements or medications?*	*Not usually. I started taking a multivitamin a couple of months ago to see if it would help improve my energy. It did seem to help, but in the past couple of months I've been feeling really tired.*
Endocrine/reproductive *Tell me about your menstrual cycle.*	*For most of my adult life it has been really regular, every 28 days. In the last couple of years it has changed and now it comes every 25 or 26 days and the bleed is much lighter and it doesn't last as long. The other thing that has changed is that in the first couple of days I get clots, but no pain.*
Stress and neurological disease *Do you feel stressed or anxious at the moment?*	*I have started to notice I'm feeling more anxious, particularly in the week before my period. That never used to happen. I'm also feeling a bit anxious about how my body is going to change after menopause.*

TABLE 5.33 **CORE**	
Analogy: Core of the apple with the seed of ill health	**Core:** Holistic assessment to understand the client
AREAS OF INVESTIGATION AND EXAMPLE QUESTIONS	CLIENT RESPONSES
Daily activities *Describe your daily routine.*	*We usually get up around 5.30 to get the vegetables ready to take to the market. Breakfast is at 7 and then we usually work around the house or farm all day if we don't have to go out. I stay home more than Rene. We eat dinner around 6 and are in bed by 9 or 9.30.*
Stress release *How do you manage your stress?*	*I don't usually feel stressed, except for the last few months. Walking or working in the gardens usually helps.*
Occupation *Do you enjoy your work?*	*Yes, we're both doing what we always wanted to do.*
Family and friends *Do you spend much time with family and friends?*	*My sister and her family live close and we have lots of friends in the local area. We have quite an active social life.*
Home life *How are things at home?*	*Rene and I have always gotten along really well, and he has always been a wonderful husband. There is a little more stress at the moment because I get tired and irritable. Sometimes I worry that he might find somebody else more attractive as I get older, but there's never been any problems like that.*
Action needed to heal *How do you think I can help you?*	*I was hoping for some dietary and lifestyle suggestions, and perhaps some herbs to help. I'm willing to try whatever you suggest.*
Long-term goals *What are your long-term goals?*	*I hope we can stay doing what we're doing for as long as possible.*

TABLE 5.34 **MAGGIE'S SIGNS AND SYMPTOMS**	
Pulse	90 bpm
Blood pressure	135/85
Temperature	36.8°C
Respiratory rate	16 resp/min
Body mass index	24.2
Waist circumference	78 cm
Face	Normal appearance, slightly anxious expression
Urinalysis	No abnormality detected (NAD)

TABLE 5.35 RESULTS OF MEDICAL INVESTIGATIONS [2, 7–11, 13]	
TEST	RESULTS
Pelvic, vaginal, abdominal examination	No bulging uterus, rebound tenderness, overactive bowel sounds, genital deformities, signs of trauma
Human chorionic gonadotropin (HCG) blood test/radioimmunoassay (RIA)	No sign of pregnancy or ectopic pregnancy
Full blood count	NAD
CRP/ESR	NAD
Blood cholesterol	Normal range
Female – progesterone level	Low serum progesterone level
Female – oestradiol (the major from of oestrogen in the blood and urine)	*Low*: PCOS, polycystic ovarian disease, ovarian failure, anorexia nervosa, weight loss, excess exercise, hypothyroidism, Cushing's syndrome, adrenal hyperplasia, menopause, Turner's syndrome, failing pregnancy, fetal death
FSH (follicle-stimulating hormone)	*Raised:* ovarian failure, menopause
LH (luteinising hormone)	*Raised:* PCOS, polycystic ovarian disease, ovarian failure, menopause
PRL (prolactin): common in secondary amenorrhoea to be raised	*Normal:* ovarian failure, anorexia, weight loss, excess exercise, adrenal tumour/hyperplasia, menopause
Testosterone	*Normal:* ovarian failure, anorexia, weight loss, excess exercise, hypothyroidism, pregnancy, menopause
Thyroid stimulating hormone	Normal range
Liver function test	Normal range
Cervical smear	Cervical cancer, request STD swabs
Basal body temperature: normally drops 24–36 hours after menses begins; a decrease indicates preovulation and an increase of 5 degrees occurs after ovulation; monitors thyroid function	Revealed pattern of biphasic temperature although temperature had only slight fluctuation

TABLE 5.36 UNLIKELY DIAGNOSTIC CONSIDERATIONS	
CONDITIONS AND CAUSES	WHY UNLIKELY
CANCER AND HEART DISEASE	
Neoplasms: vaginal, uterine cancer, ovarian, adrenal, pituitary; irregular vaginal bleeding in perimenopausal women; can be acyclic with symptoms of menopause [69]	Can be profuse menstrual flow (metrorrhagia); oestradiol was low, CRP normal

▶

INFECTION AND INFLAMMATION	
Cirrhosis or hepatitis: irregular menses, mood swings, fatigue	Liver function test NAD
SUPPLEMENTS AND SIDE EFFECTS OF MEDICATION	
Medications: vaginal bleeding	Several drugs can cause altered menstrual bleeding; Maggie is taking no medication
Progesterone-breakthrough bleeding: when a high-dose progesterone drug is administered	Low progesterone; no drug hormonal drug therapy has been taken
ENDOCRINE/REPRODUCTIVE	
Pregnancy: spotting can precede haemorrhage/spontaneous abortion, irregular periods; until complete menopause still can fall pregnant and experience complications of pregnancy	Pregnancy blood test negative, oestradiol not raised, FSH/LH was raised, prolactin levels normal
Polycystic ovarian syndrome (PCOS): irregular menstrual cycle, weight gain; can present with anovulatory irregular menstrual bleeding	Oestradiol reading was low; FSH was raised; prolactin levels normal; testosterone normal
Hypothyroidism: irregular periods, weight gain and fatigue	FSH/LH was raised; prolactin levels normal; no physical symptoms such as skin or hair changes reported; no constipation, depression, temperature intolerance or visible goitre noted; thyroid-stimulating hormone not raised
Cushing's disease: can present with anovulatory irregular menstrual bleeding and weight gain	FSH/LH was raised; prolactin levels normal; testosterone normal; no physical symptoms such as a moon-shaped face, hirsutism, acne, frontal balding of hair, hypertension, oedema; urinalysis NAD and indicating no glucose intolerance or diabetes
Diabetes: weight gain, fatigue	Urinalysis and fasting blood glucose NAD
Adult-onset adrenal hyperplasia: can present with anovulatory irregular menstrual bleeding	FSH/LH was raised; testosterone normal
Cervical dysplasia: intermenstrual spotting	Cervical smear negative
Uterine fibroids and polyps: heavy bleeding, spasmodic period pain	Often maintains normal cycle unless submucosal or nearly extruded; causes uterine enlargement; usually causes menorrhagia (blood loss of 80 mL per day and lasting more than 7 days); fibroids form due to excess oestrogen; usually symptoms of severe dysmenorrhoea, back pain and sometimes vaginal discharge

▶

Endometriosis: can have profuse or minimal bleeding; irregular menstrual cycle, intermenstrual spotting, infertility	Oestrogen dominance is more common in younger reproductive years; usually has associated symptoms such as severe episodes of pain before and during menstrual bleed, bleeding from the bowel, lower back pain; no vaginal discharge mentioned; oestradiol levels were low
Dysfunctional uterine bleeding (DUB): [69] endometrial hyperplasia, PCOS, from taking exogenous oestrogen; endocrine dysfunction (not associated with inflammation, tumour or pregnancy) anovulatory hormone related bleeding is most common; intermenstrual bleeding	Often presents with menorrhagia (heavy bleed with regular cycle) but interval between periods is shorter to appear irregular [81]; no use of exogenous oestrogen reported; usually causes bleeding that is unpredictable regarding amount and frequency; tests do not reveal an endocrine disorder; oestradiol low
Oestrogen-breakthrough bleeding – 2nd type	Oestrogen levels are well above threshold causing endometrium to become hyperplastic and outgrow blood-borne hormone supply; degeneration of endometrium with prolonged and irregular bleeding occurs; low oestradiol test
Progesterone-withdrawal bleeding: can occur when oestrogen therapy continued and progesterone stopped; also when progesterone is administered to test endogenous oestrogen	Often in PCOS; only occurs when there is an oestrogen-primed endometrium, not likely with low oestradiol; no hormonal drug therapy has been taken
Anovulatory bleeding: irregular cycle, spotting before bleed; menses can be profuse, unexpected and painless; check basal body temperature will not fluctuate (monophasic)	Maggie experiences premenstrual symptoms; slight biphasic temperature fluctuation indicated ovulation still occurring and not stopped completely

Case analysis

TABLE 5.37 **POSSIBLE DIFFERENTIAL DIAGNOSIS**		
NOT RULED OUT BY TESTS/INVESTIGATIONS ALREADY DONE [2, 7–9, 11, 13]		
CONDITIONS AND CAUSES	WHY POSSIBLE	WHY UNLIKELY
FUNCTIONAL DISEASE		
Chronic fatigue syndrome: fatigue for at least 6 months that has no physical basis, psychoses, bipolar affective disorder, eating disorder or organic brain disease	Severe disabling fatigue affects both mental and physical functioning for at least 6 months; sleeping more, depression, crying spells	Need to define whether Maggie experiences fatigue after exertion and she experiences muscular and mental fatigue for at least 24 hours before some level of recovery; need to define if fatigue improves during the day; need to define if Maggie experiences at least two neurological/cognitive manifestations of chronic fatigue syndrome such as impaired concentration and muscle weakness

▶

Functional fatigue –depression [66]	Tiredness that has lasted several months	Need to define if the feeling of fatigue improves during the day
Physiologic fatigue	Can be caused by depression, caffeine, alcohol, excess sleep, intense emotions; diagnostic studies to date are within normal limits with signs of menopause; symptoms present with changes in self-esteem, social difficulties or overall mood; perimenopausal symptoms may be associated with sleep disturbance [67]	Symptoms present as less than 14 days duration
Organic fatigue	Tired, sleep disturbances, no major physical abnormalities	Need to determine if the feeling of fatigue worsens during the day
DEGENERATIVE AND DEFICIENCY		
Osteoporosis: risk much higher after menopause [72]	Oestrogen levels dropping causing perimenopausal symptoms; asymptomatic often unless have accident to indicate low bone density	Check family history of osteoporosis
ENDOCRINE/REPRODUCTIVE		
Ovarian disease: premature menopause often due of autoimmune disease	Menses beginning to change; LH and FSH raised and oestradiol low, prolactin and testosterone levels normal; can present with symptoms of menopause	Maggie is in the typical age group for perimenopause
Ovulatory bleed: usually spotting or light bleed at time of ovulation, regular cycle	Feeling emotional, premenstrual symptoms; basal body temperature is still biphasic and fluctuates slightly, indicating ovulation has occurred	
Oestrogen-withdrawal bleeding: causes intermenstrual bleeding; the endometrium proliferates and becomes unstable when oestrogen drops below the threshold when not in the secretory phase (luteal phase) or in the absence of progesterone	Common cause of irregular bleeds in perimenopausal women due to low progesterone and oestrogen drops; bleed is not necessarily prolonged and profuse	

Oestrogen-breakthrough bleeding – 1st type: when oestrogen levels are low but constant causing sections of endometrium to degenerate	Causes spotting of blood, can be symptom of perimenopause towards complete menopause	Common when taking low-dose OCP and in PCOS
Premenstrual staining in ovulatory cycle	Gets spotting up to 7 days before menses	
STRESS AND NEUROLOGICAL DISEASE		
Mixed anxiety and depressive disorder [66]	Depressive disorder often associated with an experience of loss; grief for not having had children; feeling more emotional, anxious about her body changes, symptoms of fatigue, or intense sadness; numerous physical complaints associated with depression	Has not mentioned significant incapacity to continue daily activities

TABLE 5.38 **CONFIRMED DIAGNOSIS [3, 5, 11]**	
CONDITION	**RATIONALE**
Perimenopausal	Irregular menstrual cycle, fatigue, feeling emotional, hot flushes, weight gain
Test results	Low progesterone and oestradiol; raised FSH/LH

Working diagnosis

MAGGIE AND MENOPAUSE [2, 7–9, 11, 13, 19, 64, 65]

Maggie has been referred by her GP for natural therapies to aid symptoms of perimenopause. Blood tests have confirmed Maggie's hormone levels are dropping which is causing her symptoms of hot flushes, weight gain, fatigue and emotional changes. Maggie reveals in her consultation that not only is she experiencing physical complaints associated with the early stages of menopause, but is also experiencing enormous regret about not having had children. She blames the constant travel she and her husband Rene enjoyed over the years. She feels Rene was not ready to settle down when she was ready and still able to have a family. Maggie has also been feeling more worried about changes to her physical appearance and her attractiveness to Rene. Maggie is generally feeling uncomfortable, is going through a major life transition and is focusing on many regrets.

Menopause means the cessation of menstrual periods and usually occurs naturally between the ages of 45 and 55. During the late fourth decade FSH (follicle-stimulating hormone) and then LH (luteinising hormone) concentrations secreted by the anterior pituitary gland begin to rise as the ovarian follicle supply reduces. Oestrogen levels fall and the menstrual cycle pattern is changed to reduce the chances for ovulation to occur.

During this physical transition women either may experience irregular scanty periods that fluctuate over time, or can have a very sudden cessation of periods. Secondary causes of premature menopause may include surgical procedures to the ovaries, from ovarian disease or from radiotherapy to the ovaries. Additionally it is possible for women to experience premature menopause after a significant emotional shock or physical trauma.

Features of oestrogen deficiency include hot flushes, vaginal dryness and atrophy of the breasts, loss of libido, depression, weight gain and loss of mental focus and concentration. Postmenopausal health complications include a reduction in bone density and reduced protection against ischaemic heart disease.

Menopause is an important and completely natural life stage that often inspires reflection about the reproductive years of life. Women may experience profound changes and can feel the physiological and emotional affects of menopause to be unfamiliar and unsettling. On the other hand, menopause may also be a positive transition into a new phase of life that no longer involves the potential of child-bearing. The experience of menopause varies enormously between women and is best approached as an individual journey in which similar physiological changes are experienced.

TABLE 5.39 **DECISION TABLE FOR TREATMENT PRIOR TO REFERRAL**		
COMPLAINT	**CONTEXT**	**CORE**
Treatment for the presenting complaint and symptoms	Treatment for all associated symptoms	Treatment for mental, emotional, spiritual, constitutional, lifestyle issues and metaphysical considerations
TREATMENT PRIORITY	**TREATMENT PRIORITY**	**TREATMENT PRIORITY**
• Dietary and lifestyle recommendations to reduce severity and incidence of hot flushes and other symptoms associated with perimenopause • Physical therapy suggestions to provide relief from hot flushes and improve sleep • Herbal tea, tonic or tablet to alleviate or reduce hot flushes and improve other symptoms associated with perimenopause such as sleep disturbance and fatigue • Supplemental nutrients to reduce perimenopausal symptoms	• Dietary and lifestyle recommendations to support Maggie's general health and wellbeing, improve energy and reduce the risk of conditions such as cardiovascular disease, osteoporosis and breast cancer • Dietary and lifestyle recommendations to maintain weight within healthy BMI range • Lifestyle recommendations and herbal tonic with adaptogenic properties to help support healthy adrenal function • Herbal tonic and tablets to help reduce breast cancer risk • Supplemental nutrients to support general health and reduce the risk of cardiovascular and other disease • Supplemental minerals to support bone health and reduce the risk of osteoporosis	• Lifestyle and physical therapy recommendations to reduce the symptoms of anxiety and depression • Recommendation for Maggie to try relaxation therapies • Recommendation for Maggie to seek counselling to help her deal with issues surrounding infertility and ageing • Herbal tea, tonic or tablet with anxiolytic, antidepressant and sleep-enhancing actions

TABLE 5.40 **DECISION TABLE FOR REFERRAL [2, 7–9, 12, 13]**		
COMPLAINT	**CONTEXT**	**CORE**
Referral for presenting complaint	Referral for all associated physical, dietary and lifestyle concerns	Referral for contributing emotional, mental, spiritual, metaphysical, lifestyle and constitutional factors
REFERRAL FLAGS	**REFERRAL FLAGS**	**REFERRAL FLAGS**
Nil	• Fatigue began prior to hot flushes by several months indicating it could be from a functional disorder such as depression [67]	• Body image becoming an issue now that she is beginning menopause • Regrets about not having had children prior to menopause
ISSUES OF SIGNIFICANCE	**ISSUES OF SIGNIFICANCE**	**ISSUES OF SIGNIFICANCE**
• Hot flushes are disturbing sleep	• Reduced oestrogen increases the risk of osteoporosis	• Regrets about the impact of previous lifestyle choices on child-bearing • Indication of resentment towards Rene for not wanting to stop travelling to settle down and have children when Maggie was still able to get pregnant
REFERRAL	**REFERRAL**	**REFERRAL**
Nil	• Bone density test to assess osteoporosis risk • Mental health assessment to assess risk of depressive illness	• Counselling to address Maggie's issues of childlessness, her feelings towards Rene and going through menopause

TABLE 5.41 **FURTHER INVESTIGATIONS THAT MAY BE NECESSARY** [2, 6–8, 10, 11, 13, 71]	
TEST/INVESTIGATION	**REASON FOR TEST/INVESTIGATION**
FIRST-LINE INVESTIGATIONS:	
Referral for counselling	Emotional assessment and support
DEXA bone density test	To ascertain the health of her bones and assess what age she is likely to be when she crosses the 'fracture threshold' (this will also give an indication of how much support she needs to maintain or improve bone density)
Basal body temperature: normally drops 24–36 hours after menses begins; a decrease indicates pre-ovulation and an increase of 5 degrees occurs after ovulation; monitors thyroid function	Keep monitoring pattern of biphasic temperature to see if in some months there is a monophasic pattern emerging, although temperature had only slight fluctuation; monitor sub-clinical thyroid dysfunction

►

▶
IF NECESSARY:	
Pelvic ultrasound	Cervical cancer, uterine fibroids, PCOS
Anti-nuclear antibody blood test	Autoimmune disease causing ovarian failure
Progesterone withdrawal test	To determine whether oestrogen is still being produced
Laparoscopy	Rule out endometriosis
Endometrial, vaginal and cervical biopsies	Detect cancer; during luteal phase (10–12 days after ovulation) to determine inadequate luteal phase production or action of progesterone
Brain CT scan/MRI	Rule out pituitary adenoma

Confirmed diagnosis

Perimenopause and organic fatigue not caused by chronic depression.

PRESCRIBED MEDICATION

• Hormone replacement therapy, which Maggie has chosen not to take [68]

TABLE 5.42 **DECISION TABLE FOR TREATMENT (ONCE DIAGNOSIS IS CONFIRMED)**		
COMPLAINT	**CONTEXT**	**CORE**
Treatment for the presenting complaint and symptoms	Treatment for all associated symptoms	Treatment for mental, emotional, spiritual, constitutional, lifestyle issues and metaphysical considerations
TREATMENT PRIORITY	**TREATMENT PRIORITY**	**TREATMENT PRIORITY**
• Continue with dietary and lifestyle recommendations to reduce severity and incidence of hot flushes and other symptoms associated with perimenopause • Continue with physical therapy suggestions to provide relief from hot flushes and improve sleep • Continue with herbal tea, tonic or tablet to alleviate or reduce perimenopausal symptoms • Continue with supplemental vitamins to reduce perimenopausal symptoms **NB:** If Maggie decides to take prescribed HRT the herbal tea, tablet or tonic will need to be reviewed and reformulated; Maggie's condition should be managed collaboratively with her GP to ensure her treatment program is effective and appropriate	• Continue with dietary and lifestyle recommendations to support Maggie's general health and wellbeing, and reduce the risk of cardiovascular disease, osteoporosis and breast cancer • Continue with dietary and lifestyle recommendations to maintain weight within healthy BMI range • Continue with lifestyle recommendations and herbal tonic to support adrenal function and reduce breast cancer risk • Continue with supplemental nutrients to support general health and reduce risk of conditions such as cardiovascular disease and to support bone health	• Continue with lifestyle and physical therapy recommendations to reduce symptoms of anxiety and depression • Continue to recommend relaxation therapies and counselling • Continue with herbal tea, tonic or tablet to help with anxiety, depression and sleep

Treatment aims

- Minimise the impact of reduced oestrogen on Maggie's physical and mental health [14–17, 19].
- Provide relief from or reduction of Maggie's physical symptoms: fatigue, hot flushes, sleep disturbance and vaginal dryness [14–17].
- Support Maggie's adrenal glands. Her adrenal glands will be involved in oestrogen production following menopause [15, 17, 18] so it is important to ensure their continuing healthy function.
- Support Maggie's bone health and reduce her risk of developing osteoporosis [14–17].
- Support Maggie's cardiovascular health and reduce her risk of developing cardiovascular disease [14–17].
- Assist Maggie to maintain her BMI within normal range.
- Support Maggie's mental and emotional health during her transition to menopause [17, 19, 26].
- Support Maggie's health and wellbeing during the perimenopausal period and focus on wellness and disease prevention in her postmenopausal years [14–17].

Lifestyle alterations/considerations

- Encourage Maggie to be physically active every day. Daily physical activity reduces her risk of breast cancer [20]. Daily exercise is also associated with reduced depression and anxiety [14, 16, 21, 22, 29], improved sleep [15, 23] and reduced risk of cardiovascular disease [24]. Exercise may also reduce hot flushes [16, 31].
- Encourage Maggie to include weight-bearing exercise such as walking or strength training in her daily routine. Weight-bearing exercise supports bone health [16, 17, 25], reduces bone mineral loss [17, 25] and reduces fracture risk [25], and can help her to maintain healthy weight [43].
- Encourage Maggie not to eat a very low calorie diet in an effort to lose weight. It may reduce her metabolic rate as the body seeks to conserve energy [4, 16]. Instead encourage her to increase exercise to help maintain her weight in the normal BMI range [43].
- Maggie may gain benefit from relaxation and stress-management therapies such as meditation, yoga and autogenic (self-relaxation) training [28, 56].
- Encourage Maggie to work through her issues surrounding infertility and ageing. Perimenopausal and menopausal women are at significantly greater risk of experiencing depression and anxiety [19, 26] and she is likely to gain benefit from psychological counselling [27, 28, 30].

Dietary suggestions

- Encourage Maggie to increase her intake of dietary phyto-oestrogens [14–17, 55]. Chickpeas and soybeans are particularly good sources of isoflavones [14] along with split peas, mung beans, lentils, broad beans, alfalfa, flax seed and rye. Consuming isoflavone-rich food is associated with reduced hot flushes [17, 34, 36, 37] and vaginal dryness [17, 34, 37] as well as a lower risk for breast cancer [17, 35–37] and cardiovascular disease [14, 36, 37, 40]. Soy has a positive effect on bone health and can help prevent osteoporosis [14, 17, 36, 37, 39].
- Maggie's diet should include sufficient amounts of essential minerals for bone health including calcium, magnesium, silica, boron, zinc, manganese, copper and vitamins C, D and A [14–17].
- Maggie will benefit from a mostly vegetarian Mediterranean diet comprising a high consumption of legumes, fruits, vegetables and whole grains, moderate consumption of alcohol and low consumption of animal protein [16, 17, 38, 42].

- Maggie should ensure she consumes a wide variety of antioxidant-rich whole foods [14–17, 38, 62].
- Maggie should minimise consumption of saturated fats and avoid *trans* fats [15, 16, 38]. She should increase consumption of omega-3 fatty acids to promote cardiovascular, mental and bone health [14–17, 41].

Physical treatment suggestions

- Maggie may find massage helpful to improve her emotional health and sense of wellbeing [32].
- Acupuncture may reduce Maggie's anxiety [28, 33], improve her sleep [33, 44] and reduce hot flushes [44].
- Hydrotherapy: tread in cold water daily (especially first thing in morning and just before bed) [56, 58]. Kneel or briefly sit in cold water to decrease hot flushes and increase energy [56]. Cold sock treatment at night to bring down heat from the upper body [57]. A salt-water hot sponge bath before bed [56]. Neutral baths [57].
- Constitutional hydrotherapy for balancing internal heat in the body [57, 59, 60].

TABLE 5.43 **HERBAL TEA**		
Alternative to herbal liquid tonic if Maggie prefers a herbal tea		
HERB	**FORMULA**	**RATIONALE**
Sage leaf *Salvia officinalis*	1 part	Antihidrotic [17, 36, 46]; traditionally used to reduce sweating [17, 36]; beneficial for night sweats and hot flushes [17, 36]
Passionflower *Passiflora incarnata*	1 part	Anxiolytic [36, 46, 48]; sedative [36, 48]; hypnotic [36, 46, 48]
Zizyphus seed *Zizyphus spinosa*	2 parts	Sedative [17, 49]; hypnotic [49]; traditionally used for night sweats accompanied by anxiety and insomnia [17, 49]
Infusion: 1 tsp per cup – 1 cup 3–4 times daily; may be consumed cold if preferred		

TABLE 5.44 **HERBAL FORMULA (1:2 LIQUID EXTRACTS)**		
HERB	**FORMULA**	**RATIONALE**
Black cohosh *Cimicifuga racemosa*	30 mL	Reduces hot flushes [17, 36, 45, 51]; improves menopausal symptoms [36, 45, 51]; protective against breast cancer [51]
St John's wort *Hypericum perforatum*	60 mL	Nervine [17, 36, 45]; antidepressant [17, 36, 45]; beneficial in emotional symptoms associated with menopause [17, 51]; superior results in alleviating menopausal mood disorders when combined with black cohosh [51]
Shatavari *Asparagus racemosus*	60 mL	Tonic [48, 61]; adaptogenic [48, 61]; sexual tonic [48, 61]; traditionally used in menopause [61]
Zizyphus *Zizyphus spinosa*	50 mL	See above
Supply:	200 mL	Dose: 8 mL twice daily

TABLE 5.45 **TABLET ALTERNATIVE TO HERBAL LIQUID: MAY IMPROVE COMPLIANCE**

HERB	DOSE PER TABLET	RATIONALE
Black cohosh *Cimicifuga racemosa*	250 mg	See above
St John's wort *Hypericum perforatum*	700 mg	See above
Wild yam *Dioscorea villosa*	800 mg	Oestrogenic action [36, 53]; steroidal saponins in wild yam may help alleviate symptoms of oestrogen withdrawal [36, 53]
Lavender *Lavandula angustifolia*	300 mg	Anxiolytic [36, 48]; improves sleep [36]; antidepressant [46, 48]
Dose: 1 tablet at lunchtime, two in the evening		

TABLE 5.46 **NUTRITIONAL SUPPLEMENTS**

SUPPLEMENT AND DOSE	RATIONALE
High-potency practitioner-strength **mineral supplement** for bone health containing calcium, magnesium, zinc, manganese, boron, silica, vitamins D and K Dose as per manufacturer's recommendation, taking into account dietary intake	To provide essential nutrients for bone health [14–17]; particularly indicated if bone densiometry indicates reduced bone density [14, 36, 47]
High-potency practitioner-strength **multivitamin, mineral and antioxidant supplement** providing therapeutic levels of essential micronutrients Dose as per manufacturer's recommendation	To ensure Maggie has optimal levels of essential nutrients and antioxidants to support general health and wellbeing and help reduce the risk of conditions more likely to occur in the postmenopausal years such as cardiovascular disease and cancer [62, 63]
Vitamin E 800 IU daily [36, 54]	Reduces menopausal hot flushes [16, 36, 54]; reduces cardiovascular risk [14, 36, 47, 50]

References

[1] N.J. Talley, S. O'Connor, Pocket Clinical Examination, third edn, Churchill Livingstone Elsevier, Australia, 2009.

[2] P. Kumar, C. Clark, Clinical Medicine, sixth edn, Elsevier Saunders, London, 2005.

[3] J. Silverman, S. Kurtz, J. Draper, Skills for Communicating with Patients, second edn, Radcliff Publishing, Oxford, 2000.

[4] R. Neighbour, The Inner Consultation: how to develop an effective and intuitive consulting style, Radcliff Publishing, Oxon, 2005.

[5] M. Lloyd, R. Bor, Communication Skills For Medicine, third edn, Churchill Livingstone Elsevier, Edinburgh, 2009.

[6] G. Douglas, F. Nicol, C. Robertson, Macleod's Clinical Examination, twelfth edn, Churchill Livingstone Elsevier, Edinburgh, 2009.

[7] J. Jamison, Differential Diagnosis for Primary Care, second edn, Churchill Livingstone Elsevier, London, 2006.

[8] A. Polmear (Ed.), Evidence-Based Diagnosis in Primary Care, Churchill Livingstone Elsevier, Edinburgh, 2008, pp. 274–283.

[9] R.D. Collins, Differential Diagnosis in Primary Care, fourth edn, Lippincott Williams & Wilkins, Philadelphia, 2008.

[10] K.D. Pagna, T.J. Pagna, Mosby's Diagnostic and Laboratory Test reference, third edn, Mosby, USA, 1997 (later edition).

[11] R. Berkow, A.J. Fletcher, M.H. Beers, The Merck Manual, sixteenth edn, Merck Research Laboratories, Rathway, N.J, 1993 (later edition).

[12] D. Peters, L. Chaitow, G. Harris, S. Morrison, Integrating Complementary Therapies in Primary Care, London, Churchill Livingstone, 2002.

[13] R.H. Seller, Differential Diagnosis of Common Complaints, fourth edn, Saunders Elsevier, Philadelphia, 2007.

[14] J. Jamison, Clinical Guide to Nutrition & Dietary Supplements in Disease Management, Churchill Livingstone, Edinburgh, 2003.

[15] H. Osiecki, The Physicians Handbook of Clinical Nutrition, seventh edn, Eagle Farm: Bioconcepts, 2000.

[16] J.E. Pizzorno, M.T. Murray, H. Joiner-Bey, The Clinicians Handbook of Natural Medicine, second edn, Churchill Livingstone, St Louis, 2008.

[17] R. Trickey, Women, Hormones & The Menstrual Cycle, second edn, Allen & Unwin, Sydney, 2003.

[18] F. Al-Azzawi, Endocrinological aspects of the menopause, British Medical Bulletin 48 (2) (1992) 262–275.

[19] E.W. Freeman, M.D. Sammel, L. Liu, C.R. Gracia, D.B. Nelson, L. Hollander, Hormones and Menopausal Status as Predictors of Depression in Women in Transition to Menopause, Archives of General Psychiatry 61 (2004) 62–70.

[20] I. Thune, T. Brenn, E. Lund, M. Gaard, Physical Activity and the Risk of Breast Cancer, The N Engl J Med 336 (18) (1997) 1269–1275.

[21] P. Salmon, Effects of physical exercise on anxiety, depression, and sensitivity to stress: A unifying theory, Clinical Psychology Review 21 (1) (2001) 33–61.

[22] S. El-Hashemy, Naturopathic Standards of Primary Care, CCNM Press Inc, Toronto, 2007.

[23] K. Morgan, Daytime activity and risk factors for late-life insomnia, Journal of Sleep Research 12 (2003) 231–238.

[24] P.D. Thompson, D.B. Buchner, I.L. Pina, G.J. Balady, M.A. Williams, B.H. Marcus, K. Berra, et al., Exercise and Physical Activity in the Prevention and Treatment of Atherosclerotic Cardiovascular Disease A Statement From the Council on Clinical Cardiology (Subcommittee on Exercise, Rehabilitation, and Prevention) and the Council on Nutrition, Physical Activity, and Metabolism (Subcommittee on Physical Activity), Arteriosclerosis, Thrombosis and Vascular Biology 23 (2003) e42–e49.

[25] J. Etherington, P.A. Harris, D. Nandra, D.J. Hart, R.L. Wolman, D.V. Doyle, T.D. Spector, The Effect of Weight-Bearing Exercise on Bone Mineral Density: A Study of Female Ex-Elite Athletes and the General Population, Journal of Bone and Mineral Research 11 (9) (1996) 1333–1338.

[26] N. Sagsoz, O. Oguzturk, M. Bayram, M. Makaci, Anxiety and depression before and after the menopause, Archives of Gynecology and Obstetrics 264 (2001) 199–202.

[27] E. Ward, M. King, M. Lloyd, P. Bower, B. Sibbald, S. Farrelly, M. Gabbay, N. Tarrier, J. Addington-Hall, Randomised controlled trial of nondirective counselling, cognitive behaviour therapy, and usual general practitioner care for patients with depression. I: Clinical effectiveness, British Medical Journal 321 (2000) 1383–1388.

[28] A.F. Jorm, H. Christensen, K.M. Griffiths, R.A. Parslow, B. Rodgers, K.A. Blewitt, Effectiveness of complementary and self-help treatments for anxiety disorders, Medical Journal of Australia 181 (7) (2004) S29–S46.

[29] A. Byrne, G.D. Byrne, The effect of exercise on depression, anxiety and other mood states: A review, J Psychosom Res 37 (6) (1993) 565–574.

[30] I.M. Blackburn, S. Bishop, A.I. Glen, L.J. Whalley, J.E. Christie, The efficacy of cognitive therapy in depression: a treatment trial using cognitive therapy and pharmacotherapy, each alone and in combination, British Journal of Psychiatry 139 (1981) 181–189.

[31] J.R. Guthrie, L. Dennerstein, J.R. Taffe, P. Lehert, H.G. Burger, Hot flushes during the menopause transition: a longitudinal study in Australian-born women, Menopause 12 (4) (2005) 460–467.

[32] T. Field, G. Robinson, F. Scafidi, R. Nawrocki, A. Goncalves, Massage therapy reduces anxiety and enhances EEG pattern of alertness and math computations, International Journal of Neuroscience 86 (1996) 197–205.

[33] D.W. Spence, L. Kayumov, A. Chen, A. Lowe, U. Jain, M.A. Katzman, et al., Acupuncture increases nocturnal melatonin secretion and reduces insomnia and anxiety: A preliminary report, Journal of Neuropsychiatry and Clinical Neurosciences 16 (1) (2004) 19–28.

[34] G. Wilcox, M.L. Tahlqvist, H.G. Burger, G. Medley, Oestrogenic effects of plant foods in postmenopausal women, British Medical Journal 301 (1990) 905–906.

[35] S. Yamamoto, T. Sobue, M. Koboyashi, S. Sasaki, S. Tsugane, Soy, Isoflavones, and Breast Cancer Risk in Japan, Journal of the National Cancer Institute 95 (12) (2003) 906–913.

[36] L. Braun, M. Cohen, Herbs & Natural Supplements: An evidence based guide, second edn, Elsevier, Sydney, 2007.

[37] K.R. Setchell, A. Cassidy, Dietary Isoflavones: Biological Effects and Relevance to Human Health, The Journal of Nutrition 129 (1999) 758S–767S.

[38] S. El-Hashemy, Naturopathic Standards of Primary Care, CCNM Press Inc, Toronto, 2007 pp. 86–93.

[39] F. Branca, Dietary Phytoestrogens and Bone Health, Proceedings of the Nutrition Society 62 (2003): 877–887.

[40] P.A. Kris-Etherton, New Role for Diet in Reducing the Incidence of Cardiovascular Disease: Evidence from Recent Studies, Current Atherosclerosis Reports 1 (1999) 185–187.

[41] B.A. Watkins, Y. Li, H.E. Lippman, M.F. Seifert, Omega-3 Polyunsaturated Fatty Acids and Skeletal Health, Experimental Biology and Medicine 226 (6) (2001) 485–497.

[42] L. Mosca, C.L. Banka, E.J. Benjamin, K. Berra, C. Bushnell, R.J. Dolor, T.G. Ganiats, et al., Evidence-Based Guidelines for Cardiovascular Disease Prevention in Women: 2007 Update, Circulation 115 (2007) 1481–1501.

[43] D.L. Elliot, L. Goldberg, K.S. Kuehl, W.M. Bennett, Sustained depression of the resting metabolic rate after massive weight loss, The American Journal of Clinical Nutrition 49 (1989) 93–96.

[44] M.I. Huang, Y. Nir, B. Chen, R. Schnyer, R. Manber, A randomized controlled pilot study of acupuncture for postmenopausal hot flashes: effect on nocturnal hot flashes and sleep quality, Fertility and Sterility 86 (3) (2006) 700–710.

[45] S. Mills, K. Bone, Principles & Practice of Phytotherapy: Modern Herbal Medicine, Churchill Livingstone, Edinburgh, London, 2000.

[46] British Herbal Medicine Association, British Herbal Pharmacopoeia, BHMAA, Edinburgh, 1983.

[47] H. Osiecki, The Nutrient Bible, seventh edn, Eagle Farm: BioConcepts Publishing, 2008.

[48] S. Mills, K. Bone, The Essential Guide to Herbal Safety, Churchill Livingstone, St Louis, 2005.

[49] K. Bone, Clinical Applications of Chinese and Ayurvedic Herbs: Monographs for the Western Herbal Practitioners, Phytotherapy Press, Warwick, 1996.

[50] J. Higdon, An Evidence Based Approach to Vitamins and Minerals, Thieme, New York, 2003.

[51] V. Briesea, U. Stammwitz, M. Friedec, H. Henneicke-von Zepelin, Black cohosh with or without St. John's wort for symptom-specific climacteric treatment—Results of a large-scale, controlled, observational study, Maturitas 57 (4) (2007) 405–414.

[52] T.R. Rebbeck, A.B. Troxel, S. Norman, G.R. Bunin, A. DeMichele, M. Baumgarten, M. Berlin, et al., A retrospective case-control study of the use of hormone-related supplements and association with breast cancer, International Journal of Cancer 120 (2007) 1523–1528.

[53] M. Morgan, Herbs for the treatment of the symptoms of menopause, A Phytotherapist's Perspective 51 (2009) 1.

[54] T.D. Shanafelt, D.L. Barton, A.A. Adjei, C.L. Loprinzi, Pathophysiology and Treatment of Hot Flashes, Mayo Clinic Proceedings 77 (2002) 1207–1218.

[55] K.M. Newton, D.S. Buist, N.L. Keenan, L.A. Anderson, A.Z. LaCroix, Use of Alternative Therapies for Menopause Symptoms: Results of a Population-Based Survey, Obstetrics and Gynecology 100 (2002) 18–25.

[56] D.D. Buchman, The complete book of water healing, Contemporary Books, McGraw-Hill Companies, New York, 2001.

[57] L. Chaitow, Hydrotherapy, water therapy for health and beauty, Element, Dorset, 1999.

[58] R. Newman Turner, Naturopathic Medicine Treating the Whole Person: The principles and practice of Naturopathy, Herts: HeALL, 2000.

[59] E. Blake, in: L. Chaitow, E. Blake, P. Orrock, M. Wallden, P. Snider, J. Zeff (Eds.), Naturopathic Physical Medicine: Theory and Practice for Manual Therapists and Naturopaths, Philadelphia, Churchill Livingstone Elsevier, 2008.

[60] W. Boyle, A. Saine, Lectures in Naturopathic Hydrotherapy, Oregon: Eclectic Medical Publications, 1988.

[61] K. Bone, M. Morgan, Alternatives to False Unicorn root: Shatavari, Mediherb Professional Review 77 (2001) 3–4.

[62] M.J. Stampfer, F.B. Hu, J.E. Manson, E.B. Rimm, W.C. Willett, Primary prevention of coronary heart disease in women through diet and lifestyle, The N Engl J Med 343 (2000) 16–22.

[63] E. Giovanucci, M.J. Stampfer, G.A. Colditz, D.J. Hunter, C. Fuchs, B.A. Rosner, et al., Multivitamin Use, Folate, and Colon Cancer in Women in the Nurses' Health Study, Annals of Internal Medicine 129 (7) (1998) 517–524.

[64] G.A. Greendale, N.P. Lee, E.R. Arriola, The menopause, Lancet 353 (1999) 571–580.

[65] F. Al-Azzawi, Endocrinological aspects of the menopause, British Medical Bulletin 48 (2) (1992) 262–275.

[66] G.W. Pien, et al., Predictors of sleep quality in menopausal women, SLEEP 31 (7) (2008) 1071–1078.

[67] C.G. Solomon, R.G. Dluhy, Rethinking post-menopausal hormone therapy, N Engl J Med 348 (2003) 579–580.

[68] H. Critchley, P. Warner, A. Lee, et al., Evaluation of abnormal uterine bleeding: comparison of three outpatient procedures within cohorts defined by age and menopausal status, Health Technol Assess 8 (34) (2004) 1–139.

[69] E. Farrell, Dysfunctional Uterine Bleeding, Aust Fam Physician 33 (11) (2004) 906–908.

[70] N. Britten, N.O. O'Flynn, Menorrhagia in general practice – disease or illness?, Social Sci Med 50 (2000) 651–661.

[71] M.G. Dodson, Use of transvaginal ultrasound in diagnosing the etiology of menometrorrhagia, J Reprod Med 39 (1994) 362–372.

[72] J.A. Kanis, Diagnosis of osteoporosis and assessment of fracture risk, Lancet 359 (2002) 1929–1936.

Fertility

Case history

Katie Donaldson and her partner, Adam, are in their early 30s. Katie and Adam have been actively trying to get pregnant for nearly two years and are starting to wonder whether it will ever happen. Katie has come to the clinic by herself on the recommendation of a friend who suggested a natural therapist might be able to help them get pregnant before they need to seek medical intervention. Katie has avoided seeing any complementary therapists because she knows they will tell her to stop smoking; at the moment she is going through a pack a day. Katie tells you that Adam doesn't smoke and is always at her to quit. It seems that the longer it takes her to get pregnant the stronger her cigarette cravings are.

Adam works on an offshore oil rig, and is away for three weeks at a time before coming home for a week. He finds his work mentally and physically draining and would like to find work nearer home. Right now they are saving as much money as they can so they can buy a house and prepare for a baby.

Katie has just completed her law degree and is looking forward to earning a good wage after having been a student for so many years. She wants to have a baby before she gets too old, but she would also like to get on with the career she has worked so hard towards. She says she will put her energy into whatever comes first, although she is aware that her chances of becoming pregnant will reduce once she gets into her mid 30s.

Katie was previously taking the oral contraceptive pill but stopped taking it two and a half years ago when she and Adam decided to start trying for a baby. Her periods have not been regular since she stopped the pill and recently she didn't have a period for four months. During that time she had several pregnancy tests but they were always negative. Katie tells you she has been dieting and exercising because she is concerned about gaining weight. She mentions that she is concerned about the impact pregnancy will have on her weight as she already feels too big (she is actually very slender).

Towards the end of the consultation Katie confides that she has had two abortions: one when she was 16 and the second when she was in her early 30s. She is now wondering whether the abortions may be affecting her ability to get pregnant. She says she hasn't told Adam about the abortions because the first one occurred after she was sexually abused. She hasn't thought about it for a long time but is now concerned that it may be linked with her inability to conceive.

TABLE 5.47 **COMPLAINT**	
Analogy: Skin of the apple	**Complaint:** Define the presenting complaint and symptoms; understand the complaint *Infertility*
AREAS OF INVESTIGATION AND EXAMPLE QUESTIONS	**CLIENT RESPONSES**
Understanding the cause (client) *What do you think is the cause of your fertility problems?*	*I don't really know, but I have read that smoking doesn't help. I also read that sometimes if you've had an abortion it can affect future pregnancies.*
Timing *Do you ever chart your cycle to work out when you are ovulating and most likely to conceive?*	*No. We just try a lot whenever Adam is home from the rig.*

▶

▶ | **Y**our practitioner impression Katie is obviously underweight, with a BMI of 18, which could be contributing to her fertility problems. | |
|---|---|

TABLE 5.48 **CONTEXT**	
Analogy: Flesh of the apple	**Context:** Put the presenting complaint into context to understand the disease
AREAS OF INVESTIGATION AND EXAMPLE QUESTIONS	**CLIENT RESPONSES**
Family health *Is there anyone else in your family who has had fertility problems?*	*I don't think so. My brother and his wife have two children.*
Recreational drug use *Do you ever take recreational drugs? How much alcohol do you usually drink?*	*Not since Adam and I have been trying for a baby. Maybe 3 or 4 drinks on the weekend when Adam is home or if I go out with friends.*
Surgery and hospitalisation *Have you ever had surgery or been hospitalised?*	*Only the abortions I mentioned earlier.*
Infection and inflammation *Have you ever had infections in your urinary or reproductive system?*	*Sometimes I get cystitis or thrush, but not for ages.*
Supplements and side effects of medication *Do you take any supplements or medicines from the pharmacy or prescribed by the doctor?*	*I'm taking a pregnancy multivitamin at the moment, not that it's doing much for me.*
Endocrine/reproductive *Can you tell me about your menstrual cycle?*	Katie describes irregular cycles, with a bleed coming every 6–8 weeks. A few months ago she didn't bleed for 4 months and thought she might be pregnant, but she wasn't.
Stress and neurological disease *Do you feel you are stressed?* *Tell me about your concerns about weight.*	*Yes, I do. I'm really stressed about getting pregnant and if I should get on with my career now. If I get pregnant I worry that I might not be able to lose weight afterwards.* *Well, I work really hard to keep myself slim and lots of people tell me that you can get really fat after you get pregnant.*
Eating habits and energy *Tell me about your diet and energy levels.*	Katie's diet is low in whole foods, fruit and vegetables. She admits she should eat better but often doesn't bother to cook if it is only her at home. When Adam is back she says she eats better. She often skips meals and drinks coffee or Diet Coke to help keep her energy up.

TABLE 5.49 **CORE**	
Analogy: Core of the apple with the seed of ill health	**Core:** Holistic assessment to understand the client
AREAS OF INVESTIGATION AND EXAMPLE QUESTIONS	**CLIENT RESPONSES**
Emotional health *Do you ever feel depressed or anxious?*	*I don't think I'm depressed, but sometimes I worry about what things will be like if we have a baby, and then I worry about how I will ever get a career started.*
Daily activities *Tell me about your daily routine.*	*When I'm home by myself I get up early and go to the gym, then if I'm working I go to work. On the days I'm not working now that I don't have to study I do things around the house or go jogging; sometimes I visit friends.*
Education and learning *Do you understand the factors involved with fertility?*	*I always thought it would just happen with me and Adam since I got pregnant twice before. Maybe he has a problem, I don't know. I have read that you need to be healthy and I'm very fit although I don't always eat properly.*
Action needed to heal *How do you think natural therapies can help you?* *Would you be willing to make dietary and lifestyle changes to help achieve a pregnancy?*	*My friend told me that you have helped other people get pregnant. She said you got them to change their diet and take herbs and tablets and also gave them acupuncture.* *Yes, I think so.*
Long-term goals *What do you see yourself doing in five years?*	*I'd like to have a child and maybe be working part time.*
Time to heal *Sometimes it can take a while for natural therapies to work, will you be OK with that?*	*What do you mean by a while? I would like to have a baby soon.*

TABLE 5.50 **KATIE'S SIGNS AND SYMPTOMS**	
Pulse	85 bpm
Blood pressure	110/70
Temperature	36.9°C
Respiratory rate	14 resp/min
Body mass index	18
Waist circumference	66.5
Face	Pale
Urinalysis	No abnormality detected (NAD)

Results of medical investigations

No investigations have been carried out at this stage.

TABLE 5.51 **UNLIKELY DIAGNOSTIC CONSIDERATIONS** [2, 6–9, 11, 13]	
CONDITIONS AND CAUSES	**WHY UNLIKELY**
CANCER AND HEART DISEASE	
Adult onset and congenital adrenal hyperplasia/adrenal tumour: can present with anovulatory irregular menstrual bleeding; can cause primary and secondary amenorrhoea; anovulatory cycles	Usually presents with severe acne and hirsutism
TRAUMA AND PRE-EXISTING ILLNESS	
Turner's syndrome: no ovaries from birth; congenital condition for females causing no production of eggs for conception; sex chromosome abnormalities	It is likely this would have been reconised in childhood; Katie would never have had a menstrual period and the associated physical features of short statue and a webbed neck are not apparent
Klinefelter's syndrome (Adam): congenital condition for men that causes infertility; sex chromosome abnormalities	It is likely this would have been recognised in childhood, with Adam having physical symptoms of testicular atrophy, gynomastia and learning difficulties
INFECTION AND INFLAMMATION	
Causal factor: **Acute illness:** anovulatory cycles	No fever, full blood count NAD
Chronic salpingo-oophoritis: inability to conceive, irregular cycle; can be minimal or excessive menstrual bleed	Usually congestive dysmenorrhoea is the predominant symptom; associated with purulent discharge, fever, period pain and abdominal pain
ENDOCRINE/REPRODUCTIVE	
Polycystic ovarian syndrome (PCOS): irregular cycle, inability to conceive; extremely common cause of secondary amenorrhoea; anovulatory cycles	No secondary symptoms of skin breakouts (acne), excess facial or body hair (hirsutism), hypertension, insulin resistance or diabetes or weight gain not reported; cannot rule out completely without blood tests and further investigations
Ovulatory bleed: a mid-cycle bleed as well as regular menses; ovulation has occurred	Feels emotional, premenstrual symptoms such as ovulation pain (mittelschmerz) and mood changes; usually spotting or light bleed at time of ovulation, regular cycle; check basal body temperature – it will be biphasic and fluctuate, indicating ovulation has occurred
Diabetes: anovulatory cycles	Urinalysis NAD
Addison's disease: low weight, amenorrhoea	Urinalysis NAD; no sign of skin pigmentation or loss of body hair; no significant digestion disorders reported such as diarrhoea; need to determine if Katie is experiencing lack of appetite and weight loss

▶

Hyperthyroid: low weight, irregular menstrual cycle	No sign of bulging eye signs (exophthalmos); no diarrhoea, difficulty sleeping or hypertension reported; check appetite; no sign of goitre or muscle wasting as in Graves' disease
Hypothyroidism: cause of secondary amenorrhoea due to hyperprolactinaemia and endocrine disorder; anovulatory cycles	No weight gain, signficant fatigue, skin or hair changes reported; no constipation, depression, temperature intolerance or visible goitre noted
Cushing's syndrome: causing amenorrhoea, irregular menstrual cycles	Katie's face is not moon shaped; there is no weight gain, hirsutism, acne, frontal balding of hair, hypertension, oedema; urinalysis NAD and indicating no glucose intolerance or diabetes
Prolactinoma: may present as primary or secondary amenorrhoea	Usually presents with galactorrhoea

Case analysis

TABLE 5.52 **POSSIBLE DIFFERENTIAL DIAGNOSIS**		
Not ruled out by tests/investigations already done [2, 6–9, 11, 13, 66, 73, 74]		
CONDITIONS AND CAUSES	**WHY POSSIBLE**	**WHY UNLIKELY**
ALLERGIES AND IRRITANTS		
Causal factor: **Use of lubricants**	Need to check whether Katie and Adam use lubricants during sexual intercourse. it is possible one or both of them are allergic to lubricants or Adam's sperm is intolerant to lubricants	
CANCER AND HEART DISEASE		
Pituitary tumour	Can cause primary amenorrhoea and irregular periods; anovulatory cycles	No mention of headaches, or changes in smell or taste
Ovarian cancer	Potential organic reason for low weight; usually primary and secondary amenorrhoea	Can present with no menstrual disturbances; may causes menorrhagia or excessive menstrual bleed with a regular cycle
Lesions that cause metrorrhagia: cervical and uterine cancer, endometritis	Irregular cycle, bleeding or spotting	Check if Katie experiences bleeding or pain after intercourse
RECREATIONAL DRUG USE		
Causal factor: **Smoking cigarettes**	Katie is smoking a pack a day; passive smoking from Katie may also affect Adam's fertility status	
Causal factor: **Alcohol:** known to adversely affect both male and female fertility	Check Katie's and Adam's level of alcohol consumption	

SURGERY AND HOSPITALISATION		
Asherman's syndrome: destruction of basal layer of endometrium and formation of adhesions following badly managed uterine curettage; adhesions and fibroids form due to scars	Katie has had two abortions; can cause secondary amenorrhoea; the endometrium can fail to respond to oestrogen	
OCCUPATIONAL TOXINS AND HAZARDS		
Causal factor: **Occupational exposure to chemicals, heavy metals etc.** [70]	Check if Adam is exposed to metal fumes, solvents or pesticides in his workplace, as these can affect fertility	
FUNCTIONAL DISEASE		
Causal factor: **Underweight:** BMI of 20 and under is associated with amenorrhoea and infertility	Can cause primary and secondary amenorrhoea; Katie's BMI is 18; low body weight can affect menstrual cycle due to low body fat and hormonal metabolism; anovulatory cycles	Check Katie's weight history and determine whether her weight has fluctuated
SUPPLEMENTS AND SIDE EFFECTS OF MEDICATIONS		
Causal factor: **Drugs** e.g. diet drugs, post oral contraceptive pill (OCP)	Can cause primary and secondary amenorrhoea; Katie is concerned about weight and has taken the OCP in the past	More than two years since Katie has taken the OCP
Causal factor: **Drug taking:** steroids, cannabis and cocaine can affect fertility in men	Need to check if Adam has a history of drug taking	
Causal factor: **Medications:** sulfasalazines, tetracyclines or allopurinol as can affect fertility	Check if Adam and Katie are taking any medications	
ENDOCRINE/REPRODUCTIVE		
Causal factor: **Pregnancy** and complications of [74]	Irregular periods; missed periods; most common cause of secondary amenorrhoea	Can present with fever, vaginal discharge and pelvic/abdominal pain; Katie may have signs of breast tenderness and may have morning sickness
Causal factor: **Ectopic pregnancy**	Irregular periods; can present with no pain (rare) and can leak over several days slowly; may be missed; previous history of abortion can be a risk factor; common cause of secondary amenorrhoea	Usually associated with severe and acute abdominal pain, abdominal fullness, increased desire to urinate, purulent vaginal discharge, may have signs of fever and dull headaches
Early menopause	Inability to conceive, irregular periods	Katie has not reported experiencing hot flushes

▶

Endometriosis: fertility may be a secondary issue from endometriosis due to distortion of pelvic cavity, impaired ovum pick-up and tubal transport mechanisms, increased incidence of luteal phase dysfunction, trapped oocyte, increased peritoneal prostaglandin production and/or increased peritoneal macrophage activity	Inability to conceive, irregular cycle; can present with minimal or excessive menstrual bleeding	Usually has associated symptoms such as severe episodes of pain before and during menstrual bleed, bleeding from the bowel, lower back pain; no vaginal discharge mentioned
Female infertility [67]	Irregularity of menstrual cycle, previous terminations; alcohol intake and smoking; and adequacy of body weight	
Causal factor: **Retroverted uterus/deformity**	Can hinder the passage of sperm and reduce the chance of conception	
Ovarian cysts: may cause ovaries to not produce an egg; ovarian cysts almost never cause heavy menstrual bleeding	Irregular periods	No significant period pain mentioned; check volume of blood; need to determine the volume of Katie's menstrual bleed when it does occur
Ovarian failure: often due to autoimmune disease; can cause early menopause	Can cause primary or secondary amenorrhoea	No hot flushes
Dysfunctional uterine bleeding (DUB): endometrial hyperplasia, PCOS from taking exogenous oestrogen; endocrine dysfunction (not associated with inflammation, tumour or pregnancy); anovulatory hormone-related bleeding is most common	Intermenstrual bleeding; usually causes bleeding with unpredictable volume and frequency	No use of exogenous oestrogen reported; often associated with menorrhagia (heavy bleed with regular cycle) but the interval between periods is shorter, which makes the period appear irregular
Anovulatory bleeding: irregular bleed that appears menstrual although no ovulation has occurred; can be associated with both short and long cycles	Irregular cycle; no significant premenstrual symptoms reported to show evidence of regular association with menses cycle	Rare; check if Katie experiences premenstrual symptoms associated with her cycle; check if her bleed is unexpected and painless; blood volume can be excessive but irregular; check whether Katie's basal body temperature fluctuates; it would not fluctuate (monophasic) with anovulatory bleeding; physical findings often include obesity, hypertension, hirsutism, acne, possibly diabetes and indicate PCOS

▶

Oestrogen-withdrawal bleeding: causes intermenstrual bleeding when the endometrium proliferates and becomes unstable with oestrogen; drops below the threshold when not in the secretory phase or in the absence of progesterone	Common cause of irregular periods in reproductive years, especially if ovulation has not occurred; painless bleeding	Need to investigate whether Katie's bleeding is prolonged and profuse when it occurs
Progesterone-withdrawal bleeding: only occurs when there is an oestrogen-primed endometrium; can occur when oestrogen therapy continues and progesterone is stopped; also when progesterone is administered to test endogenous oestrogen	Irregular menstrual bleed	Often occurs in PCOS – need to investigate
Oestrogen-breakthrough bleeding – 1st type: when oestrogen levels are low but constant causing sections of the endometrium to degenerate	Intermenstrual bleed	Common when taking the low-dose OCP and with PCOS; need to investigate these two areas more; check if Katie experiences any spotting of blood
Male infertility [67]	Previous testicular damage due to trauma/local surgery; history of mumps; venereal problems causing vas deferens obstruction, prostatitis or prostate disease; abnormalities of the urethra, impotence, chemical exposure and alcohol/drug use	Adam would need a consultation to determine if any of these conditions apply to him
Impotence: erectile dysfunction can be caused by cancer, peripheral nerve disorders, spinal cord disorders, brain disorders, pituitary and endocrine disorders and for psychological reasons; drug and alcohol influences	Can occur if Adam is feeling pressure to perform sexually when he comes home from an extended time away	
Causal factor: **Inadequate sexual intercourse:** timing of intercourse for fertility is best starting a week before ovulation and up to and including ovulation	Adam is away for extended periods of time; Adam and Katie may not be together at optimal ovulation and fertile time	

STRESS AND NEUROLOGICAL DISEASE		
Causal factor: **Stress**	Can cause primary and secondary amenorrhoea; not being with her partner some of the time and at being conflicted about whether to put her energy into a career or family; past history of abortions are worrying Katie; previous history of sexual abuse and not being able to talk about it to Adam in case is has a bearing on her fertility	
Anorexia nervosa [71]	Can cause primary and secondary amenorrhoea (have experienced menstruation and then stopped); inability to conceive, concerned about physical appearance; anovulatory cycles	Check if Katie has signs of body dysmorphic disorder (BDD)
Causal factor: **Excessive sport or exercise** [73]	Can cause primary and secondary amenorrhoea; can cause menstrual irregularities when BMI is in normal range but body fat is low; anovulatory cycles	Question how much exercise Katie does during the week
Causal factor: **Emotional stress about conception difficulties**	Anxiety and strong emotions can affect intercourse and fertility success between couples	
EATING HABITS AND ENERGY		
Causal factor: **Caffeine intake:** known to affect fertility in both men and women	Check if Katie and Adam are consuming excessive amounts of coffee, tea, chocolate and other caffeine-containing foods or drinks	

TABLE 5.53 **DECISION TABLE FOR REFERRAL [2, 6–9, 11, 12]**		
COMPLAINT	CONTEXT	CORE
Referral for presenting complaint	Referral for all associated physical, dietary and lifestyle concerns	Referral for contributing emotional, mental, spiritual, metaphysical, lifestyle and constitutional factors

REFERRAL FLAGS	REFERRAL FLAGS	REFERRAL FLAGS
• Unexplained infertility	• Katie's previous terminations – possible adhesions and scars affecting fertility • Katie's low BMI • Irregular menstrual cycle – possible anovulatory cycle • Smoking • Detrimental effects on general health and fertility	• Katie's history of sexual abuse • Katie's concerns about weight gain when she is obviously underweight • Stress affecting both Katie and Adam
ISSUES OF SIGNIFICANCE	**ISSUES OF SIGNIFICANCE**	**ISSUES OF SIGNIFICANCE**
	• Adam is often away, which may be occurring during Katie's optimal time for intercourse to result in conception	• Katie is unsure whether she wants to start a career or family first
REFERRAL	**REFERRAL**	**REFERRAL**
• Medical investigations investigate physical causes of infertility for both partners [70]	• Referral to determine any underlying conditions for low BMI and irregular menses • Physical examination to determine whether there is a link with previous terminations with difficulty conceiving	• Referral for therapy for underlying emotional issues regarding past abuse • Referral for mental health assessment and counselling to address body image problems • Referral for career counselling, life coaching

TABLE 5.54 **FURTHER INVESTIGATIONS THAT MAY BE NECESSARY** [1, 2, 6, 9–11, 13, 71]	
TEST/INVESTIGATION	**REASON FOR TEST/INVESTIGATION**
FIRST-LINE INVESTIGATIONS:	
Both partners **Examine genitalia and note secondary sex characteristics**	May indicate functional or endocrine disorder; Turner's syndrome, gonadal dysgenesis and testicular feminisation will be identified due to the size and shape of genitalia
Both partners **Pelvic, vaginal, abdominal examination**	No bulging uterus for Kaite or rebound tenderness, no overactive bowel sounds, genital deformities or signs of trauma for either Katie or Adam
Female **Human chorionic gonadotropin (HCG) blood test/radioimmunoassay (RIA)**	Pregnancy, ectopic pregnancy
Female **Vaginal smear**	Evaluation of cervical mucous will indicate if ovarian oestrogen is being produced
Female **Cervical smear**	Routine check important and to evaluate in preparation of healthy conception; detect cervical cancer

Female **Papanicolaou test**	Detect cancer
Female **CA-125 serum marker**	Ovarian cancer, endometriosis, pelvic inflammatory disease
Both partners **Chlamydia cervical culture** **Cervical gonorrhoea culture**	Sexually transmitted diseases that could contribute to infertility
Male **Semen analysis**	Check volume, pH, concentration, sperm number, motility, vitality, formation and white blood cells
Female **Basal body temperature**	Normally drops 24–36 hours after menses begins; with endometriosis there is often a delay in basal body temperature to the second or third day of menses [13]; a decrease indicates preovulation and an increase of 5 degrees occurs after ovulation; monitors thyroid function
Both partners **Full blood count**	Rule out infection, tumour, inflammation, anaemia
Female **Reticulocyte count:** immature red blood cells (test bone marrow function and anaemias)	Increased in pregnancy, haemorrhage (3–4 days later)
Female **Platelet count:** essential to blood clotting	Decrease in haemorrhage
Both partners **Coagulation studies:** blood clotting *Female* **Progesterone level**	Decreased in congenital deficiency, autoimmune disease Take 7 days before menstruation to determine if ovulation has occurred; low serum progesterone level in anovulatory cycles
Both partners **Oestradiol**	*Normal:* PCOS, weight loss, excess exercise *Raised:* pregnancy, ovarian tumour, testicular tumour, adrenal tumour *Low:* PCOS, polycystic ovarian disease, ovarian failure, anorexia nervosa, weight loss, excess exercise, hypothyroidism, Cushing's syndrome, adrenal hyperplasia, menopause, Turner's syndrome, failing pregnancy, fetal death
Female **FSH** (follicle-stimulating hormone)	*Normal:* PCOS, pregnancy, anorexia, weight loss, excess exercise *Raised:* ovarian failure, menopause *Low:* polycystic ovarian disease, anorexia, weight loss, excess exercise, hypothyroidism, Cushing's syndrome, adrenal tumour/hyperplasia

▶

Female **LH** (luteinising hormone)	*Normal:* pregnancy, anorexia, weight loss, excess exercise *Raised:* PCOS, polycystic ovarian disease, ovarian failure, menopause *Low:* anorexia, weight loss, excess exercise, hypothyroidism, Cushing's syndrome, adrenal tumour/hyperplasia
Female **PRL** (prolactin): common in secondary amenorrhoea to be raised	*Normal:* ovarian failure, anorexia, weight loss, excess exercise, adrenal tumour/hyperplasia *Raised:* PCOS, hypothyroidism, Cushing's syndrome, pregnancy, amenorrhoea *Low:* pituitary destruction from tumour
Both partners **Testosterone**	*Normal:* ovarian failure, anorexia, weight loss, excess exercise, hypothyroidism, pregnancy *Raised:* PCOS, Cushing's syndrome, adrenal tumour/hyperplasia, testicular tumour, ovarian tumour *Low:* male hormonal imbalance, Klinefelter's syndrome, corticosteriod use
Female **SHBG** (sex hormone-binding globulin)	Low SHBG would indicate the presence of elevated levels of free androgens
Both partners **Thyroid function test** **TSH, T4, T3**	TSH (thyroid-stimulating hormone) suppressed in hyperthyroidism; thyroid-specific antibodies, to confirm autoimmune cause of hyperthyroidism (Graves')
Female **Fasting blood glucose test**	Raised levels can indicate diabetes mellitus, Addison's disease or Cushing's syndrome
Both partners **Rubella status**	Need to check in preparation of healthy conception
Female **Ovulation prediction kits**	Designed to detect an increase in urinary luteinising hormone (LH) excretion 24–36 hours prior to ovulation
IF NECESSARY:	
Female **Progesterone withdrawal test**	To determine whether Katie's body is producing oestrogen
Female **Abdominal and pelvic x-ray/ultrasound**	Most accurate diagnosis of PCOS, ovarian mass, ovarian cyst or tumour, retroverted uterus, tubo-ovarian abscesses, fibroids, trauma
Female **Laparoscopy and biopsy/culdoscopy**	Primary diagnostic technique for endometriosis by visualising the lesions
Female **Endometrial, vaginal and cervical biopsies**	Detect cancer; during luteal phase (10–12 days after ovulation) to determine inadequate luteal phase production or action of progesterone
Male **Testicular biopsy**	Testicular disease or blockage

▶

▶

Female Transvaginal ultrasonography	To determine cause of excess and random menstrual bleeding (menometrorrhagia) such as dysfunctional uterine bleeding, cancer
Female Brain scan CT/MRI	Pituitary tumour
Both partners Testing for heavy metal or chemical exposure	Environmental toxins can have an adverse effect on fertility [25–27]

Confirmed diagnosis

KATIE AND SUBFERTILITY

Katie and her partner Adam are both just over 30 years of age and are seeking help to conceive a child. They have been trying to fall pregnant for more than two years during which time Katie has finished her law degree and Adam has been working away from home three weeks out of four. Katie is currently smoking a pack of cigarettes a day and maintains a strict exercise regimen because she is concerned about gaining weight. Katie is concerned about weight gain in pregnancy. Katie has shared her history of sexual abuse and pregnancy terminations, something she has not yet discussed with Adam.

Infertility is now often termed 'subfertility' [68] and is defined as the inability for a couple to conceive after one year of unprotected intercourse. Infertility is diagnosed when a couple has been unable to conceive for at least two years of regular unprotected intercourse. Katie has been diagnosed with subfertility issues because she and Adam have not been living together consistently for intercourse to be regular over the past two years. Subfertility can be caused by factors of male physiology such as problems with sperm count due to lack of normal production, potency or a blockage. Female factors include tubal problems, ovulatory disorders, hostile cervical mucus, vaginal factors and idiopathic reasons.

Semen can be affected by a history of the mumps, from testicular injury, exposure to industrial or environmental toxins, excessive heat exposure, acute illness, prolonged fever within the previous three months, recreational drug use, alcohol intake or exposure to steroids. Anatomic abnormalities can be caused by varicocele or conditions such as prostatitis. Endocrine disorders affecting sperm count are more uncommon, but may include hypothyroidism, adrenal disorders or hypogonadism.

Female factors include irregular or absent ovulation. Amenorrhoea is defined as primary when it occurs in a girl of prepuberty, during pregnancy and early lactation and after menopause. Secondary amenorrhoea is when there is an absence of menstruation for more than three months in women who have previously menstruated. Menstruation can be affected by emotional and mental challenges, dietary and exercise habits, lifestyle and emotional stresses, family history of genetic problems. Additionally amenorrhoea can develop from abnormal growth and development, CNS-hypothalamic-pituitary dysfunction, polycystic ovarian syndrome, thyroid or adrenal disorders, premature ovarian failure, Asherman's syndrome or disorders of sexual differentiation. Women aged 35–39 have half the chance of conceiving than women between the ages of 19 and 26 years [68].

General references used in this diagnosis: 2, 7–9, 11, 13, 67, 73

PRESCRIBED MEDICATION

None at this stage.

TABLE 5.55 **DECISION TABLE FOR TREATMENT (ONCE DIAGNOSIS IS CONFIRMED)**		
COMPLAINT	**CONTEXT**	**CORE**
Treatment for the presenting complaint and symptoms	Treatment for all associated symptoms	Treatment for mental, emotional, spiritual, constitutional, lifestyle issues and metaphysical considerations
TREATMENT PRIORITY	**TREATMENT PRIORITY**	**TREATMENT PRIORITY**
• Preconception care program incorporating lifestyle and dietary measures to improve the general health and nutrition of Katie and Adam to help improve their fertility • Herbal tonic to help normalise Katie's menstrual cycle and improve her fertility • Lifestyle recommendations to reduce exposure to environmental pollutants, which may be adversely affecting both Katie's and Adam's fertility • Recommendation for Katie to chart her cycle to help her identify her time of greatest fertility • Specific dietary intervention and supplements to improve Katie's and Adam's general health and fertility **NB:** Supplemental herbs and nutrients for Adam should only be prescribed once he has attended the clinic for a consultation; prior to that appropriate lifestyle and dietary suggestions can be recommended • Physical therapy suggestions to enhance Katie's and Adam's fertility • Herbal tonic for both Adam and Katie with tonic, adaptogenic and specific herbal support for male and female reproductive function **NB:** Katie should cease taking her tonic if she becomes pregnant. Treatment recommendations for both Katie and Adam are aimed to improve general health and fertility; should specific causes of their fertility problems be discovered, treatments would need to be reformulated to take this into account	• Bring Katie into a normal weight range to improve her chance of conceiving • Recommend testing for chemical and heavy metal exposure to determine whether this is implicated; additional supplemental may be recommended based on the results of the tests and a detoxification program may be also recommended based on results of the hair tissue mineral test • Support Katie to quit smoking; Katie's herbal tonic has antioxidant action and will help support detoxification of toxins from cigarettes; Katie's herbal tea formula will help support her nervous system as she withdraws from nicotine **NB:** A heavy metal or chemical detoxification program should be undertaken as part of a preconception program and should not be done while Katie and Adam are actively trying for conception [27]	• Lifestyle recommendations for both partners to improve stress management • Physical therapy suggestions to help improve stress management • Herbal tea to help relax Katie's nervous system • Recommendation for Katie to have counselling to deal with the issues surrounding her history of sexual abuse and abortions as well as addressing Katie's body image problems

Treatment aims

- Help Adam and Katie to live a healthy lifestyle and achieve optimal health to improve their chances of conceiving and carrying a healthy baby to full term [14, 26].
- Get Katie to quit smoking [15].
- Both Katie and Adam should avoid smoking, exposure to cigarette smoke [15], alcohol [16, 35, 37] and recreational drugs during the preconception period [17].
- Get Katie's BMI back into normal range [18].
- Improve Katie's general health and nutritional status [19, 37].
- Normalise Katie's menstrual cycle.
- Assist Katie to recognise the signs of fertility (Billings or symptothermal method) to ensure she and Adam are trying for conception at the correct time in her cycle [20].
- Determine whether Katie may have a problem with intestinal dysbiosis and *Candida albicans* overgrowth [21]. Treat if necessary.
- Improve Adam's general health [14] and reduce oxidative [22] and psychological stress [23].
- Reduce Adam's and Katie's exposure to and levels of environmental toxins [22, 25, 27, 39].
- Design a preconception care program for both Katie and Adam [24]. The first two to three months include a detoxification phase during which toxic chemicals and heavy metals are cleared from the body [25], nutritional deficiencies are corrected [26] and general health and lifestyle improvements are made [14, 26]. This is followed by a four-month preparation for conception phase in which lifestyle and health improvements are enhanced, leading to conception attempts [27].

Lifestyle alterations/considerations

- Herbal formula and nutritional supplements should only be provided following a comprehensive consultation with Adam to ensure there are no contraindications to any recommended treatments.
- Hair tissue mineral analysis may be helpful to determine the status of toxic minerals and nutrient minerals [39, 47].
- Both Adam and Katie may benefit from stress-management and stress-reduction techniques. Stress is associated with a reduction in male fertility [23] and affects fertility in women [55].
- Katie may benefit from counselling to help her deal with her history of sexual abuse and pregnancy terminations.
- Encourage Katie to gain sufficient weight to put her in a healthy BMI weight range [18].
- Encourage Katie to chart her cycle using the Billings or symptothermal method to help her identify peak times of fertility [20].
- Both Katie and Adam should avoid wherever possible or minimise exposure to all forms of radiation, particularly ionising radiation as well as electromagnetic radiation from mobile phones and other electrical devices [27, 58, 59].

Dietary suggestions

- Eliminate highly processed and refined foods from Katie's and Adam's diets [19].
- Encourage them to eat a whole-food diet including plenty of legumes, fresh organic fruit and vegetables and foods containing high levels of antioxidants [22, 27, 38, 51].
- Encourage Katie and Adam to choose organic foods wherever possible to reduce their exposure to pesticides and herbicides and other environmental chemicals, which can adversely affect fertility and fetal development [27, 38, 39].

- Anti-candida diet if Katie has problems with *Candida* overgrowth [21].
- Eliminate alcohol consumption [16, 37].
- Eliminate consumption of tea and coffee and caffeine containing beverages [16, 35].
- Remove *trans* fats from the diet. Consumption of *trans* fats increases the risk of ovulatory infertility [36].
- Ensure sufficient intake of filtered or spring water.
- Encourage Katie and Adam to consume more omega-3-rich foods [40] and use olive oil for cooking in preference to seed oils [41]. Due to the possibility of mercury exposure, limit their intake of tuna and swordfish and choose canned mackerel, sardines and salmon in preference to tuna [42, 43].

Physical treatment suggestions

- Acupuncture could be helpful for both Adam and Katie. Acupuncture may improve sperm quality in subfertile men [52]. Acupuncture has benefits for clients undergoing IVF [53] and may enhance fertility through its effect on uterine blood flow [54].
- Massage therapy may help reduce stress [56] thereby increasing fertility for both Katie and Adam [23, 55].
- Hydrotherapy: constitutional hydrotherapy for overall health, stress release and increase immune function [60–62].
- Hot foot bath to stimulate menstrual bleed [63].
- Hot sitz bath to stimulate menstrual bleed [63, 64].
- Weekly contrasting treatments between periods, with hot fomentation on the back and abdomen for 15 minutes, followed by 30-second cold mitten friction. Next, apply heat to the pelvic area and back for another 15 minutes, repeat cold mitten friction with the client in the side lying position (repeat alternating procedure three times). Follow with an abdominal massage [62].

TABLE 5.56 HERBAL TEA FOR KATIE

Alternative to tea and coffee

HERB	FORMULA	RATIONALE
Lavender *Lavandula angustifolia*	1 part	Anxiolytic [28, 31]; sedative [28, 31]; antidepressant [28, 31]
Lemon balm *Melissa officinalis*	2 parts	Anxiolytic [28]; sedative [28, 31]; antioxidant [28]
Oats seed *Avena sativa*	2 parts	Nervine tonic [28, 66]; tonic [28, 66]; nutritive [66]; antidepressant [34]

Infusion: 1 tsp per cup – 1 cup 3 times daily

TABLE 5.57 KATIE'S HERBAL FORMULA 1:2 LIQUID EXTRACTS

Made with ethanolic extract herbal liquids (alcohol removed)

HERB	FORMULA	RATIONALE
Dong quai *Angelica sinensis*	40 mL	Traditionally used for irregular menstruation and as a female tonic [28, 30, 33]; used for infertility [28, 30, 33]

▶

Shatavari *Asparagus racemosus*	60 mL	Tonic [31, 57]; adaptogenic [31, 57]; sexual tonic [31, 58]; traditionally used to improve fertility and promote conception for both males and females [31, 32, 57]
Withania *Withania somnifera*	60 mL	Adaptogen [28, 29]; anxiolytic [28]; antioxidant [28]; antidepressant [28]; tonic [28, 29]; mild sedative [29, 30]; traditionally used for improving stress adaptation response [28]; promotes weight gain [28]; traditionally used as a tonic, aphrodisiac and to promote conception [29]
St Mary's thistle *Silybum marianum*	40 mL	Hepatoprotective [28, 29]; hepatic trophorestorative [28, 29]; antioxidant [28, 29]; indicated for use in exposure to chemical pollutants such as cigarettes [28, 29]
Supply:	200 mL	Dose: 5 mL 3 times daily

Chaste tree (*Vitex agnus castus*) 2 g dried fruit in tablet form or equivalent in liquid form [28]; normalises menstrual cycle [28, 29]; used to enhance fertility where there are luteal phases or progesterone defects [28, 29]; indicated for menstrual disorders including secondary amenorrhoea and infertility due to decreased progesterone levels [28, 29]

TABLE 5.58 **ADAM'S HERBAL FORMULA (1:2 LIQUID EXTRACTS)**		
Made with ethanolic extract herbal liquids (alcohol removed)		
HERB	**FORMULA**	**RATIONALE**
Shatavari *Asparagus racemosus*	60 mL	Tonic [31, 57]; adaptogen [31, 57]; sexual tonic [31, 57]; traditionally used to improve fertility and promote conception for both males and females [31, 32, 57]
Tribulus *Tribulus terrestris*	70 mL	Aphrodisiac [28, 31]; enhances sexual function [28]; tonic [31]; indirectly androgenic in males [31]; beneficial for the treatment of male infertility [31, 33]
Siberian ginseng *Eleutherococcus senticosus*	30 mL	Adaptogen [28, 29]; immunomodulator [28, 29]; tonic [28, 29]; increases vitality [29]
Saint Mary's thistle *Silybum marianum*	40 mL	Hepatoprotective [28, 29]; hepatic trophorestorative [28, 29]; antioxidant [28, 29]; indicated for use in exposure to chemical pollutants such as cigarettes [28, 29]
Supply:	200 mL	Dose: 5 mL 3 times daily

Nutritional supplements

TABLE 5.59 **KATIE'S NUTRITIONAL SUPPLEMENTS**	
SUPPLEMENT AND DOSE	**RATIONALE**
Zinc supplement containing 25–30 mg elemental zinc [44, 48, 50]	Adequate zinc levels are required for normal function of the female reproductive system and are essential for metabolism of reproductive hormones [28]; inadequate maternal zinc status is associated with fetal growth retardation, low birth weight and preterm delivery [45]
High-potency practitioner-strength **multivitamin and mineral supplement** designed for preconception/pregnancy which provides therapeutic levels of important vitamins and minerals and ensuring an intake of 500 μg folate [48] daily	To provide additional micronutrients and assist in improving chances of conception and healthy pregnancy outcome [27, 47]
Omega-3 fish oil At least 3000 mg daily providing 100–300 mg DHA daily [28]	Supplementation with omega-3 fatty acids during pregnancy lowers the risk of premature birth [40, 41] and increase birth weight, promoting fetal growth by increasing placental blood flow [40]; WHO and FAO guidelines recommend pregnant women consume at least 2.6 g of omega-3 fatty acids daily [28]

TABLE 5.60 **ADAM'S NUTRITIONAL SUPPLEMENTS**	
SUPPLEMENT AND DOSE	**RATIONALE**
Zinc supplement containing 25–30 mg elemental zinc [44, 48, 50]	Adequate zinc levels are required for formation and maturation of spermatozoa [28]; zinc deficiency leads to impaired male fertility and decreased spermatogenesis [28]; total sperm count increases in both subfertile and fertile men following supplementation with zinc and folic acid [46]
High-potency practitioner-strength **multivitamin supplement** providing therapeutic levels of essential micronutrients and antioxidants	Antioxidant intake is associated with higher sperm quantity and motility [49]; reducing levels of seminal oxidative stress is important for male fertility [22]
Omega-3 fish oil 2000 mg daily [50]	Essential for ensuring sperm plasma membrane has sufficient fluidity to achieve fertilisation [51]

References

[1] N.J. Talley, S. O'Connor, Pocket Clinical Examination, third edn, Churchill Livingstone Elsevier, Australia, 2009.

[2] P. Kumar, C. Clark, Clinical Medicine, sixth edn, Elsevier Saunders, London, 2005.

[3] J. Silverman, S. Kurtz, J. Draper, Skills for Communicating with Patients, second edn, Radcliff Publishing, Oxford, 2000.

[4] R. Neighbour, The Inner Consultation; how to develop an effective and intuitive consulting style, Radcliff Publishing, Oxon, 2005.

[5] M. Lloyd, R. Bor, Communication Skills For Medicine, third edn, Churchill Livingstone Elsevier, Edinburgh, 2009.

[6] G. Douglas, F. Nicol, C. Robertson, Macleod's Clinical Examination, twelfth edn, Churchill Livingstone Elsevier, Edinburgh, 2009.

[7] J. Jamison, Differential Diagnosis for Primary Care, second edn, Churchill Livingstone Elsevier, London, 2006.

[8] A. Polmear (Ed.), Evidence-Based Diagnosis in Primary Care, Churchill Livingstone Elsevier, Edinburgh, 2008, pp. 274–283.

[9] R.D. Collins, Differential Diagnosis in Primary Care, fourth edn, Lippincott Williams & Wilkins, Philadelphia, 2008.

[10] K.D. Pagna, T.J. Pagna, Mosby's Diagnostic and Laboratory Test reference, third edn, Mosby, USA, 1997 (later edition).

[11] R. Berkow, A.J. Fletcher, M.H. Beers, The Merck Manual, sixteenth edn, Rathway, N.J: Merck Research Laboratories, 1993. (later edition)

[12] D. Peters, L.Chaitow, G.Harris, S.Morrison, Integrating Complementary Therapies in Primary Care, Churchill Livingstone, London, 2002.

[13] R.H. Seller, Differential Diagnosis of Common Complaints, fifth edn, Saunders Elsevier, Philadelphia, 2007.

[14] M.A. Hassan, S.R. Killick, Negative lifestyle is associated with a significant reduction in fecundity, Fertility and Sterility 81 (2) (2004) 384–392.

[15] D. Baird, A.J. Wilcox, Cigarette Smoking Associated with Delayed Conception, Journal of the American Medical Association 253 (20) (1985) 2979–2983.

[16] R.B. Hakim, R.H. Gray, H. Zacur, Alcohol and caffeine consumption and decreased fertility, Fertility and Sterility 70 (4) (1998) 632–637.

[17] G.M. Buck, L.E. Sever, R.E. Batt, P. Mendola, Epidemiology, Life-Style Factors and Female Infertility 8 (4) (1997) 435.

[18] R.E. Frische, Body fat, menarche, fitness and fertility, Human Reproduction 12 (6) (1987) 521–533.

[19] J. Chavarro, J. Rich-Edwards, B. Rosner, W. Willett, Diet and Lifestyle in the Prevention of Ovulatory Disorder Infertility, Obstetrics & Gynecology 110 (5) (2007) 1050–1058.

[20] R.H. Gray, R.T. Kambic, Epidemiological studies of natural family planning, Human Reproduction 3 (5) (1988) 693–698.

[21] J.P. Tuttle, E.R. Bannister, F.C. Derrick, Interference of human spermatozoal motility and spermatozoal agglutination by Candida albicans, Journal of Urology 118 (5) (1977) 797–799.

[22] R.A. Saleh, A. Agarwal, Oxidative Stress and Male Infertility: From Research Bench to Clinical Practice, Journal of Andrology 23 (6) (2002) 737–751.

[23] L. Fenster, D.F. Katz, A.J. Wyrobek, C. Pieper, D.M. Rempel, D. Oman, S.H. Swan, Effects of psychological stress on human semen quality, Journal of Andrology 18 (2) (1997) 194–202.

[24] C.C. Korenbrot, A. Steinberg, C. Bender, S. Newberry, Preconception Care: A Systematic Review, Maternal and Child Health Journal 6 (2) (2002) 75–87.

[25] E.M. Smith, M. Hammonds-Ehlers, M.K. Clark, H.L. Kirchner, L. Fuortes, Occupational Exposures and Risk of Female Infertility, Journal of Occupation & Environmental Medicine 39 (2) (1997) 138–147.

[26] R.E. Chaplin, W.A. Robbins, L.A. Schieve, A.M. Sweeney, S.A. Tabacova, K.M. Tomashek, Off to a Good Start: The Influence of Pre- and Periconceptional Exposures, Parental Fertility, and Nutrition on Children's Health, Environmental Health Perspectives 112 (1) (2004) 69–78.

[27] F. Naish, J. Roberts, The Natural Way to Better Babies, Random House, Sydney, 1996.

[28] L. Braun, M. Cohen, Herbs & Natural Supplements: An evidence based guide, second edn, Elsevier, Sydney, 2007.

[29] S. Mills, K. Bone, Principles & Practice of Phytotherapy; Modern Herbal Medicine, Churchill Livingstone, Edinburgh: London, 2000.

[30] K. Bone, Clinical Applications of Chinese and Ayurvedic Herbs: Monographs for the Western Herbal Practitioners, Phytotherapy Press, Warwick, 1996.

[31] S. Mills, K. Bone, The Essential Guide to Herbal Safety, Elsevier Churchill Livingstone, St Louis, 2005.

[32] P.S. Pataki, The Role of Indigenous Drugs in the Management of Male Sexual Disorders, Probe 28 (1) (1988) 25–28.

[33] R. Trickey, Women, Hormones & The Menstrual Cycle, second edn, Allen & Unwin, Sydney, 2003.

[34] British Herbal Medicine Association, British Herbal Pharmacopoeia, BHMA, Surrey, 1983.

[35] R.B. Hakim, R.H. Gray, H. Zacur, Alcohol and caffeine consumption and decreased fertility, Fertility and Sterility 70 (4) (1998) 632–637.

[36] J.E. Chavarro, J.W. Rich-Edwards, B.A. Rosner, W. Willett, Dietary fatty acid intakes and the risk of ovulatory infertility, The American Journal of Clinical Nutrition 85 (2007) 231–237.

[37] T.K. Jensen, N.H. Hjollund, T.B. Henriksen, T. Schieke, H. Kolstad, A. Giwercman, E. Ernst, et al., Does moderate alcohol consumption affect fertility? Follow up study among couples planning first pregnancy, British Medical Journal 317 (1998) 505–510.

[38] A. Agarwal, Oxidative stress and its implications in female infertility – a clinician's perspective, Reproductive BioMedicine Online 11 (5) (2005) 641–650.

[39] R.M. Sharpe, D.S. Irvine, How strong is the evidence of a link between environmental chemicals and adverse effects on human reproductive health? British Medical Journal 328 (2004) 447–451.

[40] P. Saldeen, T. Saldeen, Women and omega-3 Fatty acids, Obstetrical Gynecological Survey 59 (10) (2004) 722–730.

[41] A.P. Simopoulos, The importance of the ratio of omega-6/omega-3 essential fatty acids, Biomedicine and Pharmacotherapy 56 (2002) 365–379.

[42] J.M. Hightower, D. Moore, Mercury Levels in High-End Consumers of Fish, Environmental Health Perspectives 111 (4) (2003) 604–608.

[43] S.M. Shim, L.E. Dorworth, J.A. Lasrado, C.R. Santerre, Mercury and Fatty Acids in Canned Tuna, Salmon, and Mackerel, Journal of Food Science 69 (9) (2004) C681–C684.

[44] J. Jamison, Clinical Guide to Nutrition & Dietary Supplements in Disease Management, Churchill Livingstone, Edinburgh, 2003.

[45] S. Jameson, Zinc Therapy in Pregnancy: The Effect of Zinc Therapy on Perinatal Mortality, Prematurity and Placental Ablation, Annals of the New York Academy of Sciences 678 (Maternal Nutrition and Pregnancy Outcome) (1993) 178–192.

[46] W.Y. Wong, H.M. Merkus, C.M. Thomas, R. Menkveld, G.A. Zielhuis, P.M. Steegers-Theunissen, Effects of folic acid and zinc sulfate on male factor subfertility: a double-blind, randomized, placebo-controlled trial, Fertility and Sterility 77 (3) (2002) 491–498.

[47] C.L. Keen, M.S. Clegg, L.A. Hanna, L. Lanoue, J.M. Rogers, G.P. Daston, P. Oteiza, et al., The Plausibility of Micronutrient Deficiencies Being a Significant Contributing Factor to the Occurrence of Pregnancy Complications, The Journal of Nutrition 133 (2003) 1597S–1605S.

[48] J. Higdon, An Evidence-Based Approach to Vitamins and Minerals. Health Benefits and Intake Recommendations, Thieme, New York, 2003.

[49] B. Eskenazi, S.A. Kidd, A.R. Marks, E. Sloter, G. Block, A.J. Wyrobek, Antioxidant intake is associated with semen quality in healthy men, Human Reproduction 20 (4) (2005) 1006–1012.

[50] H. Osiecki, The Nutrient Bible, seventh edn, BioConcepts Publishing, Eagle Farm, 2008.

[51] C. Wathes, R.E. Abayasekara, J. Aitken, Polyunsaturated Fatty Acids in Male and Female Reproduction, Biology of Reproduction 77 (2007) 190–201.

[52] S. Siterman, F. Eltes, V. Wolfson, N. Zabludovsky, B. Bartoov, Effect of acupuncture on sperm parameters of males suffering from subfertility related to low sperm quality, Archives of Andrology 39 (2) (1997) 155–161.

[53] W.E. Paulus, M. Zhang, E. Strehler, I. El-Danasouri, K. Sterzik, Influence of acupuncture on the pregnancy rate in patients who undergo assisted reproduction therapy, Fertility and Sterility 77 (4) (2002) 721–724.

[54] R. Chang, P.H. Chung, Z. Rosenwaks, Role of acupuncture in the treatment of female infertility, Fertility and Sterility 78 (6) (2002) 1149–1153.

[55] K.A. Sanders, N.W. Bruce, A prospective study of psychosocial stress and fertility in women, Human Reproduction 12 (10) (1997) 2324–2329.

[56] C.A. Moyer, J. Rounds, J.W. Hannum, A Meta-Analysis of Massage Therapy Research, Psychological Bulletin 130 (1) (2004) 3–18.

[57] K. Bone, M. Morgan, Alternatives to False Unicorn root: Shatavari, Mediherb Professional Review 77 (2001) 3–4.

[58] R.J. Aitken, L.E. Bennetts, D. Sawyer, A.M. Wiklendt, B.V. King, Impact of radio frequency electromagnetic radiation on DNA integrity in the male germline, International Journal of Andrology 28 (2005) 171–179.

[59] G.M. Shaw, L.A. Croen, Human Adverse Reproductive Outcomes and Electromagnetic Field Exposures: Review of Epidemiologic Studies, Environmental Health Perspectives 101 (suppl. 4) (2003) 107–119.

[60] W. Boyle, A. Saine, Lectures in Naturopathic Hydrotherapy, Oregon: Eclectic Medical Publications, 1988.

[61] E. Blake, in: L. Chaitow, E. Blake, P. Orrock, M. Wallden, P. Snider, J. Zeff (Eds.), Naturopathic Physical Medicine: Theory and Practice for Manual Therapists and Naturopaths, Churchill Livingstone Elsevier, Philadelphia, 2008.

[62] M. Sinclair, Modern Hydrotherapy for the Massage Therapist, Lippincott Williams & Wilkins, Baltimore, 2008.

[63] D.D. Buchman, The complete book of water healing, Contemporary Books, McGraw-Hill Companies, New York, 2001.

[64] L. Chaitow, Hydrotherapy, water therapy for health and beauty, Element, Dorset, 1999.

[65] D. Hoffman, The New Holistic Herbal, Element Books Ltd, Shaftesbury, Dorset, 1990.

[66] D.T. Baird, Amenorrhoea, Lancet 350 (1997) 275–279.

[67] A. Taylor, ABC of subfertility: extent of the problem, BMJ 327 (2003) 434–436.

[68] D. Dunson, B. Colombo, D. Baird, Changes with age in the level and duration of fertility in the menstrual cycle, Hum Reprod 17 (2002) 1399–1403.

[69] I. Figa-Talamanca, M. Traina, E. Urbani, Occupational exposures to metals, solvents and pesticides: recent evidence on male reproductive effects and biological markers, Occup Med 51 (2001) 174–188.

[70] P. Warner, H. Critchley, M. Lumsden, et al., Referral for menstrual problems: cross sectional survey of symptoms, reasons for referral, and management, BMJ 323 (2001) 24–28.

[71] L.A. Mitan, Menstrual dysfunction in anorexia nervosa, J Pediatr Adolesc Gynecol 17 (2) (2004) 81–85.

[72] M.P. Warren, L.R. Goodman, Exercise-induced endocrine pathologies, J Endocrinol Invest 26 (9) (2003) 873–878.

[73] R.B. Kiningham, B.S. Apgar, T.L. Schwenk, Evaluation of amenorrhoea, Am Fam Physican 53 (1996) 1185–1194.

[74] P.I. Wathen, M.C. Henderson, C.A. Witz, Abnormal uterine bleeding, Med Clin North Am 79 (1995) 329–343.

Benign prostatic enlargement

Case history

Bill Anderson is 59 years old. He and his wife have recently moved to Australia from Glasgow, Scotland. Bill is very happy about the move and feels he can finally relax having retired from his newsagency after running it for nearly 32 years. Ten years ago he decided he wanted to spend his retirement years somewhere warm and sunny, and both he and his wife are looking forward to this new phase of their life. Bill says two of his children live in Los Angeles and one in London, and they are all excited about visiting their parents in their new home in Australia.

Bill originally booked into the clinic for a massage to alleviate pain in his right shoulder, which he thinks is probably due to all the lifting he did during his recent move. He then tells you he has been experiencing difficulty in passing urine over the past six months or so, and that it is gradually getting worse. He is getting up more frequently during the night to urinate and has noticed a tendency to dribble urine at the end of voiding. Bill had intended to do something about it before now, but has been so preoccupied with selling his house and business in Glasgow and moving to Australia he just hasn't gotten around to it yet. A couple of days ago Bill noticed a large amount of blood in his urine, and because he had already booked in for a massage he thought he would discuss it with you at the massage appointment.

Bill has not seen a medical doctor for years. He and his family have used complementary and alternative medicine for generations and he has great faith in the power of herbs, homeopathy and nutrition to promote healing. He would like some advice about his diet to see whether there are any things he can do to improve it. He enjoys two or three glasses of red wine at the end of the day, and when he was running his newsagency, it was often the only thing that would relax him at the end of a busy day. Bill loves curries and spicy food and enjoys cheese and biscuits with his red wine. Bill and his wife eat red meat, fish and chicken and enjoy eating a wide variety of vegetables.

You get the impression that Bill is not particularly concerned about his symptoms, and is expecting you can provide him with a magical herbal potion that will fix him up and let him get on with enjoying his new life!

TABLE 5.61 **COMPLAINT**	
Analogy: Skin of the apple	**Complaint:** Define the presenting complaint and symptoms; understand the complaint *Difficulty passing urine* *Right shoulder pain*
AREAS OF INVESTIGATION AND EXAMPLE QUESTIONS	**CLIENT RESPONSES**
Onset *When did you first notice changes to your urinary flow?* *When did you first notice your shoulder pain?*	*When I think about it, it has probably been happening over the last few years and gradually getting worse.* *I noticed the shoulder pain when we finished packing up the house in Glasgow. I ignored it then thinking it would settle down but when we started unpacking here in Australia it got worse again.*
Understanding the cause (client) *You don't seem concerned that your symptoms may be very serious. Do you have any theories about what might be causing your symptoms?*	*I don't really know, but I think it probably has something to do with getting older.* *I was a little concerned about the blood and thought maybe something needed checking out so I thought you could tell me what the problem is.*
Timing *Is there a time your urinary symptoms are more problematic?*	*It is a nuisance that I have to go to the toilet more often these days, but it is more of a problem at night because I keep having to get up.*
Location *Can you describe the exact location of your shoulder pain?*	Bill points to the lateral part of his right shoulder.

TABLE 5.62 **CONTEXT**	
Analogy: Flesh of the apple	**Context:** Put the presenting complaint into context to understand the disease
AREAS OF INVESTIGATION AND EXAMPLE QUESTIONS	**CLIENT RESPONSES**
Family health *Is there a history of this type of urinary problem in your family?*	*I don't think so, although my dad wouldn't have talked about that sort of thing with me.*
Obstruction and foreign body *Do you experience back pain that radiates to the groin?* (bladder stones, kidney infection)	*No, the pain is usually in the back and shoulders.*
Surgery and hospitalisation *Have you ever had surgery or been in hospital?*	*No.*

▶

Infection and inflammation *Have you ever experienced pain and blood with urination that has come on suddenly?* (bacterial infection)	*I don't think so.*
Supplements and side effects of medication *Have you been taking any medicines, either conventional or natural?*	*Only fish oil and a multivitamin.*
Stress and neurological *Are you able to voluntarily inhibit the dribbling of urine when aware?* (stress incontinence)	*No, when that happens I just need to let it pass.*
Eating habits and energy *How are your energy levels at the moment?*	*I am a little tired, but I think that's because my shoulder is interfering with my sleep and also I keep having to get up during the night to go to the toilet.*

TABLE 5.63 CORE

Analogy: Core of the apple with the seed of ill health	**Core:** Holistic assessment to understand the client
AREAS OF INVESTIGATION AND EXAMPLE QUESTIONS	**CLIENT RESPONSES**
Occupation *Now that you're settling in to your new home, what plans do you have?*	*Taking things a bit slower, learning to surf and having plenty of time for fishing.*
Family and friends *How do you feel about being so far away from your children?* *Do you have any friends in Australia?*	*They are all grown up now and have their own lives, two of them are in LA which is a long way from Glasgow. They will probably visit once a year and Lorna and I will go and visit them once a year, so I think we might even see them more often.* *We've already met some people so I don't think it'll be difficult to make new friends.*
Action needed to heal *What do you think is necessary for you to get better?*	*I think my shoulder will fix with a bit of rest and massage, and I'm hoping you can give me a brew to fix the waterworks.*

TABLE 5.64 BILL'S SIGNS AND SYMPTOMS

Pulse	86 bpm
Blood pressure	130/80
Temperature	36.7°C
Respiratory rate	16 resp/min
Body mass index	24
Waist circumference	90 cm
Face	Pale
Urinalysis	Macroscopic blood

Results of medical investigations

No medical tests have been done.

TABLE 5.65 **UNLIKELY DIAGNOSTIC CONSIDERATIONS** [3–8]	
CONDITIONS AND CAUSES	WHY UNLIKELY
CANCER AND HEART DISEASE	
Heart failure	No advanced hypertension
OBSTRUCTION AND FOREIGN BODY	
Polycystic kidney disease	No protein in urinalysis
INFECTION AND INFLAMMATION	
Acute kidney infection	No fever, absence of leucocytes or protein in the urine
Acute prostatitis	No fever, absence of leucocytes in the urine
Urinary tract infection (UTI)	No fever, absence of leucocytes or nitrates in the urine, normal pH
ENDOCRINE/REPRODUCTIVE	
Diabetes mellitus	No glucose or ketones in urine

Case analysis

TABLE 5.66 **POSSIBLE DIFFERENTIAL DIAGNOSIS**		
Not ruled out by tests/investigations already done [1–12]		
CONDITIONS AND CAUSES	WHY POSSIBLE	WHY UNLIKELY
CANCER AND HEART DISEASE		
Early prostate cancer [53]	Difficulty with urination, dribbling urine after voiding, reduced forcefulness of urine, possible metastasis spread in bone, blood in urine	Common in men aged 80 years and over; early prostate cancer may not necessarily reveal symptoms of lower urinary tract problems until developed further [54]
Metastatic bone cancer	Ache in right shoulder and arm	Common in men aged 80 years and over; no chronic lower backache due to spinal metastasis; has not mentioned weight loss; no swelling of lymph nodes in neck, groin or abdomen has been mentioned

►

Renal/uretic cancer	Blood in urine, no pain on urination, > 55 years old; can have bone metastases; men in Bill's age group have shown high risk of developing urological cancer when large amount of blood presents in the urine [57]	No weight loss, fatigue, fever
Bladder carcinoma	Blood in urine, no pain on urination; symptoms of prostatism	
TRAUMA AND PRE-EXISTING ILLNESS		
Causal factor: **Trauma** (strains, sprains, tear, neuralgia)	Shoulder strain from recent lifting and moving	
OBSTRUCTION AND FOREIGN BODY		
Renal calculi/kidney stones	Blood in urine	No back, abdominal, loin or groin referred pain noted in Bill's case history as a predominant symptom; no loss of appetite; blood pH normal
Bladder obstruction/ stones Neck hypertrophy	Difficulty in passing urine, diminished force, stream diminished, dribbling, urine flow intermittent; blood in urine; can occur with BPH	No pain on urination
FUNCTIONAL DISEASE		
Prostatism: obstructive and irritative symptoms	*Obstructive symptoms:* hesitancy to urinate, weak urinary stream, prolonged urination, terminal dribbling, urinary retention, overflow incontinence *Irritative symptoms:* urgency, frequency, nocturia, urge to urinate and incontinence, small urine void, pelvic pain and pain on urination	
Benign prostatic enlargement (BPH)	Urination during the night, difficult urination, decreased force of stream, dribbling of urine after voiding and blood in urine; both obstructive and storage symptoms; common in men aged 60 years and over	
Lower urinary tract symptoms (LUTS): voiding and filling symptoms [51]	*Voiding symptoms:* hesitancy, weak stream, straining to void, terminal dribbling, a sensation of incomplete emptying of bladder, overflow incontinence, acute retention *Filling symptoms:* nocturia, frequency, urgency, urge incontinence	

▶

Referred shoulder pain: myocardial infarction, angina pectoris, pneumothorax, bronchogenic carcinoma, peptic ulceration, cholecystitis	Bill is in the common age group for these conditions, shoulder pain	No specific shoulder tip pain reported with associated heart, gut or lung signs or symptoms at this stage; no hypertension
Sleep apnoea	Nocturia	No reports of daytime sleepiness, unrefreshed sleep or nocturnal choking
Causal factor: **Stress incontinence**	LUTS symptoms	Usually no nocturia in stress incontinence
Nocturnal polyuria syndrome	Nocturia, increased volume of urine	Usually occurs in the elderly from conditions such as diabetes, heart disease or from medications
DEGENERATIVE AND DEFICIENCY		
Degenerative and deficiency diseases (osteoarthritis)	Pain in shoulder, physical strain; Bill is in the common age group for such conditions	
INFECTION AND INFLAMMATION		
Chronic prostatitis	Blood in urine, LUTS symptoms	Common in men aged 20–40 years from gonorrhoea or other bacterial infection; no pain reported in lower back, penis, testicles, rectum, abdomen and no fever; no recurrent UTI reported; symptoms are usually more bothersome than those of BPH; no indications of infection in urinalysis
Prostatic abscess	Difficult voiding, blood in urine, diagnosis can be undetected	No perineal pain, no fever, no recurrent UTIs, no urethral discharge
STRESS AND NEUROLOGICAL DISEASE		
Neurologic disease: multiple sclerosis (MS), spinal cord injury, cauda equina syndrome	Symptoms of LUTS	Urinary symptoms are usually advanced stages of MS; no significant trauma or injury mentioned in health history so far; no lower back pain reported; no numbness, weakness or tingling in lower limbs

TABLE 5.67 DECISION TABLE FOR REFERRAL [3, 5, 7, 12]

COMPLAINT	CONTEXT	CORE
Referral for presenting complaint	Referral for all associated physical, dietary and lifestyle concerns	Referral for contributing emotional, mental, spiritual, metaphysical, lifestyle and constitutional factors
REFERRAL FLAGS	**REFERRAL FLAGS**	**REFERRAL FLAGS**
• Increasing difficulty in urination flow with nocturia • Urine symptoms worsening • Painless macroscopic blood in urine	• Shoulder pain is associated with urinary symptoms • Bill has not had a medical check-up for many years	• Bill has just gone through a major life change moving from another country
ISSUES OF SIGNIFICANCE	**ISSUES OF SIGNIFICANCE**	**ISSUES OF SIGNIFICANCE**
Nil	• Bill's BMI is on the higher end of normal and his waist circumference is 90 cm • Bill is drinking 2–3 glasses of red wine daily	• Misses children who live in a different part of the world • Has retired from owning a business for over 30 years
REFERRAL	**REFERRAL**	**REFERRAL**
• Referral for immediate medical investigation and diagnosis	• General health check-up • Dietary evaluation	• Recommend social activities to meet people and feel part of new community if desired

TABLE 5.68 FURTHER INVESTIGATIONS THAT MAY BE NECESSARY [1–8, 13, 56, 59]

TEST/INVESTIGATION	REASON FOR TEST/INVESTIGATION
FIRST-LINE INVESTIGATIONS:	
Rectal physical examination	Benign prostate feels smooth, soft, from plum size to orange; prostatitis, prostatic abscess feels large and boggy; cancerous prostate gland feels hard and irregular nodular enlargement
Abdominal examination	Distended bladder
Prostate-specific antigen (if rectal examination shows possible malignant gland) [59]	Raised in prostatic cancer, benign prostatic hypertrophy, prostatitis
Urinary diary	Record time, quantity of each voiding; how many times and volume of urine over 24 hours/3–5 days
Full blood count	Check for infections and/or anaemia
ESR/CRP blood test	Check for inflammation, tumour detection, bacteria and viral detection
Urinalysis: repeat test	Kidney infection, stones, diabetes, blood

▶

Urine microscopy	To eliminate possibility of renal disease; will give information about specific white blood cells (the presence of 10 or more indicates an inflammatory reaction in urinary tract), red blood cells, casts (clumps of materials or cells and can indicate renal disease) and crystals (indicate renal stone formation is imminent)
Cholesterol blood test	Test for cardiac markers; adverse affects from dietary or alcohol intake
IF NECESSARY:	
Neurological examination: flexion and extension of ankle, knee and hip against resistance	Second to fourth sacral nerves to check sensory and motor function of bladder
Musculoskeletal assessment	Physical signs of mechanical or inflammatory, compression or degeneration of upper spine, shoulder
Urodynamic studies (invasive tests): cystometry, measure filling pressures and stream [61]; can be helpful tool when preparing a client for surgery if necessary [62]	Evaluate bladder function
Q-tip/stress test: mobility of urethrovesical junction and coughing in certain positions with a full bladder	Test for stress incontinence
Urea, creatinine and electrolytes (sodium, potassium, chloride, bicarbonate) blood test	Signal muscle breakdown and tissue damage and gives an indicator for renal excretory function as urea and blood creatinine is excreted entirely by the kidneys; this will show in renal abnormalities and diabetes; creatinine may be high in clients with BPH
Estimated glomerular filtration rate (eGFR)	Kidney function
Fasting blood glucose test	Test for diabetes
Transrectal ultrasound	Detect prostatic cancer
Prostatic biopsy [55]	Determine prostatic cancer
Cystoscopy of bladder and pelvic lymph nodes/retrograde pyelography	Visualisation of bladder wall/determine urethral obstruction, node metastasis
Renal ultrasound	If renal disease is suspected; ultrasound will give information about renal size, failure, stones, mass formation, lesions
Plain abdominal x-ray	Determine bladder tract involvement, kidney stones
Liver function test	To detect signs of hepatitis, which can cause increased nocturnal urination; drinking alcohol every night
Skeletal survey	Metastatic carcinoma

Confirmed diagnosis

BILL AND BENIGN ENLARGEMENT OF THE PROSTATE GLAND

Bill is 59 years old, retired and has recently moved from Glasgow to Australia with his wife. Bill is enjoying life in Australia and looking forward to his children's forthcoming visit. Bill came to the clinic for help with a sore shoulder, but during the consultation he revealed he was been having some significant genitourinary symptoms. The symptoms were indicative of benign prostatic hyperplasia (BPH).

A diagnosis of BPH was confirmed by the GP to whom Bill was referred. BPH is a condition that occurs mostly in men over the age of 60 and is less common in individuals of African and Asian descent. Now called 'LUTS', lower urinary tract symptoms are very common and is a term used to describe symptoms that are experienced with diagnosis such as benign prostatic hyperplasia, bladder outflow and prostatism [51]. The connective tissue of the prostate enlarges the gland, stretching and distorting the urethra and obstructing bladder outflow. The bladder muscle then also enlarges resulting in higher than normal pressure in the bladder to compensate for the obstruction and allow voiding of the urine. Eventually the bladder can become dilated and the muscles lose tone. Upper urinary tract infections can occur as a consequence.

Clinical features of benign enlargement of the prostate gland include symptoms of LUTS and prostatism. Voiding, filling, obstructive and irritative symptoms include frequent urination, increased urination at night, difficulty and delay in initiating urination with reduced force of urine stream. Postvoid dribbling can be common and pain can be experienced if a bacterial infection or stone develops in the bladder. Occasionally blood in the urine can occur from the rupture of prostatic veins and if left untreated there is the potential for renal failure to develop. All of the above symptoms can cause men a great deal of distress with urinary incontinence being a particularly concerning daily symptom [52]. Indeed one study suggests that symptom severity may correlate more with overall health status and wellbeing, therefore holistic forms of assessing may be required rather than just by testing commonly used physiological and anatomical measures to rate the severity of BPH [60].

General references used in this diagnosis: 3–8, 51, 58

PRESCRIBED MEDICATION

• 5-alpha reductase inhibitor

Bill does not want to take any medication for his prostate at this stage preferring to try natural therapies first. He has agreed to be monitored by his doctor and will consider medication or surgery if his symptoms do not improve within six weeks, or if they worsen during that time.

TABLE 5.69 **DECISION TABLE FOR TREATMENT (ONCE DIAGNOSIS IS CONFIRMED)**		
COMPLAINT	**CONTEXT**	**CORE**
Treatment for the presenting complaint and symptoms	Treatment for all associated symptoms	Treatment for mental, emotional, spiritual, constitutional, lifestyle issues and metaphysical considerations

TREATMENT PRIORITY	TREATMENT PRIORITY	TREATMENT PRIORITY
• Lifestyle recommendations to reduce nocturia and improve other urinary tract symptoms as well as slowing down or preventing further enlargement of the prostate • Dietary recommendations to help reduce symptoms and further progression of prostate enlargement as well as improving prostate health • Physical therapy recommendations to improve symptoms • Herbal tonic or tablets and tea to help reduce symptoms and progression of prostate enlargement • Nutritional supplements to help reduce symptoms and progression of prostate enlargement **NB:** Plasma zinc levels should be monitored to ensure Bill's zinc levels stay within normal range [32]; it is important that Bill's case is collaboratively managed with a primary care physician to ensure his treatment program is effectively and properly targeted	• Lifestyle recommendations to enhance general health and wellbeing • Dietary recommendations to support general health and wellbeing and ensure ongoing good health and to reduce the risk of prostate cancer • Supplemental nutrients to support optimal nutritional status and to reduce the risk of prostate cancer • Physical therapy recommendations to help improve Bill's shoulder pain	• Advice for healthy lifestyle practices to help Bill maintain good physical, mental and emotional health in his retirement years

Treatment aims

- Reduce symptom severity and slow down or prevent further enlargement [14].
- Increase blood flow to the prostate [14].
- Correct nutritional deficiencies that may be contributing to his condition [14].
- Restore steroid hormones to normal levels and inhibit excessive conversion of testosterone to dihydrotestosterone (DHT) [14].
- Modulate hormonal and autonomic nervous system balance in the prostate [25].
- Inhibit DHT binding [14].
- Limit exposure to substances that promote prostate hyperplasia [14].
- Endeavour to slow down or stop enlargement of the prostate.

Lifestyle alterations/considerations

- Encourage Bill to take up regular exercise [14]. Men who are more physically active have a reduced frequency of lower urinary tract symptoms [25]. Men who walk 2–3 hours a week reduce their risk of BPH by 25 per cent [25].

- Bill may experience benefit from exercises to strengthen the muscles of his pelvic floor [40].
- To reduce the chance of urinary retention Bill should urinate once every three hours or so, and 'double-void' after urinating (wait a few moments after urinating and try again) [40].
- If Bill avoids drinking fluids after his evening meal he may not have to get up as frequently to urinate during the night [40].
- Encourage Bill to avoid cigarette smoke [14, 15, 29], environmental pesticide exposure and pesticide residues in food [14, 15, 29].
- Encourage Bill to maintain healthy cholesterol levels [14, 15, 29].

Dietary suggestions

- Encourage Bill to reduce consumption of animal protein and increase consumption of protein from vegetable sources [14, 15]. He should reduce consumption of saturated fats [14] and carbohydrates [14]. There is a direct relationship between BPH and starch intake [34]. Once Bill's symptoms improve a less stringent dietary regimen can be adopted that incorporates organic whole foods [14].
- Encourage Bill to choose organic, pesticide-free food [14, 15, 29].
- Encourage Bill to reduce consumption of saturated fat [14, 29], avoid margarine and *trans* fats [14] and increase consumption of foods containing omega-3 fatty acids such as cold-water fish, nuts and seeds [14, 15, 29, 34].
- Encourage Bill to eat a handful of pumpkin seeds each day [26, 29]. Pumpkin seeds contain phytosterols, which have an inhibitory effect on testosterone [26].
- Encourage Bill to consume zinc-rich foods [14, 32], particularly once he is no longer taking a zinc supplement [32].
- Encourage Bill to increase consumption of cooked tomatoes. Lycopene from tomato products is a powerful antioxidant [16] and consumption of lycopene from tomatoes and tomato products reduces the risk of prostate cancer [27].
- Encourage Bill to increase consumption of flavonoids from apples and onions [26, 29], isoflavones from soy products [26, 29, 35] and lignans in flaxseed, cereals, whole grains, fruit and vegetables [26, 29]. Consumption of phyto-oestrogens can reduce the risk of development and progression of prostate cancer [14, 30, 35].
- Encourage Bill to reduce or eliminate alcohol consumption [14, 15, 25]. High intake of alcohol increases the risk of high prostate cancer [28] and negates the effect of finasteride in reducing prostate cancer risk [28].
- Encourage Bill to reduce consumption of coffee [14, 26]. Green tea is a better choice due to its antioxidant properties and the ability of the polyphenol EGCG to modulate the production and actions of androgens [32].
- Encourage Bill to increase consumption of foods containing the amino acids alanine, glycine and glutamic acid [32]. Sources of these amino acids include legumes, eggs, wheatgerm, whey protein, nuts, beans, oats, animal meat, fish and other seafood [33]. Vegetarian sources, fish and seafood are the preferred sources of these amino acids [14].
- Encourage Bill to increase consumption of dietary fibre [29, 32]. Dietary fibre binds steroid hormones and can be used to modify hormonal status by altering enterohepatic circulation of hormones [31]. A low fat and flaxseed-enriched diet has been demonstrated to significantly decrease PSA levels [32].

Physical treatment suggestions

- Therapeutic massage of the abdominal integuments is likely to improve micturition and Bill's quality of life [37].

- Hydrotherapy: constitutional hydrotherapy [45]. Alternating hot/cold sitz bath [45]. Cold water adaptive showers to improve the immune system [46]. Hot (no more than 110°F or 43°C) shower treatment over the shoulder joint for three minutes followed by a cold treatment (no less than 55°F or 12°C) for one minute; repeat for three rounds daily [47]. Contrast treatment for the shoulder with moist heat over the joint for three minutes, followed by an ice pack/ice cold compress for 30 seconds. Repeat [47].
- Acupuncture may improve Bill's shoulder pain [38].
- Bill may find massage therapy is beneficial for his shoulder pain [39].

TABLE 5.70 HERBAL FORMULA (1:2 LIQUID EXTRACTS)

HERB	FORMULA	RATIONALE
Saw palmetto *Serenoa repens* Standardised to contain 85%–95% fatty acids and sterols [15]	60 mL	Inhibits 5-alpha reductase activity [18, 41], thereby preventing conversion of testosterone to dihydrotestosterone [18]; inhibits binding of dihydrotestosterone and testosterone to androgen receptors [16]; inhibits trophic effect of prolactin on the prostate gland [19]; anti-inflammtory [16]; antiproliferative [16]; effective treatment for stages 1 and 2 BPH [16]; similar and faster effect to the anti-androgenic drug finasteride [17]
Pygeum *Pygeum africanum* Standardised to contain 14% triterpenes [15] (cultivated/plantation source)	60 mL	Reduces presenting symptoms and clinical signs of BPH [15, 16]; the phytochemicals in pygeum are thought to counteract the structural and biochemical changes of BPH [16]; inhibits prostatic fibroblast proliferation [17]; lowers blood cholesterol [16]
Stinging nettle root *Urtica dioica*	80 mL	Inhibits cellular proliferation in BPH [20, 21], inhibits binding activity of sex hormone-binding globulin [20]; combining stinging nettle root with saw palmetto improves pathological findings and obstructive and irritative symptoms in BPH [22]
Supply:	200 mL	Dose: 10 mL twice daily

If difficulties in obtaining **pygeum** as a liquid extract are encountered it may need to be provided in tablet form.
The recommended daily dose of liposterolic extract of **saw palmetto** for BPH is 160 mg twice daily [16]; this may be easier and more convenient to provide to Bill in tablet or capsule form

TABLE 5.71 **HERBAL TEA**		
Alternative to tea and coffee		
HERB	**FORMULA**	**RATIONALE**
Crataeva bark *Crataeva nurvala*	2 parts	Traditionally used in ayurvedic medicine to treat disorders of the urinary system and is considered a bladder tonic [24]; relieves frequency incontinence, pain and urinary retention in people with hypotonic bladder due to BPH [24]; useful to treat BPH in combination with pygeum [24]
Horsetail *Equisetum arvense*	1 part	Genitourinary astringent [23]; antihaemorrhagic [23]; indicated for inflammation or benign enlargement of the prostate [23]
Willow herb *Epilobium parviflorum*	2 parts	Diuretic [50]; anti-inflammatory [50]; antineoplastic [50]; immunostimulating [50]; inhibits prostatic cell proliferation [48, 49, 50]; indicated for use in BPH [49, 50]
Decoction: 1 tsp per cup – 1 cup 3 times daily Stinging nettle root could be added to this tea formula (at 2 parts) if saw palmetto and pygeum are given to Bill in tablet or capsule form rather than liquid extract		

TABLE 5.72 **NUTRITIONAL SUPPLEMENTS**	
SUPPLEMENT AND DOSE	**RATIONALE**
Zinc 50 mg daily for a maximum of 6 months [14, 32]; 2 mg daily of copper should be included if zinc supplement is taken for more than 1 month [26]	Antioxidant [16, 26, 33]; zinc alters hormonal binding in the prostate and inhibits activity of 5-alpha-reductase [14, 26]; zinc supplementation may be beneficial in the prevention of prostate cancer [32, 44]
Omega-3 fish oil 6000–8000 mg daily in divided doses [29]	Omega-3 fatty acids may provide protective benefit against prostate cancer [42, 43]
High-potency practitioner-strength **multivitamin, mineral and antioxidant supplement** providing therapeutic doses of antioxidant vitamins and minerals [29]	Increased oxidative stress resulting from lowered antioxidant levels may play a role in the development of prostate cancer [14, 36]

References

[1] G. Douglas, F. Nicol, C. Robertson, Macleod's Clinical Examination, twelth edn, Churchill Livingstone Elsevier, Edinburgh, 2009.

[2] N.J. Talley, S. O'Connor, Pocket Clinical Examination, third edn, Churchill Livingstone Elsevier, Australia, 2009.

[3] P. Kumar, C. Clark, Clinical Medicine, sixth edn, Elsevier Saunders, London, 2005.

[4] R.M.D. Berkow, A.J.M.D. Fletcher, M.H.M.D. Beers, The Merck Manual, sixteenth edn., Merck Research Laboratories, Rathway, N.J, 1993 (later edition).

[5] J. Jamison, Differential Diagnosis for Primary Care, second edn, Churchill Livingstone Elsevier, London, 2006.

[6] A. Polmea (Ed.), Evidence-Based Diagnosis in Primary Care, Churchill Livingstone Elsevier, Edinburgh, 2008.

[7] R.H. Seller, Differential Diagnosis of Common Complaints, fifth edn, Saunders Elsevier, Philadelphia, 2007.

[8] R.D. Collins, Differential Diagnosis in Primary Care, fourth edn, Lippincott Williams & Wilkins, Philadelphia, 2008.

[9] J. Silverman, S. Kurtz, J. Draper, Skills for Communicating with Patients, second edn, Radcliff Publishing, Oxford, 2000.

[10] R. Neighbour, The Inner Consultation; how to develop an effective and intuitive consulting style, Radcliff Publishing, Oxon, 2005.

[11] M. Lloyd, R. Bor, Communication Skills For Medicine, third edn, Churchill Livingstone Elsevier, Edinburgh, 2009.

[12] D. Peters, L. Chaitow, G. Harris, S. Morrison, Integrating Complementary Therapies in Primary Care, Churchill Livingstone, London, 2002.

[13] K.D. Pagna, T.J. Pagna, Mosby's Diagnostic and Laboratory Test reference, third edn, Mosby, USA, 1997 (later edition).

[14] J.E. Pizzorno, M.T. Murray, H. Joiner-Bey, The Clinicians Handbook of Natural Medicine, second edn, Churchill Livingstone, St Louis, 2008.

[15] S. El-Hashemy, Naturopathic Standards of Primary Care, CCNM Press Inc, Toronto, 2007.

[16] L. Braun, M. Cohen, Herbs & Natural Supplements: An evidence based guide, second edn, Elsevier, Sydney, 2007.

[17] F. Yablonski, V. Nicolas, J.P. Riffaud, F. Bellamy, Antiproliferative Effect of Pygeum Africanum Extract on Rat Prostatic Fibroblasts, The Journal of Urology 157 (6) (1997) 2381–2387.

[18] C.W. Bayne, M. Ross, F. Donnelly, F.K. Habib, The selectivity and specificity of the actions of the lipido-sterolic extract of Serenoa repens (Permixon) on the prostate, The Journal of Urology 164 (3 pt. 1) (2000) 876–881.

[19] F. VanCoppenolle, X. LeBourhis, F. Carpentier, G. Delaby, D. Cousse, J.P. Raynaud, J.P. Dupouy, N. Prevarskaya, Pharmacological Effects of the Lipidosterolic Extract of Serenoa repens (PermixonT) on Rat Prostate Hyperplasia Induced by Hyperprolactinemia: Comparison With Finasteride, The Prostate 43 (2000) 49–58.

[20] S. Mills, K. Bone, Principles & Practice of Phytotherapy; Modern Herbal Medicine, Churchill Livingstone, Edinburgh: London, 2000.

[21] T. Hirano, M. Homma, K. Oka, Effects of stinging nettle root extracts and their steroidal components on the Na+, K(+)-ATPase of the benign prostatic hyperplasia, Planta Med 60 (1) (1994) 30–33.

[22] H.J. Schneider, E. Honold, T. Masuhr: in S. Mills, K. Bone, Principles & Practice of Phytotherapy; Modern Herbal Medicine, Churchill Livingstone, Edinburgh: London, 2000, pp. 490–498.

[23] British Herbal Medicine Association, British Herbal Pharmacopoeia, BHMAA, 1983.

[24] K. Bone, Clinical Applications of Chinese and Ayurvedic Herbs: Monographs for the Western Herbal Practitioners, Phytotherapy Press, Warwick, 1996.

[25] E.A. Platz, I. Kawachi, E.B. Rimm, G.A. Colditz, M.J. Stampfer, W.C. Willett, E. Giovannucci, Physical Activity and Benign Prostatic Hyperplasia, Archives of Internal Medicine 158 (1998) 2349–2356.

[26] J. Jamison, Clinical Guide to Nutrition & Dietary Supplements in Disease Management, Churchill Livingstone, Edinburgh, 2003.

[27] E. Giovanucci, A Review of Epidemiologic Studies of Tomatoes, Lycopene, and Prostate Cancer, Experimental Biology and Medicine 227 (2002) 852–859.

[28] Z. Gong, A.R. Kristal, J.M. Schenk, C.M. Tangen, P.J. Goodman, I.M. Thompson, Alcohol Consumption, Finasteride, and Prostate Cancer Risk, Cancer 115 (2009) 3661–3669.

[29] H. Osiecki, The Physicians Handbook of Clinical Nutrition, seventh ed., Bioconcepts, Eagle Farm, 2000.

[30] F.S. Dalais, An. Meliala, N. Wattanapenpaiboon, M. Frydenberg, D.A. Suter, W.K. Thomson, M.L. Wahlqvist, Effects Of A Diet Rich In Phytoestrogens on Prostate-Specific Antigen And Sex Hormones In Men Diagnosed With Prostate Cancer, Urology 64 (3) (2004) 510–515.

[31] C.F. Whitten, T.D. Schultz, Binding of steroid hormones in vitro by water-insoluble dietary fiber, Nutrition Research 8 (11) (1988) 1223–1235.

[32] P. Ranjan, D. Dalela, S.N. Sankhwar, Diet and Benign Prostatic Hyperplasia: Implications for Prevention, Urology 68 (2006) 470–476.

[33] H. Osiecki, The Nutrient Bible, seventh edn, BioConcepts Publishing,Eagle Farm , 2008.

[34] F. Bravi, C. Bosetti, L. DalMaso, R. Talamini, M. Montella, E. Negri, V. Ramazzotti, et al., Macronutrients, fatty acids, cholesterol, and risk of benign prostatic hyperplasia, Urology 67 (2006) 1205–1211.

[35] E. Deutsch, L. Maggiorella, P. Eschwege, J. Bourhis, J.C. Soria, B. Abhulkarim, Environmental, genetic, and molecular features of prostate cancer, Lancet Oncology 5 (5) (2004) 303–313.

[36] A. Aydin, Z. Arsova-Sarafinovska, A. Sayal, A. Eken, O. Erdem, K. Erten, Y. Ozgok, A. Dimovski, Oxidative stress and antioxidant status in non-metastatic prostate cancer and benign prostatic hyperplasia, Clinical Biochemistry 39 (2006) 176–179.

[37] K. Kassolik, W. Andrzejewski, M. Brzozowski, E. Trzesicka, W. Apoznanski, T. Szydelko, A. Steciwko, et al., Medical massage as a physiotherapeutic method in benign prostatic hyperplasia in men, Journal of Bodywork and Movement Therapies 11 (2007) 121–128.

[38] J.A. Guerra de Hoyos, M. Martin, E.B. deLeon, M.V. Lopez, T.M. Lopez, F.A. Morilla, M.J. Gonzalez Moreno, Randomised trial of long term effect of acupuncture for shoulder pain, Pain 112 (2004) 289–298.

[39] P.A. van den Dolder, D.L. Roberts, A trial into the effectiveness of soft tissue massage in the treatment of shoulder pain, Australian Journal of Physiotherapy 49 (2003) 183–188.

[40] H. Simon, D. Zieve, reviewers. Enlarged Prostate; Lifestyle Changes. A.D.A.M. Inc. 2009. Retrieved 24 July 2009 from http://health.nytimes.com/health/guides/disease/enlarged-prostate/lifestyle-changes.html

[41] A.C. Buck, Phytotherapy for the prostate, British Journal of Urology 78 (3) (1996) 325–336.

[42] W.J. Aronson, J.A. Glaspy, S.T. Reddy, D. Reese, D. Heber, D. Bagga, Modulation Of Omega-3/Omega-6 Polyunsaturated Ratios With Dietary Fish Oils In Men With Prostate Cancer, Urology 58 (2001) 283–288.

[43] M.F. Leitzmann, M.J. Stampfer, D.S. Michaud, K. Augustsson, G.C. Coltitz, W.C. Willett, et al., Dietary intake of n-3 and n-6 fatty acids and the risk of prostate cancer, American Journal of Clinical Nutrition 80 (2004) 204–216.

[44] L.C. Costello, R.B. Franklin, P. Feng, M. Tan, O. Bagasra, Zinc and prostate cancer: a critical scientific, medical, and public interest issue (United States), Cancer Causes and Control 16 (2005) 901–915.

[45] W. Boyle, A. Saine, Lectures in Naturopathic Hydrotherapy, Eclectic Medical Publications, Oregon, 1988.

[46] N. Schevchuk, S. Radoja, Possible stimulation of anti-tumour immunity using repeated cold stress: a hypothesis, Infect Agent-Cancer 2 (2007) 20.

[47] M. Sinclair, Modern Hydrotherapy for the Massage Therapist, Lippincott Williams & Wilkins, Baltimore, 2008.

[48] A. Vitalone, M. Guizetti, L.G. Costa, B. Tita, Extracts of various species of Epilobium inhibit proliferation of human prostate cells, Journal of Pharmacy and Pharmacology 55 (2003) 683–690.

[49] A. Vitalone, F. Bordi, G. Baldazzi, L. Mazzanti, B. Saso, B. Tita, Anti-proliferative effect on a prostatic epithelial cell line (PZ-HPV-7) by Epilobium angustifolium L, Il Farmaco 56 (2001) 483–489.

[50] Z. Marczyński, M. Zgoda, The effect of auxiliary substances on pharmaceutical availability of medicinal substances contained in dry extract from small-flowered willow herb (Epilobium parviflorum Schreb.), Herba Polonica 51 (1–2) (2005) 29–36.

[51] C.T. Brown, G. Das, Assessment, diagnosis, and management of lower urinary tract symptoms in men, Int J Clin Pract 56 (2002) 591–603.

[52] G. Engstrom, M.-L. Walker-Engstrom, L. Henningsohn, et al., Prevalence of distress and symptom severity from the lower urinary tract in men: a population-based study with the DAN-PSS questionnaire, Fam Pract 21 (2004) 617–622.

[53] W. Hamilton, D. Sharp, T. Peters, et al., Clinical features of prostate cancer before diagnosis: a population-based, case-control study, Br J Gen Pract 56 (2006) 756–762.

[54] W. Hamilton, D. Sharp, Symptomatic diagnosis of prostate cancer in primary care: a structured review, Br J Gen Pract 54 (2004) 617–621.

[55] M. McNaughton-Collins, F.J. Fowler, J. Caubet, et al., Psychological effects of a suspicious prostate cancer screening test followed by a benign biopsy result, Am J Med 117 (2004) 719–725.

[56] I. Thompson, D. Ankerst, C. Chi, et al., Assessing prostate cancer risk: results from the prostate cancer prevention trial, J Natl Cancer Inst 98 (2006) 529–534.

[57] R. Bruyninckx, F. Buntinx, B. Aertgeerts, et al., The diagnostic value of macroscopic haematuria for the diagnosis of urological cancer in general practice, Br J Gen Pract 53 (2003) 31–35.

[58] J.M. Fitzpatrick, The natural history of benign prostatic hyperplasia, BJU Int 97 (Suppl) (2006) 3–6.

[59] C.G. Roehrborn, P. Boyle, A.L. Gould, et al., Serum prostate-specific antigen as a predictor of prostate volume in men with benign prostatic hyperplasia, Urology 53 (1999) 581–589.

[60] M.J. Barry, A.T. Cockett, H.L. Holtgrewe, et al., Relationship of symptoms of prostatism to commonly used physiological and anatomical measures of the severity of benign prostatic hyperplasia, J Urol 150 (1993) 351–358.

[61] J. Bosch, R. Kranse, R. Van Mastrigt, et al., Reasons for the weak correlation between prostate volume and urethral resistance parameters in patients with prostatism, J Urol 153 (1995) 689–693.

[62] K.M. Jensen, R.C. Bruskewitz, P. Iversen, P.O. Madsen, Spontaneous uroflowmetry in prostatism, Urology 24 (1984) 403–409.

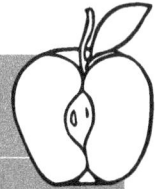

CHAPTER 6

Respiratory/ENT system

Asthma

Case history

Eleven-year-old Jake Watson has been brought to the clinic for help with a productive cough that has been present for nearly four weeks. Jake's cough is associated with clear, thick mucus.

Jake is sports mad and loves playing all sports, however, he has been doing less recently because the cough gets worse when he runs around in cold weather. Jake says he is running out of breath much more quickly when he plays sport and he needs to stop in order to breathe normally again. Jake is involved with his local junior athletics club and tends to get anxious before big competitions. Five weeks ago Jake developed an upper respiratory tract infection. His doctor prescribed a course of antibiotics, but the cough has persisted and is becoming worse, particularly at night. Because it's winter, Jake's parents would like to help boost his immune system – he seems to get a lot of coughs in the colder months. He had bronchitis three months ago, which was treated successfully with a course of antibiotics. Jake's cousin is asthmatic, but his parents tell you they are not aware of anyone else in the family who is.

Jake loves food but does not always eat vegetables and fruit. He usually has Weet-Bix and milk for breakfast and loves cheese and white-bread sandwiches for lunch. His mum tells you she always packs fruit in his lunchbox, but it often comes home uneaten. He eats whatever is served for dinner but often leaves the vegetables uneaten unless he is made to eat them. Jake loves chocolate and McDonald's, which his parents allow occasionally as a treat. Neither parent has ever smoked.

Jake's mother confides that she and Jake's dad have been arguing more recently and she thinks Jake has overheard things when he is supposed to be asleep at night. Jake lives in the country with his mum and dad and has no siblings. His mother would like to move closer to the city to be nearer her family. This has been a catalyst for tension in the household because Jake's father is happy where they are living now and doesn't want to move.

TABLE 6.1 **COMPLAINT**	
Analogy: Skin of the apple	**Complaint:** Define the presenting complaint and symptoms; understand the complaint *Chronic cough*
AREAS OF INVESTIGATION AND EXAMPLE QUESTIONS	**CLIENT RESPONSES**
Onset *When did you first notice the cough?*	*After I had a cold last month.*
Timing *How often do you cough?*	*Every day.*
Exacerbating factors *What makes it worse?*	*When I run around and at night.*
Relieving factors *What makes it better?*	*When I stay inside and during the day.*
Examination and inspection	Physical examination reveals bilateral tenderness of cervical lymph nodes.

TABLE 6.2 **CONTEXT**	
Analogy: Flesh of the apple	**Context:** Put the presenting complaint into context to understand the disease
AREAS OF INVESTIGATION AND EXAMPLE QUESTIONS	**CLIENT RESPONSES**
Family health To Jake's mum: *Is there a family history of asthma?*	*Jake's cousin has asthma.*
Allergies and irritants *Are there symptoms of sneezing or nose discharge, conjunctivitis and itching on the roof of the mouth with the cough?* (allergies)	Jake's mum answers: *No, not much in terms of sneezing or runny nose or eye symptoms.*
Infection and inflammation *Is the cough ever worse in the morning?* (PND, chronic bronchitis)	Jake's mum answers: *It seems to be getting worse during the night, but he doesn't cough more in the morning.*
Stress and neurological disease *So if I understand correctly, the cough is disturbing sleep and does* not *improve at night?* (may rule out psychogenic, habit cough, Tourette's syndrome)	Jake's mum answers: *Yes, that's right, it seems to definitely worsen during the night but I'm not sure if that's because of how cold his room gets at night sometimes.*

▶

Eating habits and energy *Tell me about Jake's diet and his energy levels.*	Jake's mum answers: *He eats whatever I give him, but doesn't like vegetables very much. He has Weet-Bix and milk for breakfast and usually a cheese sandwich for lunch. I send fruit to school every day but he usually brings it home. He would eat McDonald's every day if we let him, but we don't.* *He is usually full of energy, but he seems to be a bit lethargic recently.*

TABLE 6.3 **CORE**	
Analogy: Core of the apple with the seed of ill health	**Core:** Holistic assessment to understand the client
AREAS OF INVESTIGATION AND EXAMPLE QUESTIONS	**CLIENT RESPONSES**
Emotional health To Jake's mother: *Do you think Jake might be a bit stressed? Can you tell me about that?*	*There has been a bit of conflict between Jake's dad and myself. I would like to live closer to my family, but he really loves it where we are and wants to stay.*
Daily activities To Jake: *Tell me what you do every day.*	*I go to school and when I get home I muck around with my friends or watch TV.*
Family and friends To Jake: *Tell me about your friends and family.*	*Tim and Ryan live up the road so we hang out a lot. My cousins live in the city so I see them sometimes on the weekend or in the holidays.*
Action needed to heal To Jake: *I know you'd like to get rid of your cough and have more energy again. Do you think you'd be willing to take some medicine and do some things I suggest to help you get better?*	*Depends if I like it.*

TABLE 6.4 **JAKE'S SIGNS AND SYMPTOMS** [1–3]	
Pulse	100 bpm (normal pulse for a child is 80–120 bpm)
Blood pressure	110/77 sitting with child cuff
Temperature	37°C
Respiratory rate	14 resp/min (15–30 resp/min is usual for a child)
Body mass index	20 (85th percentile for an 11-year-old boy)
Face	Red
Physical examination	Cervical nodes small and tender on both right and left sides
Urinalysis	No abnormality detected (NAD)

Results of medical investigations

No investigations have been carried out.

TABLE 6.5 **UNLIKELY DIAGNOSTIC CONSIDERATIONS** [2–4, 63]	
CONDITIONS AND CAUSES	**WHY UNLIKELY**
INFECTION AND INFLAMMATION	
Acute viral upper respiratory tract infection	No fever, cough has been present for more than 2 weeks
Acute bronchitis	No fever, cough has been present for more than 2 weeks
Tuberculosis	No fever, cough has been present for more than 2 weeks
Pneumonia	No fever, cough has been present for more than 2 weeks

Case analysis

TABLE 6.6 **POSSIBLE DIFFERENTIAL DIAGNOSIS**		
Not ruled out by tests/investigations already done [2, 4, 5, 10–13, 63, 64, 66–68, 76, 77]		
CONDITION	**WHY POSSIBLE**	**WHY UNLIKELY**
ALLERGIES AND IRRITANTS		
Chronic allergies, irritants [64, 65]	Lives in the country, could be near irritants and pollutants such as pollens, dust and farming practices or chemicals that could trigger allergies or bronchial irritation; Jake may be exposed to chlorine and swimming pools	No history of hay fever, sinus or seasonal allergies

▶

CANCER AND HEART DISEASE		
Carcinoma: leukaemia, carcinoma of oesophagus, larynx, trachea, bronchi, alveoli, pleura	Persistent cough	Rare
TRAUMA AND PRE-EXISTING ILLNESS		
Causal factor: **Trauma/physical abuse:** from rib fracture, laceration, haemorrhage, inhalation of foreign object	Persistent cough, stress at home	No signs or symptoms of associated body pain or trauma as yet
FUNCTIONAL DISEASE		
Cystic fibrosis	Can present in school-aged children, breathlessness, recurrent chest infections	No sign of sinusitis, mucus in bowel motions, blood in sputum
Gastro-oesophageal reflux	Common cause of persistent recurrent cough; can be worse after eating chocolate or caffeinated foods/drink can be exercise induced	Usually occurs in adults and presents with a non-productive cough; usually worse on waking and after eating
INFECTION AND INFLAMMATION		
Asthma: postviral	Children with recurrent cough are often asthmatic; Jake's recent upper respiratory tract infection was most probably viral (antibiotics did not completely resolve it); family history of asthma; productive cough that is persistent and subacute with clear thick mucus; cough is worse at night, in the cold and on exertion; stressful time at home with parents fighting; shortness of breath is associated with the cough in cold weather	
Chronic bronchitis: viral, bacterial, allergen based	Jake's cough has lasted longer than 3 weeks; productive sputum, recurrent episodes, worse with exercise, lymph nodes raised; often due to dry air in winter months in school-aged children; persistent cough irritated by nonspecific bronchial irritants; shortness of breath on exertion	No exposure to cigarette smoke in the household; Jake's cough does not produce yellow mucus; he doesn't have a headache, fever, chills or abdominal pain; usually more likely for chronic bronchitis to develop in adults; often cough is worse in the morning

▶

Causal factor: **Recurrent viral upper respiratory tract infections**	Viruses are the most common cause of coughs in children who are in contact with other children; can exacerbate asthma symptoms	No current fever or sign of viral infection
Parasites or fungi in alveoli	Cause inflammatory cough	Rare
Enlarged adenoids	Common cause of persistent cough in children	No mention of sinus or throat concerns in the case history
STRESS AND NEUROLOGICAL DISEASE		
Causal factor: **Psychogenic cough**	Stress at home from parents arguing	Jakes cough does not usually improve during the night or with sleep

TABLE 6.7 DECISION TABLE FOR REFERRAL [2, 5, 8, 9]

COMPLAINT	CONTEXT	CORE
Referral for presenting complaint	Referral for all associated physical, dietary and lifestyle concerns	Referral for contributing emotional, mental, spiritual, metaphysical, lifestyle and constitutional factors
REFERRAL FLAGS	**REFERRAL FLAGS**	**REFERRAL FLAGS**
• Persistent cough that is worse at night and after exercise	• Recent upper respiratory tract infection treated with antibiotics • Possible underlying allergies or intolerances • Lowered immunity	Nil
ISSUES OF SIGNIFICANCE	**ISSUES OF SIGNIFICANCE**	**ISSUES OF SIGNIFICANCE**
Nil	• Inadequate nutritional status (does not always eat vegetables) • Recent use of antibiotics may have negatively affected intestinal microflora	• Tendency to anxiety • Stress and anxiety from hearing parents arguing
REFERRAL	**REFERRAL**	**REFERRAL**
• Referral for medical assessment and diagnosis and management plan [70, 76]	• Dietary assessment • Food allergy and intolerance assessment	• Massage for relaxation • Counsellor specialising in children's psychology to assess anxiety levels

TABLE 6.8 **FURTHER INVESTIGATIONS THAT MAY BE NECESSARY** [1, 2, 4, 5, 10–13, 75]	
TEST/INVESTIGATION	**REASON FOR TEST/INVESTIGATION**
FIRST-LINE INVESTIGATIONS:	
Ear, nose, throat physical examination	Infection and allergic signs
Chest examination: auscultation, percussion	Signs of asthma, obstruction, infection, foreign body, heart failure
Sputum test: histology, microbiology	Detect presence of eosinophils (sign for asthma), eliminate bronchitis and pneumonia, TB, fungal origin
Lung function tests: forced expiratory volume (FEV), peak expiratory flow rate (PEF)	Will be reduced in asthma and chronic bronchitis
Exercise test	Asthma
Differential white cell count	Detection of eosinophils to confirm allergic triggers for asthma
Full blood count and IgE [74]	Infection, inflammation, anaemia, allergies
ESR/CRP	Pneumonia, infection, cancer
IF NECESSARY:	
Chest x-ray	Lung abscess or tumour
Histamine/methacholine bronchial provocation test [71, 72]	Asthma
Capnometer/pulmonary gas exchange during orthostatic Tests/Nijmegen questionnaire	Hyperventilation syndrome [43–46]
Skin prick test [73]	For extrinsic allergies connected to asthma in young children
RAST [74]	To identify allergies
Food diary	To help determine any foods that may be triggering or aggravating symptoms
Sweat test	Cystic fibrosis

Confirmed diagnosis

JAKE AND ASTHMA

Jake is an only child who has presented to the clinic with asthmatic symptoms following a respiratory tract infection, which was treated with antibiotics. Jake is generally a healthy and active child, although his diet appears to be lacking in a number of nutrients essential for healthy immune and lung function. Jake is also showing signs of anxiety, which may have had an effect on his immunity and respiratory health.

Asthma is a chronic inflammatory condition of the airways. Symptoms include wheezing, chest tightness, shortness of breath on expiration, a cough that is worse at night and on exertion, and production of thick clear-coloured phlegm. Onset commonly occurs in childhood and young adulthood when asthma attacks can last from hours to days. Asthma is categorised as mild, moderate or severe depending on symptom frequency and lung function tests. The condition is often initiated by a viral upper respiratory tract infection in children and may be temporary although it can often become a permanent condition. The main defining medical features of asthma include airway limitation, airway hyperresponsiveness and inflammation of the bronchi. There are both extrinsic (definite external causes such as allergies) and intrinsic (causative agents not medically identified) reasons for why asthma is triggered and develops. Precipitating factors include allergies, atmospheric and occupational pollutants [64, 65], irritants (such as cigarette smoke), medication (NSAIDs, beta-blockers), drugs, cold air, exercise, diet and emotion. Theories suggest that more exposure to allergens and illness in early years helps children boost immune response and ward off triggers for developing asthma [60, 69].

Causes of asthma include:

- elevated eosinophils in submucosa and airway exudates – these continue the inflammatory response even when the upper respiratory infection has cleared
- mucosal oedema
- production of thick mucus by airway mucosa
- increased levels of IgE – allergy.

General references used in this diagnosis: 2, 4, 10, 11, 13, 59, 61, 62, 68, 69

PRESCRIBED MEDICATION

- Combined reliever and preventer medication

TABLE 6.9 **DECISION TABLE FOR TREATMENT (ONCE DIAGNOSIS IS CONFIRMED)**		
COMPLAINT	**CONTEXT**	**CORE**
Treatment for the presenting complaint and symptoms	Treatment for all associated symptoms	Treatment for mental, emotional, spiritual, constitutional, lifestyle issues and metaphysical considerations
TREATMENT PRIORITY	**TREATMENT PRIORITY**	**TREATMENT PRIORITY**
• Lifestyle recommendations to reduce symptom severity and improve cardiopulmonary fitness • Recommendation for breathing exercises that may reduce the frequency and severity of asthma attacks • Lifestyle recommendations to identify and manage asthma triggers • Physical therapy suggestions to improve pulmonary function	• Lifestyle recommendation to reduce exposure to known and suspected environmental triggers • Physical therapy recommendations to improve general health and immune function • Dietary recommendations to increase consumption of foods that will improve Jake's general health, nutrition and respiratory health	• Lifestyle recommendations to reduce Jake's physical symptoms • Recommendation for counselling and stress-management techniques to reduce stress and anxiety-related symptom aggravation • Recommendation for Jake's parents to talk to him regarding his anxieties about their arguing

▶

• Dietary recommendations to identify and manage food allergies or sensitivities that may be triggering asthma and to increase consumption of foods with anti-inflammatory action • Herbal tonic or tea with bronchospasmolytic, bronchodilatory, antimicrobial, expectorant anti-inflammatory and antiallergic actions • Nutritional supplements to reduce inflammation and improve bronchial tone and lung function **NB:** Herbal formula and nutritional supplements should be reviewed once Jake's symptoms are under control; it is important for Jake's condition to be collaboratively managed with his GP to ensure optimal treatment outcome	• Dietary recommendations to identify and manage food allergies or sensitivities • Herbal tonic or tea with adaptogenic, antioxidant, immunomodulatory and tonic action to improve Jake's vitality and immunity • Supplemental nutrients to improve Jake's levels of essential nutrients, reduce inflammation, allergic response, modulate immune function and restore intestinal microflora to improve general health and reduce asthma symptoms **NB:** Supplements have been recommended in order of priority to help improve compliance and take financial considerations into account	• Recommendation to keep physically active to improve physical and emotional health • Physical therapy suggestions to help reduce Jake's stress and anxiety • Herbal tonic or tea with anxiolytic and adaptogenic action to support Jake's nervous system and stress response • Nutritional support for stress and nervous system

Treatment aims

- Reduce inflammation [14], bronchial hyperreactivity [14] and bronchial smooth muscle contraction [15].
- Modulate immune-based inflammatory responses [14].
- Identify and eliminate or reduce exposure to allergies and/or sensitivities that are triggering Jake's asthma [12, 15, 16, 50].
- Identify and reduce or eliminate underlying causative or sustaining factors such as:
  - food allergies or intolerances [17, 50]
  - compromised digestive function, hypochlorhydria [15], increased intestinal permeability [15, 51]
  - underlying infection (possibly low-grade, unresolved infection) [15, 50]
  - emotional stress [15]
  - environmental triggers such as air pollution, cigarette smoke, cold dry air [16, 50].
- Improve Jake's diet and nutritional status [17].

Lifestyle alterations/considerations

- Jake may benefit from controlled breathing exercises that emphasise slow regular breathing in which the ratio of inhalation to exhalation is 1:2 (e.g. yogic breathing) [16, 28]. Breathing exercises may reduce the frequency of asthma attacks [28]. Inhaling hot, moist air during breathing exercises can enhance the benefits [28].
- Encourage Jake to keep exercising as asthma symptoms are easier to control in people who are physically fit [28]. Improved cardiopulmonary fitness improves emotional status and decreases the intensity of wheezing attacks [33].
- If it is determined that Jake has environmental allergies (e.g. house dust mites, pets, etc.), it is important to manipulate his environment to reduce his exposure to environmental allergens [28].

- Encourage Jake to avoid or minimise his exposure to environmental triggers such as cold, dry air and airborne pollutants such as cigarette smoke, smoke from wood heaters, diesel fumes, etc. [16, 53, 54].
- Stress-management techniques, such as meditation, progressive muscle relaxation and autogenic training, can help manage stress and improve pulmonary function [28]. There is considerable evidence for a link between emotional or stress responses and asthma [32]. Helping Jake to cope with his stress and emotions may help improve his asthma symptoms [32].
- Jake needs to get an asthma-management plan from his doctor. Asthma-management plans are designed to help children and parents identify early signs of worsening asthma and intervene early with appropriate treatment strategies to prevent symptoms worsening. Written asthma-management plans are strongly associated with a reduced risk of adverse outcomes among children with asthma [34].
- Jake may benefit from counselling to help him learn helpful coping strategies to deal with his anxiety [35].
- Encourage Jake's parents to talk to him about his anxieties, particularly relating to him overhearing them arguing. Reassurance from his parents is important.

Dietary suggestions

For compliance reasons, these are listed in order of priority. Jake may not be happy with an immediate radical change to his diet. The authors' clinical experience has shown that gradual dietary change is more likely to be permanent than immediate radical dietary change.

- Jake should increase dietary intake of omega-3 fatty acids from cold-water fish, almonds, walnuts, pumpkin and flaxseed [28, 47] and reduce omega-6 [48] and *trans*-fatty acids [49]. Consumption of fresh oily fish is associated with a significantly reduced risk of asthma and improved pulmonary function [28, 47].
- Check for food sensitivities, intolerances or allergies and avoid foods that may precipitate an asthma attack [12, 15–17]. Some asthmatics experience significant improvement when excluding known reactive foods [17]. Foods most commonly found to be reactive include eggs, dairy food, wheat, fish, citrus fruits, peanuts and soya [17].
- Avoid exposure to food additives [16, 55, 56].
- Encourage Jake to consume more antioxidant-containing whole foods (vegetables, fruit, whole grains, legumes, etc.) [15, 17] and reduce consumption of refined carbohydrates and sugar. Jake needs to increase his intake of essential nutrients [17].
- Include onions and garlic in Jake's diet. Compounds found in onions reduce leukotriene synthesis and can reduce bronchoconstriction [28].
- Avoid excessive salt intake; it may increase bronchial reactivity [14].

Physical treatment suggestions

- Acupuncture may improve Jake's quality of life and reduce his need for bronchodilator medication [25, 37]. When combined with conventional treatment, acupuncture performed in accordance with traditional Chinese medicine principles has significant immune modulating effects [26].
- Massage therapy may be beneficial to Jake. It may help to improved his pulmonary function [27, 36] and massage may help reduce his stress and anxiety [36].
- Hydrotherapy: constitutional hydrotherapy [38–40]. Back and front contrast treatment with cold mitten friction on the trunk when symptoms begin to ease [40, 41]. A hot chest shower [41]. Smear a mustard plaster on the chest consisting of one part mustard powder to three parts flour with enough water to make a paste [42]. A steam vapouriser will assist breathing [42].

TABLE 6.10 HERBAL FORMULA (1:2 LIQUID EXTRACTS)

Made with ethanolic extract herbal liquids (alcohol removed)

HERB	FORMULA	RATIONALE
Ginkgo *Ginkgo biloba* 50:1 Standardised extract equivalent to 4–8 g leaf [18]	40 mL	Anti-PAF activity [18]; antioxidant [18, 19]; immunostimulant [19]; anti-inflammatory [19]; anxiolytic [19]; reduces airway hyperreactivity [19]; protective against exercise induced bronchospasm [20]
Euphorbia *Euphorbia hirta*	10 mL	Expectorant [23, 24]; anti-asthmatic [23, 24]; traditionally used for bronchial asthma [23, 24]
Adhatoda *Adhatoda vasica*	40 mL	Expectorant [21]; bronchodilator [21]; anti-asthmatic [21]; protects against histamine induced bronchospasm [21]; traditionally used to treat bronchitis and asthma [22] and considered to be a sedative expectorant [22]
Baical scullcap *Scutellaria baicalensis*	80 mL	Antiallergic [19, 21]; antioxidant [19]; anti-inflammatory [19, 21]; antimicrobial [19, 21]; anxiolytic [19]
Licorice *Glycyrrhiza glabra*	30 mL	Expectorant [18, 19]; antitussive [19]; antioxidant [19]; anti-inflammatory [18, 19]; antibacterial [18, 19]; immunomodulator [19]; adaptogen [18, 19]; adrenal tonic [18, 19]; also useful to include in Jake's formula to help improve the taste
Supply:	200 mL	Dose: 5 mL twice daily

TABLE 6.11 HERBAL TEA

Alternative to herbal tonic if a tea improves compliance

HERB	FORMULA	RATIONALE
Licorice root *Glycyrrhiza glabra*	2 parts	See above
Thyme leaf *Thymus vulgarus*	2 parts	Antispasmodic [18, 19]; antimicrobial [18, 19]; expectorant [18]; antitussive [19]; anti-inflammatory [19]; antioxidant [19]; traditionally used in bronchitis and asthma and upper respiratory tract inflammation [18]; approved by Commission E for the treatment of bronchitis, whooping cough and upper respiratory tract catarrh [19]
Fennel seed *Foeniculum officinale*	½ part	Spasmolytic [18, 23]; antimicrobial [18, 23]; expectorant [18, 23]; traditional European use for upper respiratory tract conditions in children [23]
Grindelia *Grindelia camporum*	1 part	Expectorant [23, 24]; antispasmodic [23, 24]; bronchospasmolytic [23]; traditionally used for asthma, bronchitis and whooping cough [23]; BHP indication to combine with licorice in asthma and bronchitis [24]
Decoction: 1 tsp per cup – 1 cup twice daily		

Nutritional supplements

Listed in order of priority. Jake's parents may only want to take one or two supplements initially due to financial reasons, or because of concerns regarding compliance.

TABLE 6.12	
SUPPLEMENT AND DOSE	**RATIONALE**
Omega-3 fish oil 3000 mg daily in divided doses [14, 19]	Anti-inflammatory [14, 16, 19]; when taken in combination with dietary changes, improvements in asthma symptoms and lung function measurements are seen [19]
High-potency practitioner-strength **probiotic supplement** containing *Lactobacillus GG* [52] Dosage as directed by the manufacturer for a child of Jake's age and weight	Immune system modulator [19, 37, 52]; immune stimulant [19]; important for the development and maintenance of a healthy immune system [19] and supplementation may be beneficial in atopic conditions [51]; may help prevent disruption to intestinal microflora following antibiotic therapy [31]
Vitamin C Approx. 1500 mg daily in divided doses [14, 16]	Protects against exercise induced asthma [14, 16]; antioxidant [14, 19]; immunostimulant [14, 19]; antihistamine [19]
Magnesium citrate supplement providing a daily dose of 290 mg elemental magnesium [19]	Influences bronchial vasomotor tone and pulmonary vascular muscle contractility [19]; magnesium supplementation can improve asthma symptoms in children [19, 29, 57] [58], reduce bronchial reactivity [29] and reduce bronchodilator use [58]

References

[1] G. Douglas, F. Nicol, C. Robertson, Macleod's Clinical Examination, twelfth edn, Churchill Livingstone Elsevier, Edinburgh 2009.

[2] P. Kumar, C. Clark, Clinical Medicine, sixth edn, Elsevier Saunders, London, 2005.

[3] N.J. Talley, S. O'Connor, Pocket Clinical Examination, third edn, Churchill Livingstone Elsevier, Australia, 2009.

[4] A. Polmear (Ed.), Evidence-Based Diagnosis in Primary Care, Churchill Livingstone Elsevier, Edinburgh, 2008.

[5] R.D. Collins, Differential Diagnosis in Primary Care, fourth edn, Lippincott Williams & Wilkins, Philadelphia, 2008.

[6] J. Silverman, S. Kurtz, J. Draper, Skills for Communicating with Patients, second edn, Radcliff Publishing, Oxford, 2000.

[7] R. Neighbour, The Inner Consultation; how to develop an effective and intuitive consulting style, Radcliff Publishing, Oxon, 2005.

[8] D. Peters, L. Chaitow, G. Harris, S. Morrison, Integrating Complementary Therapies in Primary Care, Churchill Livingstone, London, 2002.

[9] M. Lloyd, R. Bor, Communication Skills For Medicine, third edn, Churchill Livingstone Elsevier, Edinburgh, 2009.

[10] R.H. Seller, Differential Diagnosis of Common Complaints, fifth edn, Saunders Elsevier, Philadelphia, 2007.

[11] J. Jamison, Differential Diagnosis for Primary Care, second edn, Churchill Livingstone Elsevier, London, 2006.

[12] S.E. El-Hashemy, Naturopathic Standards of Primary Care, CCNM Press, Toronto, 2008.

[13] R.M.D. Berkow, A.J.M.D. Fletcher, M.H.M.D. Beers, The Meck Manual, sixteenth edn, Merck Research Laboratories, Rathway, N.J, 1993 (later edition).

[14] J. Jamison, Clinical Guide to Nutrition & Dietary Supplements in Disease Management, Churchill Livingstone, Edinburgh, 2003.

[15] J.E. Pizzorno, M.T. Murray, H. Joiner-Bey, The Clinicians Handbook of Natural Medicine, second edn, Churchill Livingstone, St Louis, 2008 p. 63.

[16] H. Osiecki, The Physicians Handbook of Clinical Nutrition, seventh edn, Bioconcepts, Eagle Farm, 2000.

[17] J.C. Baker, J.G. Ayres, Diet and asthma, Respiratory Medicine 94 (2000) 925–934.

[18] S. Mills, K. Bone, Principles & Practice of Phytotherapy; Modern Herbal Medicine. Edinburgh, Churchill Livingstone, London, 2000.

[19] L. Braun, M. Cohen, Herbs & Natural Supplements: An evidence based guide, second edn, Elsevier, Sydney, 2007.

[20] J.H. Wilkens, H. Wilkens, J. Uffmann, J. Bovers, J. Fabel, J.C. Frolich, Effects of a PAF-antagonist (BN 52063) on bronchoconstriction and platelet activation during exercise induced asthma, British Journal of Clinical Pharmacology 29 (1990) 85–91.

[21] K. Bone, Clinical Applications of Chinese and Ayurvedic Herbs: Monographs for the Western Herbal Practitioners, Phytotherapy Press, Warwick, 1996.

[22] J.N. Dhuley, Antitussive effect of Adhatoda vasica extract on mechanical or chemical stimulation-induced coughing in animals, Journal of Ethnopharmacology 67 (1999) 361–365.

[23] S. Mills, K. Bone, The Essential Guide to Herbal Safety, Churchill Livingstone, St Louis, 2005.

[24] British Herbal Medicine Association, British Herbal Pharmacopoeia, BHMAA, 1983.

[25] W. Biernacki, M.D. Peake, Acupuncture in treatment of stable asthma, Respiratory Medicine 92 (1998) 1143–1145.

[26] S. Joos, C. Schott, H. Zhou, V. Daniel, E. Martin, Immunomodulatory effects of acupuncture in the treatment of allergic asthma: a randomized controlled study, J Altern Complement Med 6 (6) (2000) 519–525.

[27] T. Field, T. Henteleff, M. Hernandez-Reif, E. Martinez, K. Mavunda, C. Kuhn, S. Schanberg, Children with asthma have improved pulmonary functions after massage therapy, Journal of Pediatrics 132 (5) (1998) 854–858.

[28] K.J. Kemper, M.R. Lester, Alternative asthma therapies: An evidence-based review, Contemporary Pediatrics 16 (3) (1999) 162–195.

[29] C. Gontijo-Amaral, M. Ribeiro, L. Gontijo, A. Condino-Neto1, J. Ribeiro, Oral magnesium supplementation in asthmatic children: a double-blind randomized placebo controlled trial, European Journal of Clinical Nutrition 61 (2007) 54–60.

[30] J. Higdon, An Evidence Based Approach to Vitamins and Minerals, Thieme, New York, 2003.

[31] J.A. Madden, S.F. Plummer, J. Tang, I. Garaiova, N.T. Plummer, M. Herbison, J.O. Hunter, et al., Effect of probiotics on preventing disruption of the intestinal microflora following antibiotic therapy: A double-blind, placebo-controlled pilot study, International Immunopharmacology 5 (2005) 1091–1097.

[32] P.M. Lehrer, Emotionally Triggered Asthma: A Review of Research Literature and Some Hypotheses for Self-Regulation Therapies, Applied Psychophysiology and Biofeedback 23 (1) (1998) 13–41.

[33] S.R. Lucas, T.A. Platts-Mills, Physical activity and exercise in asthma: Relevance to etiology and treatment, Journal of Allergy and Clinical Immunolog 115 (5) (2005) 928–934.

[34] R.A. Lieu, C.P. Quesenberry, A.M. Capra, M.E. Sorel, K.E. Martin, G.R. Mendoza, Outpatient management practices associated with reduced risk of pediatric asthma hospitalization and emergency department visits, Pediatrics 100 (3 pt. 1) (1997) 334–341.

[35] C.L. Donovan, S.H. Spence, Prevention Of Childhood Anxiety Disorders, Clinical Psychology Review 20 (4) (2000) 509–531.

[36] S. Beider, C.A. Moyer, Randomized Controlled Trials of Pediatric Massage: A Review, ECAM 4 (1) (2007) 23–34.

[37] B. Blazek-O'Neill, Complementary and Alternative Medicine in Allergy, Otitis Media, and Asthma, Current Allergy and Asthma Reports 5 (2005) 313–318.

[38] W. Boyle, A. Saine, Lectures in Naturopathic Hydrotherapy, Eclectic Medical Publications, Oregon, 1988.

[39] L.M. Watrous, Constitutional hydrotherapy: from nature cure to advanced naturopathic medicine, Journal of Naturopathic Medicine 7 (2), (1997) 72–79.

[40] E. Blake, in: L. Chaitow, E. Blake, P. Orrock, M. Wallden, P. Snider, J. Zeff (Eds.), Naturopathic Physical Medicine: Theory and Practice for Manual Therapists and Naturopaths, Churchill Livingstone Elsevier, Philadelphia, 2008.

[41] M. Sinclair, Modern Hydrotherapy for the Massage Therapist, Lippincott Williams & Wilkins, Baltimore, 2008.

[42] D.D. Buchman, The complete book of water healing, Contemporary Books, McGraw-Hill Companies, New York, 2001.

[43] L.P. Malmberg, K. Tamminen, A.R.A. Sovijärvi, Orthostatic increase of respiratory gas exchange in hyperventilation syndrome, Thorax 55 (4) (2000) 295–301.

[44] D. Hess, Capnometry and capnography: Technical aspects, physiologic aspects, and clinical applications, Respir Care 35 (1990) 557–573.

[45] D. O'Flaherty, Capnometry, BMJ Publishing Group, London, 1994.

[46] L. Chaitow, E. Blake, P. Orrock, M. Wallden, P. Snider, J. Zeff, Natropathic Physical Medicine: Theory and Practice for Manual Therapists and Naturopaths, Churchill Livingstone Elsevier, Philadelphia, 2008.

[47] T. Nagakura, S. Matsuda, K. Shichijyo, H. Subimoti, K. Hata, Dietary supplementation with fish oil rich in n-3 polyunsaturated fatty acids in children with bronchial asthma, European Respiratory Journal 16 (2000) 861–865.

[48] W.H. Oddy, N.H. deKlerk, G.E. Kandall, S. Mihrshahi, J.K. Peat, Ratio of omega-6 to omega-3 fatty acids and childhood asthma, Journal of Asthma 41 (3) (2004) 319–326.

[49] S.K. Weiland, E. von Mutis, A. Husing, et al., Intake of trans fatty acids and prevalence of childhood asthma and allergies in Europe, Lancet 353 (1999) 2040–2041.

[50] S. Lau, S. Illi, C. Sommerfeld, B. Niggermann, R. Bergmann, E. von Mutis, et al., Early exposure to house-dust mite and cat allergens and development of childhood asthma: a cohort study, Lancet 356 (2000) 1392–1397.

[51] M. Kalliomäki, E. Isolauri, Role of Intestinal Flora in the Development of Allergy, Current Opinion in Allergy and Clinical Immunology 3 (1) (2003) 15–20.

[52] M. Kalliomäki, S. Salminen, H. Arvilommi, P. Kero, P. Koskinen, E. Isolauri, Probiotics in primary prevention of atopic disease: a randomised placebo-controlled trial, Lancet 357 (2001) 1076–1079.

[53] G. D'Amato, G. Liccardi, M. D'Amato, S. Holgate, Environmental risk factors and allergic bronchial asthma, Clin Exp Allergy 35 (2005) 1113–1124.

[54] J. Ring, B. Eberlein-Koenig, H. Behrendt, Environmental pollution and allergy, Ann Allergy Asthma Immunol 87 (6 Suppl. 3) (2001) 2–6.

[55] G. Fugslang, G. Madsen, S. Halken, S. Jorgensen, P. Ostergaard, O. Osterballe, Adverse Reactions to food additives in children with atopic symptoms, Allergy 49 (1) (1994) 31–37.

[56] M. Hannuksela, T. Haahtela, Hypersensitivity reactions to food additives, Allergy 42 (1987) 561–575.

[57] L. Ciarallo, A.H. Sauer, M.W. Shannon, Intravenous magnesium therapy for moderate to severe pediatric asthma: Results of a randomized, placebo-controlled trial, The Journal of Pediatrics 129 (6) (1996) 809–814.

[58] O. Bede, Efficacy of magnesium in children with bronchial asthma, European Journal of Clinical Nutrition 63 (2009) 589–590.

[59] J. Bousquet, et al., Asthma: from bronchoconstriction to airways inflammation and remodelling, American Journal of Respiratory and Critical Care Medicine 161 (2000) 1720–1745.

[60] S.C. Christiansen, Day care siblings and asthma – please sneeze on my child, N Engl J Med 343 (2000) 574–575.

[61] S. T. Holgate, Lessons learnt from the epidemic of asthma, Quarterly Journal of Medicine 91 (2004) 247.

[62] A.E. Tattersfield, et al., Asthma, Lancet 360 (2002) 1313–1322.

[63] R.S. Irwin, J.M. Madison, The diagnosis and treatment of cough, N Engl J Med 343 (2000) 1715–1721.

[64] F.J. Kelly, Oxidative stress: its role in air pollution and adverse health effects, Occupational and Environmental Medicine 60 (2003) 612–616.

[65] J.Q. Koenig, Air pollution and asthma, Journal of Allergy and Clinical Immunology 104 (1999) 717–722.

[66] A. Morice, The diagnosis and management of chronic cough, Eur Respir J 24 (2004) 481–492.

[67] G. Currie, R. Gray, J. McKay, Chronic cough, BMJ 326 (2003) 261.

[68] J. Marchant, I. Masters, S. Taylor, et.al., Evaluation and outcome of young children with chronic cough, Chest 129 (2006) 1132–1141.

[69] J. Rees, A.B.C. of asthma: prevalence, BMJ 331 (2005) 443–445.

[70] P. Montnemery, L. Hansson, J. Lanke, et al., Accuracy of a first diagnosis of asthma in primary healthcare, Fam Pract 19 (2002) 365–368.

[71] M. Goldstein, B. Veza, E. Dunsky, et al., Comparisons of peak diurnal expiratory flow variation, postbronchodilator FEV1 responses, and methacholine inhalation challenges in the evaluation of suspected asthma, Chest 119 (2001) 1001–1010.

[72] S. Lewis, S. Weiss, J. Britton, Airway responsiveness and peak flow variability in the diagnosis of asthma for epidemiological studies, Eur Respir J 18 (2001) 921–927.

[73] Y. Graif, M. Yigla, N. Tov, M. Kramer, Value of negative aeroallergen skin-prick test result in the diagnosis of asthma in young adults, Chest 122 (2002) 821–825.

[74] P. Eysink, G. Ter Riet, R. Aalberse, et al., Accuracy of specific IgE in the prediction of asthma: development of a scoring formula for general practice, Br J Gen Pract 55 (2005) 125–131.

[75] F. Martinez, Development of wheezing disorders and asthma in preschool children, Pediatrics 109 (2002) 362–367.

[76] H.J. Fardy, A coughing child: could it be asthma? Aust Fam Physician 33 (5) (2004) 312–315.

[77] J.C. De Jongste, M.D. Sheilds, Chronic cough in children, Thorax 58 (2003) 998–1003.

Otitis media

Case history

Tyler Narran is five years old. His parents have brought him to the clinic for help with a recurrent ear infection that usually develops in his right ear when acute. Tyler has been having problems with discomfort and hearing problems in both ears for the past 10 months. Tyler's mum, Deborah, is concerned because his ENT doctor is talking about surgery to insert a grommet to release the fluid in the middle ear. She and Tyler's dad,

Jeremy, are hoping natural therapies might be able to help Tyler so he doesn't have to have surgery.

Tyler is quiet and shy initially as he clutches his favourite teddy called 'Woof Woof', although he becomes relaxed and talkative as the consultation progresses. Deborah tells you that Tyler is the youngest of three children and has had problems with recurrent respiratory infections over the past year or so. Tyler's ear problems started earlier in the year and he has had repeated courses of antibiotics, but the earaches keep coming back. They took Tyler for a hearing test two weeks ago and were told his hearing is not as good as it was the year before.

Tyler is usually a happy and active child who loves running around and playing sport at school and with his siblings and cousins. He hasn't had quite as much energy this year since he has been having so many infections. When you ask Deborah about her pregnancy with Tyler, his birth and infancy, she tells you she had a good pregnancy and birth and she breastfed him exclusively for the first five months. When she started him on solid food he developed a rash and seemed to get some congestion in his nose. Her mother suggested she stop giving Tyler dairy and wheat. When she did his rash and congestion cleared up. Deborah tells you Tyler is a picky eater and she has to work hard to get him to eat vegetables. His favourite foods are instant noodles and grilled cheese sandwiches and, if he could, he would eat them all day every day. Tyler's parents did not have an opportunity to discuss any of the dietary issues with their GP or ENT specialist.

When you ask Tyler how he feels about doing some new things to help him get better he seems positive, although he says he doesn't know if he will like different food. Both Deborah and Jeremy say they will try whatever you recommend because they want Tyler to get better.

TABLE 6.13 **COMPLAINT**	
Analogy: Skin of the apple	**Complaint:** Define the presenting complaint and symptoms; understand the complaint *Recurrent earache*
AREAS OF INVESTIGATION AND EXAMPLE QUESTIONS	**CLIENT RESPONSES**
Onset *When did Tyler first start having problems with his ears?*	Tyler's mum answers: *Not quite a year ago. The earaches have been happening on and off, whenever he gets a cold.*
Exacerbating factors *What makes the ears feel worse?*	Tyler's mum answers: *They seem to be worse at night and always a couple of days after he starts with a head cold.*
Relieving factors *What makes the ears feel better?*	Tyler's mum answers: *Panadol seems to help and he has had antibiotics a few times, but they always come back.*
Location and radiation *Where does the ear hurt and does the pain stay in one area or does it move?*	Tyler points to his right ear. Tyler's mum explains that the pain usually occurs in his right ear but also sometimes in his left ear. She says Tyler sometimes says he has a headache in his forehead when his ear hurts.

TABLE 6.14 **CONTEXT**	
Analogy: Flesh of the apple	**Context:** Put the presenting complaint into context to understand the disease
AREAS OF INVESTIGATION AND EXAMPLE QUESTIONS	**CLIENT RESPONSES**
Family health *Is there anyone else in the family who has had problems with their ears?*	Tyler's mum answers: *Tyler's older sister had some problems with earaches when she was younger but not as bad as Tyler gets it.*
Allergies and irritants *Do you experience any associated symptoms such as sneezing, nose discharge, conjunctivitis, skin rashes or itching on roof of mouth with a cough?* (allergies)	Tyler's mum answers: *I don't think so. When he was a baby he got a skin rash and when I stopped giving him wheat and dairy it went away. He doesn't seem to have any problems with wheat and dairy now.*
Obstruction and foreign body *Did the ear pain developed after swimming, cleaning or from Tyler picking the ear?* (otitis externa)	*He did begin swimming lessons when the whole cycle of infections began, but we soon stopped them. It's a shame because he was enjoying it.*
Functional disease *Has Tyler presented with any speech complications from having ear discomfort that has interfered with hearing?* (chronic serous otitis media)	*He doesn't seem to hear us as well these days, which makes us yell more when we talk to him. He seems to talk less now, but not sure if that's because he can't hear or because he's scared of us raising our voices!*
Infection and inflammation *Is there a throbbing pain in your ear that is better when you chew on food and when you swallow?* (acute otitis media)	Tyler's mum answers: *A couple of weeks ago, he had an earache – that got better when he was eating.* *The doctor says if he gets one more acute flare up he will probably need to have surgery.*
Supplements and side effects of medication *Has Tyler been taking any supplements or medicine?*	Tyler's mum answers: *He just had antibiotics for his last earache.*
Eating habits and energy *Tell me about Tyler's diet.*	Tyler's mum answers: *He has a grilled cheese sandwich or porridge and milk for breakfast. If he's at home he usually has noodles for lunch, otherwise he gets a sandwich with cheese or polony. He doesn't like vegetables and fruit, but I try and make him have them.*

TABLE 6.15 **CORE**	
Analogy: Core of the apple with the seed of ill health	**Core:** Holistic assessment to understand the client
AREAS OF INVESTIGATION AND EXAMPLE QUESTIONS	**CLIENT RESPONSES**
Family and friends *How do you get on with your brother and sister and your friends, Tyler?*	Tyler answers: *Good, sometimes Danny doesn't let me do things when I want to.*
Home life *How are things at home?*	Tyler's mum answers: *There's always something happening at home. Lots of children, cousins and friends always in and out of the house. Tyler has his own friends to play but also tags along with his older sister and brother and cousins. There are the usual problems and fights that children have, but no real problems.*
Action needed to heal *Tyler, if I give you some medicine and ask you to eat some different food do you think you will do it?*	Tyler answers: *I don't know. Does it taste bad?* Tyler's mum answers: *We'll do whatever it takes to get Tyler better.*

TABLE 6.16 **TYLER'S SIGNS AND SYMPTOMS** [4–6]	
Pulse	100 beats per minute
Blood pressure	100/60
Temperature	37.8°C
Respiratory rate	25 breaths per minute
Face	Relaxed, smiling
Body posture	Sitting, not restless, quiet, not crying, content
Percentile	75th
Weight	20 kg
Urinalysis	NAD

TABLE 6.17 **RESULTS OF MEDICAL INVESTIGATIONS** [1–6, 10, 12]	
TEST	**RESULTS**
Examination of external ear and ear drum [49, 51, 52]	No excess wax, foreign objects or skin disorder in the outer ear canal; no external discharge or swelling of the outer ear; no tenderness over the mastoid process; slightly red and dull tympanic membrane that appears retracted, red blood vessels are visible and membrane appears immobile

▶

Hearing test (Rinne and Weber): vibrating prong on external auditory meatus and mastoid process and on forehead; whispered voice test	Sound heard best in left ear; positive conduction deafness
TMJ examination	No clicking of the jaw when he opens and closes his mouth; no tenderness
Throat examination/throat swab	No swelling or redness
Nose examination/nose swab	No infection causing referred pain to ear
Chest examination: auscultation, percussion	No signs of asthma, obstruction or infection

TABLE 6.18 UNLIKELY DIAGNOSTIC CONSIDERATIONS [1–6, 10, 12, 44]

CONDITIONS AND CAUSES	WHY UNLIKELY
TRAUMA AND PRE-EXISTING ILLNESS	
Causal factor: **Traumatic perforation of tympanic ear drum**	When ear is hit, slapped or from ear picking
OBSTRUCTION AND FOREIGN BODY	
Causal factor: **Impacted cerumen:** can have pain and impaired hearing	External ears are clean
Causal factor: **Foreign bodies:** unilateral, vague pain and discomfort, which can then become severe	Examination revealed no foreign bodies in external ear or sign of trauma
FUNCTIONAL DISEASE	
Causal factor: **TMJ dysfunction**	Usually comes and goes and worse in the morning from teeth grinding; no headache or jaw click
Causal factor: **Dental pathology:** common cause of referred pain to the ear	Recent dental check revealed no abnormalities
Gastro-oesophageal reflux: rare cause of ear pain in infants and children	No symptoms of abdominal pain or discomfort after eating
Asthma: postviral children with recurrent cough are often asthmatic; recent upper respiratory tract infection most probably viral (antibiotics did not completely resolve)	Chest examination did not reveal significant wheeze; ask more about shortness of breath and cough
Causal factor: **Referred pain:** to the ear when ear examination and hearing test is normal	Ear drum examination was not normal and conductive hearing loss is present

INFECTION AND INFLAMMATION	
Otitis externa: bilateral pain more common	More common in adults, clients with diabetes, swimmer's ear, when people have seborrheic dermatitis or psoriasis of the scalp; movement or pressure on the outer ear is not painful; there has been no discharge from the ear
Primary otalgia: chronic otitis media with effusion (middle ear infection) common in children under 8 years old; unilateral, which rules out referred pain to ear	The tympanic membrane is not perforated and no discharge present for more than 1 month
Mastoiditis: can have acute otitis media ear infection prior to mastoiditis developing by 2 weeks	Severe pain not behind the ear and no tenderness on mastoid process; no current fever or discharge from ear
Myringitis: viral, bacterial (common *Streptococcus pneumoniae*) mycoplasma infection aggravated by recurrent URIs, pain occurs in cycles	No bullae or vesicles on tympanic membrane and usually a diagnosis seen in adults; precipitated by cough and pneumonia; viral will present with watery rhinitis or a pink eardrum; if fever and hearing loss present, it's more likely to be bacterial
Acute otitic barotraumas: aggravated by recurrent URIs	No recent air flights or hay fever; need to check if pain is relieved by chewing
Upper aerodigestive tract (larynx, hypopharynx, oropharynx, base of tongue) infection or malignancy	More common in adults and elderly; tumours rarely cause pain
Impetigo: can cause pain in the ear	No skin rash

TABLE 6.19 **CONFIRMED DIAGNOSIS** [1–3, 5, 6]	
CONDITION	**RATIONALE**
Serous otitis media (glue ear): can be asymptomatic and aggravated by recurrent URIs and pharyngitis; common in children under 8 years old due to their short eustachian tube; develops due to eustachian tube dysfunction	Can be bilateral; slightly red and dull tympanic membrane that appears retracted, red blood vessels are visible and membrane appears immobile; sound heard best in the left ear; positive conduction hearing loss; no pain experienced at the time of consultation, common condition in children; children can present as healthy and still have glue ear
Recurrent acute otitis media: middle ear infection; more common to be viral origin, which antibiotic may not resolve	Unilateral; Tyler has had episodes of acute ear pain that resolves within 3 weeks; associated symptoms of fever, runny nose and upper respiratory tract infections; when in the acute stage the tympanic membrane is very red, cloudy, bulging and immobile; no perforation has occurred to date

Case analysis

TABLE 6.20 POSSIBLE FURTHER DIFFERENTIAL DIAGNOSIS

Not ruled out by tests/investigations already done [1–6, 10, 11]

CONDITIONS AND CAUSES	WHY POSSIBLE	WHY UNLIKELY
ALLERGIES AND IRRITANTS		
Atopic eczema: the word 'atopy' means to react to common environmental factors; can be caused and aggravated by diet, genetic factors, heat, humidity, drying of the skin, contact with woollen clothing or animal saliva touching the skin; house dust mites are thought to be an important factor in facial eczema	Skin rash and nasal congestion as a baby when first introduced to dairy and wheat	No significant skin rash presenting at time of consultation
Food allergy: typically to cow's milk, egg, soya, peanut, wheat and fish	Reaction of skin rash and nasal congestion to dairy and wheat	Often presents with a swelling of the lips and tongue, urticaria, skin rash, conjunctivitis, rhinitis, anaphylaxis and difficulty breathing
Coeliac disease	Can be associated with lactose intolerance; having more wheat and dairy	Ask if Tyler has experienced diarrhoea or pain in the abdomen from a change in diet
FUNCTIONAL DISEASE		
Causal factor: **Low immune function**	Recurrent upper respiratory tract infections, ear infections, inadequate diet and not balanced with food groups; less energy	
DEGENERATIVE AND DEFICIENCY		
Anaemia	Not eating balanced diet and Tyler doesn't have as much energy as used to	
INFECTION AND INFLAMMATION		
Eustachitis: inflammation of mucous membrane of eustachian tube; can be aggravated by recurrent URIs and pharyngitis	Not associated with severe earache usually; ear drum usually retracted	Check if the pain is relieved by chewing
Dermatitis herpetiformis	This condition is usually associated with gluten-sensitive enteropathy, which can be asymptomatic; rash that appeared as a baby when first ate solids	Usually associated with bullae (fluid filled palpable mass); more common to present on trunk of body

Working diagnosis

TYLER AND SEROUS OTITIS MEDIA (GLUE EAR) WITH RECURRENT ACUTE OTITIS MEDIA

Deborah and Jeremy have brought their five-year-old son, Tyler, to the clinic after being told he may need surgery to insert a grommet into his ear [32] to prevent recurrent ear infections. Tyler has been diagnosed with 'glue ear', which is beginning to affect his hearing and has precipitated several acute ear infections over the past year. Tyler is the youngest of three children and is usually a happy and active child who loves playing sports with his siblings and cousins. As the consultation progresses Tyler's parents reveal that as a baby Tyler developed nasal congestion and a skin rash when first introduced to dairy and wheat products and when these foods were taken out of his diet the symptoms resolved. Tyler now eats these foods as they don't seem to give him a skin rash anymore.

Tyler is experiencing two conditions of **otitis media** as chronic **serous otitis media** (glue ear) and episodes of **acute otitis media** (middle ear infection).

SEROUS OTITIS MEDIA (GLUE EAR)

This is a condition where fluid accumulates in the eustachian tube in the ear causing a dysfunction in the pressure of the middle ear along with conductive hearing difficulties. Glue ear is a chronic condition where the mucus has become thick and tacky like glue. This form of chronic otitis media often has an allergic cause. Infants and children are more prone to developing this because the eustachian tube is shorter in young children and gradually grows. Glue ear usually has recurrent episodes and periods of remission but will often resolve over time. Referral for surgery to insert a 'grommet' may be one option to prevent ear infections and perforation of the tympanic membrane. A grommet is essentially a tube that is inserted into the tympanic membrane and takes over the role of the eustachian tube while the membrane heals (lasts from six months to two years). A child with glue ear may develop complications including hearing impairment, delayed learning and speech development, chronic blocked ears, transient earache and the predisposition to develop acute otitis media (middle ear infection).

ACUTE OTITIS MEDIA (MIDDLE EAR INFECTION)

This condition produces symptoms of severe earache, vomiting, fever, hearing loss, runny nose and is often initiated by an upper respiratory tract infection. Mucus blocks the eustachian tube and consequently infection develops leading to swelling, redness and pain in the ear. The risk of a perforated ear drum and chronic otitis media is increased with recurrent acute otitis media.

General references used in this diagnosis: 1–3, 5, 6

Confirmed diagnosis

Serous otitis media (glue ear) with recurrent acute otitis media and dairy protein allergy.

PRESCRIBED MEDICATION
- Oral antibiotic therapy as required [46, 47]
- Oral analgesics as required
- Referral for surgery to insert a 'grommet'

TABLE 6.21 DECISION TABLE FOR TREATMENT PRIOR TO REFERRAL		
COMPLAINT	**CONTEXT**	**CORE**
Treatment for the presenting complaint and symptoms	Treatment for all associated symptoms	Treatment for mental, emotional, spiritual, constitutional, lifestyle issues and metaphysical considerations
TREATMENT PRIORITY	**TREATMENT PRIORITY**	**TREATMENT PRIORITY**
• Physical treatment recommendations to provide relief from acute symptoms and to reduce symptom recurrence • Lifestyle recommendations to provide relief from acute symptoms • Symptomatic relief with herbal ear drops • Herbal tea or tonic to reduce the accumulation of mucus and support drainage via the eustachian tube • Nutritional supplements to reduce inflammation and allergic response, which is leading to mucus accumulation in the middle ear **NB:** Caution should be taken when prescribing herbal or nutritional therapies to ensure Tyler is not given herbs or foods to which he may react because of allergies to herbs or foods from the same botanical family [14]	• Lifestyle recommendations to reduce Tyler's exposure to environmental allergens and other triggers • Dietary recommendations to identify and eliminate foods to which Tyler is allergic or intolerant • Dietary recommendations and nutritional supplements to improve Tyler's general health and immunity and reduce recurrence of upper respiratory tract infections • Herbal tea or tonic to support Tyler's immune system and reduce the allergic response	• Encourage Tyler to participate in the process of healing and to help deal with his concerns about changing his diet • Recommendation for reward chart or other motivation to help Tyler be more cooperative and motivated to participate in his treatment • Recommendation to include Tyler in decisions and implementation of dietary, lifestyle and physical treatments

TABLE 6.22 DECISION TABLE FOR REFERRAL [1–6, 10–13]		
COMPLAINT	**CONTEXT**	**CORE**
Referral for presenting complaint	Referral for all associated physical, dietary and lifestyle concerns	Referral for contributing emotional, mental, spiritual, metaphysical, lifestyle and constitutional factors
REFERRAL FLAGS	**REFERRAL FLAGS**	**REFERRAL FLAGS**
• Tyler's parents have not consulted a GP or specialist and are seeking complementary therapies instead of pursuing the surgery option • It may be considered child abuse for Tyler if he was to experience recurrent and ongoing ear pain without suitable pain relief	• Possible elimination and ongoing restriction of food groups from Tyler's diet may be unnecessary • Recurrent URIs may lead to childhood asthma	Nil

▶

ISSUES OF SIGNIFICANCE	ISSUES OF SIGNIFICANCE	ISSUES OF SIGNIFICANCE
Nil	• Tyler developed a skin rash and nasal congestion as a baby when first introduced to wheat and dairy	• Dietary and lifestyle changes may cause Tyler stress or anxiety • Physical treatment recommendations may cause Tyler stress or anxiety • Resistance to taking herbal tea or tonic and supplements
REFERRAL DECISION	**REFERRAL DECISION**	**REFERRAL DECISION**
• Tyler needs collaborative care – his ear and hearing loss needs regular monitoring between an orthodox and a complementary practitioner • Deborah and Jeremy need education regarding hearing damage and delayed learning that can develop from ear infections that are not managed carefully [48, 50]	• Food assessment and challenge to identify food triggers • Monitor asthma and lung assessment	Nil

TABLE 6.23 FURTHER INVESTIGATIONS THAT MAY BE NECESSARY [1–6, 10, 12]

TEST/INVESTIGATION	REASON FOR TEST/INVESTIGATION
FIRST-LINE INVESTIGATIONS:	
Full blood count	Infection, allergies, anaemia
Serum IgE blood test	Atopic eczema and allergic triggers for asthma
Food diary	To help determine any foods that may be triggering or aggravating symptoms
IF NECESSARY:	
RAST and/or skin prick test	To determine whether Tyler has allergies to foods or environmental antigens
Radiograph of ear	Confirms otitis media diagnosis
Tympanometry/impedance audiometry [45]	Test otitis media with effusion as compliance of the eardrum is measured during changes in pressure in air canal
CT and MRI of ear	Tumours causing primary and secondary ear pain (otalgia)
Antigliadin antibody blood test	Definitive test for gluten allergy

TABLE 6.24 **DECISION TABLE FOR TREATMENT (ONCE DIAGNOSIS IS CONFIRMED)**		
COMPLAINT	**CONTEXT**	**CORE**
Treatment for the presenting complaint and symptoms	Treatment for all associated symptoms	Treatment for mental, emotional, spiritual, constitutional, lifestyle issues and metaphysical considerations
TREATMENT PRIORITY	**TREATMENT PRIORITY**	**TREATMENT PRIORITY**
• Continue with lifestyle and physical treatment recommendations as required for relief from symptoms and to reduce symptom recurrence • Continue with use of herbal ear drops for symptomatic relief as required • Continue with herbal tea or tonic • Continue with nutritional supplements **NB**: Tyler's case should be collaboratively managed with his medical practitioners to ensure his treatment program is effective and appropriate; his case should be reviewed in 2–3 weeks and again at 6–8 weeks to assess the effectiveness of the program	• Continue with lifestyle recommendations to reduce Tyler's exposure to environmental triggers • Continue with dietary recommendations to eliminate allergic or intolerant foods • Continue with dietary recommendations and nutritional supplements to improve Tyler's general health and immunity and reduce recurrence of upper respiratory tract infections • Continue with herbal tea or tonic to support Tyler's immune system and reduce the allergic response	• Continue to encourage Tyler to participate in the process of healing and to be involved in decisions and the implementation of the dietary and lifestyle change • Continue with motivational and reward activities to encourage Tyler's continued participation in the process

Treatment aims

- Provide symptomatic relief [14, 15].
- Support eustachian tube drainage [14, 15].
- Identify and manage underlying allergies or intolerances that are likely to be contributing to Tyler's problems [14, 15, 22, 23].
- Enhance Tyler's immune function [14, 15] and modulate his allergic response [14, 15].
- Reduce the requirement for antibiotics, which may be contributing to the recurrence of middle ear infections [15, 25].
- Improve Tyler's diet and nutritional status [14, 15, 42].
- Protect Tyler's hearing and prevent hearing loss and associated speech and developmental problems, which may result from impaired hearing [14, 15].

Lifestyle alterations/considerations

- Encourage Tyler's parents to ensure he is not exposed to cigarette smoke [14, 15] and other airborne environmental irritants such as smoke from wood fires [20].
- Tyler's parents should be aware that waiting for 24 hours before instituting antibiotic therapy when Tyler has an acute aggravation of otitis media is advisable [16, 18]. If his symptoms are resolving after 24 hours, antibiotic therapy may not be necessary [15, 16, 18].

- Tyler may benefit from the use of homeopathic medicines to manage acute episodes of otitis media [14, 17].
- Tyler may benefit from chewing Xylitol chewing gum. Xylitol may reduce the incidence of acute episodes of otitis media [15, 19].
- It is likely that Tyler has food and/or environmental allergies [14, 15, 22–24]. If allergy tests indicate environmental allergies, Tyler's parents should reduce his exposure through the use of mould- and dust-reducing cleaning techniques such as a HEPA filter vacuum cleaner and damp dusting, etc. [20, 21]. Even if Tyler does not test positive to environmental allergens, they should ensure their home environment is healthy and free from mould [20].
- Tyler may benefit from the use of a room humidifier [15].
- In order to help Tyler cooperate with the recommended dietary, lifestyle and treatment measures, it may be helpful to use a reward chart or similar motivation to help improve compliance.
- Deborah and Jeremy should discuss Tyler's treatment recommendations with him and involve him in the selection and preparation of recommended foods as well as the preparation and administration of recommended herbal and nutritional products. Tyler is more likely to be compliant if he feels involved in the process.
- Where practical, Deborah and Jeremy should include Tyler in decisions about trying particular physical therapies and become actively involved in implementing lifestyle changes and some physical therapies. By making Tyler feel involved in the process he is less likely to feel anxious and more likely to be compliant.

Dietary suggestions

- Encourage food allergies to be tested for and managed appropriately [14, 15, 22–24]. Commonly implicated foods include dairy products, wheat, eggs, soy, corn, oranges, strawberries and peanuts [14, 15]. The use of an elimination and rotation diet should be recommended [14, 15, 23, 24].
- Encourage Tyler to eat plenty of fresh fruit and vegetables, whole grains, beans and legumes, lean meat and fish to improve his intake of essential nutrients [14, 42].
- Increasing consumption of bioflavanoid-rich foods can help reduce allergic and inflammatory responses and consequent mucus production [14, 26].
- Encourage Tyler to minimise consumption of concentrated simple carbohydrates such as sugar, honey, dried fruit and concentrated fruit juice as excessive consumption may have a negative effect on his immune system [15, 43].
- Encourage Tyler to avoid consuming potentially mucus-forming foods such as wheat, dairy and orange juice [14].

Physical treatment suggestions

- Tyler may find benefit from local application of heat to the affected ear in acute exacerbations of otitis media [15].
- Hydrotherapy: hot salt bag application to affected ear to draw out catarrhal blockage and relieve pain [36].
- Hot leg bath, hot foot bath, hot foot wrappings to bring heat away from ear down to feet [36].
- Hot moist cloths on the mastoid bone applied simultaneously with an ice bag placed over the carotid artery on the same side as the ear pain (up to 30 minutes). Follow this with cold mitten friction on the trunk and limbs [36].
- A cold throat compress on the throat to draw heat away from the ear [36, 40].

- Constitutional hydrotherapy to strengthen Tyler's immune system and tonify his lungs [37–39].
- For recurrent chest infections: back and front contrast treatment with cold mitten friction on the trunk when symptoms begin to ease [39, 41]. Hot chest shower [41]. Smear a mustard plaster over the chest made with one part mustard powder to three parts flour and enough water to make a paste [36]. A steam vapouriser will assist breathing [36].
- Laser acupuncture or acupressure may be beneficial to Tyler [14].
- Blowing into Tyler's affected ear with hot air from a hair dryer directed through a straw may help reduce middle ear pressure and promote drainage [15].

TABLE 6.25 HERBAL EAR DROP FORMULA; OLIVE OIL INFUSION

HERB	FORMULA	RATIONALE
Garlic oil *Allium sativum*	1 part	Anti-inflammatory [26]; antimicrobial [26, 30]
Mullein *Verbascum thapsus* (infused oil)	4 parts	Demulcent [26, 30]; emollient [26]; antimicrobial [26]; anticatarrhal [30]
Calendula flowers *Calendula officinalis* (infused oil)	2 parts	Antimicrobial [26, 30]; anti-inflammatory [26, 30]
St John's wort *Hypericum perforatum* (infused oil)	2 parts	Antimicrobial [26, 27]; anti-inflammatory [26]; analgesic [26]
Lavender flowers *Lavandula angustifolia* (essential oil)	½ part	Antimicrobial [26]

5 drops in the affected ear 3 times daily [15]
These 5 herbs administered as an eardrop preparation are effective in relieving the symptoms of otitis media [19, 25, 26]

TABLE 6.26 HERBAL TEA

Alternative to herbal liquid tonic if there are compliance problems

HERB	FORMULA	RATIONALE
Elder flower *Sambucus nigra*	2 parts	Anticatarrhal [30]; anti-inflammatory [33]; immune stimulator with benefit in treating otitis media [14]
Eyebright *Euphrasia officinalis*	2 parts	Anticatarrhal [26, 28, 30]; astringent [26, 28, 30]; anti-inflammatory [26, 30]; mucous membrane tonic [30]; reduces upper respiratory tract secretions [26]
Echinacea *Echinacea purpurea*	2 parts	Immunomodulator [26, 27]; immunostimulant [26, 27]; anti-inflammatory [26, 27]; lymphatic [27]; beneficial for upper respiratory tract infections [26, 27, 34]

▶

Chamomile *Matricaria recutita*	1 part	Anti-inflammatory [14, 26, 27]; antimicrobial [14, 26, 27]; immunostimulant [26]
Licorice root powder *Glycyrrhiza glabra*	½ part	Anti-inflammatory [26, 27]; antimicrobial [26, 27]; immunomodulator [26, 27]; mucoprotective [27]; expectorant [26, 27]; beneficial in upper respiratory tract infections [26, 27]; also helpful as a sweet flavouring agent [26]
Infusion: 1 tsp per cup – 2 cups daily		

TABLE 6.27 **HERBAL FORMULA (1:2 LIQUID EXTRACTS)**
Made with ethanolic extract herbal liquids (alcohol removed)

HERB	FORMULA	RATIONALE
Echinacea *Echinacea purpurea*	25 mL	See above
Eyebright *Euphrasia officinalis*	20 mL	See above
Elder flower *Sambucus nigra*	15 mL	See above
Licorice root *Glycyrrhiza glabra*	10 mL	See above
Albizia *Albizia lebbek*	30 mL	Antiallergic [26, 31]; stabilises mast cells [26, 31]; antimicrobial [26, 31]; traditionally used for respiratory diseases [31]
Supply:	100 mL	Dose: 2 mL 3 times daily

TABLE 6.28 **NUTRITIONAL SUPPLEMENTS**

SUPPLEMENT AND DOSE	RATIONALE
High-potency practitioner-strength **probiotic supplement** containing a range of human strain organisms including *Lactobacillus GG* [26]	Immune system modulator [26]; immune stimulant [26]; important for the development and maintenance of a healthy immune system [26]; may help prevent disruption to intestinal microflora following antibiotic therapy [35]
High-potency practitioner-strength **children's multivitamin and mineral** supplement containing therapeutic doses of essential micronutrients Dose: as directed by the manufacturer for a child of Tyler's weight and age	Poor nutritional status is associated with increased risk of lowered immunity and infection [42, 43]; Tyler's current diet is nutritionally deficient and supplementation will help improve his nutritional status

Cod liver oil Dose: approx. 3 mL to provide no more than 2500 IU of vitamin A daily [26, 29]	Vitamin A, D and omega-3 supplement; vitamin A is essential for immune function and maintenance of epithelial tissue [26, 29] and is beneficial in treating upper respiratory tract infections [26, 29]; omega-3 fatty acids are anti-inflammatory [26, 29, 32]
Vitamin C and bioflavanoid complex providing 250 mg vitamin C and 250 mg bioflavanoids (containing quercetin) 3 times daily [15]	Vitamin C is antihistaminic [26, 29, 32]; immunostimulant [26, 29, 32] and an antioxidant [26, 29, 32]; quercetin is antiallergic [26, 29], antioxidant [26, 29, 32]; immunomodulator [26]; anti-inflammatory [26, 29, 32]; quercetin inhibits inflammatory enzymes, prostaglandins and leukotrienes [26], stabilises mast cells [26] and inhibits mast cell release of histamine [29]

References

[1] R.H. Seller, Differential Diagnosis of Common Complaints, fifth edn, Saunders Elsevier, Philadelphia, 2007.

[2] A. Polmear (Ed.), Evidence-Based Diagnosis in Primary Care, Churchill Livingstone Elsevier, 2008, pp. 274–283.

[3] J. Jamison, Differential Diagnosis for Primary Care, second edn, Churchill Livingstone Elsevier, London, 2006.

[4] N.J. Talley, S. O'Connor, Pocket Clinical Examination, third edn, Churchill Livingstone Elsevier, Australia, 2009.

[5] G. Douglas, F. Nicol, C. Robertson, Macleod's Clinical Examination, twelfth edn, Churchill Livingstone Elsevier, 2009.

[6] P. Kumar, C. Clark, Clinical Medicine, sixth edn, Elsevier Saunders, London, 2005.

[7] J. Silverman, S. Kurtz, J. Draper, Skills for Communicating with Patients, second ed, Radcliff Publishing, Oxford, 2000.

[8] R. Neighbour, The Inner Consultation; how to develop an effective and intuitive consulting style, Radcliff Publishing, Oxon, 2005.

[9] M. Lloyd, R. Bor, Communication Skills For Medicine, third edn, Churchill Livingstone Elsevier, Edinburgh, 2009.

[10] R.D. Collins, Differential Diagnosis in Primary Care, fourth edn, Lippincott Williams & Wilkins, Philadelphia, 2008.

[11] R.M.D. Berkow, A.J.M.D. Fletcher, M.H.M.D. Beers, The Merck Manual, sixteenth edn, Merck Research Laboratories, Rathway, N.J, 1993 (later edition).

[12] K.D. Pagna, T.J. Pagna, Mosby's Diagnostic and Laboratory Test reference, third edn, Mosby, USA, 1997 (later edition).

[13] D. Peters, L. Chaitow, G. Harris, S. Morrison, Integrating Complementary Therapies in Primary Care. London: Churchill Livingstone, 2002.

[14] S. El-Hashemy, Naturopathic Standards of Primary Care, CCNM Press Inc, Toronto, 2007.

[15] J.E. Pizzorno, M.T. Murray, H. Joiner-Bey, The Clinicians Handbook of Natural Medicine, second edn, Churchill Livingstone, St Louis, 2008.

[16] P. Little, C. Gould, I. Williamson, M. Moore, G. Warner, J. Dunleavey, Pragmatic randomised controlled trial of two prescribing strategies for childhood acute otitis media, British Medical Journal 322 (2001) 336–342.

[17] J. Jacobs, D.A. Springer, D. Crothers, Homeopathic treatment of acute otitis media in children: a preliminary randomized placebo-controlled trial, Pediatric Infectious Disease Journal 29 (2) (2001) 177–183.

[18] D.M. Spiro, K.Y. Tay, D.H. Arnold, J.D. Dziura, M.D. Baker, E.D. Shapiro, Wait-and-See Prescription for the Treatment of Acute Otitis Media: A Randomized Controlled Trial, Journal of the American Medical Association 296 (2006) 1235–1241.

[19] B. Blazek-O'Neill, Complementary and Alternative Medicine in Allergy, Otitis Media, and Asthma, Current Allergy and Asthma Reports 5 (2005) 313–318.

[20] M. Kilpeläinen, E.O. Terho, H. Helenius, M. Koskenvuo, Home dampness, current allergic diseases, and respiratory infections among young adults, Thorax 56 (2001) 462–467.

[21] M.S. Dykewicz, Rhinitis and sinusitis, Journal of Allergy and Clinical Immunology 111 (Suppl. 2) (2003) S520–S529.

[22] R. Alles, A. Parikh, L. Hawk, Y. Darby, J.N. Romero, G. Scadding, The prevalence of atopic disorders in children with chronic otitis media with effusion, Pediatric Allergy and Immunology 12 (2) (2001) 102–106.

[23] T.M. Nsouli, S.M. Nsouli, R.E. Linde, F. O'Mara, R.T. Scanlon, J.A. Bellanti, Role of food allergy in serous otitis media, Annals of Allergy 73 (3) (1994) 215–219.

[24] C.M. Arroyave, Recurrent otitis media with effusion and food allergy in pediatric patients (article in Spanish), Rev. Alerg Mex 48 (5) (2001) 141–144.

[25] E.M. Sarrell, H.A. Choen, E. Kahan, Naturopathic Treatment for Ear Pain in Children, Pediatrics 111 (2003) e574–e579.

[26] L. Braun, M. Cohen, Herbs & Natural Supplements: An evidence based guide, second edn, Elsevier, Sydney, 2007.

[27] S. Mills, K. Bone, Principles & Practice of Phytotherapy; Modern Herbal Medicine, Churchill Livingstone, Edinburgh : London, 2000.

[28] British Herbal Medicine Association, British Herbal Pharmacopoeia, BHMAA, 1983.

[29] H. Osiecki, The Nutrient Bible, seventh edn, BioConcepts Publishing, Eagle Farm, 2008.

[30] S. Mills, K. Bone, The Essential Guide to Herbal Safety, Churchill Livingstone, St Louis, 2005.

[31] K. Bone, Clinical Applications of Chinese and Ayurvedic Herbs: Monographs for the Western Herbal Practitioners, Phytotherapy Press, Warwick, 1996.

[32] J. Jamison, Clinical Guide to Nutrition & Dietary Supplements in Disease Management, Churchill Livingstone, Edinburgh, 2003.

[33] E. Harokopakis, M.H. Albzreh, E.M. Haase, F.A. Scannapieco, G. Hajishengallis, Inhibition of proinflammatory activities of major periodontal pathogens by aqueous extracts from elder flower (Sambucus nigra), Journal of Periodontology 77 (2) (2006) 271–279.

[34] V. Goel, R. Lovlin, C. Chang, J.V. Slama, R. Barton, R. Gahler, R. Bauer, et al., A proprietary extract from the echinacea plant (Echinacea purpurea) enhances systemic immune response during a common cold, Phytotherapy Research 19 (8) (2005) 689–694.

[35] J.A. Madden, S.F. Plummer, J. Tang, I. Garaiova, N.T. Plummer, M. Herbison, J.O. Hunter, et al., Effect of probiotics on preventing disruption of the intestinal microflora following antibiotic therapy: A double-blind, placebo-controlled pilot study, International Immunopharmacology 5 (2005) 1091–1097.

[36] D.D. Buchman, The complete book of water healing, Contemporary Books, McGraw-Hill Companies, New York, 2001.

[37] W. Boyle, A. Saine, Lectures in Naturopathic Hydrotherapy, Eclectic Medical Publications, Oregon, 1988.

[38] L.M. Watrous, Constitutional hydrotherapy: from nature cure to advanced naturopathic medicine, Journal of Naturopathic Medicine 7 (2) (1997) 72–79.

[39] E. Blake, in: L. Chaitow, E. Blake, P. Orrock, M. Wallden, P. Snider, J. Zeff, Naturopathic Physical Medicine (Eds.), Theory and Practice for Manual Therapists and Naturopaths, Churchill Livingstone Elsevier, Philadelphia, 2008.

[40] L. Chaitow, Hydrotherapy, water therapy for health and beauty, Element, Dorset, 1999.

[41] M. Sinclair, Modern Hydrotherapy for the Massage Therapist, Lippincott Williams & Wilkins, Baltimore, 2008.

[42] N.S. Scrimshaw, J.P. SanGiovanni, Synergism of nutrition, infection and immunity: an overview, The American Journal of Clinical Nutrition 66 (1997) 464S–477S.

[43] R.A. Chandra, Nutrition and the immune system, Proceedings of the Nutrition Society 52 (1993) 77–84.

[44] A.K. Leung, J.H. Fong, A.G. Leong, Otalgia in children, J Natl Med Assoc 92 (5) (2000) 254–260.

[45] K. Blomgren, A. Pitkaranta, Current challenges in diagnosis of acute otitis media, International Journal of Pediatric Otorhinolaryngol 69 (3) (2005) 295–299.

[46] P. Glasziou, C. Del Mar, S. Sanders, M. Haymen, Antibiotics for acute otitis media in children, The Cochrane Database of Systematic Reviews, 2004. (Issue 1. Art No: CD000219. DOI:10.1002/14651858. CD000219.pub2)

[47] P. Burke, J. Bain, D. Robinson, Acute red ear in children: controlled trial of non-antibiotic treatment in general practice, BMJ 303 (1991) 558–562.

[48] E. Asher, E. Leibovitz, J. Press, et al., Accuracy of acute otitis media diagnosis in community and hospital settings, Acta Paediatr 94 (2005) 423–428.

[49] T. Heikkinen, O. Ruuskanen, Signs and symptoms predicting acute otitis media, Arch Pediatr Adolesc Med 149 (1995) 26–29.

[50] M. Niemela, M. Uhari, K. Jounio-Ervasti, et al., Lack of specific symptomatology in children with acute otitis media, Paediatr Infect Dis J 13 (1994) 765–768.

[51] P. Karma, M. Penttila, M. Siplia, et al., Otoscopic diagnosis of middle ear effusions in acute and non-acute otitis media. I. The value of different otoscopic findings, Int J Pediatr Otorhinolaryngol 17 (1989) 37–49.

[52] R. Rothman, T. Owens, D. Simel, Does this child have acute otitis media? JAMA 290 (2003) 1633–1640.

Chronic bronchitis

Case history

Tara Pietrowski is 31 years old and has come to the clinic for help with a cough she has had for the past three months. Tara is in the middle of an around Australia road trip with her husband, something they have been planning for a number of years. They had both hoped they would have children by now but, despite trying for four years, Tara has never fallen pregnant. Two years ago they made the decision that if Tara wasn't pregnant by the beginning of this year they would take time off and go travelling.

Tara tells you they started travelling six months ago, and since then she feels as if she has been sick most of the time. Tara has been having what she thinks are recurrent upper respiratory tract infections for almost the whole time they have been away, with a cough that is worse in the morning. When the cough is particularly bad Tara coughs up yellow-green sputum, particularly in the mornings. The cough can disturb Tara's sleep.

Tara has experienced this type of thing in the past and as recently as last year during winter. In her late teens and early 20s she experienced frequent episodes of the cough. Whenever she gets run down or sick, it seems to go straight to her chest and she gets a cough that can take months to resolve. Tara thinks she is finding exercise more difficult in recent years because of shortness of breath, although she has never been diagnosed with asthma. Tara remembers that she used to cough a lot as a child and her mother said she was just like her grandfather, coughing away and spreading germs!

Tara gave up smoking for four years while she was trying to get pregnant and says she felt really good during that time. She started smoking again when they started travelling, partly because she couldn't see the point in not smoking since she had lost faith that she will ever become pregnant and also because she enjoys smoking and the positive effect it has on her mood.

Tara and her husband have been eating a wide range of different food, depending on where they are and what is available. She loves food and will eat just about anything. Tara's weight has increased by a couple of kilograms since they began travelling, which she attributes to spending less time exercising and more time sitting down and looking out the window of their kombivan. Tara feels she is in a significant point of change in her life, and is excited about the possibilities although she is a little confused about what is ahead for her and her husband. What she does want right now is something natural to help her stop coughing!

TABLE 6.29 **COMPLAINT**	
Analogy: Skin of the apple	**Complaint:** Define the presenting complaint and symptoms; understand the complaint *Chronic cough*
AREAS OF INVESTIGATION AND EXAMPLE QUESTIONS	**CLIENT RESPONSES**
Onset *When did you notice the cough?*	*About five months ago, we had been travelling for about a month and I got sick and started coughing. I've been coughing on and off since then.*

▶

Understanding the cause (client) *What do you think is causing your cough?*	*I think it's caused by colds. Whenever I get sick I start coughing almost straight away.*
Exacerbating factors *What makes the cough worse?*	*Cold air. It seems to be worse first thing in the morning and sometimes at night when I'm in bed.*
Relieving factors *What makes it better?*	*Being well and the warmer weather. It's not as bad during the day.*
Examination and inspection	Tara's breathing is audible and wheezy. You notice her elevating her shoulders slightly when she breathes in. Her cough sounds rattly. She looks pale and clammy.

TABLE 6.30 **CONTEXT**	
Analogy: Flesh of the apple	**Context:** Put the presenting complaint into context to understand the disease
Family health *Is there anyone else in your family who has had problems with their lungs?*	*My mum says my grandfather was always coughing. He ended up with emphysema.*
Allergies and irritants *Are there particular days in the week your cough is worse?* (exposure to possible allergen)	*Not that I know of.*
Recreational drug use *How many cigarettes are you smoking daily?* *How much alcohol are you drinking a week?*	*Probably about 15 or 20.* *It depends on where we are, but I think on average about 5 or 6 drinks each week.*
Functional disease *Do you experience a sour taste in the mouth and heartburn with the cough?* (gastro-oesophageal reflux)	*Not really, but I do get a sore chest from so much coughing.*
Infection and inflammation *How often have you been sick in the last six months?* *Have you noticed the purulent sputum associated with the cough is foul smelling?* (lung abscess)	*It feels like almost all the time. I feel like I have a cold or the flu every two or three weeks and then I cough for a couple of weeks before the next one comes along. Certainly get a lot of mucus, but it is not too bad smelling.*
Supplements and side effects of medication *Are you taking any supplements or medicines?*	*I'm taking a multivitamin to try and help my immune system. I've had a couple of courses of antibiotics.*

Endocrine/reproductive *Tell me about your menstrual cycle.*	Tara describes a 28–30 day cycle, with a 5–7 day bleed which is heaviest on days 1–3. She doesn't experience any pain, but gets a little anxious and irritable in the week before her period.
Stress and neurological disease *You mentioned your cough is worse in the mornings, does it ever stop altogether during the night?* (psychogenic, habit cough, Tourette's syndrome)	*I cough during the night too. But when I get up I can have some really major coughing fits with a lot of mucus.*
Eating habits and energy *Tell me about your diet and energy levels.*	*We eat whatever we can get hold of; it depends on where we are and what's available. I try to get fresh fruit and vegetables, but they can be hard to get in some places. We mostly eat out of cans at the moment.*

TABLE 6.31 CORE

Analogy: Core of the apple with the seed of ill health	**Core:** Holistic assessment to understand the client
AREAS OF INVESTIGATION AND EXAMPLE QUESTIONS	**CLIENT RESPONSES**
Emotional health *How do you feel about your problems conceiving?*	*When I think we might never have a baby I can get quite sad.*
Family and friends *Are you staying in contact with family and friends while you're travelling?*	*We send postcards and call them. We've got some friends house-sitting for us at the moment.*
Action needed to heal *Are you willing to make dietary and lifestyle changes if I recommend them?*	*Yes, I really want to get better. I know you're going to tell me to stop smoking.*
Long-term goals *Where do you see yourself in five years?*	*I'd like to see myself with one or two children, but maybe I'll be doing something completely different.*

TABLE 6.32 TARA'S SIGNS AND SYMPTOMS [1–3]

Pulse	80 bpm
Blood pressure	130/70
Temperature	37.4°C
Respiratory rate	18 resp/min; elevation of shoulders on inspiration
Cough sound	Noisy breathing reduced by coughing
Body mass index	23
Waist circumference	77.6 cm
Face	Pale
Fingers	Tobacco stained
Urinalysis	No abnormality detected (NAD)

Results of medical investigations

No tests have been carried out.

TABLE 6.33 **UNLIKELY DIAGNOSTIC CONSIDERATIONS [3–7]**	
CONDITIONS AND CAUSES	**WHY UNLIKELY**
CANCER AND HEART DISEASE	
Heart failure: persistent chronic cough can be the first symptom of heart failure; shortness of breath; history of smoking	No tachycardia or hypertension; usually occurs in older age groups; often presents with a nocturnal cough; Tara has not reported chest pain on exertion
OBSTRUCTION AND FOREIGN BODY	
Pulmonary embolism: can lodge in large pulmonary artery, medium-sized artery, terminal arteries; differing severity of symptoms depending on where it lodges and the size of the emboli; persistent cough can be an early symptom; small emboli may cause gradual progression of shortness of breath	Usually accompanied by a dry cough and with sudden onset of symptoms of fever, chest pain and tachycardia
INFECTION AND INFLAMMATION	
Acute bronchitis [59]	No significant fever
Pneumonia [60]	No significant fever
Acute legionnaire's disease	No significant fever
Acute tuberculosis	No significant fever
AUTOIMMUNE DISEASE	
Autoimmune disease e.g. Wegener's granulomatosis; persistent cough from lesions in the upper respiratory tract	Usually begins with severe nasal symptoms before a cough and then chest pain; Tara has not reported any kidney-related symptoms; urinalysis clear of abnormalities

Case analysis

TABLE 6.34 **POSSIBLE DIFFERENTIAL DIAGNOSIS**		
Not ruled out by tests/investigations already done [1, 3–9, 55]		
CONDITION	**WHY POSSIBLE**	**WHY UNLIKELY**
ALLERGIES AND IRRITANTS		
Causal factor: **Chronic allergies** [58]	Recurrent cough, travelling, potential exposure to irritants	Tara has not reported any significant nasal symptoms; her eyes are not red and do not have dark circles underneath
Causal factor: **Smoker's cough** [55, 56, 62, 71]	Chronic cough; worse in the morning; smoking again over the past 6 months; history of smoking	Usually minimum sputum production

▶

CANCER AND HEART DISEASE		
Bronchial carcinoma [68, 72]	Cough, recurrent chest infection, immune compromised; history of cigarette smoking; shortness of breath	No weight loss, Tara has not reported blood in her sputum, no chest pain; no additional bone pain indicating metastases; no signs of nail clubbing; usually presents with reduced breath sounds
OBSTRUCTION AND FOREIGN BODY		
Chronic obstructive pulmonary disease (COPD): chronic bronchitis, emphysema, chronic asthma, mixed; a condition of airway limitation that is not fully reversible [55, 74]	Chronic cough present for more than 3 months; cigarette smoking is a major risk factor; long history of chest infections; shortness of breath; family history of chronic cough (grandfather)	Usually in elderly age group, more often in men
FUNCTIONAL DISEASE		
Causal factor: Vocal cord dysfunction/ vocal cord polyps	Persistent chronic cough	Tara has not reported any changes in her voice or any difficulty eating; no blood in the sputum reported
Gastro-oesophageal reflux (GORD) [54]	Common cause of persistent recurrent cough; can be worse after eating chocolate or caffeine foods/ drink; worse in the morning or during the night	Usually non-productive cough; no heartburn reported
Causal factor: Postnasal drip (PND) [54]	Persistent chronic cough; worse in the morning; cough can disturb sleep	Tara has not reported any nasal symptoms
DEGENERATIVE AND DEFICIENCY		
Emphysema	Chronic cough present for more than 3 months; cigarette smoking is a major risk factor; history of chest infections; shortness of breath	Tara doesn't have the typical signs of emphysema: pink appearance to skin, weight loss, pursed lips, barrel chest, decreased breath sounds; no severe breathlessness reported
INFECTION AND INFLAMMATION		
Asthma [65]	Recurrent cough, recent infection, long-term history of chest infections, history of smoking; shortness of breath; can develop into chronic asthmatic bronchitis	Exercise intolerance occurs more often during acute episodes of asthma and is better between episodes of asthma; usually asthma has no mucus or if present will be clear thick mucus rather than yellow-green mucus; no history of allergy reported; no wheeze reported; only appears pale/blue in skin appearance in stages of attack

Chronic bronchitis	Recurrent episodes of cough, productive cough for 3 months, smokes cigarettes, long history of chest infections; had similar cough within the past 2 years; gradual exercise intolerance with shortness of breath; most common cause of chronic cough in adults; can be accompanied by bacterial infection producing yellow/green mucus; signs of chronic bronchitis: pale / blue appearance to skin, productive cough, purulent sputum, noisy breathing reduced by coughing	
Chronic sinusitis/rhinitis	Persistent chronic cough; cough can disturb sleep; shortness of breath	Tara has not reported any nasal symptoms
Causal factor: **Recurrent upper respiratory tract infections:** secondary bacterial infection causing chronic bronchitis [69, 71, 73]	Persistent cough; can exacerbate asthma symptoms; presence of yellow-green mucus	No fever at present
Causal factor: **Postviral cough**	Persistent cough; recent recurrent upper respiratory tract infections	Usually presents as a dry cough
STRESS AND NEUROLOGICAL DISEASE		
Causal factor: **Emotional stress psychogenic cough**	Not being able to fall pregnant; stress and grief; persistent cough, shortness of breath	Does not usually disturb sleep; does not usually present with a productive cough accompanied by yellow-green mucus showing signs of bacterial infection

TABLE 6.35 **DECISION TABLE FOR REFERRAL** [3–8, 12]		
COMPLAINT	**CONTEXT**	**CORE**
Referral for presenting complaint	Referral for all associated physical, dietary and lifestyle concerns	Referral for contributing emotional, mental, spiritual, metaphysical, lifestyle and constitutional factors
REFERRAL FLAGS	**REFERRAL FLAGS**	**REFERRAL FLAGS**
• Persistent productive cough lasting for more than 3 months	• Cigarette smoking • Family history of respiratory problems (grandfather) • Recurrent respiratory infections/low immunity • History of chronic respiratory tract infections • Unexplained infertility	• Grief and loss associated with fertility problems

ISSUES OF SIGNIFICANCE	ISSUES OF SIGNIFICANCE	ISSUES OF SIGNIFICANCE
• Lack of oxygen due to chronic cough	• Diet is often unbalanced due to availability of food while travelling • Reduced levels of physical activity	• Increase in respiratory infections associated with Tara's decision to give up trying to have a baby
REFERRAL DECISION	**REFERRAL DECISION**	**REFERRAL DECISION**
• Tara must be referred for medical assessment and management of lung disease [63]	• Dietary assessment	• Assessment for depression and emotional status

TABLE 6.36 **FURTHER INVESTIGATIONS THAT MAY BE NECESSARY [1, 2, 4–9]**	
TEST/INVESTIGATION	**REASON FOR TEST/INVESTIGATION**
FIRST-LINE INVESTIGATIONS:	
Ear, nose, throat physical examination	Infection and allergic signs
Chest examination: auscultation, percussion	Signs of asthma, obstruction, infection, foreign body, heart failure
Full blood count	Haemoglobin level may be elevated in bronchitis; the main function of haemoglobin for red cells is to carry oxygen to the tissues and return CO_2 to the lungs; white cell count high in infection
Differential white cell count	Detection of eosinophils to confirm allergic triggers for cough
CRP (C-reactive protein)	Infection, cancer, inflammation raised in chronic bronchitis
Sputum test: histology, microbiology	Detect presence of eosinophils, eliminate bronchitis, pneumonia, TB
Peak expiratory flow rate (PEFR) test: used often to monitor progression of disease [64, 66]	Will be reduced in chronic bronchitis, asthma
Spirometry-FEV (forced expiratory volume), **FVC** (forced vital capacity): test best used for assessment of airflow limitation [64, 66]	Will be reduced in chronic bronchitis, COPD, asthma
Total lung capacity (TLC) [66]	May be normal or increased in chronic bronchitis as will alleviate asthma symptoms more effectively
Hyperresonance reactivity test: salbutamol	Distinguish between asthma and chronic bronchitis
Blood gases: CO_2 gas transfer	Reduced in emphysema

Chest x-ray [60]	Detect presence of bronchitis and pneumonia; chronic bronchitis may show over inflation of lungs with low and flattened diaphragm; hypertranslucent lung fields; rule out bronchial carcinoma, TB, pneumonia, legionnaires' disease
IF NECESSARY:	
Skin prick test	For extrinsic allergies
Antineutrophil cytoplasmic antibody (ANCA)	Wegener's granulomatosis and autoimmune disease affecting lungs
IgM and IgG antibodies	Mycoplasma infection, viral respiratory tract infection

Confirmed diagnosis

TARA AND CHRONIC BRONCHITIS

Tara is a 31-year-old woman who has come to your clinic for help with a recurrent cough she has been having problems with since she started travelling around Australia with her husband; Tara has a longstanding history of chest infections and cigarette smoking. Over the past four years she and her husband have been trying to fall pregnant. When their attempts to have a child did not succeed, they decided to travel extensively around Australia. Recently Tara began smoking again after having given up for several years while she was trying to fall pregnant. Tara would like relief from her persistent cough, which has developed into chronic bronchitis.

The condition 'chronic bronchitis' is categorised under the term 'chronic obstructive pulmonary disease' (COPD) along with chronic asthma and emphysema. All syndromes are involved in the destruction of lung and airflow capability that is not fully reversible. Although the three syndromes are linked together because they can often overlap and coexist with one another, there are some differentiating features between each syndrome. Chronic bronchitis specifically has a productive cough with sputum that is experienced most days for at least three months of the year for more than one year. There are often recurrent episodes, a long history of chest infections and cigarette smoking in the health history [55, 62, 71]. The most consistent pathological finding in chronic bronchitis is hypertrophy of the mucus-secreting glands of the bronchial tree. The number of mucus-secreting glands is increased, which leads to increased mucus production and expectoration. In more advanced cases the bronchi can become inflamed leading to ulceration and narrowing of the airways.

The characteristic symptoms of chronic bronchitis are cough with productive sputum, wheeze, breathlessness and often a smoker's cough. Frequent infections with every cold 'going to the chest' and breathlessness are other common characteristics. Airway limitation is a long-term consequence of chronic bronchitis [67].

General references used in this diagnosis: 3–7, 57, 62, 67, 69, 73, 74, 76, 77

PRESCRIBED MEDICATION
- Antibiotics [61]
- Inhaled bronchodilator and corticosteroid [70, 75]

TABLE 6.37 **DECISION TABLE FOR TREATMENT (ONCE DIAGNOSIS IS CONFIRMED)**		
COMPLAINT	**CONTEXT**	**CORE**
Treatment for the presenting complaint and symptoms	Treatment for all associated symptoms	Treatment for mental, emotional, spiritual, constitutional, lifestyle issues and metaphysical considerations
TREATMENT PRIORITY	**TREATMENT PRIORITY**	**TREATMENT PRIORITY**
• Lifestyle recommendations to reduce congestion and improve clearance of mucus from Tara's lungs • Recommendation for Tara to quit smoking • Lifestyle recommendations to avoid exposure to air pollution, increase exercise and do breathing exercises to improve Tara's respiratory function • Physical therapy recommendations to reduce congestion and improve clearance of mucus from Tara's lungs • Physical therapy recommendations to improve respiratory function • Herbal tonic or tea with immunostimulant, antimicrobial, expectorant and anti-inflammatory action • Nutritional supplements to enhance immune function and support respiratory health **NB:** Vitamin A at high dose should not be taken long term [36] but only for the duration of the current infection and then reduced [8]; Tara's case should be collaboratively managed with conventional medical practitioners to ensure optimal management and treatment outcomes [61]	• Lifestyle recommendations to quit smoking and reduce exposure to air pollution and other environmental triggers to improve respiratory function and reduce the incidence of infection • Lifestyle recommendations to improve general health, fitness and respiratory health • Lifestyle recommendations to avoid or minimise triggers or aggravating factors • Physical therapy suggestions to enhance respiratory health • Dietary recommendations to improve general health, immunity and nutritional status • Dietary recommendations to identify and manage any food allergies or sensitivities • Herbal tonic or tea with immunostimulant, antioxidant, adaptogenic and tonic action to enhance general health and wellbeing • Nutritional supplements to enhance general health, wellbeing and respiratory health	• Lifestyle and physical therapy recommendations to improve Tara's emotional health • Lifestyle and dietary recommendations to improve the chances of a successful pregnancy • Recommendation to investigate the underlying causes of infertility • Dietary recommendation to drink herbal teas with nervine action instead of coffee • Herbal tea formula with nervine action

►

	• Dietary recommendations to improve intake of essential nutrients to improve general health and respiratory function as well as fertility • Dietary supplements to improve general health **NB:** Tara's vitamin and mineral levels should be monitored to ensure she stays within normal range; recommendation to use beta carotene instead of vitamin A in the longer term to avoid toxicity and any adverse affects of vitamin A supplementation on a future pregnancy [36]	

Treatment aims

- Get Tara to quit smoking [8, 14, 16, 23, 37, 38].
- Eliminate Tara's current bronchial infection [14, 38].
- Enhance Tara's immunity to reduce the incidence of infection [8, 14, 16].
- Improve Tara's lung function [8, 15, 16, 38].
- Reduce hypersecretion of mucus and support drainage of secretions from the respiratory tract [14, 38].
- Improve Tara's symptoms, quality of life and prevent or minimise progression of the condition and further lung damage [16, 38].
- Reduce oxidative stress [16, 52, 53].
- Identify and manage allergies that may be contributing to the problem [8, 14, 16].
- Improve Tara's diet and nutritional status [8, 14, 16, 38].
- Improve Tara's lifestyle, diet, general health, fitness and vitality with the long-term goal of achieving and maintaining a healthy pregnancy [24–26].

Lifestyle alterations/considerations

- Tara must quit smoking [8, 14, 16, 23, 37, 38]; it has a negative effect on Tara's respiratory [8, 23, 37, 38] and reproductive health [24].
- Encourage Tara to avoid exposure to air pollution wherever possible [38, 40].
- Twelve drops of eucalyptus oil in boiling water as a steam inhalation or five drops in a nebuliser can help alleviate symptoms of congestion [18]. Eucalyptus has antitussive, antimicrobial, decongestant and anti-inflammatory properties [18].
- Tara may find taking hot showers or baths soothes bronchial irritation [8].
- Breathing exercises, such as active expiration, slow and deep breathing and diaphragmatic breathing, may improve Tara's respiratory function and increase the strength of her respiratory muscles [27, 38].
- Tara may find applying liniments containing menthol or peppermint to her chest can help soothe her cough and enhance expectoration [18, 19].
- 'Bottle blowing' may help Tara improve the clearance of infected secretions, decrease the impairment of pulmonary function and increase total lung capacity [14]. This technique involves blowing through a plastic tube inserted into a bottle containing 10 cm water to create bubbles. The recommended frequency is 20 times on 10 occasions daily [14].

- Regular exercise will help improve Tara's respiratory health [15, 23, 38].
- Educating Tara about her condition and ways to manage and reduce symptoms is important to ensure her compliance to treatment and to reduce progression [23, 38]. A specific respiratory rehabilitation program may be of particular benefit to her [23, 38].
- Tara and her husband may want to seek medical investigations into the reasons for their unexplained infertility.
- Because Tara is still travelling it is unlikely she will attend the clinic on more than a couple of occasions. Treatment protocols and referrals must be provided in written form so other complementary therapists and medical practitioners can be informed of the treatments you have recommended.

Dietary suggestions

- Encourage Tara to increase consumption of nutrient-dense, antioxidant and flavanoid-rich whole foods: vegetables, fish, fresh fruit, whole grains, nuts and seeds, etc. They have a positive effect on respiratory health [16, 28, 29, 31, 32, 53]. High intake of vegetables and fruit is associated with enhanced ventilatory function, which reduces the risk of COPD [39] while low intake of vegetables (particularly cruciferous vegetables) and fruit is a risk factor for COPD [39].
- Encourage Tara to increase her intake of dietary fibre from vegetables, legumes, whole grains and fruit [16, 39].
- Encourage Tara to reduce or eliminate consumption of alcohol. Alcohol consumption is a risk factor for COPD [16, 28, 38].
- Encourage Tara to increase consumption of foods rich in omega-3 fatty acids and reduce consumption of omega-6 fatty acids [29]. Increased consumption of omega-3 fatty acids has been associated with improved lung function in COPD [30] and reduced risk for COPD [40].
- Encourage Tara to significantly reduce or eliminate consumption of refined carbohydrates, red meat, processed meat and fried foods [16, 31].
- Identify and eliminate food allergens or sensitivities and have Tara follow a hypoallergenic diet for two to three weeks [8]. Dairy products and wheat should be eliminated during this time [8].
- Encourage Tara to increase her fluid consumption [8, 16]. Vegetable broths, chicken soup and ginger tea with honey and lemon are good choices [8]. Herbal teas with a nervine and relaxation action such as passionflower [18, 20] or chamomile [18, 19] would also be a good choice.
- Encourage Tara to consume 2–5 g fresh raw garlic each day [18]. It has antioxidant, antimicrobial and immune-enhancing properties [18].

Physical treatment suggestions

- Tara may find reflexology is helpful [41].
- Massage therapy may be beneficial for Tara's emotional health [42, 43, 44].
- Acupuncture can help reduce dyspnoea [45] and may improve airway mucociliary clearance [33].
- Hydrotherapy: constitutional hydrotherapy [46–48]. Back and front contrast treatment with cold mitten friction on the trunk when symptoms begin to ease [48, 49]. Hot chest showers [49]. Smear a mustard plaster on the chest made with one part mustard powder to three parts flour and enough water to make a paste [50].
  A steam vapouriser will assist breathing [50].

TABLE 6.38 HERBAL FORMULA (1:2 LIQUID EXTRACTS)

HERB	FORMULA	RATIONALE
Echinacea root *Echinacea angustifolia/purpurea*	50 mL	Immunostimulant [18, 19]; anti-inflammatory [18, 19]; antioxidant [18]; increases resistance to infection [19]
Thyme *Thymus vulgaris*	30 mL	Expectorant [18, 19]; spasmolytic [18, 19]; respiratory antiseptic [18]; traditionally used for the treatment of bronchitis [18, 19, 20]; approved for use by Commision E for treating bronchitis [18]
Mullein *Verbascum thapsus*	55 mL	Respiratory demulcent [18]; antimicrobial [18]; traditionally used for bronchitis [18, 20]; approved for use by Commission E for treating respiratory catarrh [18]
Astragalus *Astragalus membranaceus*	60 mL	Immunostimulant [18, 19, 51]; tonic [18, 19, 51]; adaptogen [19, 51]; indicated for use with chronic infections [51]
Ginger *Zingiber officinalis*	5 mL	Anti-inflammatory [18, 19]; antimicrobial [18, 19]; antioxidant [18, 19]; immunomodulator [18]; anxiolytic [18]; traditionally used as a warming or diaphoretic herb [19]
Supply:	200 mL	Dose: 5 mL four times daily until bronchitis has resolved

TABLE 6.39 HERBAL TEA

Alternative to herbal liquid if Tara prefers a tea

HERB	FORMULA	RATIONALE
Elecampane root *Inula helenium*	2 parts	Expectorant [20, 21, 22]; antibacterial [20, 21, 22]; traditionally used for bronchitis [22, 23]
Thyme herb or flower *Thymus vulgaris*	1½ parts	See above
Echinacea root *Echinacea angustifolia/ purpurea*	2 parts	See above
Peppermint herb *Mentha × piperita*	1 part	Antimicrobial [18, 19]; antioxidant [18]; sedative [19]; traditionally used for respiratory infections [18, 19]
Ginger root *Zingiber officinalis*	¼ part	See above
Decoction: 1 cup four times daily		

TABLE 6.40 **NUTRITIONAL SUPPLEMENTS**	
SUPPLEMENT AND DOSE	RATIONALE
Quercetin 1500 mg daily in divided doses [16, 34]	May play a role in decreasing damage to lung tissue [16, 17]
Vitamin C 1000 mg twice daily [8]	Antioxidant [34, 35]; smokers have an increased requirement for vitamin C [34, 35]; possible link between vitamin C deficiency and COPD [38, 40]
Vitamin A 25000 IU twice daily until current infection resolves [8]; the dose should be reduced to no more than 2500 IU daily [35] thereafter or swap to a 6 mg beta carotene supplement daily [18] to ensure there are no adverse effects to the fetus from vitamin A should Tara become pregnant [36]	Antioxidant [34, 35]; deficiency is associated with low immunity [34, 35]; enhances resistance to infection [34] and maintains mucosal barrier to infection [34]
Zinc sulphate or citrate [36] 30 mg elemental zinc twice daily [8] 1 hour before or 2 hours after food [36] and taken at least 2 hours away from antibiotics and other supplements [36] 2 mg daily of copper should be included if zinc supplement is taken for more than 1 month [36] Dosage should be reviewed once the current infection resolves	Antioxidant [18]; plays an important role in immunity [36]; deficiency may be associated with low immunity [34]; and reproductive disorders [18, 34]; zinc supplementation may reduce the incidence of lower respiratory tract infections [35]
Omega-3 fish oil 4000 mg daily in divided doses [18, 36]	Anti-inflammatory [34]; may improve respiratory function in COPD [29, 30]
High-potency practitioner-strength **multivitamin, mineral and antioxidant supplement** providing therapeutic doses of essential micronutrients and antioxidants Dosage as per the manufacturer's instructions	To ensure Tara's intake of essential nutrients and antioxidants is sufficient; people with COPD often have lower intakes of essential vitamins and antioxidants [28, 29]; particularly important when Tara is unable to find fresh fruit and vegetables

References

[1] G. Douglas, F. Nicol, C. Robertson, Macleod's Clinical Examination, twelfth edn, Churchill Livingstone Elsevier, Edinburgh, 2009.
[2] N.J. Talley, S. O'Connor, Pocket Clinical Examination, third edn, Churchill Livingstone Elsevier, Australia, 2009.
[3] P. Kumar, C. Clark, Clinical Medicine, sixth edn, Elsevier Saunders, London, 2005 pp. 900–906.
[4] A. Polmear (Ed.), Evidence-Based Diagnosis in Primary Care, Churchill Livingstone Elsevier, Edinburgh, 2008.
[5] R.D. Collins, Differential Diagnosis in Primary Care, fourth edn, Lippincott Williams and Wilkins, Philadelphia, 2008.
[6] R.H. Seller, Differential Diagnosis of Common Complaints, fifth edn, Saunders Elsevier, Philadelphia, 2007.
[7] J. Jamison, Differential Diagnosis for Primary Care, second edn, Churchill Livingstone Elsevier, London, 2006.
[8] S.E. El-Hashemy, Naturopathic Standards of Primary Care, CCNM Press, Toronto, 2008.
[9] R.M.D. Berkow, A.J.M.D. Fletcher, M.H.M.D. Beers, The Merck Manual, sixteenth edn, Merck Research Laboratories, Rathway, N.J, 1993 (later edition).
[10] J. Silverman, S. Kurtz, J. Draper, Skills for Communicating with Patients, second edn, Radcliff Publishing, Oxford, 2000.

[11] R. Neighbour, The Inner Consultation: how to develop an effective and intuitive consulting style, Radcliff Publishing, Oxon, 2005.

[12] D. Peters, L. Chaitow, G. Harris, S. Morrison, Integrating Complementary Therapies in Primary Care, Churchill Livingstone, London, 2002.

[13] M. Lloyd, R. Bor, Communication Skills For Medicine, third edn, Churchill Livingstone Elsevier, Edinburgh, 2009.

[14] J.E. Pizzorno, M.T. Murray, H. Joiner-Bey, The Clinicians Handbook of Natural Medicine, second edn, Churchill Livingstone, St Louis, 2008.

[15] Y. Lacasse, E. Wong, G.H. Guyatt, D. King, D.J. Cook, R.S. Goldstein, Meta-analysis of respiratory rehabilitation in chronic obstructive pulmonary disease, Lancet 348 (1996) 1115–1119.

[16] H. Osiecki, The Physicians Handbook of Clinical Nutrition, seventh edn, Bioconcepts, Eagle Farm, 2000.

[17] C. Pagonia, A.I. Tauber, N. Pavlotsky, E.R. Simons, Flavonoid impairment of neutrophil response, Biochemical Pharmacology 35 (2) (1986) 237–245.

[18] L. Braun, M. Cohen, Herbs & Natural Supplements: An evidence based guide, second edn, Elsevier, Sydney, 2007.

[19] S. Mills, K. Bone, Principles & Practice of Phytotherapy: Modern Herbal Medicine. Edinburgh, 2000.

[20] British Herbal Medicine Association, British Herbal Pharmacopoeia, BHMAA, 1983.

[21] D. Hoffman, The New Holistic Herbal, third edn, Element Books Limited, Brisbane, 1996.

[22] S. Mills, K. Bone, The Essential Guide to Herbal Safety, Churchill Livingstone, St Louis, 2005.

[23] B.W. Willemse, N.H. ten Hacken, B. Rutgers, I.G. Lesman-Leegte, W. Timens, D.S. Postma, Smoking cessation improves both direct and indirect airway hyperresponsiveness in COPD, European Respiratory Journal 24 (2004) 391–396.

[24] D. Baird, A.J. Wilcox, Cigarette Smoking Associated with Delayed Conception, Journal of the American Medical Association 253 (20) (1985) 2979–2983.

[25] G.M. Buck, L.E. Sever, R.E. Batt, P. Mendola, Life-Style Factors and Female Infertility, Epidemiology 8 (4) (1997) 435.

[26] C.C. Korenbrot, A. Steinberg, C. Bender, S. Newberry, Preconception Care: A Systematic Review, Maternal and Child Health Journal 6 (2) (2002) 75–87.

[27] R. Gosselink, Breathing techniques in patients with chronic obstructive pulmonary disease (COPD), Chronic Respiratory Disease 1 (2004) 163–172.

[28] C. Tabak, H.A. Smit, D. Heederik, M.C. Ocke, D. Kromhouts, Diet and Chronic Obstructive, Pulmonary Disease: independent beneficial effects of fruits, whole grains and alcohol (the MORGEN study), Clinical and Experimental Allergy 31 (2001) 747–755.

[29] I. Romieu, C. Trenga, Diet and Obstructive Lung Diseases, Epidemiological Reviews 23 (2) (2001) 268–287.

[30] W. Matsuyama, H. Mitsuyama, M. Watanabe, K. Oonakahara, I. Higashimoto, M. Osame, K. Arimura, Effects of Omega-3 Polyunsaturated Fatty Acids on Inflammatory Markers in COPD, Chest 128 (2005) 3817–3827.

[31] R. Varraso, T.T. Fung, F.R. Hu, W. Willett, C.A. Camargo, Prospective study of dietary patterns and chronic obstructive pulmonary disease among US men, Thorax 62 (9) (2007) 786–791.

[32] L. Watson, B. Margetts, P. Howarth, M. Dorward, R. Thompson, P. Little, The association between diet and chronic obstructive pulmonary disease in subjects selected from general practice, European Respiratory Journal 20 (2002) 313–318.

[33] S. Tai, J. Wang, F. Sun, S. Xutian, T. Wang, M. King, Effect of needle puncture and electro-acupuncture on mucociliary clearance in anesthetized quails BMC Complementary and Alternative Medicine (4) (2006) 6.

[34] H. Osiecki, The Nutrient Bible, seventh ed, BioConcepts Publishing, Eagle Farm, 2008, pp. 33.

[35] J. Higdon, An Evidence Based Approach to Vitamins and Minerals, Thieme, New York, 2003, pp. 65–72.

[36] J. Jamison, Clinical Guide to Nutrition & Dietary Supplements in Disease Management, Churchill Livingstone, Edinburgh, 2003, pp. 677–683.

[37] B.W. Willemse, D.S. Postma, W. Timens, N.H. ten Hacken, The impact of smoking cessation on respiratory symptoms, lung function, airway hyperresponsiveness and inflammation, European Respiratory Journal 23 (2004) 464–476.

[38] N.M. Siafakas, P. Vermeire, N.B. Pride, P. Paoletti, J. Gibson, P. Howard, J.C. Yernault, et al., Optimal assessment and management of chronic obstructive pulmonary disease (COPD), European Respiratory Journal 8 (1995) 1398–1420.

[39] F. Celik, F. Topcu, Nutritional risk factors for the development of chronic obstructive pulmonary disease (COPD) in male smokers, Clinical Nutrition 25 (2006) 955–961.

[40] G. Viegi, Epidemiology of Chronic Obstructive Pulmonary Disease (COPD), European Respiratory Journal 8 (1995) 1398–1420.

[41] I.S. Wilkinson, S. Prigmore, C.F. Rayner, A randomised-controlled trial examining the effects of reflexology of patients with chronic obstructive pulmonary disease (COPD), Complementary Therapies in Clinical Practice 12 (2006) 141–147.

[42] A.F. Jorm, H. Christensen, K.M. Griffiths, B. Rodgers, Effectiveness of complementary and self-help treatments for depression, Medical Journal of Australia 176 (2002) S84–S96.

[43] C.A. Moyer, J. Rounds, J.W. Hannum, A Meta-Analysis of Massage Research, Psychological Bulletin 130 (1) (2004) 3–18.

[44] T. Field, M. Hernandez-Reif, M. Diego, Cortisol decreases and serotonin and dopamine increase following massage therapy, International Journal of Neuroscience 115 (2005) 1397–1413.

[45] M. Suzuki, K. Namura, Y. Ohno, H. Tanaka, M. Egawa, Y. Yokoyama, et al., The Effect of Acupuncture in the Treatment of Chronic Obstructive Pulmonary Disease, The J Altern Complement Med 14 (9) (2008) 1097–1105.

[46] W. Boyle, A. Saine, Lectures in Naturopathic Hydrotherapy, Eclectic Medical Publications, Oregon, 1988.

[47] L.M. Watrous, Constitutional hydrotherapy: from nature cure to advanced naturopathic medicine, Journal of Naturopathic Medicine 7 (2) (1997) 72–79.

[48] E. Blake, in: L. Chaitow, E. Blake, P. Orrock, M. Wallden, P. Snider, J. Zeff, (Eds.), Naturopathic Physical Medicine Theory and Practice for Manual Therapists and Naturopaths, Churchill Livingstone Elsevier, Philadelphia, 2008.

[49] M. Sinclair, Modern Hydrotherapy for the Massage Therapist, Lippincott Williams & Wilkins, Baltimore, 2008.

[50] D.D. Buchman, The complete book of water healing, Contemporary Books, McGraw-Hill Companies, New York, 2001.

[51] K. Bone, Clinical Applications of Chinese and Ayurvedic Herbs: Monographs for the Western Herbal Practitioners, Phytotherapy Press, Warwick, 1996.

[52] I. Rahman, D. Morrison, K. Donaldson, W. MacNee, Systemic oxidative stress in asthma, COPD and smokers, American Journal of Respiratory and Critical Care Medicine 154 (4) (1996) 1055–1060.

[53] I. Rahman, I.M. Adcock, Oxidative stress and redox regulation of lung inflammation in COPD, European Respiratory Journal 28 (2006) 219–242.

[54] M. Pratter, Overview of common causes of chronic cough, Chest 129 (Suppl. 1) (2006) S59–S62.

[55] E.G. Tzortzaki, N.M. Siafakas, A hypothesis for the initiation of COPD, Eur Respir J 34 (2009) 310–315.

[56] P.J. Barnes, Small airways in COPD, N Engl J Med 350 (2004) 2635–2637.

[57] P.M.A. Calverley, P. Walker, Chronic obstructive pulmonary disease, Lancet 362 (2003) 1053–1061.

[58] Mike Thomas, David Price, Andrew M Ross, Douglas M Fleming, Peter B Graves, Yvonne Doyle, G N Malavige, Chronic cough, BMJ 2003;326:1036, doi: 10.1136/bmj.326.7397.1036

[59] J. Macfarlane, W. Holmes, P. Gard, et al., Prospective study of the incidence, aetiology and outcome of adult lower respiratory tract illness in the community, Thorax 56 (2001) 109–114.

[60] D. Liebermann, P. Shvartzman, I. Korsonsky, et al., Diagnosis of ambulatory community-acquired pneumonia. Comparison of clinical assessment versus chest x-ray, Scand J Prim Healthcare 21 (2003) 57–60.

[61] R. Hopstaken, S. Coenen, C. Butler, Treating patients not diagnoses: challenging assumptions underlying the investigations and management of LRTI in general practice, J Antimicrob Chemother 56 (2005) 941–943.

[62] A. Lokke, P. Lange, H. Scharling, et al., Developing COPD: a 25 year follow up study of the general population, Thorax 61 (2006) 935–939.

[63] S. Straus, F. McAlister, D. Sackett, et al., Accuracy of history, wheezing, and forced expiratory time in diagnosis of chronic obstructive pulmonary disease, J Gen Intern Med 17 (2002) 684–688.

[64] H. Jackson, R. Hubbard, Detecting chronic obstructive pulmonary disease using peak flow rate: cross sectional survey, BMJ 327 (2003) 653–654.

[65] P.G. Gibson, J.L. Simpson, The overlap syndrome of asthma and COPD: what are its features and how important is it? Thorax 64 (2009) 728–735.

[66] S.H. Loring, M. Garcia-Jacques, A. Malhotra, Pulmonary characteristics in COPD and mechanisms of increased work of breathing, J Appl Physiol 107 (2009) 309–314.

[67] M.G. Cosio, M. Saetta, A. Agusti, Immunologic Aspects of Chronic Obstructive Pulmonary Disease, NEJM 360 (2009) 2445–2454.

[68] A. Punturieri, E. Szabo, T.L. Croxton, S.D. Shapiro, S.M. Dubinett, Lung Cancer and Chronic Obstructive Pulmonary Disease: Needs and Opportunities for Integrated Research, J Natl Cancer Inst 101 (2009) 554–559.

[69] G.J. Gaschler, M. Skrtic, C.C.J. Zavitz, M. Lindahl, P.-O. Onnervik, T.F. Murphy, S. Sethi, M.R. Stampfli, Bacteria Challenge in Smoke-exposed Mice Exacerbates Inflammation and Skews the Inflammatory Profile, Am J Respir Crit Care Med 179 (2009) 666–675.

[70] D.E. O'Donnell, P. Laveneziana, J. Ora, K.A. Webb, Y.-M. Lam, D. Ofir, Evaluation of acute bronchodilator reversibility in patients with symptoms of GOLD stage I COPD, Thorax 64 (2009) 216–223.

[71] C. Herr, C. Beisswenger, C. Hess, K. Kandler, N. Suttorp, T. Welte, J.-M. Schroeder, C. Vogelmeier, R.B.f.t.C.S Group, Suppression of pulmonary innate host defence in smokers, Thorax 64 (2009) 144–149.

[72] T. Walser, X. Cui, J. Yanagawa, J.M. Lee, E. Heinrich, G. Lee, S. Sharma, S.M. Dubinett, Smoking and Lung Cancer: The Role of Inflammation, Proc Am Thorac Soc 5 (2008) 811–815.

[73] S. Sethi, T.F. Murphy, Infection in the Pathogenesis and Course of Chronic Obstructive Pulmonary Disease, NEJM 359 (2008) 2355–2365.

[74] S.M. Dubinett, D.R. Aberle, D.P. Tashkin, J.T. Mao, The Partners – Airflow Obstruction, Emphysema, and Lung Cancer, Am J Respir Crit Care Med 178 (2008) 665–666.

[75] J.A. Falk, O.A. Minai, Z. Mosenifar, Inhaled and Systemic Corticosteroids in Chronic Obstructive Pulmonary Disease, Proc Am Thorac Soc 5 (2008) 506–512.

[76] W. MacNee, Update in Chronic Obstructive Pulmonary Disease 2007, Am J Respir Crit Care Med 177 (2008) 820–829.

[77] K.H. Groenewegen, D.S. Postma, W.C.J. Hop, P.L.M.L. Wielders, N.J.J. Schlosser, E.F.M. Wouters, Increased Systemic Inflammation Is a Risk Factor for COPD Exacerbations*, Chest 133 (2008) 350–357 for the COSMIC Study Group.

Allergic rhinitis

Case history

Andrew Donovan, 28, has come to the clinic to get some help for an ongoing problem with what he thinks is hay fever, except he has it all year round. Andrew has experienced an aggravation of his symptoms in the past week with itchy eyes, sneezing and a constantly runny nose, which he is finding exhausting. This recent aggravation is what has driven Andrew to seek help at the clinic – he will be a guest speaker at a major national conference next week and doesn't want to be sneezing and blowing his nose all the way through his presentation. Andrew tells you when he is really bad his eyes become very itchy and quite bloodshot. He has noticed his symptoms are often worse at the office, although he isn't sure why. He is also badly affected by cats and if he visits someone who owns a cat he always ends up sneezing.

Andrew smokes around 20 cigarettes a day and enjoys partying hard on the weekend. He tends to get 'stuck into' alcohol on the weekends but avoids drinking during the week. He occasionally smokes marijuana, and sometimes takes something 'with a bit more of a kick' when he is with his friends. He only does this on the weekends because he wants to keep his head clear for work during the week. Andrew tells you he is extremely ambitious and his five-year goal is to become a senior manager at the insurance-broking company where he is working. Andrew is in a relationship at the moment but isn't sure if it is going to be long term. He tells you he is a little wary of commitment. His older brother is married with three children and a big mortgage and it doesn't look like much fun to Andrew.

Andrew enjoys the inner-city lifestyle his income provides and he usually eats out, rarely cooking at home. He particularly likes Thai, Japanese and Italian food. During the day he will have up to five cups of coffee, at least three of which are cappuccinos from the local coffee shop. He sometimes remembers to drink a glass or two of water during the day but often forgets. Andrew's job involves long hours in an air-conditioned office sitting behind his desk and he doesn't have as much time for surfing and cycling as he used to, which he thinks is why he has put on weight in the past few years. He is hoping to go away with some mates for a weekend surfing trip after the big conference is over.

Andrew tells you he usually has a lot of energy and doesn't slow down much. He is close with his family but hasn't spent a lot of time with them lately because his work and social life take up nearly all of his time. His mother was diagnosed with breast cancer two years ago and has had a couple of operations. He admits he hasn't made much effort to visit his parents because even though his mother is doing very well, he feels like things aren't quite the same as they used to be. He sends her lots of cards, and emails and phones her at least twice a week to let her know he is thinking of her. He also finds that visiting his parents' farm during spring and summer makes his sneezing worse because of all the grasses and pollen, and because of that he hasn't visited as much as he probably should have.

TABLE 6.41 **COMPLAINT**	
Analogy: Skin of the apple	**Complaint:** Define the presenting complaint and symptoms; understand the complaint *Hayfever*
AREAS OF INVESTIGATION AND EXAMPLE QUESTIONS	**CLIENT RESPONSES**
Onset *When did you notice your symptoms getting worse?*	*About a week ago.*
Understanding the cause (client) *What do you think might have caused this?*	*Well, I know pollens, dust and animals can set me off so I suppose there must be something in the air at the office at the moment.*
Timing *How long do your exacerbations last for and how often does it happen?*	*Recently as soon as I get to the office. It lasts till the medicine from the chemist kicks in. It seems to be happening every day.*
Exacerbating factors *What makes it worse?*	*Spending time in the office definitely seems to make my symptoms worse. Maybe I'm allergic to work!*
Relieving factors *What makes it better?*	*The tablets from the pharmacy. They are not supposed to make you drowsy, but I feel a little groggy after a while when I take them. That's why I'm looking for something different to help me.*

TABLE 6.42 **CONTEXT**	
Analogy: Flesh of the apple	**Context:** Put the presenting complaint into context to understand the disease
AREAS OF INVESTIGATION AND EXAMPLE QUESTIONS	**CLIENT RESPONSES**
Family health *Does anyone else in your family have hayfever?*	*My sister does, but she doesn't get it as bad as I do.*
Allergies and irritants *Are you confident you are aware of everything you are allergic to?*	*Grass, pollen and cats. I think I must be allergic to something at work also.*
Trauma and pre-existing illness *Have you experienced any trauma to your eyes or head recently that may have triggered the red eyes?*	*No. This is a usual response when I begin sneezing.*
Recreational drug use *How much alcohol do you consume in a week?* *Do you ever take recreational drugs?*	*A fair bit on the weekend but not during the week.* *Sometimes on the weekend with my mates, but never during the week.*

▶

Functional disease *Have you noticed needing to swallow a lot of mucus?* (postnasal drip. PND)	*Yes. In the morning it seems to be worse and seems to make me cough for a while.*
Infection and inflammation *Do you feel pain when you sneeze?* (sinusitis)	*Not at the moment, but I have had that before when I have had a flare up.*
Supplements and side effects of medication *Are you taking any supplements or medication at the moment?*	*Antihistamine tablets every day.*
Eating habits and energy *Tell me about what you eat and your energy levels.*	Andrew tells you he mostly eats out, preferring Thai, Japanese and Italian food. He has about 5 cups of coffee every day.

TABLE 6.43 **CORE**	
Analogy: Core of the apple with the seed of ill health	**Core:** Holistic assessment to understand the client
AREAS OF INVESTIGATION AND EXAMPLE QUESTIONS	**CLIENT RESPONSES**
Daily activities *Tell me about your daily routine.*	Andrew gets up at around 6.30 am and gets breakfast on the way to work. He is usually at the office by 8 am and leaves around 6 or 6.30 pm. He either goes out to a restaurant for dinner or gets takeaway and eats it at home. He is usually in bed by midnight. He rarely has the time to exercise, although he does try to be active on the weekends.
Stress release *How do you manage your stress?*	*I try to blow off steam on the weekends when I'm out with my friends.*
Action needed to heal *How are you hoping I can help you?* *Would you consider making some dietary and lifestyle changes if that helped improve your symptoms?*	*I'm hoping you can give me something to help with my symptoms that won't make me feel tired.* *Maybe, it depends on what they are.*

TABLE 6.44 **ANDREW'S SIGNS AND SYMPTOMS** [1–3]	
Pulse	70 bpm
Blood pressure	130/75 sitting
Temperature	36.7°C
Respiratory rate	12 resp/min
Body mass index	28
Waist circumference	98 cm
Face	Dark under the eyes, which are red; pale waxy skin on the face, apart from around the nose where the skin is red and raw looking
Urinalysis	No abnormality detected (NAD)

Results of medical investigations

No investigations have been carried out.

TABLE 6.45 **UNLIKELY DIAGNOSTIC CONSIDERATIONS** [3, 4, 49]	
CONDITIONS AND CAUSES	**WHY UNLIKELY**
TRAUMA AND PRE-EXISTING CONDITIONS	
Subconjunctival haemorrhage: broken blood vessels in the conjunctiva causing red eye	Andrew has not experienced any eye trauma or foreign objects in the eye; usually more likely to occur in one eye only; clarify if Andrew experiences pain in the eyes; usually no eye discharge; redness can be localised to one area of eye(s); photophobia is usually a symptom but no visual changes
INFECTION AND INFLAMMATION	
Acute upper respiratory tract infection	No fever
Acute viral infection	No fever

Case analysis

TABLE 6.46 **POSSIBLE DIFFERENTIAL DIAGNOSIS**		
Not ruled out by tests/investigations already done [1, 3–6, 11, 49]		
CONDITION	**WHY POSSIBLE**	**WHY UNLIKELY**
ALLERGIES AND IRRITANTS		
Allergic rhinitis: seasonal 'hay fever' lasts for days/ weeks at a time [51, 53]	Attacks of sneezing, runny nose, itchy eyes, affected by grasses, pollens; red eyes and dark under eyes; seasonal variation	Need to define if Andrew has persistent watery nasal and eye discharge; clarify if the onset of his symptoms developed before the age of 20 years; check if he has smell disturbance (common); can have seasonal attacks of asthma; can get itchy throat and ears
Allergic rhinitis: perennial, lasts months/years at a time [51, 53]	Nasal congestion, runny nose, itchy nose; cat allergy; worse in the air-conditioning from dust mite allergy; symptoms are all year round; more common during 20s and 30s and decreases with age; cigarette smoke is an irritant; there is family history of symptoms	Andrew has noticed seasonal variation in the past at parents' farm; need to determine if Andrew has persistent watery nasal discharge; sneezing is variable; unsure if Andrew has smell disturbance (common); eye and throat symptoms are rare; asthma is common
Causal factor: **Food allergy/intolerance**	Nasal congestion, dark under eyes	Can cause rhinitis and asthma [14] as well as sinusitis [12]

▶

CANCER AND HEART DISEASE		
Nasal polyps/nasal tumour [55]	Runny nose, nasal congestion; associated with allergic and non-allergic rhinitis (more common)	Nasal discharge can be blood stained; symptoms are often unilateral; nose bleeds are common; can cause loss of smell and taste
OBSTRUCTION AND FOREIGN BODY		
Nasal obstruction: foreign body, deviated septum	Nasal discharge, congestion	Usually unilateral where obstruction is; nasal discharge can be blood stained; nose bleeds common
RECREATIONAL DRUG USE		
Drug abuse/induced psychoses: cocaine use or alcoholism, cannabis	Wakefulness, restlessness	Not clear whether Andrew has experienced delusions or hallucinations
Causal factor: **Liver damage:** binge drinking and use of recreational drugs	Can cause sneezing; alcohol, caffeine, nicotine and recreational drug intake	No jaundice, significant fatigue or gastrointestinal disturbances reported
OCCUPATIONAL TOXINS AND HAZARDS		
Causal factor: **Occupational rhinitis/sick building syndrome** [48]	Nasal and eye symptoms worse in the office	If Andrew has this condition he may not have allergy symptoms such as itchy eyes (unless allergic to dust mites from the air-conditioner)
FUNCTIONAL DISEASE		
Causal factor: **Postnasal drip (PND)**	Persistent nasal symptoms, common in allergic rhinitis	Andrew experiences increased mucus in the morning when he wakes up, which makes him cough; need to determine if Andrew experiences a cough during the night
Obstructive sleep apnoea	Low immune function from a lack of deep sleep could cause nasal symptoms	Need to determine if Andrew doesn't feel well rested in the morning and if he snores during the night; would complain of fatigue or exhaustion when nasal symptoms are present
DEGENERATIVE AND DEFICIENCY		
Anaemia	Cause pale skin; Andrew's eating pattern may be erratic; binge drinking and recreational drug use can affect nutrient status	No significant fatigue, shortness of breath or palpitations reported

INFECTION AND INFLAMMATION		
Non-allergic rhinitis with eosinophila (NARES): no allergic response but eosinophils still present in a nasal smear [50, 51, 58]	Runny nose, sneezing	This condition does not present with itchy eyes or nose symptoms common to allergic response; clarify if has aspirin or NSAID intolerance (common)
Chronic rhinitis: idiopathic, vasomotor (non-specific nasal hyperactivity due to imbalance of autonomic nervous system) [51]	Nasal congestion, mild conjunctival irritation, sneezing, runny nose; can be exacerbated by allergies, stress, chemical irritants, odours, temperature variations, alcohol, spicy foods; can be sporadic or perennial	Usually no specific cause; need to determine if nasal blockage changes from side to side; sneezing not common; usually no severe nasal or eye itchiness; can be significant nasal stuffiness; pain or fullness in the head not common; very unpredictable when reaction will happen; onset usually occurs after 20 years of age and can continue to stay the same for a long period of time; smell disturbance is usually not a symptom; check if there has been any previous nasal trauma
Sinusitis [52]	Nasal congestion, runny nose, common in allergic rhinitis (perennial); occasionally in allergic rhinitis (seasonal)	Need to determine if Andrew experiences pain and tenderness over the sinus area and if it is unilateral or bilateral; clarify if Andrew has a prior history of sinusitis; coughing usually present; thick yellow-green nasal discharge; no fever
Bacterial rhinosinusitis	Runny nose	Usually after an upper respiratory tract infection; associated with sinus pain, tenderness, facial or dental pain on one side of the face and blood in nasal secretions; purulent nasal discharge
Conjunctivitis: perennial allergic, seasonal	Red eyes, sneezing, nasal discharge, can be worse due to dust mites when near forced air heaters/conditioners in an office space; mild burning in the eyes; eyes are itchy	Need to determine if Andrew is experiencing significant eye discharge and if it is pale and stringy; clarify if he experiences mild eye pain; minimal photophobia and visual changes

Conjunctivitis: viral and bacterial	Red eyes, mild burning in the eyes	Need to determine if there is eye discharge and if it is watery or thick; more common if he has had a recent upper respiratory infection
Conjunctivitis: chlamydial	Prevalent in young adults, onset can be slow, mild burning in the eyes	Need to determine if Andrew is sexually active and whether he and/or his partners have been tested for STIs; scarring can be present on the eyelids; pale yellow discharge; slight pain
Episcleritis/scleritis	Red eyes, burning, itching	Need to determine if Andrew's eyes are very painful and if there has been a decrease in vision; common in systemic inflammatory conditions; large pupil; decreased vision
Superficial keratitis: corneal inflammation	Red eyes	Need to determine if Andrew ever uses contact lenses or has had the herpes simplex virus or blepharitis
Herpetic keratitis	Red eyes	Severe photophobia not reported
Blepharitis: lid margins inflamed	Common condition where symptoms may be itchy, burning eyes	Eye lids did not appear inflamed
Uveitis: inflammation of iris, ciliary body and choroid	Red eyes	Common in systemic inflammatory conditions; need to determine if Andrew is experiencing eye pain or photophobia; small pupil; decreased vision
Atrophic rhinitis: ozaena, chronic inflammation of nose and atropy of nasal mucosa	Runny nose	Clarify if Andrew has bad breath (halitosis); more common in females and during puberty; may have loss of smell; can have blood nose; rare condition
Asthma [57]	History of rhinitis of allergic origin; coughing in the morning	Need to ask more about Andrew's respiratory symptoms, if symptoms are worse upon exercise, difficulty breathing
SUPPLEMENTS AND SIDE EFFECTS OF MEDICATION		
Causal factor: **Rhinitis medicamentosa:** due to chronic use of nasal sprays or drops	Nasal congestion, runny nose	Need to clarify if Andrew has used cocaine or there is persistent use of over-the-counter nasal decongestants

Causal factor: Medication/drug induced rhinitis	Red eyes, persistent nasal symptoms, recreational drug use, smoker	Need to determine if Andrew has been using nasal sprays, antihypertensive drugs, hormones, psychotropic drugs that can cause nasal congestion; aspirin and NSAIDs can cause rhinorrhoea and nasal stuffiness; need to determine if Andrew has smoked marijuana before coming to the consultation
STRESS AND NEUROLOGICAL DISEASE		
Causal factor: Anxiety/addiction [58]	Keeps busy, recreational drug intake, caffeine intake, nicotine intake	Unsure if use of recreational drugs was triggered by an emotional event or as a way of coping with his lifestyle

Working diagnosis

ANDREW AND ALLERGIC RHINITIS

Andrew is a 28-year-old man who has come for help with symptoms of itchy eyes, sneezing, runny nose and what he thinks is all-year-round hay fever. Andrew is ambitious and has a busy lifestyle with a career as an insurance broker. He enjoys living in the city and eating out and while socialising on the weekend uses recreational drugs and alcohol to unwind. Andrew smokes cigarettes every day and enjoys several cups of coffee. Andrew is in a relationship at the moment but is unsure about his level of commitment. Although he is close to his family he has not visited them for some time. Andrew knows his symptoms are worse in the office environment, from being near cats and when he visits his parents' farm at certain times of the year. Andrew has a big presentation coming up next week and is looking for help to clear his symptoms without affecting his performance.

Andrew has symptoms of **allergic rhinitis** that present with sneezing attacks and nasal discharge that persist for more than an hour on most days both seasonally and also throughout the whole year. Rhinitis can be either seasonal or perennial in character.

Seasonal:

Often seasonal rhinitis is called 'hay fever' and is the most common of the allergic conditions. Nasal irritation, sneezing, runny nose, itchy and runny eyes and even itchy ears can be part of the symptom picture. Some people with rhinitis also have asthma and the common allergens are dust mites, pollen grains, domestic pets and moulds.

Perennial:

When symptoms are experienced all year round there is less aggravation of the eyes and throat. Those with allergic perennial rhinitis may experience sneezing and watery nose throughout the year or nasal blockage as the major concern. Because the mucosa is swollen in the sinuses in this chronic condition, it is common for sinusitis to develop. The major cause of perennial rhinitis is an allergen contained in dust mite faecal dust that can be found throughout the house, in human bedding and damp houses. Allergens also come from the saliva or urine from domestic pets, industrial dust, vapours and fumes. The long-term presence of rhinitis makes the nose more reactive to cigarette smoke, traffic fumes, strong detergents and perfumes.

Complications of both types of allergic rhinitis include associated symptoms of postnasal drip, allergic conjunctivitis, recurrent sinusitis and asthma.

General references used in this diagnosis: 3–6, 49, 51, 53, 54, 56

TABLE 6.47 **DECISION TABLE FOR TREATMENT PRIOR TO REFERRAL:**		
COMPLAINT	**CONTEXT**	**CORE**
Treatment for the presenting complaint and symptoms	Treatment for all associated symptoms	Treatment for mental, emotional, spiritual, constitutional, lifestyle issues and metaphysical considerations
TREATMENT PRIORITY	**TREATMENT PRIORITY**	**TREATMENT PRIORITY**
• Lifestyle recommendations to reduce symptom severity and exposure to known or potential allergens • Dietary recommendations to identify and manage dietary allergies or intolerances that may be causing or aggravating symptoms • Physical therapy recommendations to reduce symptom severity • Herbal tonic or tablets and tea with antiallergic, anti-inflammatory, anticatarrhal and immunomodulatory properties providing symptom relief and to modulate allergic response • Supplemental nutrients with antihistaminic properties	• Herbal tonic with immunomodulatory action to reduce immune reactivity • Supplemental nutrients to reduce inflammation and histamine response to help reduce immune reactivity and to improve Andrew's antioxidant status • Recommendation to stop binge drinking and recreational drug use • Physical therapy recommendation to support withdrawal from nicotine	Nil

TABLE 6.48 **DECISION TABLE FOR REFERRAL** [3–6, 10]		
COMPLAINT	**CONTEXT**	**CORE**
Referral for presenting complaint	Referral for all associated physical, dietary and lifestyle concerns	Referral for contributing emotional, mental, spiritual, metaphysical, lifestyle and constitutional factors
REFERRAL FLAGS	**REFERRAL FLAGS**	**REFERRAL FLAGS**
• Chronic upper respiratory symptoms, which are worsening	• Cigarette smoking • Consistent alcohol intake • Exposure to recreational drugs • Excessive consumption of coffee • Potential chronic environmental allergies	• Lack of commitment to relationships • Excessive lifestyle

▶

ISSUES OF SIGNIFICANCE	ISSUES OF SIGNIFICANCE	ISSUES OF SIGNIFICANCE
• Seminar presentation in 1 week, Andrew needs to have his symptoms under control	• Recent weight gain • Reduced physical activity	• Avoiding visiting his mother
REFERRAL	**REFERRAL**	**REFERRAL**
• Medical investigations to determine the cause of the chronic upper respiratory symptoms	• Refer to blood tests to ascertain liver function and immune status • Recreational drug use education and prevention • Dietary analysis to determine nutrient intake	• Counselling to discuss how mother's illness affected Andrew emotionally

TABLE 6.49 **FURTHER INVESTIGATIONS THAT MAY BE NECESSARY** [1–6, 54–56]

TEST/INVESTIGATION	REASON FOR TEST/INVESTIGATION
FIRST-LINE INVESTIGATIONS:	
Physical examination of nose (rhinoscopy)	Allergic rhinitis (seasonal) – pale, boggy nasal turbinates; chronic rhinitis (idiopathic) has swollen nasal turbinates; presence of nasal polyps indicates non-allergic origin
Physical examination of the eyes	Conjunctivitis, uveitis, scleritis, foreign body
Full blood count [52]	Allergies, infection, anaemia
Differential white blood cell count IgE (eosinophils antibody blood test) [54]	Definitive diagnosis for allergic triggers for rhinitis
ESR [52]	Inflammation, infection, allergy
IF NECESSARY:	
Serological radioallergosorbent testing (RAST) [56]	Detect specific IgE that binds to common allergens
Skin prick testing [56]	Test for extrinsic specific allergies
Liver function test	Alcohol and recreational drug abuse
Nasal smear	Allergic rhinitis (eosinophils), rhinitis medicamentosa (no eosinophils)
Sinus CT scan	Sinusitis

Confirmed diagnosis

ANDREW HAS ALLERGIC RHINITIS (SEASONAL AND PERENNIAL)

PRESCRIBED MEDICATION

• 24-hour non-drowsy antihistamine tablets to be taken daily until symptom control is achieved
• Steroid nasal spray

Andrew is not keen on taking a steroid nasal spray but will take antihistamine tablets to get his symptoms under control before the conference. He would like to see whether there is a natural way of controlling his symptoms.

TABLE 6.50 **DECISION TABLE FOR TREATMENT (ONCE DIAGNOSIS IS CONFIRMED)**		
COMPLAINT	**CONTEXT**	**CORE**
Treatment for the presenting complaint and symptoms	Treatment for all associated symptoms	Treatment for mental, emotional, spiritual, constitutional, lifestyle issues and metaphysical considerations
TREATMENT PRIORITY	**TREATMENT PRIORITY**	**TREATMENT PRIORITY**
• Continue with lifestyle recommendations to reduce symptom severity and exposure to allergens • Recommendation for testing to determine specific allergies • Continue with dietary recommendations to manage food allergies or intolerances • Continue with physical therapy recommendations to reduce symptom severity • Continue with herbal tonic or tablets and tea with antiallergic, anti-inflammatory, anticatarrhal and immunomodulatory properties providing symptom relief and to modulate allergic response • Continue with supplemental nutrients with antihistaminic properties **NB:** Herbal and nutritional therapy should be reviewed after 2 months	• Recommendation to consider desensitisation therapy to reduce symptom severity • Dietary recommendations to increase status of essential nutrients and antioxidants • Continue with herbal tonic with immunomodulatory action to reduce immune reactivity • Continue with supplemental nutrients • Supplemental probiotics to help modulate immune response • Recommendation to stop binge drinking and recreation drug use • Physical therapy recommendations to support withdrawal from nicotine	• Recommendation to improve lifestyle and negotiate a treatment contract to reduce/quit alcohol, cigarette and recreational drug consumption • Encourage more discussion and/or professional counselling for intimacy and commitment concerns • Recommendation for counselling if withdrawal from drug and stimulant intake causes anxiety

Treatment aims

- Provide symptomatic relief and reduce swelling and inflammation in nasal mucosa [13].
- Reduce the allergic response [13, 14] and normalise the immune response [15].
- Reduce the inflammatory response [13, 14].
- Prevent complications or progression of allergic rhinitis to asthma or sinusitis [13, 14].
- Prevent development of nasal polyps [13].
- Identify allergens or irritants and reduce or eliminate exposure to them [13, 14].
- Change Andrew's work and home environments where possible to reduce exposure to allergens [13, 14].
- Improve Andrew's general health and lifestyle.

Lifestyle alterations/considerations

- Encourage Andrew to quit smoking cigarettes and marijuana. Exposure to cigarette smoke worsens respiratory symptoms [28] and increases his risk of developing asthma [29].
- Encourage Andrew to avoid aspirin; aspirin sensitivity is linked to the development of nasal polyps [14, 42, 43].
- If Andrew is sensitive to dust mites or mould spores he should ensure air-conditioner filters are regularly cleaned at home and work. Vacuum cleaners that filter air should be used at home and work and he should discuss office air quality with his employer to see whether it can be improved.
- Encourage Andrew to be tested for allergies to determine what he is reacting to, and avoid exposure to allergens where he can.
- Andrew may benefit from a course of desensitisation therapy [30].
- Encourage Andrew to be encouraged to live a healthier lifestyle. Encourage him to reduce alcohol consumption and to quit using cigarette and recreational drugs. He may find it easier to stop one thing at a time rather than stopping all at the same time [37].
- Andrew may find counselling helpful if he experiences difficulties reducing alcohol and quitting drugs and cigarettes [14, 37].
- Andrew may benefit from exploring the reasons for his aversion to commitment and avoidance of his family.

Dietary suggestions

- Encourage Andrew to increase his water intake. He may find it easier to remember to drink more water if he keeps an 800 mL or 1 L water bottle on his desk and replace some of his daily coffees with the prescribed herbal tea or water.
- Food allergies and intolerances should be identified and managed appropriately [13, 14].
- Encourage Andrew to reduce consumption of saturated fats [46], omega-6 fatty acids [14, 27] and *trans*-fatty acids [14, 46, 47].
- Encourage Andrew to increase consumption of nutrient and antioxidant-rich whole foods [26, 44] and reduce consumption of refined carbohydrates [44].
- Andrew may benefit from avoiding dairy products [14, 44, 45].
- Encourage Andrew to increase dietary consumption of omega-3 fatty acids. They are helpful to reduce inflammation in the respiratory tract [13, 16].

Physical treatment suggestions

- Andrew may benefit from a course of acupuncture. Acupuncture is effective in the symptomatic treatment of both seasonal [20] and perennial [21] allergic rhinitis.
- Andrew may also find acupuncture is beneficial to help him quit smoking [31, 32].
- Encourage Andrew to use a saline solution twice or three times daily to irrigate his nasal and sinus passages. Nasal irrigation can dramatically reduce symptoms of allergic rhinitis [22, 23].
- Andrew may find relief from his allergic conjunctivitis by washing his eyes with cool chamomile tea or by placing cooled chamomile teabags on his eyes to reduce inflammation and irritation. Chamomile has an anti-inflammatory [16, 19] and antipruritic [16] action.
- Hydrotherapy: alternating hot (two minutes) and cold (one minute) local compresses to the sinus area with a wash cloth for three rounds [33, 34]. Constitutional hydrotherapy [35]. A mustard foot bath and/or hot leg baths to draw congestion away from the head [34, 35]. Short cold applications to the back of the neck for mucous membrane vasoconstriction of the nose [36]. Steam inhalation for 15 minutes to clear congestion [33, 36]. Cold shower up to two minutes after a hot shower daily for more than three months has been shown to improve immunity [36].

TABLE 6.51 HERBAL FORMULA (1:2 LIQUID EXTRACTS)

HERB	FORMULA	RATIONALE
Baical scullcap *Scutellaria baicalensis*	50 mL	Anti-allergic [16, 17]; anti-inflammatory [16, 17]; antioxidant [16, 17]; antimicrobial [16, 17]
Albizia *Albizia lebbek*	50 mL	Antiallergic [16, 17]; antimicrobial [16, 17]; stabilises mast cells [16]
Eyebright *Euphrasia officinalis*	40 mL	Anti-catarrhal [18, 19]; anti-inflammatory [18, 19]; astringent [18, 19]; traditionally used for nasal catarrh [18, 19]
Echinacea *Echinacea angustifolia/purpurea*	40 mL	Immunomodulator [16, 18]; anti-inflammatory [16, 18]; antimicrobial [16, 18]; indicated for use in naso-pharyngeal catarrh in BHP [19]
Licorice *Glycyrrhiza glabra*	20 mL	Anti-inflammatory [16, 18]; antimicrobial [16, 18]; immunomodulator [16, 18]; demulcent [19]
Supply:	200 mL	Dose: 10 mL 3–4 times daily when symptoms are acute, reduce to 10 mL twice as symptoms improve

TABLE 6.52 TABLET ALTERNATIVE TO HERBAL LIQUID: MAY IMPROVE COMPLIANCE

HERB	DOSE PER TABLET	RATIONALE
Baical scullcap *Scutellaria baicalensis*	800 mg	See above
Albizia *Albizia lebbek*	500 mg	See above
Eyebright *Euphrasia officinalis*	500 mg	See above
Golden rod *Solidago virgaurea*	500 mg	Anti-inflammatory [16]; traditionally used for nasopharyngeal catarrh [16, 19]; specific indication in BHP for low-grade inflammation of the naso-pharynx with persistent catarrh [19]

Dose: 2 tablets twice daily

TABLE 6.53 HERBAL TEA

In addition to herbal liquid or tablets – alternative to coffee

HERB	FORMULA	RATIONALE
Elder flowers *Sambucus nigra*	1 part	Anticatarrhal [19, 38, 39]
Nettle leaf *Urtica dioica/urens*	1 part	Antiallergic [18, 38]; anti-inflammatory [18]
Peppermint leaves *Mentha × piperita*	1 part	Antiallergic [16]; antimicrobial [16, 18]; may help reduce symptoms of allergic rhinitis [40]; the pleasant taste of peppermint in the blend will help improve compliance

Infusion: 1 tsp per cup, 1 cup 2–3 times daily to replace coffee

TABLE 6.54 **NUTRITIONAL SUPPLEMENTS**	
SUPPLEMENT AND DOSE	**RATIONALE**
Vitamin C 1000 mg 3 times daily [13, 14]	Modulates inflammation [13, 14]; antioxidant [13, 14]; antihistamine [14, 24]; smokers have a higher need for vitamin C [13]; beneficial to reduce symptoms of allergic rhinitis [13, 14, 24]
2000 mg **quercetin** [14, 16] daily and 1500 mg **bromelain** [13] daily in divided doses	Bromelain is mucolytic [13, 14] and anti-inflammatory [13, 14]; quercetin is anti-inflammatory [16, 24], anti-allergic [16, 24] and an immunomodulator [16]; quercetin inhibits inflammatory enzymes, prostaglandins and leukotrienes [16], stabilises mast cells [16] and inhibits mast cell release of histamine [24]
High-potency practitioner-strength **multivitamin, mineral and antioxidant supplement** providing therapeutic levels of essential nutrients and antioxidants Dosage as per the manufacturer's instructions	Andrew has lower antioxidant levels because he is a smoker [25, 26]
Omega-3 fatty acids 6000 mg daily in divided doses [13, 16]	Anti-inflammatory [16, 24]; low levels of omega-3 fatty acids are associated with allergic sensitisation and allergic rhinitis [27]
High quality practitioner-strength **probiotic supplement** containing human strain organisms including *Lactobacillus rhamnosus GG* [15, 16] Dosage as per manufacturer's instructions	Moderates inflammatory and immune response [16]; strengthens intestinal barrier function [16, 41] and reduces antigen load in the gut [41]; healthy bowel microflora assists with production of regulatory T cells, which may promote anti-inflammatory and anti-allergic responses [15, 41]

References

[1] G. Douglas, F. Nicol, C. Robertson, Macleod's Clinical Examination, twelfth edn, Churchill Livingstone Elsevier, 2009.

[2] N.J. Talley, S. O'Connor, Pocket Clinical Examination, third edn, Churchill Livingstone Elsevier, Australia, 2009.

[3] P. Kumar, C. Clark, Clinical Medicine, sixth edn, Elsevier Saunders, London, 2005.

[4] J. Jamison, Differential Diagnosis for Primary Care, second edn, Churchill Livingstone Elsevier, London, 2006.

[5] R.H. Seller, Differential Diagnosis of Common Complaints, fifth edn, Saunders Elsevier, Philadelphia, 2007.

[6] A. Polmear (Ed.), Evidence-Based Diagnosis in Primary Care, Churchill Livingstone Elsevier, 2008.

[7] J. Silverman, S. Kurtz, J. Draper, Skills for Communicating with Patients, second edn, Radcliff Publishing, Oxford, 2000.

[8] R. Neighbour, The Inner Consultation: how to develop an effective and intuitive consulting style, Radcliff Publishing, Oxon, 2005.

[9] M. Lloyd, R. Bor, Communication Skills For Medicine, third edn, Churchill Livingstone Elsevier, Edinburgh, 2009.

[10] D. Peters, L. Chaitow, G. Harris, S. Morrison, Integrating Complementary Therapies in Primary Care, Churchill Livingstone, London, 2002.

[11] R.D. Collins, Differential Diagnosis in Primary Care, fourth edn, Lippincott Williams & Wilkins, Philadelphia, 2008.

[12] J.E. Pizzorno, M.T. Murray, H. Joiner-Bey, The Clinicians Handbook of Natural Medicine, second edn, Churchill Livingstone, St Louis, 2008.

[13] J. Jamison, Clinical Guide to Nutrition & Dietary Supplements in Disease Management, Churchill Livingstone, Edinburgh, 2003.

[14] H. Osiecki, The Physicians Handbook of Clinical Nutrition, seventh edn, Eagle Farm: Bioconcepts, 2000.

[15] H.H. Smits, A. Engering, D. van der Kleij, E.C. de Jong, K. Schipper, T.M. van Capel, B.A. Zaat, et al., Selective probiotic bacteria induce IL-10–producing regulatory T cells in vitro by modulating dendritic cell function through dendritic cell–specific intercellular adhesion molecule 3–grabbing nonintegrin, Journal of Allergy and Immunology 115 (6) (2005) 1260–1267.

[16] L. Braun, M. Cohen, Herbs & Natural Supplements: An evidence based guide, second edn, Elsevier, Sydney, 2007.

[17] K. Bone, Clinical Applications of Chinese and Ayurvedic Herbs: Monographs for the Western Herbal Practitioners, Phytotherapy Press, Warwick, 1996.

[18] S. Mills, K. Bone, Principles & Practice of Phytotherapy: Modern Herbal Medicine. Edinburgh, Churchill Livingstone, London, 2000.

[19] British Herbal Medicine Association, British Herbal Pharmacopoeia, BHMAA, 1983.

[20] C.C. Xue, R. English, J.J. Zhang, C. DaCosta, C.G. Li, Effect of Acupuncture in the Treatment of Seasonal Allergic Rhinitis: A Randomized Controlled Clinical Trial, The American Journal of Chinese Medicine 30 (1) (2002) 1–11.

[21] C.C. Xue, X. An, T.P. Cheung, C. DaCosta, G.B. Lenon, F.C. Thien, D.F. Story, Acupuncture for persistent allergic rhinitis: a randomised, sham-controlled trial, Medical Journal of Australia 187 (6) (2007) 337–341.

[22] W. Garavello, F. Di Berardino, M. Romagnoli, G. Sambataro, R.M. Gaini, Nasal rinsing with hypertonic solution: an adjunctive treatment for pediatric seasonal allergic rhinoconjunctivitis, International Archives of Allergy and Immunology 137 (4) (2005) 310–314.

[23] D.E. Olson, B.M. Rasgon, R.L. Hilsinger, Radiographic comparison of three methods for nasal saline irrigation, Laryngoscope 112 (8 Pt. 1) (2002) 1394–1398.

[24] H. Osiecki, The Nutrient Bible, seventh edn, BioConcepts Publishing, Eagle Farm, 2008.

[25] M.A.M. Abou Seif, Blood antioxidant status and urine sulfate and thiocyanate levels in smokers, Journal of Biochemical Toxicology 11 (3) (1996) 133–138.

[26] K. Marangon, B. Herbeth, E. Lecomte, A. Paul-Dauphin, P. Grolier, Y. Chancerelle, Y. Artur, et al., Diet, antioxidant status, and smoking habits in French men, The American Journal of Clinical Nutrition 67 (1998) 231–239.

[27] S. Hoff, H. Seiler, J. Heinrich, I. Kompauer, A. Nieters, N. Becker, G. Nagel, et al., Allergic sensitisation and allergic rhinitis are associated with n-3 polyunsaturated fatty acids in the diet and in red blood cell membranes, European Journal of Clinical Nutrition 59 (2005) 1071–1080.

[28] C. Janson, S. Chinn, D. Jarvis, J. Zock, K. Toren, P. Burney, Effect of passive smoking on respiratory symptoms, bronchial responsiveness, lung function, and total serum IgE in the European Community Respiratory Health Survey: a cross-sectional study, Lancet 358 (9299) (2001) 2103–2109.

[29] R. Polosa, J.D. Knoke, C. Russo, G. Piccillo, P. Caponnetto, M. Sarva, L. Proietti, et al., Cigarette smoking is associated with a greater risk of incident asthma in allergic rhinitis, Journal of Allergy and Clinical Immunology 121 (6) (2008) 1428–1434.

[30] M.A. Calderon, B. Alves, M. Jacobson, B. Hurwitz, A. Sheikh, S. Durham, Allergen injection immunotherapy for seasonal allergic rhinitis (Review), Cochrane Database of Systematic Reviews, 2007. Issue 1. Art. No: CD001936. DOI: 10.1002/14651858.CD001936.pub.

[31] Y. Chae, M. Yeom, J.H. Jan, H.J. Park, D.H. Hahm, I. Shim, et al., Effect of acupuncture on anxiety-like behavior during nicotine withdrawal and relevant mechanisms, Neuroscience Letters 430 (2008) 98–102.

[32] D. He, J.I. Medbo, A.T. Hostmark, Effect of Acupuncture on Smoking Cessation or Reduction: An 8-Month and 5-Year Follow-up Study, Preventive Medicine 33 (2001) 364–372.

[33] M. Sinclair, Modern Hydrotherapy for the Massage Therapist, Lippincott Williams & Wilkins, Baltimore, 2008.

[34] D.D. Buchman, The complete book of water healing, Contemporary Books, McGraw-Hill Companies, New York, 2001.

[35] L. Chaitow, Hydrotherapy, water therapy for health and beauty, Element, Dorset, 1999.

[36] E. Blake, in: L. Chaitow, E. Blake, P. Orrock, M. Wallden, P. Snider, J. Zeff, (Eds.), Naturopathic Physical Medicine Theory and Practice for Manual Therapists and Naturopaths, Churchill Livingstone Elsevier, Philadelphia, 2008.

[37] T.R. Kosten, P.G. O'Connor, Management of Drug and Alcohol Withdrawal, N Engl J Med 348 (2003) 1786–1795.

[38] S. Mills, K. Bone, The Essential Guide to Herbal Safety, Churchill Livingstone, St Louis, 2005.

[39] D. Hoffman, The New Holistic Herbal. Shaftesbury, Element Books Ltd, Dorset, 1990.

[40] T. Inoue, Y. Sugimoti, H. Masuda, C. Kamei, Effects of Peppermint (Mentha piperita L.) Extracts on Experimental Allergic Rhinitis in Rats, Biological & Pharmaceutical Bulletin 24 (1) (2001) 92–95.

[41] M. Kalliomäki, E. Isolauri, Role of Intestinal Flora in the Development of Allergy, Current Opinion in Allergy and Clinical Immunology 3 (1) (2003) 15–20.

[42] M.L. Kowalski, R. Pawliczak, J. Wozniak, K. Siuda, M. Poniatowska, et al., Differential Metabolism of Arachidonic Acid in Nasal Polyp Epithelial Cells Cultured from Aspirin-sensitive and Aspirin-tolerant Patients, American Journal of Respiratory and Critical Care Medicine 161 (2000) 391–398.

[43] G. Settipane, Epidemiology of nasal polyps, Allergy & Asthma Proceedings 17 (5) (1996) 231–236.

[44] S. Farchi, F. Forastiere, N. Agabiti, G. Corbo, R. Pistelli, C. Fortes, V. DellOrco, et al., Dietary factors associated with wheezing and allergic rhinitis in children, European Respiratory Journal 22 (2003) 772–780.

[45] P.D. Buisseret, Common manifestations of cow's milk allergy in children, Lancet 311 (8059) (1978) 304–305.

[46] D.P. Rakel, A. Rindfleisch, Inflammation: Nutritional, Botanical, and Mind-body Influences, Southern Medical Journal 98 (3) (2005) 303–310.

[47] S. Stender, J. Dyerberg, Influence of trans fatty acids on health, Annals of Nutrition and Metabolism 48 (2) (2004) 61–66.

[48] A. Drake-Lee, R. Ruckley, A. Parker, Occupational rhinitis: a poorly diagnosed condition, J Laryngol Otol 116 (2002) 580–585.

[49] J.W. Georgitis, Prevalence and differential of chronic rhinitis, Curr Allergy Asthma Rep 1 (2001) 202–206.

[50] M. Staevska, J.N. Baraniuk, Persistent nonallergic rhinosinusitis, Curr Allergy Asthma Rep 5 (3) (2005) 233–242.

[51] B. Sibbald, E. Rink, Epidemiology of seasonal and perennial rhinitis. Clinical presentation and medical history, Thorax 46 (1991) 895–901.

[52] M. Lindbaek, P. Hjortdahl, The clinical diagnosis of acute purulent sinusitis in general practice – a review, Br J Gen Pract 52 (2002) 491–495.

[53] M. Smolensky, A. Reinberg, G. Labrecque, Twenty-four hour pattern in symptom intensity of viral and allergic rhinitis: treatment implications, J Allergy Clin Immunol 95 (1995) 1084–1096.

[54] K. Gendo, E. Larson, Evidence-based diagnostic strategies for evaluating suspected allergic rhinitis, Ann Intern Med 140 (2004) 278–289.

[55] C. Grigoreas, D. Vourdas, K. Petalas, et al., Nasal polyps in patients with rhinitis and asthma, Allergy Asthma Proc 23 (2002) 169–174.

[56] M. Crobach, J. Hermans, A. Kaptein, et al., The diagnosis of allergic rhinitis: how to combine the medical history with the results of radioallergosorbent tests and skin prick tests, Scand J Prim Healthcare 16 (1998) 30–39.

[57] ARIA, Allergic rhinitis and its impact on asthma, Allergic Rhinitis and its Impact on Asthma Initiative, 2001. Online Available: www.whiar.com.

[58] S. Jaradeh, T. Smith, L. Torrico, et al., Autonomic nervous system evaluation of patients with vasomotor rhinitis, Laryngoscope 110 (2000) 1828–1831.

Tinnitus

Case history

Mr Henry Ang has come to the clinic at the suggestion of his daughter, who is an existing client. Mr Ang has been having problems with his hearing and his daughter told him you may be able to help.

Mr Ang is 73 and has recently moved in to live with his daughter and son-in-law following the death of his wife eight months ago; it has been a stressful time. Mr Ang was a ship's engineer for 40 years before retiring eight years ago. Mr Ang tells you he has had problems with noises in both ears for quite a few years and when he was tested several years ago he was told he had noise-induced hearing loss (NIHL). Recently though, his hearing has been worsening and he is finding the noise in his ears more troublesome. He describes the noise as a high-pitched sound that is there all of the time, but sometimes it seems to be worse. When it is really bad it can interfere with his ability to hear. Mr Ang goes on to tell you that as a ship's engineer he often worked in noisy engine rooms so he thinks his hearing was affected by the constant noise, but it has been the past 10 years in which he has really noticed his hearing is getting worse.

Mr Ang went to his doctor who referred him to an audiologist and an ENT specialist. The doctor told him his hearing is deteriorating and that he has tinnitus, which is causing the ringing in his ears. He has been recommended to wear hearing aids. Mr Ang hopes you may be able to help with the noise in his ears because it is affecting his sleep.

When you ask him about his diet Mr Ang tells you he eats what his daughter cooks, but she has been making a special effort to cook food he enjoys the way his wife used to make it. He particularly likes pickles and salted fish and she has used the internet to learn how to make them properly. His daughter and son-in-law have a home espresso coffee machine and he enjoys making cappuccinos and espresso coffees. He probably drinks about four each day. Apart from that Mr Ang loves eating all kinds of fruit and fresh vegetables and enjoys growing them himself. Mr Ang is slim and says he eats large meals and often feels hungry. He likes to keep busy and finds it difficult to get a full night's sleep these days.

Mr Ang is taking enalapril maleate for high blood pressure and he also takes 100 mg of aspirin daily at the recommendation of his doctor. Since he moved in with his daughter, she has been giving him a multivitamin and one fish oil capsule every day.

TABLE 6.55 **COMPLAINT**	
Analogy: Skin of the apple	**Complaint:** Define the presenting complaint and symptoms; understand the complaint *Tinnitus*
AREAS OF INVESTIGATION AND EXAMPLE QUESTIONS	**CLIENT RESPONSES**
Onset *When did you first start to have problems with your ears?*	*Many years ago. It has become much worse in the last year.*
Exacerbating factors *Is there anything that makes it worse?*	*It is worse at night and gives me problems falling asleep, but I don't know if I just notice it more at night.*
Relieving factors *Is there anything that makes it better?*	*When I am busy and try not to think about the ringing I feel better.*

TABLE 6.56 **CONTEXT**	
Analogy: Flesh of the apple	**Context:** Put the presenting complaint into context to understand the disease
AREAS OF INVESTIGATION AND EXAMPLE QUESTIONS	**CLIENT RESPONSES**
Family health *Is there anyone else in your family who has had this problem?*	*No.*
Allergies and irritants *Do you experience any symptoms such as excess sneezing or nasal discharge, or itching on roof of mouth with a cough?* (allergies)	*No, it is usually just the ears that give me the most problems.*
Trauma and pre-existing illness *Have you experienced any trauma to your ear recently?* (traumatic perforation of ear drum)	*No, not that I can think of.*

▶

Surgery and hospitalisation *Have you ever had surgery to your ears or head?*	*No.*
Degenerative and deficiency *Is the ringing in your ears continuous?* (otosclerosis, NIHL, presbyacusis, acoustic neuroma)	*Yes, I can hear it all of the time and I wonder if it is louder at night because everything else is so quiet?*
Infection and inflammation *Have you experienced any discharge from the ear?* (otitis externa, ruptured tympanic membrane from acute otitis media, mastoiditis, trauma to the ear)	*No, just the ringing.*
Supplements and side effects of medication *Are you taking any supplements or medicines?*	*Yes. My daughter gives me fish oil and a multivitamin every day. My doctor has given me these tablets for my blood pressure* (he shows you a packet of enalapril maleate) *and I take one aspirin tablet daily* (he shows you a box of 100 mg aspirin tablets).
Stress and neurological disease *Have you experienced any sensations of nausea or as the room in spinning?* (inner ear vertigo)	*Sometimes I feel dizzy, but not where the room is actually spinning, more like I am going to fall down suddenly.*
Eating habits and energy *Tell me about your diet and energy levels.*	Mr Ang tells you he eats whatever his daughter cooks and that she is making a special effort to cook what he likes. She is making him pickles and salted fish. He has about 4 cups of coffee every day.

TABLE 6.57 **CORE**	
Analogy: Core of the apple with the seed of ill health	**Core:** Holistic assessment to understand the client
AREAS OF INVESTIGATION AND EXAMPLE QUESTIONS	**CLIENT RESPONSES**
Emotional health *How are you coping since your wife passed away?*	*I am still very sad and I miss her. Sometimes at night I cry for her. I have been very stressed since my wife passed away, and it was difficult when I had to move. I am not so stressed now and my daughter and her family are very good to me.*
Daily activities *What do you do during the day?*	*I go for a walk with the dog every morning. Sometimes I look after the grandchildren when my daughter goes to work and sometimes I go out to the library or to visit with friends.*

| Family and friends
Do you have other family or friends nearby? | *Yes, I have a son near me and I have some old friends and some new friends.* |
| Action needed to heal
How would you like me to help you today? | *I hope you can give me some medicine or treatment that might help.* |

TABLE 6.58 MR ANG'S SIGNS AND SYMPTOMS

Pulse	70 bpm
Blood pressure	135/87
Temperature	37°C
Respiratory rate	14 resp/min
Body mass index	21
Waist circumference	83.8 cm
Face	Puffiness and dark rings under the eyes
Urinalysis	No abnormality detected (NAD)

TABLE 6.59 RESULTS OF MEDICAL INVESTIGATIONS [2, 6–12]

TEST	RESULTS
Examination of external ear and ear drum	No excess wax, foreign objects or skin disorder in outer ear canal; no external discharge or swelling of outer ear; no tenderness over mastoid process; no redness of tympanic membrane
Hearing test (Rinne and Weber): vibrating prong on external auditory meatus and mastoid process and on forehead; whispered voice test [66]	*Rinne test:* air conduction > bone conduction (perceptive) *Weber test:* right ear less deaf and could hear sound better indicating perceptive deafness
Audiometry/audiogram	Hearing loss in the past has been at 4000 Hz; lower frequencies shown now older age
TMJ examination	No clicking of the jaw when he opens and closes his mouth; no tenderness
Throat examination/throat swab	No swelling or redness
Nose examination/nose swab	No infection causing referred pain to ear
Chest examination: auscultation, percussion	No signs of asthma, obstruction or infection
Full blood count	NAD
Fasting blood glucose test	NAD
Fasting blood lipid test (chylomicrons are primarily trigylcerides, LDLs are primarily cholesterol, VLDLs primarily triglycerides, HDLs are predominantly proteins)	NAD
Cholesterol blood test (usually includes VLDL value)	NAD
Homocysteine blood test	NAD

TABLE 6.60 UNLIKELY DIAGNOSTIC CONSIDERATIONS [2, 6–11, 64, 68]

CONDITIONS AND CAUSES	WHY UNLIKELY
CANCER AND HEART DISEASE	
Acoustic neuromas: slow-growing benign schwannoma of vestibular nerve	Would have unilateral perceptive deafness with continuous tinnitus; would be a sudden onset of tinnitus that can be present for months or years before hearing loss or vertigo experienced
Causal factor: **Vascular disorder of the head and neck**	Objective tinnitus that is a pulsating sound [69, 70]
Hyperlipidaemia: tinnitus can be associated	Fasting blood lipid and cholesterol test within normal range
Hypertension: tinnitus can be associated	Blood pressure within normal limits and controlled by medication
TRAUMA AND PRE-EXISTING ILLNESS	
Causal factor: **Trauma/head injury:** may have perceptive deafness, tinnitus	Physical examination shows no clear signs of head injury; no neurological signs to consider internal injury
FUNCTIONAL DISEASE	
Causal factor: **Soft tissue disorder of middle ear, eustachian tube**	Tinnitus would be a clicking or banging sound; may also hear blowing sounds synchronised with breathing; can have awareness of his own voice; tinnitus can disappear when lying down with the head rested; would be positive for conductive deafness; no abnormality on inspection of the tympanic membrane
Causal factor: **Temporomandibular joint dysfunction (TMJ):** tinnitus [71]	Examination showed NAD
DEGENERATIVE AND DEFICIENCY	
Presbyacusis: age-related hearing loss and likely to be over 50 years of age [61]	Need to determine if bilateral deafness of gradual onset without long-term history of exposure to noise; it is still unclear how NIHL and presbyacusis can interrelate [13, 61]
Anaemia: B12 and iron deficiency tinnitus can be associated; iron deficiency can be connected to aspirin use in older people [63]	Full blood count NAD
Otosclerosis: middle ear [65]	Would have conductive deafness and continuous tinnitus; more often develops in the second and third decade in females; a hereditary disorder
INFECTION AND INFLAMMATION	
Causal factor: Infection of nervous system	Persistent vertigo would be experienced; no fever present

▶

Causal factor: Disorder of external auditory canal	No visible sign of foreign body, excess wax or infection of external canal on inspection; tinnitus would be an intermittent scratching sound that is worse by pressing on the ear; would be positive for conductive deafness
ENDOCRINE/REPRODUCTIVE	
Prostatism: insomnia; age related	No nocturia reported or difficulty with urination
Diabetes: tinnitus can be associated	Fasting blood glucose and urinalysis NAD; can be unilateral tinnitus due to diabetic neuropathy
STRESS AND NEUROLOGICAL DISEASE	
Ménière's disease: sensorineural hearing loss and tinnitus (inner ear)	Usually a low-pitched noise with roaring bursts of sound during attacks of vertigo; tinnitus is usually unilateral when it first develops; usually develops between second and fifth decade and tinnitus is fluctuating and not continuous; will have fluctuating deafness at low tones in later stages that leads to severe deafness; nausea and vomiting can be associated
Multiple sclerosis: tinnitus	Usually more often presents in women and initially at a younger age, no unilateral eye presentation, sudden onset vertigo
Migraine: tinnitus	No severe headache reported with tinnitus

TABLE 6.61 **CONFIRMED DIAGNOSIS** [2, 8, 61, 67]	
CONDITION	**RATIONALE**
Continuous tinnitus: with bilateral perceptive deafness noise-induced hearing loss (NIHL)	High-pitched sound; gradual onset with symptoms of deafness; Rinne and Weber test revealed sensorineural hearing loss/perceptive deafness; both ears affected; long history of working in noise due to occupation

Case analysis

TABLE 6.62 **POSSIBLE FURTHER DIFFERENTIAL DIAGNOSIS**		
Not ruled out by tests/investigations already done [2, 6–11]		
CONDITIONS AND CAUSES	**WHY POSSIBLE**	**WHY UNLIKELY**
ALLERGIES AND IRRITANTS		
Causal factor: **Salicylate intolerance:** salicylates can alter auditory nerve activity to cause tinnitus [14, 21]	Aspirin being taken for a long time; eating foods high in salicylates; tinnitus can be a symptom in highly sensitive individuals	

▶

Causal factor: **Allergies affecting the nose:** can develop nasal polyps due to aspirin intolerance [15]	Tinnitus can develop due to ongoing allergies that cause nose blockage; puffiness and dark rings under the eyes	No sneezing or runny nose reported
FUNCTIONAL DISEASE		
Insomnia: age related; requires further investigation as due to age; often has associated physical, medical and painful reasons for lack of sleep in older people	Common to present with difficulty getting to sleep, then fitful and light sleep for a short period of time; with age the body can function on as little as 4 hours' sleep a night; delayed period of going to sleep and poor sleep quality common	
SUPPLEMENTS AND SIDE EFFECTS OF MEDICATION		
Causal factor: **Ototoxic medication:** aspirin, NSAIDs, antibiotics, antiviral, cardiac drugs, diuretics, antidepressants, heavy metals; can affect hair cells, 8th cranial nerve or central nerve connections causing toxic labyrinthitis	Long-term use of aspirin can increase damage done to ears due to loud noise in the past; can have have tinnitus and hearing loss that is bilateral	Can also experience vertigo
ENDOCRINE/REPRODUCTIVE		
Hyperthyroidism	Slim build but large appetite, often hungry, not a lot of sleep, busy and appears restless	No typical Graves eye signs or goitre
STRESS AND NEUROLOGICAL DISEASE		
Causal factor: **Psychological disorder**	Genuine tinnitus that develops from a psychological disorder	History of exposure to noise; tests verify noise-related damage
Causal factor: **Adjustment disorder – psychological depression**	Insomnia; new relocation into different living environment; a change from independent living	Aspects of symptoms need to be clarified; usually adjustment disorder depression does not continue over 2 months; not considered major depression; usually a low mood due to a particular life-changing event or psychological cause; need to clarify how depressed he has been feeling since his wife passed away

▶

▶

General anxiety disorder (GAD)	Has been at least 6 months; anxiety disorder is often associated with loss or threat of a loss; weight loss, lack of sleep; can develop due to having tinnitus, not sleeping long hours; person often complains of physical symptoms without thinking there may be a mental disorder; delayed period of getting to sleep is common; new environment to live in; drinking excess tea and coffee (caffeine)	Ascertain whether there has been significant weight loss; if tension and stress has been overwhelming for at least 6 months; often associated with diarrhoea, tight chest, difficulty breathing; less common to experience frequent waking and early morning wakefulness as in depression
Chronic depression	Chronic insomnia; missing his wife, feeling lonely without her; can be undiagnosed in the elderly population; can develop due to having tinnitus, lack of sleep; due to continuous tinnitus it is important to understand mental health status	The fact that Mr Ang tends to the garden is a good sign that he is active and productive with his daily activities
Short-term insomnia (less than 3 weeks): caused by emotion, excitement life stress, change, noise, stimulation, pain, grief, anxiety, jet lag, change in working hours	Moving in with family, sleeping in unfamiliar bed, noise of grandchildren, recent travel	Need to clarify how long sleep has been disturbed
Causal factor: **Relocation to new environment**	Affect sleep and anxiety levels	
Causal factor: **Physiologic fatigue:** caused by depression, caffeine, alcohol, excess sleep, poor sleep due to uncomfortable mattress or pillow, being too hot or cold when trying to sleep, hunger during the night, excess exercise and intense emotions	Common to have a delay in falling asleep; diagnostic studies are within normal limits	Symptoms present as less than 14 days' duration and not usually associated with changes in self-esteem, social difficulties or overall mood
EATING HABITS AND ENERGY		
Causal factor: **High intake of salicylate foods**	Affect salicylate intolerance; tea, pickles, salted fish, several fruit and vegetables [15]	
Causal factor: **Excess caffeine intake**	Mr Ang is having excess tea and coffee intake; common to have a delay in falling asleep if consuming caffeine prior to going to sleep; for some individuals having caffeine 6 hours before bed can affect sleep	

Working diagnosis

MR ANG AND TINNITUS WITH BILATERAL PERCEPTIVE DEAFNESS NOISE-INDUCED HEARING LOSS (NIHL)

Mr Ang is 73 years old and has come to the clinic with his daughter after having had a confirmed diagnosis of tinnitus and hearing loss in both ears. He is hoping to gain help with reducing the sound in his ears so he can get better sleep. Mr Ang recently moved in with his daughter's family as it was becoming difficult to live independently after the death of his wife eight months ago. There has been enormous change during the past year and at times great stress. Mr Ang likes to keep active growing vegetables and enjoys drinking espresso coffee and eating a variety of foods during the day. Mr Ang takes blood pressure medication daily and is fit and slim for his age.

Tinnitus is a sensation of sound in the ear which is usually bilateral and when there is no specific auditory stimulus involved. Tinnitus may develop for individuals with no hearing loss. The hissing or ringing sound can be extremely stressful and vascular conditions may be associated. There are several causes of the symptom of tinnitus ranging from age-related hearing loss, noise-induced damage to the ear, trauma and injury-related conditions, nerve and vascular dysfunction, systemic disease and infection.

Mr Ang has experienced NIHL for some years, which is characteristic of bilateral hearing loss of gradual onset due to long-term exposure to noise. If tinnitus is due to the NIHL from long exposure to noise, it is more likely to be continuous.

It is most important to assess what the mental health status of a person is who experiences tinnitus because the symptom can be very distressing, with a possible psychological nature to the cause. Because Mr Ang has experienced great change over the past year with significant grief and symptoms such as lack of sleep developing, it was important to refer him for further physical and emotional assessments.

A dietary assessment was also crucial for Mr Ang because he was ingesting several foods that contained high levels of salicylate in his diet. Salicylates can cause auditory nerve dysfunction and either cause or exacerbate the symptom of tinnitus. For this reason Mr Ang was referred back to his doctor to additionally assess the level of salicylate intake included in long-term prescriptive cardiac medication such as aspirin.

General references used in this diagnosis: 2, 7–9, 11, 62, 67

TABLE 6.63 **DECISION TABLE FOR TREATMENT PRIOR TO REFERRAL**		
COMPLAINT	**CONTEXT**	**CORE**
Treatment for the presenting complaint and symptoms	Treatment for all associated symptoms	Treatment for mental, emotional, spiritual, constitutional, lifestyle issues and metaphysical considerations

▶

TREATMENT PRIORITY	TREATMENT PRIORITY	TREATMENT PRIORITY
• Lifestyle recommendations to reduce exposure to triggering or aggravating factors • Dietary recommendations to reduce or eliminate consumption of foods which may be aggravating his symptoms • Dietary recommendations to increase consumption of essential nutrients to address deficiencies that may be affecting his symptoms • Dietary recommendations to increase consumption of foods with a reduced inflammatory response • Physical treatment suggestions to reduce or improve tolerance to symptoms • *Ginkgo biloba* herbal supplement, which may reduce or alleviate symptoms • Nutritional supplements to reduce symptoms and improve or protect hearing	• Lifestyle recommendations to enhance health and wellbeing • Dietary recommendation to increase consumption of essential nutrients and enhance health and wellbeing • Dietary recommendations to ensure Mr Ang does not miss out on essential nutrients due to reduction/ elimination of salicylate-containing foods • *Ginkgo biloba* herbal tablet to enhance cognition and general wellbeing • Nutritional supplements to enhance nutritional status, health and wellbeing • Lifestyle recommendation to exercise daily to enhance health, wellbeing and reduce blood pressure	• Recommendation to exercise daily to support positive mental health

TABLE 6.64 **DECISION TABLE FOR REFERRAL** [2, 8, 11, 16]		
COMPLAINT	**CONTEXT**	**CORE**
Referral for presenting complaint	Referral for all associated physical, dietary and lifestyle concerns	Referral for contributing emotional, mental, spiritual, metaphysical, lifestyle and constitutional factors
REFERRAL FLAGS	**REFERRAL FLAGS**	**REFERRAL FLAGS**
• Long-term ingestion of aspirin [21] and current use of antihypertensive medication [58] • Tinnitus with hearing loss that would benefit from a hearing aid	• High intake of salicylate-containing foods • High caffeine intake	• Recent death of wife • Recent relocation was stressful
ISSUES OF SIGNIFICANCE	**ISSUES OF SIGNIFICANCE**	**ISSUES OF SIGNIFICANCE**
• Tinnitus is affecting his sleep • Tinnitus that interferes with his daily activity	• Increased hunger and slim build • Lack of sleep	• Moved in with daughter

REFERRAL DECISION	REFERRAL DECISION	REFERRAL DECISION
• To see his doctor again to assess patterns of sleep and activities and regarding a hearing aid • Referral to consider alternative heart medication other than salicylate-containing drugs • Referral to doctor to review the potential for Mr Ang's antihypertensive medication to be causing and/or aggravating his tinnitus [58]	• Dietary assessment and reduction/elimination of salicylate-containing foods	• Grief counselling • Stress release such as massage

TABLE 6.65 **FURTHER INVESTIGATIONS THAT MAY BE NECESSARY** [2, 7, 8, 11, 12]	
TEST/INVESTIGATION	**REASON FOR TEST/INVESTIGATION**
FIRST-LINE MEDICAL INVESTIGATIONS:	
Counselling/psychiatry consultation: mental health assessment	Bereavement, new lifestyle
Thyroid function test TSH, T4, T3	TSH (thyroid-stimulating hormone) suppressed in hyperthyroidism; thyroid-specific antibodies, to confirm auto-immune cause of hyperthyroidism (Graves')
Sleep diary for one week	See patterns of sleep and activities prior to sleep; note the time Mr Ang goes to bed, how long it takes for him to get to sleep, how many times he wakes during the night, the last time of waking up before morning, any dreams or nightmares that were experienced, need to urinate during the night; writing down thoughts before bed and when waking is also helpful
Diet diary for one week	Have a more detailed look at what foods Mr Ang is eating, what times he is eating, how he is preparing the food and amounts of food being ingested
IF NECESSARY:	
X-ray of skull	Head trauma may cause tinnitus
Rectal physical examination	Benign prostate feels smooth, soft, from plum size to orange; prostatitis, prostatic abscess feels large and boggy; cancerous prostate gland feels hard and irregular nodular enlargement

Confirmed diagnosis

Mr Ang has tinnitus with bilateral perceptive deafness NIHL and salicylate intolerance.

PRESCRIBED MEDICATION/TREATMENTS
- Captopril (antihypertensive medication to replace enalapril maleate)
- Hearing aid

TABLE 6.66 **DECISION TABLE FOR TREATMENT**		
COMPLAINT	CONTEXT	CORE
Treatment for the presenting complaint and symptoms	Treatment for all associated symptoms	Treatment for mental, emotional, spiritual, constitutional, lifestyle issues and metaphysical considerations
TREATMENT PRIORITY	TREATMENT PRIORITY	TREATMENT PRIORITY
• Continue with lifestyle recommendations to reduce exposure to triggering or aggravating factors • Continue with dietary recommendations • Continue with physical treatment suggestions • Continue with *Ginkgo biloba* supplement. Ginkgo treatment should be reviewed after 3 months [49] • Continue with nutritional supplements	• Continue with lifestyle and dietary recommendations to enhance health and wellbeing • Continue with dietary recommendations to ensure intake of essential nutrients while reducing salicylate-containing foods • Continue with *Ginkgo biloba* to enhance cognition and general wellbeing • Continue with nutritional supplements	• Continue with exercise recommendations • Recommendation for Mr Ang to get involved in a supportive social network as he is going through a time of significant life change

Treatment aims
- Reduce or eliminate tinnitus symptoms.
- Support/protect hearing [20, 24].
- Identify and manage any environmental or food allergies/sensitivities that may be contributing to Mr Ang's hearing problems [19, 21].
- Identify and correct any nutritional deficiencies that may be contributing to Mr Ang's problem [22–24].
- Enhance Mr Ang's antioxidant and nutritional status [20, 22–24].
- Improve Mr Ang's sleep.
- Improve Mr Ang's diet and lifestyle to enhance his health and wellbeing [33–36].
- Support Mr Ang's mental health as he deals with recent life-changing events.

Lifestyle alterations/considerations
- Encourage Mr Ang to consider eliminating aspirin. Salicylates are known to induce tinnitus in some people and ceasing the aspirin may result in significant improvements in his symptoms [17, 21].

- Encourage Mr Ang to stop smoking if he is a smoker. Nicotine can cause or aggravate symptoms [25].
- Encourage Mr Ang to reduce his exposure to excessive noise as it may exacerbate his symptoms [25].
- Encourage Mr Ang to ensure his hypertension continues to be properly managed [32].
- Encourage Mr Ang to be physically active. Regular physical activity in older adults improves wellbeing and psychological health [34, 36] as well as helping reduce blood pressure [47, 48].
- Mr Ang may benefit from getting involved in a supportive social network such as a community or social group with other people with similar interests and/or background. This is particularly important as Mr Ang is entering a new phase of his life with the death of his wife and moving in with his daughter and son-in-law.

Dietary suggestions

- Encourage Mr Ang to reduce consumption of salicylate-containing foods [21, 25]. Dietary recommendations to reduce salicylates ensures Mr Ang does not miss out on essential nutrients.
- Food sensitivities or allergies should be identified and managed accordingly [19].
- Encourage Mr Ang to eliminate sugar, alcohol and caffeine-containing foods and drinks, as well as products made from cocoa [25, 26]. These can increase uric acid levels, which has been implicated in the development of tinnitus [32].
- Encourage Mr Ang to replace coffee with green tea for its antioxidant and health-enhancing properties [40]. Mr Ang should take his vitamin and mineral supplements two hours either before or after drinking green tea to ensure their absorption is not reduced [40].
- Encourage Mr Ang to reduce consumption of sodium [17, 27].
- Encourage Mr Ang to increase consumption of manganese-rich foods such as avocados, blueberries, nuts and seeds, seaweed, egg yolks, whole grains, legumes, dried peas and green leafy vegetables [17, 23]. Manganese deficiency has been associated with tinnitus [23].
- Encourage Mr Ang to increase consumption of foods rich in omega-3 fatty acids. Omega-3 fatty acids are beneficial for Mr Ang's cardiovascular health [18, 40].
- Encourage Mr Ang to increase water consumption [17, 32].
- Encourage Mr Ang to consume a whole-food, Mediterranean-type diet to enhance his general health and wellbeing [33, 35].

Physical treatment suggestions

- Mr Ang may find acupuncture improves both his symptoms of tinnitus and his sleep quality [28, 29].
- Transcutaneous electrical nerve stimulation (TENS) therapy is likely to improve Mr Ang's quality of life [28, 30, 31].
- Mr Ang may find vibrational therapy or phase shift therapy is helpful in alleviating his symptoms [23, 38].
- Tinnitus retraining therapy may prove helpful. This therapy involves counselling and sound therapy [23, 25, 37].
- Constitutional hydrotherapy for overall immune health, circulation and nervous system support [50–53].
- Alternating hot and cold showers daily [50, 54].
- To help sleep at night – a hot hydrotherapy shower 2–10 minutes twice a day [51, 55], followed by treading in cold foot bath and cold stomach rub or cold compress to heat the body prior to sleep at night [50, 51, 56, 57].

TABLE 6.67 HERBAL FORMULA

HERB	FORMULA	RATIONALE
Ginkgo 2:1 liquid extract *Ginkgo biloba* Standardised extract providing 14.4mg ginkgo flavonglycosides and 3.6 mg ginkgolides and bilobalide	80 mL	Enhances cerebral blood flow [40, 41, 43]; circulatory stimulant [40, 41, 43]; antioxidant [40, 41, 43]; may be of benefit in salicylate-induced tinnitus [39]; some studies have shown ginkgo is of benefit in tinnitus [23, 40]; enhances cognitive function in the elderly [41, 43]; enhances quality of life [43]
Rehmannia 1:2 liquid extract *Rehmannia glutinosa*	120 mL	Anti-inflammatory [49, 59]; adrenal tonic [49, 59]; may be beneficial in treating tinnitus [60]; adrenal tonic properties may help Mr Ang adjust to his new lifestyle
Supply:	200 mL	Dose: 7 mL twice daily

TABLE 6.68 NUTRITIONAL SUPPLEMENTS

SUPPLEMENT AND DOSE	RATIONALE
Magnesium citrate supplement providing a daily dose of 600 mg elemental magnesium [40]	Protective against NIHL [20, 42]; supplementation can reduce noise sensitivity and improve tinnitus symptoms [17, 22, 23]; antihypertensive [18, 40, 42, 46]
Coenzyme Q10 100 mg daily [18, 40]	Improves auditory hair energetics [44]; prevents respiratory metabolic impairment of hair cells due to hypoxia [44]; antioxidant [18, 40]; antihypertensive [40]
Natural vitamin E 800 IU daily [40]	Antioxidant [18, 40, 42, 46]; alternative to aspirin for prevention of cardiovascular disease [40, 50]
Zinc citrate supplement providing 30 mg elemental zinc daily [45]	Zinc supplementation in elderly tinnitus clients with dietary zinc deficiency can relieve symptoms [23, 45]
High-potency practitioner-strength **multivitamin, mineral and antioxidant supplement** containing therapeutic levels of B-group vitamins and manganese [23] Dose as directed by the manufacturer	To enhance nutritional and antioxidant status; antioxidant supplementation may be beneficial for NIHL [22]; supplementation with B-group vitamins, minerals and antioxidants can be beneficial in tinnitus [23]
Omega-3 fish oil 2 × 1000 mg capsules twice daily [18, 40]	Anti-inflammatory [18, 40, 42]; modulates leukotriene synthesis and inflammatory responses [18, 42]; prostaglandin precursor [42]; suppresses production of pro-inflammatory cytokines [18, 40]; beneficial in the prevention of cardiovascular disease [18, 40]; hypotensive [40]

References

[1] N.J. Talley, S. O'Connor, Pocket clinical examination, third edn, Churchill Livingstone Elsevier, Australia, 2009.

[2] P. Kumar, C. Clark, Clinical Medicine, sixth edn, Elsevier Saunders, London, 2005.

[3] J. Silverman, S. Kurtz, J. Draper, Skills for Communicating with Patients, second edn, Radcliff Publishing, Oxford, 2000.

[4] R. Neighbour, The Inner Consultation; how to develop an effective and intuitive consulting style, Radcliff Publishing, Oxon, 2005.

[5] M. Lloyd, R. Bor, Communication Skills For Medicine, third edn, Churchill Livingstone Elsevier, Edinburgh, 2009.

[6] G. Douglas, F. Nicol, C. Robertson, Macleod's Clinical Examination, twelfth edn, Churchill Livingstone Elsevier, 2009.

[7] J. Jamison, Differential Diagnosis for Primary Care, second edn, Churchill Livingstone Elsevier, London, 2006.

[8] A. Polmear (Ed.), Evidence-Based Diagnosis in Primary Care, Churchill Livingstone Elsevier, Edinburgh, 2008, pp. 274–283.

[9] R.M.D. Berkow, A.J.M.D. Fletcher, M.H.M.D. Beers, The Merck Manual, sixteenth edn, Merck Research Laboratories, Rathway, N.J, 1993 (later edition).

[10] R.H. Seller, Differential Diagnosis of Common Complaints, fifth edn, Saunders Elsevier, Philadelphia, 2007.

[11] R.D. Collins, Differential Diagnosis in Primary Care, fourth edn, Lippincott Williams & Wilkins, Philadelphia, 2008.

[12] K.D. Pagna, T.J. Pagna, Mosby's Diagnostic and Laboratory Test reference, third edn, Mosby, USA, 1997 (later edition).

[13] U. Rosenhall, The influence of ageing on noise-induced hearing loss, Noise Health 5 (2003) 47–53.

[14] M. Knipper, U. Zimmermann, M. Muller, Molecular aspects of tinnitus, Hearing Research, (2009). DOI:10.1016/j.heares.2009.07.013.

[15] R. McEvoy, Allergies and other Environmental Illnesses. A practice handbook for doctors. Mount Lawley, Western Australia: The Environmental Allergy Centre, 1992.

[16] D. Peters, L. Chaitow, G. Harris, S. Morrison, Integrating Complementary Therapies in Primary Care. London: Churchill Livingstone, 2002.

[17] H. Osiecki, The Physicians Handbook of Clinical Nutrition, seventh edn, Eagle Farm: Bioconcepts, 2000.

[18] J. Jamison, Clinical Guide to Nutrition & Dietary Supplements in Disease Management, Churchill Livingstone, Edinburgh, 2003.

[19] M.J. Derebery, Allergic management of Meniere's disease: An outcome study, Otolaryngolic Head and Neck Surgery 122 (2000) 174–182.

[20] D. Parasher, New strategies for prevention and treatment of noise-induced hearing loss, Lancet 352 (1998) 1240–1242.

[21] M.J. Guitton, J. Caston, J. Ruel, R.M. Johnson, R. Pujol, J.L. Puel, Salicylate Induces Tinnitus through activation of Cochlear NMDA Receptors, The Journal of Neuroscience 23 (9) (2003) 3944–3952.

[22] C.G. Le Prell, L.F. Hughes, J.M. Miller, Free radical scavengers, vitamins A, C, and E, plus magnesium reduces noise trauma, Free Radic Biol Med 42 (9) (2007) 1454–1463.

[23] M.D. Seidman, S. Babu, Alternative medications and other treatments for tinnitus: facts from fiction, Otolaryngolic Clinics of North America 36 (2003) 359–381.

[24] C.G. Le Press, D. Yamashita, S. Minami, T. Yamasoba, J.M. Miller, Mechanisms of Noise-Induced Hearing Loss Indicate Multiple Methods of Prevention, Hearing Research 226 (1–2) (2007) 22–43.

[25] B.S. Richmond, Tinnitus: Prevalence, Causes and Treatment Approaches, Geriatric Times 4 (4) 2003. http://www.cmellc.com/geriatrictimes/g030821.html.

[26] P. Nawrot, S. Jordan, J. Eastwood, J. Rotstein, A. Hugenholtz, M. Feeley, Effects of caffeine on human health, Food Additives and Contaminants 20 (1) (2003) 1–30.

[27] A.R. Moller, Pathophysiology of Tinnitus, Otolaryngolic Clinics of North America 36 (2) (2003) 249–266.

[28] R.A. Dobie, A Review of Randomized Clinical Trials in Tinnitus, The Laryngoscope 109 (1999) 1202–1211.

[29] A. Jackson, H. MacPherson, S. Hahn, Acupuncture for tinnitus: A series of six n=1 controlled trials, Complementary Therapies in Medicine 14 (2006) 39–46.

[30] C. Herraiz, A. Toledano, I. Diges, Trans-electrical nerve stimulation (TENS) for somatic tinnitus, Progress in Brain Research 166 (2007) 389–394.

[31] G. Aydemir, M.S. Tezer, P. Borman, H. Bodur, A. Unal, Treatment of tinnitus with transcutaneous electrical nerve stimulation improves patients' quality of life, Journal of Laryngology and Otology 120 (6) (2006) 442–445.

[32] P.E. Newman, Can idiopathic tinnitus be caused by hyperuricemia? Medical Hypotheses 50 (1998) 535–536.

[33] A. Trichopoulou, E. Vasilopoulou, Mediterranean diet and longevity, British Journal of Nutrition 84 (S2) (2000) S205–S209.

[34] A. Stathi, K.R. Fox, J. McKenna, Physical Activity and Dimensions of Subjective Well-Being in Older Adults, Journal of Aging and Physical Activity 10 (2002) 76–92.

[35] W.C. Willett, The Mediterranean diet: science and practice, Public Health Nutrition 9 (1A) (2006) 105–110.

[36] A.H. Taylor, N.T. Cable, G. Faulkner, M. Hillsdon, M. Narici, A.K. Van Der Bij, Physical activity and older adults: a review of health benefits and the effectiveness of interventions, Journal of Sports Sciences 22 (2004) 703–725.

[37] C. Herraiz, F.J. Hernandez, A. Toledano, J.M. Aparicio, Tinnitus retraining therapy: prognosis factors, American Journal of Otolaryngology–Head and Neck Medicine and Surgery 28 (2007) 225–229.

[38] R.I. Lipman, S.P. Lipman, Phase-shift treatment for predominant tone tinnitus, Otolaryngology–Head and Neck Surgery 136 (2007) 763–768.

[39] P.J. Jastreboff, S. Zhou, M.M. Jastreboff, U. Kwapisz, U. Gryczynska, Attenuation of salicylate-induced tinnitus by Ginkgo biloba extract in rats, Audiology and Neuro-otology 2 (4) (1997) 197–212.

[40] L. Braun, M. Cohen, Herbs & Natural Supplements: An evidence based guide, second edn, Elsevier, Sydney, 2007.

[41] S. Mills, K. Bone, Principles & Practice of Phytotherapy: Modern Herbal Medicine. Edinburgh, Churchill Livingstone, London, 2000.

[42] H. Osiecki, The Nutrient Bible, seventh edn, BioConcepts Publishing, Eagle Farm, 2008.

[43] M. Morgan, Clinical Research & Applications of Standardised Ginkgo Extract, A Phytotherapist's Perspective 123 (2009) 1–8.

[44] K. Sato, Pharmacokinetics of coenzyme Q10 in recovery of acute sensorineural hearing loss due to hypoxia, Acta Otolaryngol Supplement 458 (1988) 95–102.

[45] S. Yetiser, F. Tosun, B. Satar, M. Arslanhan, T. Akcam, Y. Ozkaptan, The role of zinc in management of tinnitus. Auris, Nasus, Larynx 29 (2002) 329–333.

[46] J. Higdon, An Evidence Based Approach to Vitamins and Minerals, Thieme, New York, 2003.

[47] S.P. Whelton, A. Chin, X. Xin, J. He, Effect of Aerobic Exercise on Blood Pressure: A Meta-Analysis of Randomized, Controlled Trials, Annals of Internal Medicine 136 (2002) 493–503.

[48] S. El-Hashemy, Naturopathic Standards of Primary Care, CCNM Press Inc, Toronto (2007) 78–86.

[49] S. Mills, K. Bone, The Essential Guide to Herbal Safety, Churchill Livingstone, St Louis, 2005.

[50] W. Boyle, A. Saine, Lectures in Naturopathic Hydrotherapy, Eclectic Medical Publications, Oregon, 1988.

[51] E. Blake, in: L. Chaitow, E. Blake, P. Orrock, M. Wallden, P. Snider, J. Zeff, (Eds.), Naturopathic Physical Medicine Theory and Practice for Manual Therapists and Naturopaths, Churchill Livingstone Elsevier, Philadelhia, 2008.

[52] L.M. Watrous, Constitutional hydrotherapy: from nature cure to advanced naturopathic medicine, Journal of Naturopathic Medicine 7 (2) (1997) 72–79.

[53] L. Chaitow, Hydrotherapy, water therapy for health and beauty, Element, Dorset, 1999.

[54] M. Sinclair, Modern Hydrotherapy for the Massage Therapist, Lippincott Williams & Wilkins, Baltimore, 2008.

[55] N. Shevchuk, Hydrotherapy as a possible neuroleptic and sedative treatment, Medical Hypotheses 70 (2) (2008) 230–238.

[56] G.M. Schleinkofer, Lectures on Hydrotherapy according to S.Kneipp, Sebastian Kneipp School, Bad Worishofen, Germany, July 2008.

[57] R. Newman Turner, Naturopathic Medicine Treating the Whole Person: The principles and practice of Naturopathy, Herts: HeALL, 2000.

[58] MIMS online (2003), Enalapril maleate, Australia Pty Ltd, retrieved 21/11/09 from http://www.mims.com.au.

[59] K. Bone, Clinical Applications of Chinese and Ayurvedic Herbs: Monographs for the Western Herbal Practitioners, Phytotherapy Press, Warwick, 1996.

[60] H. Yu, Y. Kim, S. Jung, et al., Rehmannia glutinosa activates intracellular antioxidant enzyme systems in mouse auditory cells, Am J Chin Med 34 (6) (2006) 1083–1093.

[61] J.H. Macrae, Noise-Induced Hearing Loss and Presbyacusis, International Journal of Audiology 1971, 10, No. 5–6: 323–333 doi:10.3109/00206097109072569.

[62] A.H. Lockwood, Tinnitus, N Engl J Med 347 (2003) 904–910.

[63] D.A. Black, C.M. Fraser, Iron deficiency anaemia and aspirin use in old age, Br J Gen Pract 49 (446) (1999) 729–730.

[64] C. Nicolas-Puel, R.L. Faulconbridge, M. Guitto, et al., Characteristics of tinnitus and etiology of associated hearing loss: a study of 123 patients, Int Tinnitus J 8 (2002) 37–44.

[65] R.E. Gristwood, W.N. Venables, Otosclerosis and chronic tinnitus, Ann Otol Rhinol Laryngol 112 (2003) 398–403.

[66] S. Pirozzo, T. Papinczak, P. Glasziou, Whispered voice test for screening for hearing impairment in adults and children: systematic review, BMJ 327 (2003) 967–970.

[67] S. Kowalksa, W. Sulkowski, Tinnitus in noise-induced hearing impairment, Medycyna Pracy 52 (2001) 305–313.

[68] D.S. Fortune, D.S. Haynes, J.W. Hall 3rd, Tinnitus. Current evaluation and management, Med Clin North Am 83 (1999) 153–162.

[69] H.W. Mahlo, S. Kellermann, Pulsatile tinnitus. Causes, diagnostic procedures, case presentation, Laryngorhinootologie 70 (1991) 675–677.

[70] A. Daneshi, H. Hadizadeh, S. Mahmoudian, et al., Pulsatile tinnitus and carotid artery atherosclerosis, Int Tinnitus J 10 (2004) 161–164.

[71] L.G. Upton, S.J. Wijeyesakere, The incidence of Tinnitus in people with disorders of the temporomandibular joint, Int Tinnitus J 10 (2004) 174–176.

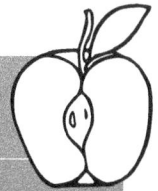

CHAPTER 7

Cardiovascular/ haematological systems

Hypertension

Case history

Tom Sanderson is 55 years old, works full time as an architect for a busy city firm and has come to the clinic for a general check-up. During the course of the consultation he tells you he thinks his health is fine, but he sometimes experiences a dull headache at the base of his head when he wakes up in the morning. Tom thinks this is probably due to his eyesight not being as good as it used to be and that he probably needs to wear glasses when working on detailed architectural plans. He notices the headache usually occurs after he has been working for three or four days in a row.

Tom works long hours, and when he is not working he prefers to be alone rather than socialising with colleagues. At home he enjoys cooking and drinking red or white wine and port in the evenings. Tom will drink a moderate amount of alcohol most nights and has done so for many years. He does not enjoy binge drinking or getting drunk because he likes to remember the experience of enjoying wines he has collected over several decades. When you question Tom about what he considers moderate he says he drinks two to three glasses of wine in the evenings during the week and up to four glasses over lunch or dinner on the weekends. Tom tells you he knows he is overweight and unfit. He recently started to get off his morning train at an earlier stop to walk further to his office in an attempt to get fit. However, he stopped doing that when he noticed his heart rate going quite fast (possibly too fast) when he walks briskly.

When Tom cooks he loves to create rich meals with plenty of dairy foods. Tom prefers savoury foods and likes to add salt. He doesn't eat a lot of red meat because he doesn't particularly like it. Tom admits he drinks at least five cups of coffee daily, at least two from the coffee shop and three from the espresso machine at work, and thinks he needs to drink more water. Tom has never smoked.

Tom's father had two heart attacks shortly after he turned 60, and is now on medication that has stabilised his blood pressure. Tom currently lives alone, has no children and has never been married. It is Tom's father who encouraged him to visit a CAM therapist because he feels his health was improved significantly by changing his lifestyle and diet to help encourage a healthy heart after his own heart attacks. Now that Tom is approaching the age his father was when he developed cardiac symptoms, Tom is keen for guidance about improving his lifestyle to prevent heart disease. Tom doesn't think there isn't anything significantly wrong with his health at the moment, so he didn't feel it was necessary to see a GP for a medical check-up. He feels dietary and lifestyle advice from a CAM practitioner is all that he needs right now.

TABLE 7.1 **COMPLAINT** [1–8, 48, 50, 51]	
Analogy: Skin of the apple	**Complaint:** Define the presenting complaint and symptoms, understand the complaint *Headaches* *Tachycardia*
AREAS OF INVESTIGATION AND EXAMPLE QUESTIONS	**CLIENT RESPONSES**
Onset *When did you first start noticing your headaches?* *When did you notice your heart racing?*	*The last 4 months. The headaches have been coming more often recently.* *When I started trying to get fit again.*
Understanding the cause (client) *What do you think might be causing the headaches?* *What do you think might be causing your heart to race?*	*Probably tension. Maybe I need to get new glasses.* *I'm unfit, I need to get my fitness back.*
Timing *When do you get the headaches?* *When does your heart race?*	*Usually in the morning after I've been working for 3–4 days on detailed plans.* *When I walk fast or try to run. It settles down pretty quickly once I slow down.*
Location *Where do you feel the headache pain?*	Tom points to the occipital region on his head.
Examination and inspection *I can see you are surprised to have a high blood pressure reading. Can I ask you some more questions so we can consider the possibilities?* *Did you feel anxious about having your blood pressure taken today?* *Were you feeling stressed before coming for your consultation today?* *Did you feel cold while I was taking your blood pressure?* *Did you experience physical pain while I was taking your blood pressure?* *Did you drink coffee just before coming in for your consultation today?*	Tom is quite overweight, his face appears red and flushed. Blood pressure is elevated. *OK.* *No, not really.* *I was running late, so I was a bit stressed about that.* *No, this room is warm.* *I am feeling a bit of pain in my neck and head today.* *Yes, about 3 cups this morning.*

TABLE 7.2 **CONTEXT**	
Analogy: Flesh of the apple	**Context:** Put the presenting complaint into context to understand the disease
AREAS OF INVESTIGATION AND EXAMPLE QUESTIONS	**CLIENT RESPONSES**
Family health *Can you tell me about your family health history?*	*My dad has had a couple of heart attacks.*

▶

Cancer and heart disease *Have you experienced swelling in the ankles or fingers?* (difficulties removing any rings on fingers?) *Does coughing and sneezing aggravate the headache?* (vascular origin) *When your heart races, does it feel like your heart misses a beat, jumps or flutters?* (ventricular or atrial extrasystoles) *Does your heart feel like it is jumping about or racing and is associated with breathlessness?* (atrial fibrillation) *Does your heart feel like it is racing or fluttering and is associated with increased urination?* (supraventricular tachycardia) (T1–T5 lesion in spine, drug induced with smoking and alcohol, anxiety induced) *When you feel your heart racing with breathlessness, do you have the feeling of wanting to faint?* (ventricular tachycardia) *Do you feel palpitations after exercise, intense emotion, stress?* (hyperdynamic circulation) *Can you tap out the beat of the palpitations on the desk for me to hear?*	*I have noticed my fingers swell a bit more than have done in the past but nothing too bad.* *Yes, I have noticed if I sneeze in the morning I can feel the dull headache come on.* *I can feel breathless when my heart races, yes.* *No, I haven't noticed this.* *I'm not sure what you mean.* *Sometimes.* *Yes, definitely after exercise.* Tom taps a beat on the desk that sounds like a fast pace flutter rather than missing a beat or jumping.
Recreational drug use *How much alcohol do you drink in a week?* *Do you smoke?* *Do you ever take recreational drugs?*	*Moderately. Two or three a night during the week, maybe four a day on the weekend.* *No, never smoke.* *Not for quite a few years.*
Functional disease *Does your headache come on after exercise, coughing or having sexual intercourse?* (exertional headache) *Is your headache aggravated by bending down?* (frontal sinusitis, temporal arteritis)	*I think there is a connection with exercise.* *Not that I have noticed.*
Infection and inflammation *Do you wake with a dull headache that worsens during the day and lessens towards evening?* (hypertension, tension headache, sinus headaches, intracranial pressure)	*Yes, that is usually the pattern.*
Supplements and side effects of medication *Are you taking any supplements or medications?*	*No.*
Stress and neurological symptoms *Do you experience any prodromal and unusual feelings/symptoms before you feel the headaches?* (epilepsy, brain tumour)	*No, just my heart racing sometimes.*

▶

Eating habits and energy *Tell me about your diet and energy levels.*	Tom tells you he enjoys food and makes an effort to cook something every day. He eats chicken a couple of times a week and has either pasta or fish once a week. He particularly enjoys gourmet cheese and prefers salt and savoury food to sweet food. He often uses cream in sauces.

TABLE 7.3 **CORE**	
Analogy: Core of the apple with the seed of ill health	**Core:** Holistic assessment to understand the client
AREAS OF INVESTIGATION AND EXAMPLE QUESTIONS	**CLIENT RESPONSES**
Emotional health *Do you ever feel sad or depressed?*	*Sometimes, not often.*
Occupation *Do you enjoy your work?* *What do you enjoy most about your work?*	*Yes, I do.* *I like the fast pace and the adrenalin of getting a job done.*
Home life *Who is at home with you?*	*Just me. At the moment I'm by myself.*
Education and learning *How long have you been collecting wines?* *What do you enjoy most about wine collecting?*	*I learned this from my father; it is sort of a family tradition to collect wines.* *I've been interested since I was a boy and it was something nice to share with my dad.*
Action needed to heal *Has anything happened in your past that may influence why you have avoided having medical check-ups?* *How were you hoping I could help you?*	*I just don't like seeing doctors – that's enough to elevate my blood pressure! I think with my dad going through his heart attack, I don't have great memories of that time. Give me some information about changing my diet and how to exercise so I don't get palpitations.*
Long-term goals *Is there anything in your life you would like to change?* *How would you like to see yourself in five years' time?*	*Perhaps it would be nice to meet someone and have some intimacy in my life.* *Feeling more healthy, maybe in a relationship, perhaps doing more travel.*

TABLE 7.4 **TOM'S SIGNS AND SYMPTOMS** [1–5]	
Pulse	100 bpm irregular
Blood pressure	160/100 (moderate hypertension)
Temperature	36.3°C
Respiratory rate	16 resp/min
Body mass index	31
Waist circumference	100.3 cm
Face	Red and flushed appearance
Urinalysis	No glucose or protein; pH normal; no blood or leucocytes detected

Results of medical investigations

No medical investigations have been carried out.

TABLE 7.5 **UNLIKELY DIAGNOSTIC CONSIDERATIONS** [3–5, 9, 12, 47, 55]	
CONDITIONS AND CAUSES	WHY UNLIKELY
CANCER AND HEART DISEASE	
Malignant hypertension: brain lesion/tumour; high blood pressure; intermittent headaches, low temperature, high diastolic reading; headache on waking	Usually symptoms of nausea, severe headache, disturbed speech, vision, unusual sensations, lack of concentration and paralysis; usually slow regular pulse rate; throbbing headache rather than dull
Phaeochromocytoma (tumours of sympathetic nervous system where 90% occur in the adrenal gland) high pulse rate, hypertension	Very rare; no sign of fever; no weight loss or diarrhoea or anxiety reported
TRAUMA AND PRE-EXISTING ILLNESS	
Renal impairment: occurs late in benign and early in malignant hypertension; can cause occipital headache	Urinalysis NAD
Subarachnoid haemorrhage: occipital headache	Usually neck stiffness reported and headache is severe with a sudden-onset, not recurrent; usually low regular pulse rate
OBSTRUCTION AND FOREIGN BODY	
Renal calculi: long-term alcohol and dairy, caffeine consumption, lack of water in diet	No significant acid/alkaline detected in urinalysis; confirm with biochemistry blood test
Vascular complications: aneurysms; high blood pressure	Would present as sudden, extreme and life-threatening; clarify whether blood pressure has suddenly increased or this has been a gradual process; no BP history known in this initial consultation
INFECTION AND INFLAMMATION	
Causal factor: **Acute viral or bacterial illness**	No signs in full blood count of recent fever or infection

▶

▶

Temporal arteritis: cause of headaches for clients over 50 years of age; visual deterioration	Uncommon, more often experienced by elderly women; usually presents as unilateral with low-grade fever; dull ache is not aggravated by bending over
Sinus headache: headache worse on waking in the morning	No upper respiratory symptoms mentioned, no frontal facial pain reported; dull ache is not aggravated by bending over
ENDOCRINE/REPRODUCTIVE	
Diabetes mellitus: overweight and increased alcohol intake are risk factors, headaches can be experienced, high diastolic reading can be associated; palpitations can be common	Urinalysis detected no excess glucose; confirm with fasting blood glucose blood test
Cushing's syndrome: overweight, high blood pressure	No glucose in urine, muscle wasting or weakness reported; typical moon-shaped face not observed
STRESS AND NEUROLOGICAL DISEASE	
Migraine headache: stress can exacerbate	Severe painful headaches; often unilateral and located in the front and temporal regions of the head; headaches not aggravated by sound or light; headaches usually improve upon waking and after sleep; no indication of nausea and vomiting associated with the headache
Cluster headaches: common to begin in males between the ages of 40 and 60; no family history associated with cluster headaches	Extremely severe headaches, stabbing and burning; usually unilateral and pain behind eye radiating to the front of the face

Case analysis

TABLE 7.6 **POSSIBLE DIFFERENTIAL DIAGNOSIS**		
Not ruled out by tests/investigations already done [1, 3–5, 8–10, 12, 46–56]		
CONDITION	**WHY POSSIBLE**	**WHY UNLIKELY**
ALLERGIES AND IRRITANTS		
Causal factor: **Food intolerance amine sensitivity**	Headaches, drinking red wine, dairy, may be delayed sensitivity	Headaches are in the morning on waking rather than after eating particular foods; usually cause migraine headaches
CANCER AND HEART DISEASE		
Congenital cardiac disorder: e.g. coarctation of the aorta	High blood pressure, headaches	No clubbing of finger nails; no nose bleeds reported or cold legs
Hyperaldosteronism: (adrenal tumour) increase sodium in blood increases blood volume	High blood pressure	No reported muscle cramps, weakness, urination at night or increased urination

▶

Causal factor: **Poor left ventricular function** [48, 49]	High blood pressure, heart racing on exertion; systemic hypertension	No breathlessness, or difficulty breathing during sleep reported
Essential systemic hypertension	High alcohol and sodium intake, obesity, stress, high systolic and diastolic reading; sustained fast irregular pulse rate (atrial fibrillation); congenital (Tom's father has a history of heart disease)	It is not common for people with hypertension to experience headaches, however, it may develop for some individuals; unknown BP history
Symptomatic arrhythmia (sustained): abnormal heart beat; ventricular or atrial; palpitations when tachycardia heart rate sustains > 100 beats per minute or bradycardia sustains < 60 beats per minute [48, 49]	Pulse is 100 beats per minute and irregular; can be due to exercise, alcohol, caffeine, anxiety; less tolerance to stimulants with age; the combination of Tom experiencing sustained palpitations with high blood pressure is a more serious indication of heart disease; atrial fibrillation common in hypertension	
TRAUMA AND PRE-EXISTING ILLNESS		
Hypertensive retinopathy	Associated with high blood pressure, eyesight strained	Usually no intermittent headaches
Causal factor: **Liver disease**	High alcohol intake, increased dairy and fatty foods, dull headaches	Usually low pulse regular rate, no jaundice or yellow sclera
OBSTRUCTION AND FOREIGN BODY		
Atherosclerosis	High alcohol intake, hypertension, heart racing on exertion	No chest pain
OCCUPATIONAL TOXINS AND HAZARDS		
Causal factor: **Sick building syndrome**	Headaches worse after working a few days in a row	Tom has not mentioned respiratory complaints or fatigue
FUNCTIONAL DISEASE		
Causal factor: **Obesity**	BMI 31, increased caloric intake with drinking alcohol; lack of exercise; usually general distribution of weight gain; can be associated with high blood pressure	Usually no other health features other than being overweight; need to determine if any familial history of obesity; need to determine if weight gain has been gradual and if oedema is present
Hyperdynamic circulation	Rapid pulse rate after exercise	Check if Tom's symptoms occur after intense emotion, stress; pulse usually rapid and regular

Causal factor: **Sleep apnoea**	High blood pressure, drinking alcohol at night, increased weight	No significant fatigue reported
Causal factor: **TMJ dysfunction**	Headache on waking	Tom did not mention pain in his jaw or ear; check if he grinds his teeth at night
Causal factor: **Postural cause**	Possible postural issues when sleeping	Check what mattress and pillow Tom is using
Causal factor: **Exertional headache**	Headache	Check if the headache also comes on after exercise, cough or sexual intercourse
Causal factor: **Eye strain**	Dull headaches at the base of the head (occiput area) typical of eye strain; Tom's work requires close vision work; headaches will generally occur after working for a few days in a row	
DEGENERATIVE AND DEFICIENCY		
Anaemia	Heart racing on exertion, no red meat in diet; headaches can be a symptom	Unsure if Tom is fatigued
Paget's disease: causes increase cardiac output and often located in the skull (rapid bone remodelling causing calcium excess)	High blood pressure, dull headache, more often seen in those over 40 years of age	Can present with alkaline urine (high pH)
INFECTION AND INFLAMMATION		
Cervical arthritis	Headache at the base of the head/neck area; more likely to develop in this age group	No specific neck pain reported
SUPPLEMENTS AND SIDE EFFECTS OF MEDICATION		
Causal factor: **Drug-induced hypertension:** NSAIDs, steroids, alcohol, thyroid medication, amphetamines, epinephrine, nasal decongestants, caffeine	High blood pressure, fast pulse rate, drinking alcohol and caffeine every day	Check if Tom is taking any stimulant drugs or medications such as amphetamines, cocaine, digitalis glycosides, psychotropic agents, thyroid hormone; check if Tom has ever taken over-the-counter weight-loss products
ENDOCRINE/REPRODUCTIVE		
Hypothyroidism	Obesity, low temperature, can sometimes have high blood pressure	Usually low regular pulse rate
Hyperthyroidism	High blood pressure, increased pulse rate that is irregular and sustained	Usually weight loss, increased heat intolerance, sweating, skin changes

STRESS AND NEUROLOGICAL DISEASE		
Causal factor: **Stress**	High blood pressure, palpitations, busy employment, working full time	
Causal factor: **Anxiety**	Working long hours, palpitations, taking many stimulants, dull headaches, fast pulse	
Causal factor: **Hyperventilation**	Anxiety, palpitations	Tom has not mentioned dizziness or tingling in his hands or feet
Causal factor: **White coat syndrome** [57]	High blood pressure in a clinical setting	Tom has other lifestyle factors that put him in the risk category for hypertension such as alcohol intake, weight gain, lack of exercise, family history of cardiac disease
Causal factor: **Muscle contraction: tension headache**	Dull headaches; usually due to a psychogenic cause influenced by work; can be caused by prolonged mental concentration, family and home issues; often occipital and on waking	Need to ask if the intensity increases during the day and lessens in the evening; more common in females
EATING HABITS AND ENERGY		
Causal factor: **Dehydration**	Lack of water in diet, dull headaches, drinking excess tea and coffee, drinking alcohol	

TABLE 7.7 **DECISION TABLE FOR REFERRAL** [3–6, 8, 9, 11]		
COMPLAINT	**CONTEXT**	**CORE**
Referral for presenting complaint	Referral for all associated physical, dietary and lifestyle concerns	Referral for contributing emotional, mental, spiritual, metaphysical, lifestyle and constitutional factors
REFERRAL FLAGS	**REFERRAL FLAGS**	**REFERRAL FLAGS**
• Recurrent headaches • Tom experiences a headache that is worse on waking and has no neck discomfort • Elevated systolic and diastolic pressure	• Tom has hypertension and visual changes • Tom describes a feeling of the heart fluttering or beating quickly on exertion • Tom is obese • Tom is unfit • Excessive consumption of alcohol, salt and caffeine • Tom's father has had two heart attacks	• Tom is living alone without someone immediately available if symptoms of more serious cardiac conditions occur

ISSUES OF SIGNIFICANCE	ISSUES OF SIGNIFICANCE	ISSUES OF SIGNIFICANCE
Nil	Nil	• Tom is working long hours and is under considerable stress • Tom has a lack of social support • Tom's lifestyle is excessive
REFERRAL DECSION	**REFERRAL DECSION**	**REFERRAL DECSION**
• Immediate referral for medical assessment by a GP to assess Tom's high systolic and diastolic blood pressure reading	• Immediate referral for medical assessment by GP to assess the reasons for the increased pulse rate; eye test	• May be helpful for Tom to see a counsellor to assess mental and emotional stability

TABLE 7.8 **FURTHER INVESTIGATIONS THAT MAY BE NECESSARY** [1–5, 9, 10, 59]	
TEST/INVESTIGATION	**REASON FOR TEST/INVESTIGATION**
FIRST-LINE INVESTIGATIONS:	
Blood pressure testing: multiple times	Definite hypertension; a persistence of hypertensive readings once all variables have been ruled out
Chest examination: auscultation, palpation	Arrhythmia
Urinalysis: multiple times	Blood and protein indicating renal cause for hypertension, diabetes
Electrocardiogram	Sinus rhythm will tell if there is cardiac arrhythmia or organic heart disease
Fasting blood lipid test	When in excess they deposit in fatty tissues and cause a risk of coronary and vascular disease; can rise with alcohol ingestion and fatty foods
Cholesterol blood test	Risk of heart disease
Fasting blood glucose test	More definitive test for risk of diabetes
Eye test	Check if degeneration of sight affecting symptoms
Full blood count	Indicates infection and anaemia; platelet count
ESR	Temporal arteritis
Urea, creatinine and electrolytes (sodium, potassium, chloride, bicarbonate) blood test	Signals muscle breakdown and tissue damage and gives an indicator for renal excretory function as urea and blood creatinine is excreted entirely by the kidneys; this will show in renal abnormalities and diabetes; impaired renal function can cause hypertension; electrolyte values can give an indication of a danger of cardiac arrest and cardiac arrhythmia

▶

Cardiac enzymes: creatine kinase, aspartate transferase, lactic dehydrogenase	Raised in silent myocardial infarction presenting as arrhythmia
Liver function test	High concentrations of biliary enzyme GGT (gamma-glutamyl transpeptidase) are found in liver and heart; can be raised in high alcohol ingestion, even at small intakes
Forced hyperventilation for 3–4 minutes in a paper bag	Check if palpitations occur after hyperventilation
Eye test	May need glasses for reading and working on the computer for long hours
Muscle testing: grade 0–5	Paralysis associated with hypertension
Headache diary	Track the pattern of the headaches more closely
IF NECESSARY:	
Stress echocardiography [59]	Exercise or pharmacologically induced
Chest x-ray	Exclusion or confirmation of organic heart disease
Neurological examination	Tumours affecting nerves and the brain
Serum cortisol blood test	Phaeochromocytoma, aldosteronism (adrenal tumour or hyperplasia)
Glucagon stimulation test	Phaeochromocytoma
Thyroid function test	Thyroid function contributing to weight gain
Radiograph of TMJ	Teeth grinding and muscle contraction in jaw
Radiograph of cervical spine	Cervical arthritis
Brain and cardiac CT scan or MRI	Signs of malignancy or tumour; to confirm or rule out brain tumour/lesion; heart muscle damage

Confirmed diagnosis

TOM AND ESSENTIAL SYSTEMIC HYPERTENSION

Tom is a 55-year-old man who has come to the CAM clinic for a general check-up and guidance to improve his lifestyle and diet to enhance his general health, and cardiac health in particular. Tom's father encouraged him to come to the clinic because he suffered two heart attacks around the age Tom is now and found CAM very helpful to improve his health and wellbeing. Tom has a busy lifestyle and lives alone. He enjoys cooking and drinking wine in the evenings. Tom has been experiencing dull early morning headaches during the working week. He knows he is overweight and unfit, but has not pursued exercise after he experienced exercise-induced palpitations on more than one occasion. Overall Tom is convinced his general health is fine and because of this has not had a medical check-up for some time. During the consultation he is very surprised to learn that his blood pressure is 160/100 and his resting pulse rate is 100 beats per minute. During the consultation it is explained why immediate referral for a medical opinion is necessary in order to rule out definitive primary and secondary causes of high blood pressure before CAM treatment or medicines can be prescribed.

Following medical investigation Tom is given a diagnosis of **essential and systemic hypertension**, which is usually a progressive disease and is significantly associated with more serious cardiovascular events. Systemic hypertension is diagnosed when a diastolic reading is 100 mmHg and/or a systolic reading is 160 mmHg. 160/100 is abnormal and called hypertensive. Additionally, Tom's doctor advised his total cholesterol is bordering on high and his triglycerides are elevated. Blood pressure is determined by the product of cardiac output and the peripheral vascular resistance. In the early stages of hypertension there is usually an increase in cardiac output that causes later changes in vascular resistance. In later stages even if the cardiac output is normal, the changes in vascular resistance causes chronic hypertension.

In hypertension the increased blood pressure does not induce a slower heart rate to compensate as would normally occur.

Causes of essential hypertension include genetics, environmental factors, stress, obesity, alcohol and salt intake. Secondary hypertension is caused by renal and endocrine diseases, congenital cardiovascular diseases, medications, pregnancy and malignancies.

It is extremely important to diagnose the cause of hypertension correctly to avoid unnecessary prescription of medication which eventuates in side effects that are better to avoid [46]. The decision to commence drug therapy may be delayed for up to six months while lifestyle and environmental changes are implemented. Regular monitoring of blood pressure occurs during this time. In other circumstances where the blood pressure is extremely elevated, it may be deemed necessary to commence drug treatment sooner while evaluating possible primary and secondary causes.

General references used in this diagnosis: 3–5, 9, 12, 46, 52–54

PRESCRIBED MEDICATION [46, 58, 60]

- Thiazide diuretic
- Statin drugs will be considered if Tom's cholesterol continues to increase
- Blood pressure monitor to check Tom's blood pressure levels on a daily basis

TABLE 7.9 **DECISION TABLE FOR TREATMENT (ONCE DIAGNOSIS IS CONFIRMED)**		
COMPLAINT	**CONTEXT**	**CORE**
Treatment for the presenting complaint and symptoms	Treatment for all associated symptoms	Treatment for mental, emotional, spiritual, constitutional, lifestyle issues and metaphysical considerations

TREATMENT PRIORITY	TREATMENT PRIORITY	TREATMENT PRIORITY
• The initial focus is to achieve acceptable blood pressure with dietary and lifestyle measures in combination with conventional medical treatment • The longer term aim is to maintain normal blood pressure through diet and lifestyle without the need for antihypertensive medication, herbs or supplements • Herbal tonic or tablets with hypotensive and antiarrhythmic action may be used as adjunctive therapy to dietary and lifestyle changes if necessary • Nutritional supplements with hypotensive action may be used as adjunctive therapy to dietary and lifestyle changes if necessary • Physical therapy suggestions to help reduce blood pressure **NB:** Tom's blood pressure should be reviewed regularly in collaboration with his GP to determine the effectiveness of his treatment program	• Lifestyle and physical therapy recommendations to improve fitness, assist weight loss and improve general health • Dietary recommendations to improve general nutrition and overall health • Dietary recommendations to reduce alcohol and coffee consumption and to replace with herbal tea and water • Dietary recommendations and supplements to normalise triglycerides and cholesterol • Herbal tonic or tablet containing herbs with antioxidant, adaptogenic, cardiotonic and hepatoprotective properties • Nutritional supplements with antioxidant, cardioprotective and cholesterol and triglyceride-lowering action	• Lifestyle and physical therapy suggestions to help reduce stress • Recommendation for Tom to engage in social interactions outside of work • Herbal tonic or tablets containing adaptogenic, anxiolytic and nervine herbs • Herbal tea to replace coffee with anxiolytic herbs to help reduce Tom's stress levels

Treatment aims

- Reduce Tom's blood pressure using DASH (dietary approaches to stop hypertension) [13, 15] and lifestyle changes [13–16].
- Prevent complications of hypertension such as stroke and myocardial infarction [15].
- Weight loss: bring Tom's BMI into normal range [14–16].
- Significantly reduce or avoid alcohol consumption [13–16].
- Reduce coffee consumption [14–16].
- Reduce dietary sodium intake [13–16] and increase dietary potassium intake [13–16].
- Support Tom's liver function (history of excessive alcohol consumption).
- Improve Tom's blood lipid profile.
- Reduce Tom's stress levels [13–16].
- Improve Tom's lifestyle, diet and fitness [13–16].

Lifestyle alterations/considerations

- Encourage Tom to make changes to his lifestyle to reduce stress [14–16] and live a more balanced lifestyle.
- Tom may find stress-reduction techniques, such as meditation, relaxation exercises and yoga, are beneficial [15, 16, 31]. Transcendental meditation has been shown to reduce blood pressure [30].

- Weight loss of 10 per cent is likely to reduce both systolic and diastolic blood pressure [13, 32, 33]; therefore, a weight-loss program aiming to bring Tom back into a normal BMI range would be most beneficial [14–16].
- Ideally Tom should try dietary modification and lifestyle measures to reduce his blood pressure [16]. He may also choose to utilise nutritional supplements and herbal therapy; however, the long-term goal is for diet and lifestyle changes to maintain his blood pressure at normal levels without the need for supplemental nutrients, herbal therapy or drug therapy [13–16].
- Encourage Tom to consider socialising with other people outside of work. He may find attending cooking classes is helpful because he can combine his love of cooking with a social activity.

Dietary suggestions

- Encourage Tom to restrict or eliminate sodium chloride (salt) intake [13–16, 32] and consume less than 2 g sodium (less than 1 tsp salt) from all sources daily [13]. Tom can replace table salt with potassium salt [15].
- Encourage Tom to reduce intake of refined sugar and refined carbohydrates [14].
- Encourage Tom to increase consumption of garlic and onions [14, 15]. Consuming 600–900 mg of fresh garlic (bruised, crushed or chewed) each day can reduce his blood pressure [14, 15, 17].
- Encourage Tom to restrict consumption of saturated fat [15, 16, 41] and avoid *trans* fats [41]. Encourage consumption of foods containing omega-3 fatty acids [15, 41] and oils from nuts, seeds and avocado [14].
- Encourage Tom to reduce consumption of dairy products [15]. If he chooses to consume dairy products, he should have low-fat or fat-free dairy products only [13, 14, 16].
- Encourage Tom to increase consumption of whole, antioxidant-rich foods from a wide range of whole foods, fruit and vegetables [13–16].
- Encourage Tom to follow the DASH recommendations [13, 16]. These include doubling the average daily serving of fruit and vegetables, and reducing consumption of fats and oils by half, red meat by two-thirds and snacks and sweets by three-quarters [13].
- Encourage Tom to include cold-pressed extra virgin olive oil in his diet every day [14, 16].
- Encourage Tom to increase consumption of soluble fibre and legumes [14, 16].
- Encourage Tom to increase consumption of foods high in potassium [13–16] and magnesium [35].
- Encourage Tom to eliminate or significantly reduce coffee consumption [14–16].
- Encourage Tom to eliminate or significantly reduce alcohol consumption [13–16].

Physical treatment suggestions

- Tom may find benefit from acupuncture to reduce both stress [26] and blood pressure [24, 25].
- Massage therapy is likely to reduce Tom's stress [27] and blood pressure [27, 28].
- Aerobic exercise reduces blood pressure [29]. Tom should exercise for 30–40 minutes at 70 per cent of his heart rate maximum (HR_{MAX}) at least three times per week [16]. Tom would be wise to undertake a supervised exercised program to ensure he does not put excessive stress on his cardiovascular system [29].
- Hydrotherapy: alternating arm and foot baths with the hot component no longer than 15 minutes and cold for five minutes – up to three times a day [37]. *Note: ice cold applications can initially increase blood pressure* [37]. Low workload, full-body water exercise [38]. Constitutional hydrotherapy [39, 40]. A hot compress (two minutes) alternating with cold compress (30 seconds) over tired eyes [37].

TABLE 7.10 **HERBAL TEA**		
Alternative to coffee		
HERB	**FORMULA**	**RATIONALE**
Passionflower *Passiflora incarnata*	2 parts	Anxiolytic [17, 23]; sedative [17, 23]; to reduce stress
Peppermint *Mentha × piperita*	1 part	CNS sedative [17, 19]; analgesic [17, 19]; antioxidant [17]; enhances cognitive performance [17]; useful to alleviate headache [17, 19]; pleasant taste helps to improve compliance
Lime flowers *Tilia cordata*	1 part	Mild sedative [20, 23]; peripheral vasodilator [20, 23]; indicated in hypertension [20, 23]
Infusion: 1 tsp per cup – 1 cup 3 times daily		

TABLE 7.11 **HERBAL FORMULA (1:2 LIQUID EXTRACTS)**		
Made with ethanolic extract herbal liquids (alcohol removed)		
HERB	**FORMULA**	**RATIONALE**
Hawthorn leaves *Crataegus* spp	50 mL	Hypotensive [17, 19]; antiarrythmic [17, 19]; cardiotonic [17, 19]; antioxidant [17, 19]; lipid lowering [17, 19]; beneficial effects are expected within 2–6 weeks of continuous use [17]
Motherwort *Leonurus cardiaca*	30 mL	Hypotensive [22]; cardiotonic [22]; antiarrhythmic [20, 22]
St Mary's thistle *Silybum marianum*	50 mL	Hepatoprotective [17, 19]; hepatic trophorestorative [17, 19]; antioxidant [17, 19]; hypolipidaemic [17, 19]; beneficial to protect against alcoholic liver damage [19]
Coleus *Coleus forskohlii*	70 mL	Hypotensive [18]; antiplatelet [18]; cardiotonic [18]
Supply:	200 mL	Dose: 10 mL twice daily

TABLE 7.12		
Tablet alternative to herbal liquid: may improve compliance		
HERB	**DOSE PER TABLET**	**RATIONALE**
Dan shen *Salvia miltiorrhiza*	500 mg	Hypotensive [18]; cardioprotective [18]; hepatoprotective [18]; anticoagulant [18]
Hawthorn *Cratageus spp*	750 mg	See above
Coleus *Coleus forskolii*	700 mg	See above
Valerian *Valeriana officinalis*	450 mg	Anxiolytic [17, 19]; relieves stress [17, 19]
Dose: 2 tablets twice daily		

TABLE 7.13 NUTRITIONAL SUPPLEMENTS	
SUPPLEMENT AND DOSE	**RATIONALE**
Coenzyme Q10 100 mg daily [13, 16, 17]	Antihypertensive [17, 21, 43]; cardioprotective [17]; antioxidant [17, 42]
Magnesium citrate Providing 600 mg elemental magnesium daily in divided doses [16, 17]	Antihypertensive [14, 16, 17]; magnesium acts as a natural calcium channel blocker, reducing vasoconstriction [16]; decreased serum magnesium levels contribute to arterial stiffness in hypertension [34]; magnesium deficiency is implicated in hypertension [35]
High-potency practitioner-quality **multivitamin, mineral and antioxidant supplement** providing therapeutic doses of essential micronutrients and antioxidants along with a daily dose of 100 mg vitamin B6, 250 mcg vitamin B12 and 500 mcg folate [14, 15, 17, 42] Dosage as recommended by manufacturer to achieve the abovementioned daily doses	A broad range of balanced nutrients and antioxidants; supplementation with a broad-spectrum multivitamin and antioxidant supplementation may lower the risk of cardiovascular disease [36]; supplemental vitamin B6, B12 and folate reduce homocysteine levels [13, 17, 21, 42]; elevated homocysteine levels are associated with hypertension and cardiovascular disease [44, 45]
Omega-3 fish oil 7000 mg daily in divided doses [14, 17]	Omega-3 oils are effective in lowering blood pressure [14–17, 22]; omega-3 oils significantly lower triglyceride levels [17, 21, 22]; beneficial for the secondary prevention of coronary heart disease [22]

References

[1] G. Douglas, F. Nicol, C. Robertson, Macleod's Clinical Examination, twelfth edn, Churchill Livingstone Elsevier, 2009.

[2] N.J. Talley, S. O'Connor, Pocket Clinical Examination, third edn, Churchill Livingstone Elsevier, Australia, 2009.

[3] P. Kumar, C. Clark, Clinical Medicine, sixth edn, Elsevier Saunders, London, 2005.

[4] J. Jamison, Differential Diagnosis for Primary Care, second edn, Churchill Livingstone Elsevier, London, 2006.

[5] R.H. Seller, Differential Diagnosis of Common Complaints, fifth edn, Saunders Elsevier, Philadelphia, 2007.

[6] J. Silverman, S. Kurtz, J. Draper, Skills for Communicating with Patients, second edn, Radcliff Publishing, Oxford, 2000.

[7] R. Neighbour, The Inner Consultation; how to develop an effective and intuitive consulting style, Radcliff Publishing, Oxon, 2005.

[8] M. Lloyd, R. Bor, Communication Skills For Medicine, third edn, Churchill Livingstone Elsevier, Edinburgh, 2009.

[9] R.D. Collins, Differential Diagnosis in Primary Care, fourth edn, Lippincott Williams & Wilkins, Philadelphia, 2008.

[10] K.D. Pagna, T.J. Pagna, Mosby's Diagnostic and Laboratory Test reference, third edn, Mosby, USA, 1997 (later edition).

[11] D. Peters, L. Chaitow, G. Harris, S. Morrison, Integrating Complementary Therapies in Primary Care, Churchill Livingstone, London, 2002.

[12] A. Polmear (Ed.), Evidence- Based Diagnosis in Primary Care, Churchill Livingstone Elsevier, 2008, pp. 274–283.

[13] J. Jamison, Clinical Guide to Nutrition & Dietary Supplements in Disease Management, Churchill Livingstone, Edinburgh, 2003.

[14] H. Osiecki, The Physicians Handbook of Clinical Nutrition, seventh edn, Bioconcepts, Eagle Farm, 2000.

[15] J.E. Pizzorno, M.T. Murray, H. Joiner-Bey, The Clinicians Handbook of Natural Medicine, second edn, Churchill Livingstone, St Louis, 2008.

[16] S. El-Hashemy, Naturopathic Standards of Primary Care, CCNM Press Inc, Toronto, 2007.

[17] L. Braun, M. Cohen, Herbs & Natural Supplements: An evidence based guide, second edn, Elsevier, Sydney, 2007.

[18] K. Bone, Clinical Applications of Chinese and Ayurvedic Herbs: Monographs for the Western Herbal Practitioners, Phytotherapy Press, Warwick, 1996.

[19] S. Mills, K. Bone, Principles & Practice of Phytotherapy; Modern Herbal Medicine. Edinburgh, Churchill Livingstone, London, 2000.

[20] British Herbal Medicine Association, British Herbal Pharmacopoeia, BHMAA, 1983.

[21] H. Osiecki, The Nutrient Bible, seventh edn, BioConcepts Publishing, Eagle Farm, 2008.

[22] T.A. Jacobson, Beyond lipids: the role of omega-3 fatty acids from fish oil in the prevention of coronary heart disease, Current Atherosclerosis Reports 9 (2) (2007) 145–153.

[23] S. Mills, K. Bone, The Essential Guide to Herbal Safety, Churchill Livingstone, St Louis, 2005.

[24] C.S. Yin, B.K. Seo, H. Park, M. Cho, W.S. Jung, R. Choue, C.H. Kim, et al., Acupuncture, a promising adjunctive therapy for essential hypertension: a double-blind, randomized, controlled trial, Neurological Research 29 (S1) (2007) 98–103.

[25] E.A. Macklin, P.M. Wayne, L.A. Kalish, P. Valaskatgis, J. Thompson, M. Pian-Smith, Q. Zhang, et al., Stop Hypertension With the Acupuncture Research Program (SHARP): Results of a Randomized, Controlled Clinical Trial, Hypertension 48 (2006) 838–845.

[26] J. Chan, D. Briscomb, E. Waterhouse, A. Cannaby, An uncontrolled pilot study of HT7 for 'stress', Acupuncture in Medicine 20 (2002) 74–77.

[27] T. Field, M. Hernandez-Reif, M. Diego, Cortisol Decreases and Serotonin and Dopamine Increase Following Massage Therapy, International Journal of Neuroscience 115 (2005) 1397–1413.

[28] M. Hernandez-Reif, T. Field, B.A. Krasnegor, Z. Hossain, B.A. Theakston, L.M.T. Burman, High blood pressure and associated symptoms were reduced by massage therapy, Journal of Bodywork and Movement Therapies 4 (1) (2000) 31–38.

[29] S.P. Whelton, A. Chin, X. Xin, J. He, Effect of Aerobic Exercise on Blood Pressure: A Meta-Analysis of Randomized, Controlled Trials, Annals of Internal Medicine 136 (2002) 493–503.

[30] R.H. Schneider, C.N. Alexander, F. Staggers, D.W. Orme-Johnson, M. Rainforth, J.W. Salerno, W. Sheppard, et al., A Randomized Controlled Trial of Stress Reduction in African Americans Treated for Hypertension for Over One Year, American Journal of Hypertension 18 (1) (2005) 88–98.

[31] P. Grossman, L. Niemann, S. Schmidt, H. Walach, Mindfulness-based stress reduction and health benefits A meta-analysis, Journal of Psychomatic Research 57 (2004) 35–43.

[32] P.K. Whelton, L.J. Appel, M.A. Espeland, W.B. Applegate, W.H. Ettinger, J.B. Kostis, S. Kumanyika, et al., Sodium Reduction and Weight Loss in the Treatment of Hypertension in Older Persons: A Randomized Controlled Trial of Nonpharmacologic Interventions in the Elderly, Journal of the American Medical Association 279 (11) (1998) 839–846.

[33] D.J. Goldstein, Beneficial health effects of modest weight loss, International Journal of Obesity Related Metabolic Disorders 16 (6) (1992) 397–415.

[34] L.M. Resnick, D. Militianu, A.J. Cunnings, J.G. Pipe, J.L. Evelhoch, R.L. Soulen, Direct Magnetic Resonance Determination of Aortic Distensibility in Essential Hypertension Relation to Age, Abdominal Visceral Fat, and In Situ Intracellular Free Magnesium, Hypertension 30 (1997) 654–659.

[35] R.M. Toyuz, Role of magnesium in the pathogenesis of hypertension, Molecular Aspects of Medicine 24 (1–3) (2003) 107–136.

[36] C.D. Morris, S. Carson, Routine Vitamin Supplementation To Prevent Cardiovascular Disease: A Summary of the Evidence for the U.S. Preventive Services Task Force, Annals of Internal Medicine 139 (2003) 56–70.

[37] M. Sinclair, Modern Hydrotherapy for the Massage Therapist, Lippincott Williams & Wilkins, Baltimore, 2008.

[38] E. Blake, in: L. Chaitow, E. Blake, P. Orrock, M. Wallden, P. Snider, J. Zeff (Eds.), Naturopathic Physical Medicine: Theory and Practice for Manual Therapists and Naturopaths, Churchill Livingstone Elsevier, Philadelphia, 2008.

[39] W. Boyle, A. Saine, Lectures in Naturopathic Hydrotherapy, Eclectic Medical Publications, Oregon, 1988.

[40] L.M. Watrous, Constitutional hydrotherapy: from nature cure to advanced naturopathic medicine, Journal of Naturopathic Medicine 7 (2) (1997) 72–79.

[41] L. Mosca, C.L. Banka, E.J. Benjamin, K. Berra, C. Bushnell, R.J. Dolor, T.G. Ganiats, et al., Evidence-Based Guidelines for Cardiovascular Disease Prevention in Women: 2007 Update, Circulation 115 (2007) 1481–1501.

[42] J. Jamison, Clinical Guide to Nutrition & Dietary Supplements in Disease Management, Churchill Livingstone, Edinburgh, 2003.

[43] F.L. Rosenfeldt, S.J. Haas, H. Krum, A. Hadj, K. Ng, J. Leong, et al., Coenzyme Q10 in the treatment of hypertension: A meta-analysis of the clinical trials, Journal of Molecular and Cellular Cardiology 42 (2007) S125–S128.

[44] K. Sutton-Tyrrell, A. Bostom, J. Selhub, C. Zeigler-Johnson, High homocysteine levels are independently related to isolated systolic hypertension in older adults, Circulation 96 (6) (1997) 1745–1749.

[45] J. Sundström, L. Sullivan, R.B. D'Agostino, P.F. Jacques, J. Selhub, I.H. Rosenberg, et al., Plasma Homocysteine, Hypertension Incidence, and Blood Pressure Tracking: The Framingham Heart Study, Hypertension 42 (2003) 1100–1105.

[46] H.-C. Diener, V. Limmroth, Medication-overuse headache: a worldwide problem, Lancet Neurol 3 (2004) 475–483.

[47] M. Maizels, The patient with daily headaches, Am Fam Physician 70 (2004) 2299–2306, 2313–2314.

[48] A.V. Abbot, Diagnostic approach to palpitations, Am Fam Physican 71 (2005) 743–750, 755–756.

[49] P. Zimetbaum, M.E. Josephson, Evaluation of patients with palpitations, N Engl J Med 338 (1998) 1369–1373.

[50] T.T. Beery, The genetics of cardiac arrhythmias, Biol Res Nurs 6 (4) (2005) 249–261.

[51] G.W. Ressel, AAFP and ACP release practice guideline on management of newly detected atrial fibrillation, Am Fam Physician 69 (10) (2004) 2474–2475.

[52] R.S. Vasan, et al., Impact of high-normal blood pressure on the risk of cardiovascular disease, N Engl J Med 345 (2001) 1291–1297.

[53] M. Jessup, S. Brozena, Heart Failure, N Engl J Med 348 (2003) 2007–2018.

[54] J.J.V. McMurray, M.A. Pfeffer, Heart Failure, Lancet 365 (2005) 1877–1889.

[55] W. Young, Minireview: primary aldosteronism-changing concepts in diagnosis and treatment, Endrocrinology 144 (2003) 2208–2213.

[56] J. Therrien, G. Webb, Clinical update on adults with congenital heart disease, Lancet 362 (2003) 1305–1313.

[57] F. Angeli, P. Verdecchia, R. Gattobigio, M. Sardone, G. Reboldi, White-coat hypertension in adults, Blood Pressure Monitoring 10 (6) (2005) 301–305.

[58] M.J. Brown, et al., Better blood pressure control: how to combine drugs. Review, Journal of Human Hypertension 17 (2) (2003) 81–86.

[59] E.A. Ashly, J. Myers, U. Froelicher, Exercise testing in clinical medicine, Lancet 356 (2000) 1592–1597.

[60] J. Staessen, E. Den Hond, H. Celis, et al., Antihypertensive treatment based on blood pressure measurement at home or in the physician's office: a randomized controlled trial, JAMA 291 (2004) 955–964.

Hypercholesterolaemia

Case history

Helene Oldham is 58 years old. She has come to the clinic after being referred by her GP to find out whether natural therapies can help her. Helene is about to retire from her job as a public servant and start a new life with her husband, Jack. They married four years ago and have been planning their retirement together ever since. Helene and Jack have purchased a semi-rural block and are preparing to move into their new house in the next couple of weeks. Helene was single for 10 years before she met Jack. She has two adult children and is expecting the arrival of her first grandchild in three months. She tells you she is looking forward to having the grandchildren over to stay, raising chickens, growing organic vegetables and travelling with Jack.

Recently Helene has been experiencing fatigue and a feeling of weakness, particularly in her legs. She went to her doctor who ran a series of blood tests. She was told that everything was fine, although her cholesterol levels were raised. This did not surprise her as her father died of a heart attack and her mother had diabetes, which later caused cardiovascular disorders.

Helene went through menopause three years ago and experienced only minor problems with hot flushes. Since then she has felt very well, until the past couple of months.

Helene has a good appetite and enjoys eating a wide range of foods. She enjoys cooking and drinks socially on the weekends but not usually during the week. Helene eats red meat three or four times per week and chicken two or three times; she rarely eats fish. Jack is a 'meat and three veg' man, so Helene's diet has changed since they married to accommodate Jack's food preferences. She eats more red meat, cheese and bread than she used to and wonders whether this may be part of the reason she has not been feeling well. She has never smoked, although her first husband was a heavy smoker.

Helene also tells you that she has been under a fair bit of stress in the past four months due to the new house being built, the forthcoming move and preparing for retirement. She feels she has probably taken less care with her diet and exercise because of this and is looking forward to being able to relax and take things more slowly once they move into the new house and she retires. She confesses she is concerned that if her symptoms of fatigue do not improve she may not be able to enjoy her new life. Helene confides to you that she did not tell her doctor she is constantly worrying about this and has had problems falling asleep at night because she is thinking so much about everything. Helene usually sleeps very well and hopes you can suggest a natural remedy to help with this.

Helene's doctor suggested she consult with a CAM therapist to see whether dietary and lifestyle changes could lower her cholesterol. He wants her to come back in three months, at which time he may have to prescribe cholesterol-lowering medication if her levels are still too high. Helene does not want to have to take medication and would like to learn how to manage her cholesterol with diet and lifestyle. Helene also wants help with her stress.

TABLE 7.14 COMPLAINT [1–5, 69]

Analogy: Skin of the apple	**Complaint:** Define the presenting complaint and symptoms; understand the complaint *Elevated cholesterol*
AREAS OF INVESTIGATION AND EXAMPLE QUESTIONS	**CLIENT RESPONSES**
Onset *When did you start to feel something was not right with you?*	*Probably about 4 or 5 months ago. I realised I was not improving so I went to the doctor who told me my cholesterol was up.*
Understanding the cause (client) *Do you understand what elevated cholesterol means and how it can occur?*	*I think so. The doctor told me it can be due to diet or family history. I need to get it down so I don't end up with heart disease.*
Exacerbating factors *Is there anything that makes your fatigue worse?*	*When I'm very busy or stressed.*
Relieving factors *Is there anything that makes your fatigue better?*	*Rest and on the weekends when I'm not quite so busy.*

TABLE 7.15 CONTEXT

Analogy: Flesh of the apple	**Context:** Put the presenting complaint into context to understand the disease
AREAS OF INVESTIGATION AND EXAMPLE QUESTIONS	**CLIENT RESPONSES**
Family health *Is there a family history of heart disease or elevated cholesterol?*	*Yes, my father died of a heart attack and my mother has diabetes and heart disease.*

▶

▶

Obstruction and foreign body *Do you experience day time sleepiness, decreased alertness and feel a desire to sleep?* (drowsiness, sleep apnoea)	No, I just feel tired during the day.
Recreational drug use *How much alcohol would you drink during the week?* *Do you smoke?*	I don't drink during the week, and maybe have 2 or 3 drinks on the weekend. I've never smoked, although my first husband was a heavy smoker.
Functional disease *Is the fatigue often present and worse in the morning?* (functional origin) *Has the fatigue been of long duration?* (functional origin, depression) *Did the fatigue begin at a time of emotional trauma or major life change?* (functional origin) *Is the fatigue always associated with periods of prolonged physical or mental activity, inadequate rest, poor sleep, dieting, sedentary lifestyle or mental stress?* (physiologic fatigue)	Only when I have not slept very well during the night. I think it has developed during the past few months really. I think the house business really brought it all on. Yes, absolutely.
Infection or inflammation *Is the fatigue improved by rest and worsen as the day progresses?* (organic origin) *Has the fatigue been gradually progressing rather than fluctuating?* (organic origin) *Is your fatigue aggravated by effort?* (organic fatigue)	Rest definitely helps, but it does not necessarily get better during the day. It tends to fluctuate depending on how full on my life is getting – but lately it has been all of the time – so it is getting worse. Yes, it does get worse with effort, but I feel like my whole health is suffering at the moment so I do not bounce back as well as I used to.
Supplements and side effects of medication *Are you taking any supplements or medicines?*	Not at the moment. I was hoping you could give me guidance as to what to take.
Stress and neurological disease *Is the fatigue associated with restlessness, irritability, increased sweating or heart palpitations?* (chronic anxiety)	I can feel irritable sometimes when I'm tired but haven't noticed sweating or palpitations.
Eating habits and energy *Tell me about your diet.*	Helene tells you she eats red meat 3–4 times a week and chicken usually 2–3 times. She has 3–4 different vegetables with her meals. Breakfast is usually porridge or wholegrain toast and honey. Lunch is usually a meat and salad sandwich.

TABLE 7.16 **CORE**	
Analogy: Core of the apple with the seed of ill health	**Core:** Holistic assessment to understand the client
AREAS OF INVESTIGATION AND EXAMPLE QUESTIONS	**CLIENT RESPONSES**
Stress release *Do you feel stressed at the moment?* *How do you manage your stress?*	*I'm very stressed. I can't wait to move into our new house and retire so I can take time out to relax.* *Not very well at the moment. I try to walk as often as I can, but haven't had the time to exercise as much as I would like. I try and take some time out every day to read a book or listen to some soothing music.*
Family and friends *Tell me about your family and friends.*	*My daughter is just about to have her first baby and we are all really looking forward to that. I can't wait to be a grandma! My son lives overseas at the moment but is talking about coming back home in the next couple of years. Jack and I have some very good friends and I'm hoping to spend more time with them soon.*
Action needed to heal *How do you hope I can help you?*	*Dietary and lifestyle advice. Maybe some natural remedies that will help my sleep and stress as well as reducing my cholesterol.*
Long-term goals *What do you hope to be doing in five years?*	*Spending time with my grandchildren, travelling with Jack, growing organic vegetables and enjoying my life.*

TABLE 7.17 **HELENE'S SIGNS AND SYMPTOMS** [1, 2, 6]	
Pulse	82 bpm (regular)
Blood pressure	125/80
Temperature	36.9°C
Respiratory rate	18 resp/min
Body mass index	27
Waist circumference	86 cm
Face	Normal appearance, good colour
Eyes	Corneal arcus around the boundary of the iris caused by cholesterol crystals; yellow cholesterol plaques around the eyelids
Urinalysis	No abnormality detected (NAD)

TABLE 7.18 **RESULTS OF MEDICAL INVESTIGATIONS** [1, 2, 6–8]	
TEST	**RESULTS**
Full blood count	NAD
ESR (erythrocyte sedimentation rate indicates inflammation in general)	NAD
CRP	NAD
Fasting blood lipid test (chylomicrons are primarily trigylcerides, LDLs are primarily cholesterol, VLDLs primarily triglycerides, HDLs are predominantly proteins)	Total cholesterol elevated; LDL high, HDL low; triglycerides slightly elevated
Cholesterol blood test (usually includes VLDL value)	Moderately raised
Homocysteine blood test	Slightly raised
Electrolyte blood test	NAD
Fasting blood glucose test	NAD
Liver function test	NAD
Thyroid function test	NAD

TABLE 7.19 **UNLIKELY DIAGNOSTIC CONSIDERATIONS** [2, 7–9, 65]	
CONDITIONS AND CAUSES	**WHY UNLIKELY**
FAMILY HEALTH	
Heterozygous familial hypercholesterolaemia: usually not many physical signs; family history of heart disease	Usually high LDL cholesterol reading (alone); can be unresponsive to dietary treatment and often associated with family history of cardiovascular disease; two clinical findings include thickening, yellow nodules (xanthomata) of Achilles tendons and extensor tendons of fingers due to deposits of lipids
Homozygous familial hypercholesterolaemia	High LDL cholesterol (alone); very rare where there are no LDL receptors in the liver; usually death in late childhood or adolescence from ischaemic heart disease
CANCER AND HEART DISEASE	
Atherosclerosis risk	No hypertension and CRP not raised
Low-density lipoprotein disorders: alone	High LDL cholesterol reading (alone)
Very low density lipoprotein disorders and chylomicrons: alone (hypertriglyceridaemia)	Excess VLDLs (alone) circulating; hypertriglyceridaemia; often family history of pancreatitis, retinal vein thrombosis and familial hypertriglyceridaemia

▶

▶

HDL disorders: normal total cholesterol and triglycerides (Tangier disease)	Low HDL (alone) concentration; total cholesterol is not usually raised; secondary complications such as cardiovascular disease, corneal opacities and polyneuropathy can occur
Combined hyperlipidaemia remnant hyperlipidaemia – raised cholesterol and triglycerides; family history	Rare disorder; diagnostic features include thickened skin (xanthoma) over palmar creases and knees, elbows
TRAUMA AND PRE-EXISTING ILLNESS	
Mutations in the apoprotein B-100 gene	High LDL cholesterol – alone; common single gene disorder
Polygenic hypercholesterolaemia	High LDL serum cholesterol (alone) without any monogenic disorders
Renal disease (nephrotic syndrome): high cholesterol	Urinalysis and electrolyte blood test NAD
Liver disease (biliary cirrhosis, hepatoma, glycogen storage disease and obstructive jaundice): high cholesterol	Liver function test NAD, no yellow sclera or signs of jaundice
SUPPLEMENTS AND SIDE EFFECTS OF MEDICATION	
Drug-induced hypercholesterol	Helene not taking exogenous oestrogen, corticosteroids, thiazides, β-adrenergic blocking agents
ENDOCRINE/REPRODUCTIVE	
Diabetes mellitus: high cholesterol common	Urinalysis and fasting blood glucose test NAD
Hypothyroid: high cholesterol, fatigue, weight gain and sore legs common	Thyroid function test NAD

TABLE 7.20 **CONFIRMED DIAGNOSIS**	
CONDITION	**RATIONALE**
Combined hyperlipidaemia: most common client group	High LDL and low HDL concentration
Familial combined hyperlipidaemia	Very common; raised cholesterol and triglycerides; family history of heart disease; no typical physical signs present

Case analysis

TABLE 7.21 **POSSIBLE FURTHER DIFFERENTIAL DIAGNOSIS**		
Not ruled out by tests/investigations already done [2, 7, 9–11, 64–68, 70–72]		
CONDITIONS AND CAUSES	**WHY POSSIBLE**	**WHY UNLIKELY**
ALLERGIES AND IRRITANTS		
Causal factor: **Food intolerance**	Fatigue, recent dietary change since feeling low; may be eating more of certain foods than she did before her marriage; taken over comfortable threshold	Need to gain more insight into Helene's previous and current diet and associated symptoms
OBSTRUCTION AND FOREIGN BODY		
Causal factor: **Sleep apnoea**	Doesn't usually complain of 'sleepiness' but rather fatigue generally	Need to determine if she wakes feeling unrefreshed and if she snores during the night
RECREATIONAL DRUG USE		
Causal factor: **Passive smoking**	Increase homocysteine levels	
FUNCTIONAL DISEASE		
Fibromyalgia	Tiredness, weakness in the legs; more common in women	No multiple sites of muscle pain reported
Causal factor: **Physiologic fatigue**	Can be caused by depression, sleep changes, intense emotions; diagnostic studies to date are mostly within normal limits	Symptoms present for less than 14 days and not usually associated with changes in self-esteem, social difficulties or overall mood
DEGENERATIVE AND DEFICIENCY		
Osteoporosis	Menopausal, weakness in legs; commonly develops in this age group	
Causal factor: **Nutritional deficiencies** (low B vitamins)	Slightly raised homocysteine levels, increase in stress and worry, history of exposure to cigarette smoke	
Causal factor: **Organic fatigue**	Tired, sleep disturbances, no major physical abnormalities	Shorter duration than functional fatigue; need to determine if Helene's fatigue worsens during the day
ENDOCRINE/REPRODUCTIVE		
Causal factor: **Passed menopause**	Increase homocysteine levels, risk of osteoporosis	

▶

STRESS AND NEUROLOGICAL DISEASE		
Depression	Tiredness that has lasted several months, began after building new house; preparing to retire	Has many aspects of her life that give her joy
Causal factor: **Hyperventilation syndrome – functional breathing concern** (causes increased CO_2, fatigue, muscle pain, digestive complaints)	Breathing quickly, fatigue; muscle weakness felt in the legs; hyperventilation syndrome can be a consequence of chronic anxiety, irritability; habitual patterns of breathing are developed to keep CO_2 levels low that leads to anxiety-provoking consequences	No significant shortness of breath reported
Causal factor: **Emotional stress**	Tired, concerns about health affecting her retirement plans, retiring soon from long-term employment and job security; longer duration than acute organic origin of tiredness; can increase cholesterol levels	No irritability or shortness of breath reported
Causal factor: **Extreme worrier**	Restlessness, difficulty sleeping; symptoms presented as significantly intense although her GP has said everything is OK	Need to determine if Helene has experienced loss of appetite
Causal factor: **Functional fatigue (depression)**	Tiredness that has lasted several months	Need to define if Helene's fatigue improves during the day
EATING HABITS AND ENERGY		
Causal factor: **Increase of saturated fatty acids and carbohydrates in diet**	Eats more red meat, cheese and bread than she used to; increased cholesterol	
Causal factor: **Lack of activity**	Increased stress, weight gain, elevated homocysteine levels; decreased fitness, disturbed sleep, increased risk of heart disease	

Working diagnosis

HELENE AND HYPERCHOLESTEROL

Helene is a 58-year-old woman who has been referred by her GP to your clinic for assistance with dietary and lifestyle strategies to reduce cholesterol levels. If Helene's cholesterol levels have not reduced sufficiently after three months of dietary and lifestyle changes, her GP will prescribe a cholesterol-lowering medication. Helene is currently in a period of major life change, as she is approaching retirement and finally fulfilling her dream of moving into a newly built home with her husband Jack. Helene originally saw her GP to discuss the increased fatigue and weakness in the legs she has been experiencing. Several investigations were performed, which revealed she has **combined hyperlipidaemia** with raised **total cholesterol**, decreased **high-density lipoproteins** (HDLs) and raised **low-density lipoproteins** (LDLs).

Cholesterol is important for the production of steroids, bile acids and cellular membranes in the body. When in excess it is also the main cause of arteriosclerosis and heart disease. The main source of cholesterol comes from foods of animal origin such as red meat and dairy products. LDLs are rich in cholesterol, which is carried by LDLs to peripheral tissues and, when in excess, cause risk of atherosclerotic heart disease.

Triglycerides are a form of fat in the blood stream that is carried by **very low density lipoproteins** (VLDLs) and **low-density lipoproteins** (LDLs). Triglycerides are produced in the liver and are important for storage of energy. When in excess they can deposit in the bloodstream as fatty tissue increasing risk of heart disease. HDLs are predominantly protein and are carriers of cholesterol. They have an important purpose of removing excess cholesterol from the peripheral tissues and transporting it to the liver for excretion.

High levels of LDLs in the bloodstream create an increased risk of heart disease. Risk factors for high cholesterol include dietary sources, genetic propensity for heart disease and hyperlipidaemia, stress and lack of exercise. Secondary causes of hyperlipidaemia/high cholesterol include conditions such as hypothyroidism, diabetes mellitus, obesity, renal impairment, liver dysfunction and from ingesting certain medications. Combined hyperlipidaemia (hypercholesterolaemia and elevated triglycerides) is a common disorder influenced greatly by lifestyle and, although it does not usually present with many physical findings, there is often a strong family history of heart disease.

General references used in this diagnosis: 2, 8, 64, 65

FURTHER INVESTIGATIONS FOR CONSIDERATION

During the course of the consultation Helene shared more detailed information about her current levels of stress and increased worry about her recently diagnosed condition and forthcoming major life change. After discussing this with her, it became apparent it was also important to support Helene with continuing collaborative referral while CAM treatment progressed.

TABLE 7.22 **DECISION TABLE FOR TREATMENT PRIOR TO REFERRAL**		
COMPLAINT	**CONTEXT**	**CORE**
Treatment for the presenting complaint and symptoms	Treatment for all associated symptoms	Treatment for mental, emotional, spiritual, constitutional, lifestyle issues and metaphysical considerations

TREATMENT PRIORITY	TREATMENT PRIORITY	TREATMENT PRIORITY
• Lifestyle and dietary recommendations to reduce LDL and total cholesterol and increase HDL • Herbal tea, tonic and tablets with hypolipidaemic action • Supplemental nutrients with hypolipidaemic action	• Dietary and supplement suggestions to increase antioxidant status and prevent or reduce oxidation of LDL and progression to atherosclerosis • Herbal tea, tonic and tablets with anti-inflammatory, antioxidant, antiplatelet and cardioprotective action • Supplemental nutrients with anti-inflammatory, antioxidant and cardioprotective action • Lifestyle and physical therapy suggestions to improve Helene's sleep • Herbal sleep tea or tablets to improve sleep and reduce anxiety • Referral to GP for mental health assessment and integrative management of Helene's anxiety and sleep problems	• Lifestyle and physical therapy suggestions to reduce anxiety • Herbal tea or tablet formula to reduce anxiety • Educating Helene about how the dietary and lifestyle changes can improve her health and reduce cardiovascular risk will help reduce her anxiety levels

TABLE 7.23 DECISION TABLE FOR REFERRAL [1, 2, 6, 7, 9, 12]

COMPLAINT	CONTEXT	CORE
Referral for presenting complaint	Referral for all associated physical, dietary and lifestyle concerns	Referral for contributing emotional, mental, spiritual, metaphysical, lifestyle and constitutional factors
REFERRAL FLAGS	**REFERRAL FLAGS**	**REFERRAL FLAGS**
• Stress levels becoming overwhelming for Helene and interrupting daily activities	• Weakness in legs	• Fatigue is continuing and may be linked to worry regarding impending retirement, indicating possible functional/depression causes for fatigue
ISSUES OF SIGNIFICANCE	**ISSUES OF SIGNIFICANCE**	**ISSUES OF SIGNIFICANCE**
Nil	• History of exposure to second-hand smoke in her first marriage • Worrying thoughts disturbing sleep • Fatigue linked to increased stress, lack of sleep and high cholesterol reading indicating possible organic and physiologic reasons for lack of energy • Lack of physical activity • Increase of high fat and carbohydrate diet	• Impending retirement • Building a new home

REFERRAL DECISION	REFERRAL DECISION	REFERRAL DECISION
• Refer back to GP for a mental health assessment	• Physical treatment for stress reduction and muscle release • Musculoskeletal assessment on the weakness in the legs	• Counselling to assist with major life changes

TABLE 7.24 FURTHER INVESTIGATIONS THAT MAY BE NECESSARY [2, 7, 8, 11]	
TEST/INVESTIGATION	REASON FOR TEST/INVESTIGATION
FIRST-LINE INVESTIGATIONS:	
Musculoskeletal assessment	Fibromyalgia, osteoporosis, neuromuscular disease
Nijmegen questionnaire	Hyperventilation
Food diary	Diet aggravating high cholesterol, food intolerances
Mental health assessment	Depression, anxiety
Vitamin D test	Vitamin D deficiency, risk of osteoporosis
Vitamin B levels	Increased anxiety and increased homocysteine levels
IF NECESSARY:	
Bone density	Check risk of osteoporosis
Ultracentrifugation of plasma	Remnant hyperlipidaemia
Capnometer/pulmonary gas exchange during orthostatic tests	Hyperventilation
Sleep clinic observation	Sleep apnoea
Epstein-Barr/Ross River virus blood test	Check for postviral infection, fatigue

Confirmed diagnosis

Hypercholesterol with associated organic fatigue/emotional stress

PRESCRIBED MEDICATION

• Statin medication will be prescribed if dietary and lifestyle measures do not bring Helene's cholesterol levels within acceptable limits

TABLE 7.25 DECISION TABLE FOR TREATMENT (ONCE DIAGNOSIS IS CONFIRMED)		
COMPLAINT	CONTEXT	CORE
Treatment for the presenting complaint and symptoms	Treatment for all associated symptoms	Treatment for mental, emotional, spiritual, constitutional, lifestyle issues and metaphysical considerations

TREATMENT PRIORITY	TREATMENT PRIORITY	TREATMENT PRIORITY
• Continue with lifestyle and dietary recommendations to reduce LDL and total cholesterol and increase HDL • Continue with herbal tea, tonic and tablets to help reduce cholesterol **NB:** Herbal tea, tonic and tablets and nutritional supplements to be reviewed in 3 months when Helene's cholesterol levels are retested • Continue with supplemental nutrients to help reduce cholesterol **NB:** Supplemental nutrients to be reviewed in 3 months when Helene's cholesterol levels are retested	• Continue with dietary and supplement suggestions to increase antioxidant status and prevent or reduce oxidation of LDL and progression to atherosclerosis • Continue with herbal tea, tonic and tablets with anti-inflammatory, antioxidant, antiplatelet and cardioprotective action • Continue with supplemental nutrients with anti-inflammatory, antioxidant, antihomocysteine and cardioprotective action • Dietary and lifestyle recommendations for weight loss • Continue with lifestyle and physical therapy suggestions to improve Helene's sleep • Continue with herbal sleep tea or tablets to improve sleep and reduce anxiety **NB:** Herbal sleep tea or tablets to be reviewed once Helene has transititioned into her new life	• Continue with lifestyle and physical therapy suggestions to reduce stress and anxiety • Continue with supplemental nutrients to support stress response

Treatment aims

- Modulate cholesterol metabolism [14, 15] and bring Helene's cholesterol levels into normal range, increasing HDL and lowering LDL and triglycerides [13–16].
- Reduce homocysteine levels [13–16].
- Improve Helene's diet and lifestyle [13–16].
- Dietary modification to reduce consumption of saturated fat and increase consumption of healthy fats and soluble fibre [13–16].
- Reduce inflammation within the vascular system to prevent or reduce the risk of atherosclerotic lesions developing [13–16].
- Reduce or prevent excessive platelet aggregation [13, 15].
- Stop or reverse the progression of any lesions already present [35].
- Reduce the risk of cardiovascular disease, stroke and other complications of atherosclerosis [13–16].
- Increase Helene's antioxidant status to help prevent oxidation of cholesterol [13–15].
- Bring Helene's weight into normal BMI range [27, 44].
- Support Helene's stress response during the next few weeks and months until she has adjusted to her new lifestyle.
- Improve Helene's sleep.

Lifestyle alterations/considerations

- Encourage Helene to increase physical activity and exercise. There is a positive correlation between increased levels of physical activity and increased HDL [24]. Without exercise, dietary interventions are less successful at lowering LDL [25]. Exercise may reduce inflammation, which is involved in the development of atherosclerotic lesions and cardiovascular disease [26, 27]. Habitual physical activity prevents development of coronary artery disease (CAD) and reduces symptoms in clients with established CAD [27].
- Increasing physical activity will assist Helene with weight loss [27, 44], reducing stress and anxiety [49, 50] and may improve her sleep patterns [53, 54].
- Reducing her stress levels will benefit Helene and reduce her risk of developing CAD [28]. Stress-management activities, such as breathing exercises, meditation and relaxation exercises, can lower CAD risk [29].
- Providing Helene with information and literature about health and lifestyle, specifically relating to elevated cholesterol and cardiovascular disease risk is important. By understanding how the recommended dietary and lifestyle changes will help her health and reduce cardiovascular risk, her anxiety levels are likely to reduce.

Dietary suggestions

- Encourage Helene to significantly reduce consumption of saturated fat [15, 16, 44].
- Encourage Helene to avoid consuming margarine, *trans*-fatty acids and partially hydrogenated oils [15, 16, 44]. She should also minimise consumption of polyunsaturated fatty acids from corn oil, safflower and cottonseed oil [16].
- Encourage Helene to increase dietary intake of omega-3 fatty acids [15, 16, 23, 44] and monounsaturated fatty acids [16]. She should consume 35 g or more of cold-water fish [13] such as sardines in olive oil.
- Encourage Helene to consume nuts and seeds [13, 15], particularly almonds and walnuts [14, 31]. Nuts are a rich source of arginine, which is beneficial in the prevention and treatment of atherosclerosis [13, 21].
- Helene would benefit from following a Mediterranean diet [16], which consists of high consumption of legumes, fruits, vegetables and whole grains, moderate consumption of alcohol and low to moderate consumption of meat and dairy products [33].
- Cold-pressed olive oil is Helene's best choice for low-temperature cooking [32] and in salad dressings [17]. Monounsaturated fats such as olive oil as part of a Mediterranean diet reduces the risk of cardiovascular disease [17, 33].
- Encourage Helene to increase consumption of whole foods that are rich in antioxidant and plant sterols [55, 56] from a wide range of whole grains, fruit and vegetables [13–16].
- Helene's weight-loss program should incorporate higher protein and lower carbohydrate intake and include adequate levels of essential fatty acids [45, 46] that comprise low GI/GL foods [47].
- Encourage Helene to minimise consumption of high GI foods [13, 14].
- Encourage Helene to consume 2–5 g of fresh garlic (bruised, crushed or chewed) [17] in her diet each day [14–16]. Garlic has a modest effect on reducing serum cholesterol levels [17, 18, 37], and has anti-inflammatory [17] and antiatherosclerotic activity [17, 37]. If Helene does not want to eat fresh garlic, she could take it in tablet form.
- Encourage Helene to increase consumption of dietary fibre, particularly soluble fibre [14, 16, 44]. Soluble fibre has a cholesterol-lowering effect [39, 40]. Whole oats are particularly beneficial due to their beta-glucan content [52].

- Encourage Helene to include ginger in her diet [14, 16]. It has hypolipidaemic [17], antiplatelet [17, 18], antioxidant [17] and anti-inflammatory [17, 18] actions.
- Helene will benefit from including 1–3 tsp of lecithin granules in her diet each day [14, 34]. Dietary lecithin modifies cholesterol homeostasis providing benefits in the prevention and treatment of cardiovascular disease [34].
- Helene will benefit from drinking green tea. She may consume the green tea as part of the prescribed herbal tea, or drink green tea on its own if she chooses to take the herbal tonic in preference to the prescribed herbal tea for its antioxidant properties [17, 36]. Green tea can reduce cholesterol [36] and protect against cardiovascular disease [17]. It may also aid weight loss [17, 48].

Physical treatment suggestions

- Helene may find massage is beneficial in reducing her stress levels [30].
- Acupuncture therapy may help reduce Helene's anxiety [49] and improve her sleep [51].
- Hydrotherapy study revealed positive results to treat high cholesterol with a program of central cooling using whole water bath immersion by decreasing temperature slowly from 22 to 14°C (increasing time from 5 to 20 minutes) over 90 days [57].
- Hydrotherapy: constitutional hydrotherapy [59, 60]. Alternating sitz bath for fatigue [58]. Cold-water arm shower for fatigue [61]. Short, cold head shower for fatigue [62]. Alternate hot and cold showers [61].

TABLE 7.26 HERBAL FORMULA (1:2 LIQUID EXTRACTS)

HERB	FORMULA	RATIONALE
Globe artichoke *Cynara scolymus*	55 mL	Antioxidant [17]; hypocholesterolaemic [17, 18]; anticholesterolaemic [18]; choleretic [17, 18]; cholagogue [17, 18]; hepatoprotective [17, 18]
Turmeric *Curcuma longa*	80 mL	Antioxidant [17, 18]; anti-inflammatory [17, 18]; hypolipidaemic [17, 18]; choleretic [18]; cholagogue [17]
Tienchi ginseng *Panax notoginseng*	50 mL	Hypocholesterolaemic [22]; anti-inflammatory [22]; cardioprotective [22]
Ginger *Zingiber officinale*	15 mL	Hypolipidaemic [17]; antiplatelet [17, 18]; antioxidant [17]; anti-inflammatory [17, 18]
Supply:	200 mL	Dose 5 mL 3 times daily

Garlic tablet containing the equivalent of 5 g fresh garlic *Allium sativum* (providing approx. 4–5 mg alliin per tablet) twice daily
Helene may prefer to take garlic in tablet form if she is not keen on eating fresh garlic every day
Antioxidant [17, 36]; hypocholesterolaemic [17, 36]; antiatherosclerotic [17, 36]; anti-inflammatory [17, 36]

TABLE 7.27 **HERBAL TEA**		
Alternative to herbal liquid if Helene prefers to drink herbal tea rather than a tonic – day formula		
HERB	**FORMULA**	**RATIONALE**
Green tea *Camellia sinensis*	3 parts	Antioxidant [17, 36]; green tea consumption is associated with a decrease in total serum cholesterol [36] and is protective against cardiovascular disease [17]; thermogenic [17, 48]; may be beneficial to aid weight loss [17, 48]
Lemon balm *Melissa officinalis*	1 part	Antioxidant [17]; anxiolytic [17, 19]; hypolipidaemic [37]; hepatoprotective [37]
Celery seed *Apium graveolens*	½ part	Anti-inflammatory [17]; cholagogue [17]; hypocholesterolaemic [38]
Cinnamon bark powder *Cinnamomum cassia*	2 parts	Antioxidant [17]; anti-inflammatory [17]; can reduce LDL and total cholesterol [41]
Ginger *Zingiber officinale*	¼ part	See above
Infusion: 1 tsp per cup – 1 cup 3–4 times daily		

TABLE 7.28 **HERBAL TEA**		
Evening formula to aid sleep		
HERB	**FORMULA**	**RATIONALE**
Skullcap *Scutellaria lateriflora*	1 part	Nervine tonic [19, 20]; mild sedative [19, 20]
Passionflower *Passiflora incarnata*	½ part	Sedative [19, 20]; hypnotic [20]
Hops *Humulus lupulus*	1 part	Hypnotic [17, 19, 20]; mild sedative [17, 19, 20]; beneficial in insomnia in combination with other sedative herbs [17]
Strong infusion: 2 tsp per cup – 1 cup in the evening before bedtime		

TABLE 7.29 **HERBAL TABLET ALTERNATIVE**		
Tablet alternative to sleep formula herbal tea if Helene prefers a tablet		
HERB	**DOSE PER TABLET**	**RATIONALE**
Valerian *Valeriana officinalis*	700 mg	Anxiolytic [17, 18]; hypnotic [17, 18]; decreases sleep latency and improves sleep quality [17, 18]
Passionflower *Passiflora incarnata*	500 mg	See above
Zizyphus *Zizyphus spinosa*	900 mg	Sedative [19, 22]; hypnotic [19, 22]; anxiolytic [19]
Dose: 2 tablets one hour before bed time		

TABLE 7.30 **NUTRITIONAL SUPPLEMENTS**	
SUPPLEMENT AND DOSE	**RATIONALE**
Omega-3 fatty acids 6000 mg daily in divided doses [13, 17]	Lowers triglycerides [17, 21]; lowers LDL [13, 15, 21]; improves HDL/trigylceride ratio in postmenopausal women [13]; anti-inflammatory [13, 17, 21]; cardioprotective [13]; beneficial for the secondary prevention of heart disease [13, 42]
High-potency practitioner-strength **multivitamin, mineral and antioxidant supplement** containing therapeutic doses of Vitamins B6, B12 and Folate [14, 15, 16]	Vitamins B6, B12 and folate reverse hyperhomocysteinaemia [15, 16]; increasing Helene's antioxidant levels helps protect against cardiovascular disease [13–15]; increased requirement for B-group vitamins during times of stress [13, 17, 21]
Vitamin E 800 IU daily [43]	Lipid soluble antioxidant [13, 17, 21, 43]; protects against LDL oxidation [15, 17]; reduces risk of cardiovascular disease [17, 43]
Policasanol 5 mg daily [17]	Lowers total cholesterol [15, 17]; increases HDL cholesterol [15, 17]; lowers LDL cholesterol [15, 17]; reduces oxidation of LDL cholesterol [17]; Helene may prefer to take policasanol as an alternative to cholesterol-lowering medications [17]
Coenzyme Q10 100 mg daily [13, 17]	Antioxidant [13, 17]; cardioprotective [17]; reduces total and LDL cholesterol [17, 63]; reduces side effects of statin drugs, which may be helpful if Helene decides to take cholesterol lowering medication [13, 17]

References

[1] N.J. Talley, S. O'Connor, Pocket Clinical Examination, third edn, Churchill Livingstone Elsevier, Australia, 2009.
[2] P. Kumar, C. Clark, Clinical Medicine, sixth edn, Elsevier Saunders, London, 2005.
[3] J. Silverman, S. Kurtz, J. Draper, Skills for Communicating with Patients, second edn, Radcliff Publishing, Oxford, 2000.
[4] R. Neighbour, The Inner Consultation; how to develop an effective and intuitive consulting style, Radcliff Publishing, Oxon, 2005.
[5] M. Lloyd, R. Bor, Communication Skills For Medicine, third edn, Churchill Livingstone Elsevier, Edinburgh, 2009.
[6] G. Douglas, F. Nicol, C. Robertson, Macleod's Clinical Examination, twelfth edn, Churchill Livingstone Elsevier, Edinburgh, 2009.
[7] R.D. Collins, Differential Diagnosis in Primary Care, fourth edn, Lippincott Williams & Wilkins, Philadelphia, 2008.
[8] K.D. Pagna, T.J. Pagna, Mosby's Diagnostic and Laboratory Test reference, third edn, Mosby, USA, 1997 (later edition).
[9] J. Jamison, Differential Diagnosis for Primary Care, second edn, Churchill Livingstone Elsevier, London, 2006.
[10] A. Polmear (Ed.), Evidence-Based Diagnosis in Primary Care, Churchill Livingstone Elsevier, Edinburgh, 2008, pp. 274–283.
[11] L. Chaitow, E. Blake, P. Orrock, M. Wallden, P. Snider, J. Zeff (Eds.), Natropathic Physical Medicine: Theory and Practice for Manual Therapists and Naturopaths, Churchill Livingstone Elsevier, Philadelphia, 2008.
[12] D. Peters, L. Chaitow, G. Harris, S. Morrison. Integrating Complementary Therapies in Primary Care. Churchill Livingstone, London, 2002.
[13] J. Jamison, Clinical Guide to Nutrition & Dietary Supplements in Disease Management, Churchill Livingstone, Edinburgh, 2003.
[14] H. Osiecki, The Physicians Handbook of Clinical Nutrition, seventh edn, Bioconcepts, Eagle Farm, 2000.
[15] J.E. Pizzorno, M.T. Murray, H. Joiner-Bey, The Clinicians Handbook of Natural Medicine, second edn, Churchill Livingstone, St Louis, 2008.

[16] S. El-Hashemy, Naturopathic Standards of Primary Care, CCNM Press Inc, Toronto, 2007.

[17] L. Braun, M. Cohen, Herbs & Natural Supplements: An evidence based guide, second edn, Elsevier, Sydney, 2007.

[18] S. Mills, K. Bone, Principles & Practice of Phytotherapy; Modern Herbal Medicine, Churchill Livingstone, Edinburgh: London, 2000.

[19] S. Mills, K. Bone, The Essential Guide to Herbal Safety, Churchill Livingstone, St Louis, 2005.

[20] British Herbal Medicine Association, British Herbal Pharmacopoeia, BHMAA, 1983.

[21] H. Osiecki, The Nutrient Bible, seventh edn, BioConcepts Publishing, Eagle Farm, 2008.

[22] K. Bone, Clinical Applications of Chinese and Ayurvedic Herbs: Monographs for the Western Herbal Practitioners, Phytotherapy Press, Warwick, 1996.

[23] T.A. Jacobson, Beyond lipids: the role of omega-3 fatty acids from fish oil in the prevention of coronary heart disease, Current Atherosclerosis Reports 9 (2) (2007) 145–153.

[24] W.L. Haskell, H.L. Taylor, P.D. Wood, H. Schrott, G. Heiss, Strenuous physical activity, treadmill exercise test performance and plasma high-density lipoprotein cholesterol. The Lipid Research Clinics Program Prevalence Study, Circulation 62 (4 Pt. 2) (1980) IV53–61.

[25] M.L. Stefanick, S. Mackey, M. Sheehan, N. Ellsworth, W.L. Haskell, P.D. Wood, Effects Of Diet And Exercise In Men And Postmenopausal Women With Low Levels Of HDL Cholesterol And High Levels of LDL Cholesterol, N Engl J Med 339 (1) (1998) 12–20.

[26] E.S. Ford, Does Exercise Reduce Inflammation? Physical Activity and C-reactive Protein Among U.S. Adults, Epidemiology 13 (5) (2002) 561–568.

[27] P.D. Thompson, D.B. Buchner, I.L. Pina, G.J. Balady, M.A. Williams, B.H. Marcus, K. Berra, et al., Exercise and Physical Activity in the Prevention and Treatment of Atherosclerotic Cardiovascular Disease: A Statement From the Council on Clinical Cardiology (Subcommittee on Exercise, Rehabilitation, and Prevention) and the Council on Nutrition, Physical Activity, and Metabolism (Subcommittee on Physical Activity), Arteriosclerosis, Thrombosis and Vascular Biology 23 (2003) e42–e49.

[28] W.L. Haskell, Cardiovascular Disease Prevention and Lifestyle Interventions: Effectiveness and Efficacy, The Journal of Cardiovascular Nursing 18 (4) (2003) 245–255.

[29] C. Patel, M.G. Marmot, D.J. Terry, M. Patel, Trial of relaxation in reducing coronary risk: Four year follow up, British Medical Journal 290 (6475) (1985) 1103–1106.

[30] T. Field, M. Hernandez-Reif, M. Diego, Cortisol Decreases and Serotonin and Dopamine Increase Following Massage Therapy, International Journal of Neuroscience 115 (2005) 1397–1413.

[31] M. Abbey, M. Noakes, G.B. Belling, P.J. Nestel, Partial replacement of saturated fatty acids with almonds or walnuts lowers total plasma cholesterol and LDL cholesterol, The American Journal of Clincal Nutrition 59 (1994) 995–999.

[32] J. Velasco, C. Dobarganes, Oxidative Stability of Virgin Olive Oil, European Journal of Lipid Science and Technology 104 (9–10) (2002) 661–676.

[33] M.A. Martinez-Gonzalez, A.S. Sanchez-Villegas, The emerging role of Mediterranean diets in cardiovascular epidemiology: Monounsaturated fats, olive oil, red wine or the whole pattern? European Journal of Epidemiology 19 (2004) 9–13.

[34] M.J. LeBlanc, S. Brunet, G. Bouchard, T. Lamireau, I.M. Yousef, V. Gavino, E. Levy, et al., Effects of dietary soybean lecithin on plasma lipid transport and hepatic cholesterol metabolism in rats, Journal of Nutritional Biochemistry 14 (2003) 40–48.

[35] J.J. Badimon, L. Badimon, V. Fuster, Regression of Atherosclerotic Lesions by High Density Lipoprotein Plasma Fraction in the Cholesterol-fed Rabbit, Journal of Clinical Investigation 85 (4) (1990) 1234–1241.

[36] K. Bone, M. Morgan, Green Tea and Garlic as Cardiovascular Life Extension Strategies, Townsend Letter for Doctors and Patients 269 (2005) 51–56.

[37] S. Bolkent, R. Yanardag, O. Karabulut-Bulan, B. Yesilyaprak, Protective role of Melissa officinalis L. extract on liver of hyperlipidemic rats: a morphological and biochemical study, Journal of Ethnopharmacology 99 (3) (2005) 391–398.

[38] D. Tsi, B.K. Tan, The mechanism underlying the hypocholesterolaemic activity of aqueous celery extract, its butanol and aqueous fractions in genetically hypercholesterolaemic rico rats, Life Sciences 66 (8) (2000) 755–767.

[39] L.P. Bell, K.J. Hectorn, H. Reynolds, D.B. Hunninghake, Cholesterol lowering effects of soluble fiber cereals as part of a prudent diet for patients with mild to moderate hypercholesterolaemia, The American Journal of Clinical Nutrition 52 (1990) 1020–1026.

[40] L. Brown, B. Rosner, W.W. Willett, F. Sacks, Cholesterol-lowering effects of dietary fiber: a meta-analysis, The American Journal of Clinical Nutrition 69 (1999) 30–42.

[41] A. Khan, M. Safdar, M.M. Khan, K.N. Khattak, R.A. Anderson, Cinnamon Improves Glucose and Lipids of People With Type 2 Diabetes, Diabetes Care 26 (12) (2003) 3215–3218.

[42] T.A. Jacobson, Beyond lipids: the role of omega-3 fatty acids from fish oil in the prevention of coronary heart disease, Current Atherosclerosis Reports 9 (2) (2007) 145–153.

[43] J. Higdon, An Evidence Based Approach to Vitamins and Minerals, Thieme, New York, 2003.

[44] L. Mosca, C.L. Banka, E.J. Benjamin, K. Berra, C. Bushnell, R.J. Dolor, T.G. Ganiats, et al., Evidence-Based Guidelines for Cardiovascular Disease Prevention in Women: 2007 Update, Circulation 115 (2007) 1481–1501.

[45] J.S. Voelk, M.J. Sharman, A.L. Gomez, D.A. Judelson, M.R. Rubin, G. Watson, B. Sokmen, et al. Comparison of energy-restricted very low-carbohydrate and low-fat diets on weight loss and body composition in overweight men and women.

[46] D.K. Layman, R.A. Boileau, D.J. Erickson, J.E. Painter, H. Shiue, C. Sather, D.D. Christou, A Reduced Ratio of Dietary Carbohydrate to Protein Improves Body Composition and Blood Lipid Profiles during Weight Loss in Adult Women, The Journal of Nutrition 133 (2) (2003) 411–417.

[47] M.A. Pereira, J. Swain, A.B. Goldfine, N. Rifai, D.S. Ludwig, Effects of a Low-Glycemic Load Diet on Resting Energy Expenditure and Heart Disease Risk Factors During Weight Loss, Journal of the American Medical Association 292 (20) (2004) 2482–2490.

[48] A.G. Dulloo, J. Seydoux, L. Girardier, P. Chantre, J. Vandermander, Green tea and thermogenesis: interactions between catechin-polyphenols, caffeine and sympathetic activity, International Journal of Obesity Related Metabolic Disorders 24 (2) (2000) 252–258.

[49] A.F. Jorm, H. Christensen, K.M. Griffiths, R.A. Parslow, B. Rodgers, K.A. Blewitt, Effectiveness of complementary and self-help treatments for anxiety disorders, Medical Journal of Australia 181 (7) (2004) S29–S46.

[50] A. Byrne, G.D. Byrne, The effect of exercise on depression, anxiety and other mood states: A review, J Psychosom Res 37 (6) (1993) 565–574.

[51] D.W. Spence, L. Kayumov, A. Chen, A. Lowe, U. Jain, M.A. Katzman, et al., Acupuncture increases nocturnal melatonin secretion and reduces insomnia and anxiety: A preliminary report, Journal of Neuropsychiatry and Clinical Neurosciences 16 (1) (2004) 19–28.

[52] K.M. Queenan, M.L. Stewart, K.N. Smith, W. Thomas, G. Fulcher, J.L. Slavin, Concentrated oat β-glucan, a fermentable fiber, lowers serum cholesterol in hypercholesterolemic adults in a randomized controlled trial, Nutrition Journal 26; 6:6 (2007).

[53] K. Morgan, Daytime activity and risk factors for late-life insomnia, Journal of Sleep Research 12 (2003) 231–238.

[54] E.J. Stepanski, J.K. Wyatt, Use of sleep hygiene in the treatment of insomnia, Sleep Medicine Reviews 7 (3) (2003) 215–225.

[55] R.S. Tilvis, T.A. Miettinen, Serum plant sterols and their relation to cholesterol absorption, The American Journal of Clinical Nutrition 43 (1986) 92–97.

[56] V. Piironen, Toivo, A.M. Lampi, Natural Sources of Dietary Plant Sterols, Journal of Food Composition and Analysis 13 (2000) 619–624.

[57] F. De Lorenzo, M. Mukherjeem, Z. Kadziolaz, R. Sherwood, V.V. Kakkar, Central cooling effects in patients with hypercholesterolaemia, Clinical Science 95 (1998) 213–217.

[58] L. Chaitow, Hydrotherapy, water therapy for health and beauty, Element, Dorset, 1999.

[59] L.M. Watrous, Constitutional hydrotherapy: from nature cure to advanced naturopathic medicine, Journal of Naturopathic Medicine 7 (2) (1997) 72–79.

[60] W. Boyle, A. Saine, Lectures in Naturopathic Hydrotherapy, Eclectic Medical Publications, Oregon, 1988.

[61] D.D. Buchman, The complete book of water healing, Contemporary Books, McGraw-Hill Companies, New York, 2001.

[62] M. Sinclair, Modern Hydrotherapy for the Massage Therapist, Lippincott Williams & Wilkins, Baltimore, 2008.

[63] R.B. Singh, N.S. Neki, K. Kartikey, D. Pella, A. Kumar, M.A. Niaz, et al., Effect of coenzyme Q10 on risk of atherosclerosis in patients with recent myocardial infarction, Molecular and Cellular Biochemistry 246 (2003) 75–82.

[64] H.B. Brewer, Increasing HDL cholesterol levels, N Engl J Med 350 (2004) 1491–1560.

[65] A.M. Scanu, Lp(13) lipoproteins, N Engl J Med 2003 (349) (2003) 2089–2156.

[66] K. Asplund, Antioxidant vitamins in the prevention of cardiovascular disease: a systematic review, Journal of Internal Medicine 251 (2002) 372–392.

[67] D.P. Vivekananthan, M.S. Penn, S.K. Sapp, et al., Use of antioxidant vitamins for the prevention of cardiovascular disease: meta-analysis of randomised trials, Lancet 361 (2003) 2017–2023.

[68] D.S. Wald, M. Law, J.K. Morris, Homocysteine and cardiovascular disease: evidence on causality from meta-analysis, British Medical Journal 325 (2002) 1202–1206.

[69] M. Ebell, What is a reasonable initial approach to the patient with fatigue? J Fam Pract 50 (16) (2001) 16–17 discussion.

[70] L. Darbishire, L. Ridsdale, P.T. Seed, Distinguishing patients with chronic fatigue from those with chronic fatigue syndrome: a diagnostic study in UK primary care, Br J Gen Pract 53 (2003) 441–445.

[71] R.D. Chervin, Sleepiness, fatigue, tiredness, and lack of energy in obstructive sleep apnea, Chest 118 (2000) 372–379.

[72] W.R. Pigeon, M.J. Sateia, R.J. Ferguson, Distinguishing between excessive daytime sleepiness and fatigue: toward improved detection and treatment, J Psychosom Res 54 (2003) 61–69.

Iron deficiency anaemia

Case history

Hannah Dalton is 24 years old and has come to the clinic with her mother Penny, who has come along to support and help Hannah answer questions because Hannah has Down syndrome (DS).

Hannah went to the family doctor a few months ago because she was feeling very tired and Penny noticed she was looking quite pale. Hannah was prescribed some iron tablets, but she is finding they make her nauseous and constipated. Penny is hoping we can prescribe some form of iron that does not make Hannah feel unwell.

With Penny's help Hannah tells you she has been feeling tired for a while and wants to feel better. Penny explains that Hannah has regular periods, which last for around seven days. They have become heavier and more painful in the past few years and she thinks this is why Hannah is feeling tired and needs iron. Penny reveals that Hannah has not been doing much exercise lately because she gets so tired easily and has consequently gained weight.

Apart from the fatigue, Hannah's health is generally good. Penny tells you Hannah has had regular medical investigations since birth and does not have visual or hearing problems and her heart is also fine. Hannah had most of the childhood illnesses you would expect any child to have and there were some problems with earache in early childhood, but she hasn't had problems with her ears for many years. Hannah does have a tendency to constipation, which has been worsened by the iron tablets and her skin has a tendency to dryness. Penny also mentions she is aware that people with Down syndrome are at higher risk of developing Alzheimer's disease, but she hasn't noticed any signs of that yet.

Hannah tells you she works in a plant nursery four days a week and volunteers at an animal shelter every Friday. She goes to Friendship Club on some Saturdays and her brothers and cousins visit her and take her out with them or play on the Wii with her. Hannah says her favourite things to do are the Wii and scrapbooking, which she does with her cousin Amy. Hannah is very excited to tell you she is moving into her own house soon. Penny explains that she and her husband are planning for Hannah to live independently in about six months. They are in the process of selling their family home and buying a duplex, with Hannah living in one side and them living in the other.

Hannah is very outgoing and communicative and obviously living a productive and happy life. Penny tells you she and her husband believe every child is a gift from God and Hannah is a wonderful person who enriches their lives in ways they never could have imagined, and she brings positive energy to all who will receive it.

TABLE 7.31 **COMPLAINT** [1–10]	
Analogy: Skin of the apple	**Complaint:** Define the presenting complaint and symptoms; understand the complaint *Fatigue*
AREAS OF INVESTIGATION AND EXAMPLE QUESTIONS	**CLIENT RESPONSES**
Onset *When did you first start feeling tired?*	Hannah answers: *For a long time.* Penny comments *I think she has been tired for at least 6 months.*

▶

▶

Exacerbating factors *Is there anything that makes you feel more tired?*	Hannah answers: *When I'm doing things.*
Relieving factors *Is there anything that makes you feel better?*	Hannah answers: *When I sit down and have a rest.*
Examination and inspection	Hannah appears quite pale, with pale conjunctiva and nail bed. Nails are spooning slightly. Hannah's skin is quite dry.

TABLE 7.32 CONTEXT

Analogy: Flesh of the apple	**Context:** Put the presenting complaint into context to understand the disease
AREAS OF INVESTIGATION AND EXAMPLE QUESTIONS	**CLIENT RESPONSES**
Family health *Does anyone else in the family have similar symptoms to Hannah?*	Penny answers: *No.*
Functional disease *Does Hannah have any other medical conditions?*	Penny answers: *Apart from Down's, no.*
Degenerative and deficiency *These blood tests indicate Hannah has low iron levels. What did the doctor tell you about that?*	Penny answers: *Yes, he told me she was anaemic and to take iron tablets. The problem is the tablets aren't really agreeing with her.* Hannah adds: *They make me feel sick and my poo is hard to get out.*
Endocrine/reproductive *Hannah, can you tell me about your periods?*	Hannah answers: *Sometimes it hurts.* Penny comments: *Her periods seem to have been getting heavier and she says her tummy hurts when she has them.*

TABLE 7.33 **CORE**	
Analogy: Core of the apple with the seed of ill health	**Core:** Holistic assessment to understand the client
AREAS OF INVESTIGATION AND EXAMPLE QUESTIONS	CLIENT RESPONSES
Daily activities *Hannah, tell me what you do every day.*	Hannah answers: *I go to work at the nursery and I go and look after the animals. On the weekend I play on the Wii with my brothers and Amy does scrapbooking with me. Sometimes I go to Friendship Club and see my friends.*
Action needed to heal *Hannah, will you take any medicine or eat things I say to help you get better?*	Hannah answers: *Yes.*
Long-term goals *Hannah, what would you like to do in the future?*	Hannah answers: *I'm moving into my own house next to Mum and Dad.*

TABLE 7.34 **HANNAH'S SIGNS AND SYMPTOMS** [1, 2, 6]	
Pulse	98 bpm
Blood pressure	135/88
Temperature	36.8°C
Respiratory rate	16
Body mass index	27 – higher prevalence of obesity in DS women than men [26]
Waist circumference	85 cm
Face	Facial skin pale, conjunctiva pale, sores on both sides of mouth; skin appears dry
Nails	Fingernails brittle, slightly concave (spoonlike) and skin around nails is dry and split, pale nail bed
Urinalysis	No abnormality detected (NAD)

TABLE 7.35 **RESULTS OF MEDICAL INVESTIGATIONS** [2, 22, 6–9, 11]	
TEST	RESULTS
Neurological examination	No sign of dementia or spinal cord compression
Cardiac examination	No sign of heart disease or mitral valve prolapse
Ophthalmologic examination	No cataracts and eyesight NAD
Pap smear	No cervical cancer

Breast examination	NAD
Full blood count	Haemoglobin – low; main function for red cell is carrying oxygen to tissues and returning CO_2 from tissues to lungs *Red cell indices:* MCV – reduced (indicates size of red blood cell)
Film comments	Film comments – microcytic hypochromic RBC *Microcytic* means the red blood cell is a small weight and generally these cells have less haemoglobin *Hypochromic* means the red blood cell has a deficiency in haemoglobin; the presence of anaemia with microcytosis and hypochromia indicate causes such as iron deficiency, thalassaemia, sideroblastic anaemia and anaemia of chronic disease
Serum ferritin	Reduced
Serum iron levels	Reduced
Total iron binding capacity	Raised
Serum soluble transfer receptors	Increased Will be raised in iron deficiency and can differentiate between other types of anaemia; reduce need for bone marrow examination
ESR (erythrocyte sedimentation rate indicates inflammation in general)	NAD
CRP	NAD
Fasting blood lipid test (chylomicrons are primarily trigylcerides, LDLs are primarily cholesterol, VLDLs primarily triglycerides, HDLs are predominantly proteins)	NAD
Cholesterol blood test (usually includes VLDL value)	NAD
Homocysteine blood test	NAD
Electrolyte blood test	NAD
Fasting blood glucose test	NAD
Liver function test	NAD
Thyroid function test (TFT)	TSH slightly raised and T3 and T4 normal range

TABLE 7.36 **UNLIKELY DIAGNOSTIC CONSIDERATIONS** [2, 7–10, 12, 22, 57, 60, 61]	
CONDITIONS AND CAUSES	**WHY UNLIKELY**
CANCER AND HEART DISEASE	
Heart disease: common for DS	No high cholesterol, BP normal range, homocysteine within normal range
Breast or cervical cancer	Examination NAD
High cholesterol: common for DS	Within normal range
DEGENERATIVE AND DEFICIENCY	
Bone marrow fibrosis	Would present with normal-sized cells along with low haemoglobin
Sideroblastic anaemia: microcytic blood cells and low haemoglobin	MCV can often be raised, serum iron will be raised, total iron-binding capacity (TIBC) would be normal; serum ferritin would be raised
Thalassaemia: microcytic blood cells and low haemoglobin	Normal results would be seen for serum iron, TIBC, serum ferritin, serum soluble transfer receptors
Anaemia of chronic diease: microcytic blood cells and low haemoglobin	Would present with normal-sized cells along with low haemoglobin; serum TIBC would be reduced, serum ferritin would be normal or raised, serum soluble transfer receptors would be normal
Folate deficiency	Would be macrocytic/megaloblastic
Pernicious anaemia: B12 deficiency	Would be macrocytic/megaloblastic due to lack of B12 absorption due to immune destruction of intrinsic factor in atrophic gastritis and loss of stomach parietal cells; can present with hypothyroidism
Haemolytic anaemias	Would present with normal size cells along with low haemoglobin
Liver disease	Liver function NAD; anaemias of liver disease more often present as macrocytic large blood cells and normoblastic
Vision disorders: common for DS	Ophthalamologic examination NAD
ENDOCRINE/REPRODUCTIVE	
Hypothyroid needs to be tested annually for DS in this age group, fatigue, heavy periods, constipation, dry skin, weight gain	T4 and T3 test within normal range; advanced endocrine disease will more often present with normal size red blood cells along with low haemoglobin; no physical signs of goitre, slow pulse, change in voice, or cold hands as would have in clinical low thyroid condition
Diabetes	Urinalysis and fasting blood glucose level NAD

▶

▶

Anovulatory bleeding	Usually irregular bleed that appears menstrual although no ovulation has occurred; bleed would be painless and unexpected; physical findings will often include hirsutism, acne
Ovarian cyst: irregular periods	Ovarian cysts almost never cause heavy menstrual bleeding

TABLE 7.37 **CONFIRMED DIAGNOSIS** [2, 7]	
CONDITION	RATIONALE
Iron deficiency anaemia	Low haemoglobin, reduced MCV, microcytic hypochromic red blood cells, serum iron reduced, serum TIBC raised, serum ferritin reduced and serum-soluble transfer receptors increased; heavy menstrual periods, feeling fatigue gradually over a period of time; anaemia and low serum ferritin can cause heavy menstrual bleeding [19]

Case analysis

TABLE 7.38 **POSSIBLE FURTHER DIFFERENTIAL DIAGNOSIS**		
Not ruled out by tests/investigations already done [2, 7–10, 12, 54, 57–61]		
CONDITION	WHY POSSIBLE	WHY UNLIKELY
CANCER AND HEART DISEASE		
Ovarian, uterine cancer	Heavy irregular bleeding; can cause iron deficiency	No vaginal discharge reported
TRAUMA AND PRE-EXISTING ILLNESS		
Causal factor: **Postviral infection**	Fatigue	Need to rule out if Hannah has had viral symptoms prior to feeling fatigued
OBSTRUCTION AND FOREIGN BODY		
Causal factor: **Obstructive sleep apnoea**	Common for people with DS to develop due to hypotonic muscles, feeling tired; fatigue during the day; more common when overweight or obese; do not usually complain of 'sleepiness' but rather fatigue generally	Need to determine if feel not well rested in the morning and if snore during the night
Causal factor: **Intestinal obstruction:** bowel cancer, adhesions, hernias, fecal impaction with overflow	Abdominal constipation	No vomiting, abdominal pain and distension

▶

FUNCTIONAL DISEASE		
Coeliac disease [22]	Constipation, can develop for people with DS; fatigue, skin changes; often has anaemia as an associated symptom	Need to gain more insight into Hannah's diet and associated symptoms
Causal factor: **Hypotonic muscles in digestive tract**	Common in DS, causes constipation	
Causal factor: **Functional constipation**	Abdominal constipation	Need to check if more than 1 in 4 bowel motions is lumpy and hard, and causes strain, a feeling of incomplete evacuation or blockage; need to check if manual help is needed to facilitate a bowel motion passing; does she have fewer than 3 evacuations in a week
INFECTION AND INFLAMMATION		
Subclinical hypothyroidism	TSH slightly raised and T3 and T4 normal range; TSH levels are higher than previous tests, indicating that Hannah may have subclinical hypothyroidism	Check if there are any reasons why her TSH may be artificially raised – potential presence of thyroid antibody, medication reaction, recovery from illness, rare congenital defect that causes clinical euthyroidism, adrenal glucocorticoid insufficiency, renal failure, undertreated hypothyroidism when thyroxine not at appropriate level
ENDOCRINE/REPRODUCTIVE		
Premenstrual syndrome	Can experience pain and fatigue before period	Need to determine if Hannah experiences premenstrual mood changes, feels teary, bloated or swollen 1–12 days before her period and whether she experiences a dull pelvic ache or abdominal bloating
Pregnancy	Can still have regular periods when pregnant, of child-bearing age, fatigue; can cause iron deficiency	Need to assess if Hannah is sexually active
Perimenopausal	Can develop at an earlier age for those with DS, heavy periods, fatigue	
Uterine fibroids and polyps: fibroids form due to excess oestrogen and can cause symptoms of heavy bleeding, uterine enlargement	Usually causes menorrhagia (blood loss of 80 mL per day and lasting more than 7 days); can cause iron deficiency	Often maintains normal cycle unless submucosal or nearly extruded

Endometriosis	Pain with heavy menstrual bleed; can cause iron deficiency	No bleeding from the bowel; usually brown discharge with associated abdominal and pelvic pain
Dysfunctional uterine bleeding (DUB): endometrial hyperplasia, PCOS, from taking exogenous oestrogen; endocrine dysfunction *(not associated with inflammation, tumour or pregnancy)*	Often menorrhagia (heavy bleed with regular cycle); can cause iron deficiency	No use of exogenous oestrogen reported; usually causes unpredictable volume and frequency of bleeding; interval between periods can be shorter to appear irregular
AUTOIMMUNE DISEASE		
Hashimoto's disease: autoimmune thyroid disease	Subclinical hypothyroid reading	No goitre visible
STRESS AND NEUROLOGICAL DISEASE		
Depression	Fatigue and depression can be common for DS	
EATING HABITS AND ENERGY		
Lack of exercise	Weight gain, fatigue, constipation	

Working diagnosis

HANNAH AND IRON DEFICIENCY ANAEMIA

Hannah is a 24-year-old woman with Down syndrome who has come with her mother Penny for help with a recently diagnosed condition of iron deficiency anaemia. Hannah had been prescribed iron supplementation from her doctor to correct the symptoms; however, the therapy has caused Hannah to have constipation and nausea. Penny is hoping to find an alternative way to help treat the iron deficiency that has developed. During the consultation it is explained that Hannah's menstrual bleed has become heavier and more painful over the past few years and she can feel very tired. She is generally prone to constipation and weight gain, which has worsened lately as Hannah no longer engages in regular exercise due to her fatigue. On a more positive note Hannah is entering into an exciting stage in her life where she is about to move into a home of her own for the first time. She is very happy about this and enjoys being socially active with family and friends.

Anaemia is not a diagnosis in itself and the cause should be investigated. The condition is characterised by low levels of haemoglobin in the blood and the three major types of anaemia are **hypochromic microcytic** (iron deficiency, thalassaemia, anaemia of chronic disease, sideroblastic), **normochromic normocytic** (acute blood loss, anaemia of chronic disease, renal failure, connective tissue disease, bone marrow fibrosis, endocrine disease and haemolytic anaemias) and **macrocytic** (vitamin B12 or folate deficiency, liver disease, excess alcohol). Due to compensatory processes in the body, haemoglobin may drop over a period of time and the anaemia may appear to be asymptomatic. However, if blood loss is more rapid then signs and symptoms of anaemia may present as more severe and include non-specific symptoms such as fatigue, headaches, feeling faint, breathless chest pain, palpitations along with signs of pale skin or a fast pulse. Causes can range from blood loss, nutritional deficiency from inadequate diet, malabsorption in the GI tract and abdominal disorders such as coeliac or Crohn's disease. Other forms of anaemia can develop from bone marrow failure, genetic dysfunction affecting red blood cells and organic diseases affecting the liver or endocrine system.

Iron deficiency anaemia is a common presentation and may develop due to lack of dietary iron intake, gastrointestinal dysfunction, blood loss due to heavy menstrual periods, blood loss due to trauma or labour and throughout pregnancy from the demands of the growing baby.

The body's iron content is usually maintained within a narrow limit with loss and intake carefully balanced. How much is absorbed is influenced by levels of stored iron. It is not possible to excrete iron once it has been absorbed. Blood loss through heavy menstruation will often result in iron deficiency as increased iron absorption from the gastrointestinal tract cannot adequately compensate for the loss. Iron deficiency anaemia can in turn be a causal factor for heavy menstrual bleeding [19, 48].

General references used in this diagnosis: 2, 7–9, 58, 61

TABLE 7.39 **DECISION TABLE FOR TREATMENT PRIOR TO REFERRAL:**		
COMPLAINT	**CONTEXT**	**CORE**
Treatment for the presenting complaint and symptoms	Treatment for all associated symptoms	Treatment for mental, emotional, spiritual, constitutional, lifestyle issues and metaphysical considerations
TREATMENT PRIORITY	**TREATMENT PRIORITY**	**TREATMENT PRIORITY**
• Dietary recommendations to increase intake and absorption of iron • Dietary recommendations to reduce inhibition of iron absorption • Recommendation to supplement iron in a more easily absorbed form that also reduces the gastrointestinal side effects • Herbal tonic to increase iron levels	• Reduce loss of iron through excessive menstrual bleeding • Improve menorrhagia by improving iron status [19, 48] • Dietary recommendations to increase consumption of antioxidants and essential fatty acids to optimise general health and cognitive function • Recommendation for a multivitamin, mineral and antioxidant supplement designed specifically for the needs of people with DS • Recommendation to increase intake of essential fatty acids via diet and supplement to enhance general health, cognitive function and reduce risk of Alziehmer's • Dietary recommendations and herbal tea to support digestive function and improve absorption of nutrients • Herbal tonic to increase iron levels, support thyroid function, reproductive hormone balance and cognitive function • Physical therapy and lifestyle recommendations for exercise to enhance thyroid function and maintain healthy weight • Hydrotherapy suggestion to support thyroid function	

TABLE 7.40 **DECISION TABLE FOR REFERRAL** [2, 7, 9, 12, 13]		
COMPLAINT	**CONTEXT**	**CORE**
Referral for presenting complaint	Referral for all associated physical, dietary and lifestyle concerns	Referral for contributing emotional, mental, spiritual, metaphysical, lifestyle and constitutional factors
REFERRAL FLAGS	**REFERRAL FLAGS**	**REFERRAL FLAGS**
• Hannah wants to try a different iron supplement after being prescribed a specific type by her GP • Looking very pale, spoon like finger nails, cheilosis around mouth	• Overweight • Heavy periods • TFT reveals subclinical hypothyroid reading	• Fatigue may be a symptom of depression
ISSUES OF SIGNIFICANCE	**ISSUES OF SIGNIFICANCE**	**ISSUES OF SIGNIFICANCE**
• Iron supplement causes nausea and constipation	• Constipation • Skin dryness • Fatigue on exertion • Lack of exercise	• Feeling tired with a move into her own house imminent
REFERRAL DECISION	**REFERRAL DECISION**	**REFERRAL DECISION**
• Discuss options given to Hannah with her GP in a collaborative manner regarding iron supplementation [62]	• Dietary assessment • Complete medical check-up for hormonal balance and pregnancy	• Referral for emotional assessment prior to moving into independent home if appropriate

TABLE 7.41 **FURTHER INVESTIGATIONS THAT MAY BE NECESSARY** [2, 7–12, 62]	
TEST/INVESTIGATION	**REASON FOR TEST/INVESTIGATION**
FIRST-LINE MEDICAL INVESTIGATIONS:	
Pelvic, vaginal, abdominal examination	Check for bulging uterus, ovaries can be palpable in PCOS, abdominal rebound tenderness, overactive bowel sounds, genital deformities, signs of trauma
Human chorionic gonadotropin (HCG) blood test/ radioimmunoassay (RIA)	Pregnancy, ectopic pregnancy
Progesterone level	Test 7 days before menstruation is due to see if ovulated; low serum progesterone level in anovulatory cycles
Oestradiol	*Normal*: PCOS, weight loss, excess exercise *Raised*: pregnancy, ovarian tumour, testicular tumour, adrenal tumour *Low*: PCOS, polycystic ovarian disease, ovarian failure, anorexia nervosa, weight loss, excess exercise, hypothyroidism, Cushing's syndrome, adrenal hyperplasia, menopause, Turner's syndrome, failing pregnancy, fetal death

►

FSH (follicle-stimulating hormone)	*Normal*: PCOS, pregnancy, anorexia, weight loss, excess exercise *Raised:* ovarian failure, menopause *Low:* polycystic ovarian disease, anorexia, weight loss, excess exercise, hypothyroidism, Cushing's syndrome, adrenal tumour/hyperplasia
LH (luteinising hormone): due to pulsatile action of this hormone it may not be accurately measured on one random sample	*Normal:* pregnancy, anorexia, weight loss, excess exercise *Raised:* PCOS, polycystic ovarian disease, ovarian failure, menopause *Low:* anorexia, weight loss, excess exercise, hypothyroidism, Cushing's syndrome, adrenal tumour/hyperplasia
Basal body temperature	Normally drops 24–36 hours after menses commences; with endometriosis there is often a delay in basal body temperature to the second or third day of menses; a decrease indicates preovulation and an increase of 5 degrees occurs after ovulation; monitors thyroid function; low temperature readings consistently over a period of days can indicate subclinical or clinical hypothyroidism
Abdominal and pelvic ultrasound	Most accurate diagnosis of PCOS, ovarian mass, ovarian cyst or tumour, retroverted uterus, tubo-ovarian abscesses, fibroids, trauma; intestinal obstruction
Diet diary	Assess caloric intake and possible food sensitivities
IF NECESSARY:	
Bone marrow examination	Differentiate iron deficiency from other forms of anaemia
Epstein-Barr virus blood test	Postviral symptoms, may show that Hannah has had this virus in the past
PRL (prolactin) common in secondary amenorrhoea to be raised	*Normal:* ovarian failure, anorexia, weight loss, excess exercise, adrenal tumour/hyperplasia *Raised:* PCOS (mildly), hypothyroidism, Cushing's syndrome, pregnancy, amenorrhoea *Low:* pituitary destruction from tumour
Testosterone	*Normal:* ovarian failure, anorexia, weight loss, excess exercise, hypothyroidism, pregnancy *Raised*: PCOS, Cushing's syndrome, adrenal tumour/hyperplasia, testicular tumour, ovarian tumour *Low:* corticosteriod use
TSH, free T4 and T3	Borderline subclinical hypothyroidism
Antithyroid antibody test	Autoimmune thyroid disease causing subclinical thyroid test result
Serum cortisol level	Adrenal insufficiency contributing to subclinical hypothyroidism
SHBG (sex hormone-binding globulin)	Low SHBG would indicate the presence of elevated levels of free androgens

Confirmed diagnosis

HANNAH AND ANAEMIA AND SUBCLINICAL HYPOTHYROIDISM

Subclinical hypothyroidism is defined as a serum thyroid-stimulating hormone (TSH) level above the defined upper limit of the reference range, with a serum-free thyroxine (T4) within the reference range [2, 53, 54]. Hannah's TSH levels are slightly raised and have increased since her last thyroid function test. This result indicates she has or is developing subclinical hypothyroidism.

PRESCRIBED MEDICATION

- OCP suggested as an option to lighten menstrual bleed
- Thyroid hormone therapy may be prescribed if Hannah's TSH levels increase further

TABLE 7.42 **DECISION TABLE FOR TREATMENT (ONCE DIAGNOSIS IS CONFIRMED)**		
COMPLAINT	**CONTEXT**	**CORE**
Treatment for the presenting complaint and symptoms	Treatment for all associated symptoms	Treatment for mental, emotional, spiritual, constitutional, lifestyle issues and metaphysical considerations
TREATMENT PRIORITY	**TREATMENT PRIORITY**	**TREATMENT PRIORITY**
• Continue with dietary recommendations to increase iron intake and absorption • Continue with dietary recommendations to reduce inhibition of iron absorption • Continue with recommended iron supplement until tests indicate Hannah's iron levels have returned to well within normal range • Continue with herbal tonic until tests indicate Hannah's iron levels have returned to well within normal range	• Continue to improve iron status to improve menorrhagia [19, 48] • Ongoing dietary recommendations to increase consumption of antioxidants and essential fatty acids • Ongoing supplementation with specific multivitamin, mineral and antioxidant supplement for DS • Ongoing maintenance of essential fatty acid intake via diet and supplement to enhance general health, cognitive function and reduce risk of Alzheimer's disease • Ongoing dietary recommendations and herbal tea to support digestive function and improve nutrient absorption • Ongoing use of herbal tonic to support thyroid function, reproductive hormone balance and cognitive function; review the formula in 3–4 months based on blood test results and changes/improvement in menstrual symptoms • Ongoing physical therapy and lifestyle recommendations for exercise to enhance thyroid function and maintain healthy weight • Ongoing hydrotherapy suggestions to support thyroid function; this can be reviewed in 3–4 months based on blood test results	• Recommendation for continuing and strengthening Hannah's social and support network • Recommendation for Hannah's parents to connect with disability support organisations and networks for assistance and support as they care for Hannah's needs now and as they plan for her future

Treatment aims

- Increase and maintain Hannah's iron levels [14, 19]. This is likely to improve menorrhagia [19, 48].
- Increase Hannah's dietary intake of iron [14, 19] and improve iron absorption [14, 19].
- Optimise Hannah's nutritional status, particularly of nutrients essential for absorption and metabolism of iron [14, 19].
- Reduce excessive menstrual bleeding, which is contributing to Hannah's anaemia [14, 19, 48].
- Optimise Hannah's thyroid function [17, 53] and minimise any potential effect of subclinical hypothyroidism on her menstrual cycle [2, 19, 20].
- Support Hannah's cognitive function and delay onset of or reduce the rate of cognitive decline [21, 22].
- Support Hannah's nutrition and general health [16, 55, 56].
- Improve Hannah's antioxidant status [16, 39].

Lifestyle alterations/considerations

- Encourage Hannah to exercise daily. Exercise stimulates thyroid hormone secretion and increases tissue sensitivity to thyroid hormone [16, 17, 23, 24].
- Encourage Penny to monitor Hannah's weight and help her maintain a normal BMI. There is a higher prevalence of obesity in people with Down syndrome [26].
- Encourage Hannah to continue and strengthen her social interactions in the friendship club and with family to ensure she has a strong social network [25].
- Refer Penny and her husband to local disability support organisations and networks for ongoing support and assistance as they care for Hannah and plan for her future needs [25].

Dietary suggestions

- Encourage Hannah to eat foods containing haem iron [15, 18, 27]. These include lean red meat, fish, poultry, liver, heart, kidney, oysters, clams and shellfish [15, 18, 27]. Haem iron is more easily absorbed than non-haem iron [18, 27].
- Encourage Hannah to also consume non-haem iron-containing foods, particularly those with higher levels of available iron such as citrus fruit, tomatoes, papaya, broccoli, pumpkin, chickpeas and cabbage [15, 18, 27].
- When she is eating non-haem iron-rich foods, Hannah should minimise consumption of foods containing non-haem iron-solubility inhibitors [15, 18, 27]. These include foods containing phytic acid, oxalic acid and calcium [15, 18, 27].
- Encourage Hannah to avoid tea, coffee or other polyphenol-containing beverages when eating iron-containing foods or iron supplements because the polyphenols can significantly inhibit iron absorption [15, 18, 27, 29].
- Encourage Hannah to add acidic dressings such as lemon juice or vinegar to non-haem iron-containing foods [18, 19, 27].
- Hannah will benefit from consuming 100 mg vitamin C with meals to maximise absorption of non-haem iron [15, 18]. Alternatively she may prefer to drink some acidic fruit juice [15, 18].
- Consumption of bitter fruit or vegetables before or during the meal can stimulate the flow of gastric juices and improve absorption of nutrients [18, 19].
- Encourage Hannah to eat an antioxidant-rich whole-food diet [16, 39, 45].
- Encourage Hannah to consume foods high in omega-3 fatty acids [16, 45].

- Hannah should eat foods containing iodine, selenium, copper, iron, zinc, B-group vitamins and tyrosine, which are essential nutrients for thyroid function [16, 17].
- Goitrogenic foods should be cooked [16, 46, 47].

Physical treatment suggestions

- Hydrotherapy: cold hydrotherapy to stimulate thyroid function may be beneficial to Hannah [17, 52]. Whole body cold mitten friction to increase circulation in anaemia [50]. Cold sitz bath or icebag between the thighs to prevent heavy menstrual bleeding [49, 50]. Cold sitz bath with simultaneous, hot foot bath to ease congestion (*note: hot foot baths can stimulate menstrual bleeding*) [49, 50]. For acute period pain, spray a hot hand shower to the pelvic area for two minutes, then alternate and spray with cold water for one minute (repeat three times) [51]. Hot compress/fomentation on the back during menstrual pain [51]. Between periods, weekly contrasting treatments with hot fomentation on the back and abdomen for 15 minutes, followed by 30-second cold mitten friction. Follow that with heat on the pelvic area and back for another 15 minutes, repeat cold mitten friction with the client in the side lying position (repeat alternating procedure three times). End with an abdominal massage [51].
- Exercise incorporating resistance training can support or improve Hannah's metabolic rate and help her maintain normal weight [16, 17, 23, 24, 28].

TABLE 7.43 **HERBAL FORMULA (1:2 LIQUID EXTRACTS)**		
HERB	**FORMULA**	**RATIONALE**
Withania *Withania somnifera*	50 mL	Adaptogen [18, 31]; tonic [31]; cognition enhancer [31]; increases haemoglobin and red cell count [31, 42]; stimulates thyroid activity [17, 40]; enhances serum T4 concentration [18, 37]
Codonopsis *Codonopsis pilosula*	50 mL	Adaptogen [38]; increases RBC and haemoglobin [38, 39]
Schisandra *Schisandra chinensis*	50 mL	Antioxidant [18, 35]; adaptogen [18, 35]; improves mental, physical and sensory performance [19, 35]; improves detoxifying capacity of the liver [18, 35]; will assist hormonal balance by enhancing hepatic hormonal clearance [19]
Ginkgo *Ginkgo biloba* 2:1 extract standardised to contain approx; 9 mg/mL Ginkgo flavone glycosides	50 mL	Cognition enhancer [18, 31]; neuroprotective [18, 31]; antioxidant [18, 31]; improves cognitive function in DS [41]
Supply:	200 mL	Dose: 8 mL twice daily

TABLE 7.44 HERBAL LIQUID TO BE TAKEN DURING MENSTRUAL BLEED (1:2 LIQUID EXTRACTS)

HERB	FORMULA	RATIONALE
Tienchi ginseng *Panax notoginseng*	60 mL	Antihaemorrhagic [19, 35]; traditionally used in excessive bleeding [19]; indicated for excessive menstrual bleeding
Yarrow *Achillea millefolium*	40 mL	Haemostatic [34]; traditionally used in the management of excessive bleeding [19, 34]
Supply:	100 mL	Dose: 5 mL 2–3 times daily as required during menstrual period

TABLE 7.45

Tablet alternative to herbal liquid for menstrual bleed if compliance is a problem

HERB	DOSE PER TABLET	RATIONALE
Tienchi ginseng *Panax notoginseng*	1000 mg	See above
Dose: 1–4 tablets daily required during menstrual period		

TABLE 7.46 HERBAL TEA

Alternative to tea and coffee

HERB	FORMULA	RATIONALE
Rose hip *Rosa canina*	2 parts	Nutrient [30]; mild laxative [30]
Nettle leaf *Urtica dioica*	2 parts	Nutritive [31, 36]; haemostatic [31, 32]; traditionally used for anaemia and conditions involving blood loss such as menorrhagia [31, 32]
Ginger root powder *Zingiber officinale*	¼ part	Digestive stimulant [18, 31]; thermogenic [18, 31]; antioxidant [18]
Licorice root powder *Glycyrrhiza glabra*	½ part	Flavouring agent [18, 31]; antioxidant [18, 31]; mild laxative [31]
Infusion: 1 tsp per cup – 2–3 cups daily		

TABLE 7.47 NUTRITIONAL SUPPLEMENTS

SUPPLEMENT AND DOSE	RATIONALE
Iron amino acid chelate or iron gluconate providing 12 mg elemental iron combined with B-group vitamins and vitamin C [15, 18, 27] in liquid form to enhance absorption [44]. Initially 1 dose twice daily until fatigue and iron status improves, then reduce to once daily [15, 18, 33]	Iron amino acid chelate and iron gluconate have higher bioavailability than iron sulphate [43, 44] and are less likely to cause gastrointestinal problems [43]; combined with nutritional cofactors essential for absorption and metabolism of iron [14, 15, 33]

▶

High-potency practitioner-strength **multivitamin, mineral and antioxidant supplement** specifically designed for the requirements of individuals with DS providing therapeutic doses of essential micronutrients Dose: As recommended by the manufacturer Taken at least 90 minutes away from iron supplement to optimise absorption of supplemental nutrients [27]	Enhancing antioxidant status is beneficial in DS [16, 39, 56] and in reducing the risk of Alzheimer's disease [39, 45]; contains nutrients essential for optimal thyroid function [16, 17]
Omega-3 fish oil 4000 mg daily in divided doses [15, 18]	Cognition enhancer [18]; EPA reduces the risk of Alzheimer's disease [18, 45]

References

[1] N.J. Talley, S. O'Connor, Pocket Clinical Examination, third edn, Churchill Livingstone Elsevier, Australia, 2009.

[2] P. Kumar, C. Clark, Clinical Medicine, sixth edn, Elsevier Saunders, London, 2005.

[3] J. Silverman, S. Kurtz, J. Draper, Skills for Communicating with Patients, second edn, Radcliff Publishing, Oxford, 2000.

[4] R. Neighbour, The Inner Consultation; how to develop an effective and intuitive consulting style, Radcliff Publishing, Oxon, 2005.

[5] M. Lloyd, R. Bor, Communication Skills For Medicine, third edn, Churchill Livingstone Elsevier, Edinburgh, 2009.

[6] G. Douglas, F. Nicol, C. Robertson, Macleod's Clinical Examination, twelfth edn, Churchill Livingstone Elsevier, 2009.

[7] J. Jamison, Differential Diagnosis for Primary Care, second edn, Churchill Livingstone Elsevier, London, 2006.

[8] R. Berkow, A.J. Fletcher, M.H. Beers, The Merck Manual, sixteenth edn, Merck Research Laboratories, Rathway, N.J, 1993 (later edition).

[9] R.D. Collins, Differential Diagnosis in Primary Care, fourth edn, Lippincott Williams & Wilkins, Philadelphia, 2008.

[10] R.H. Seller, Differential Diagnosis of Common Complaints, fifth edn, Saunders Elsevier, Philadelphia, 2007.

[11] K.D. Pagna, T.J. Pagna, Mosby's Diagnostic and Laboratory Test reference, third edn, Mosby, USA, 1997 (later edition).

[12] U.S. Department of Health and Human Services (HHS) National Institutes of Health Research Plan on Down syndrome National Institutes of Health (NIH) October 2007. Retrieved 20 September 2009 from http://www.nichd.nih.gov/publications/pubs/upload/NIH_Downsyndrome_plan.pdf

[13] D. Peters, L. Chaitow, G. Harris, S. Morrison, Integrating Complementary Therapies in Primary Care, Churchill Livingstone: London 2002.

[14] S. El-Hashemy, Naturopathic Standards of Primary Care, CCNM Press Inc, Toronto, 2007.

[15] J. Jamison, Clinical Guide to Nutrition & Dietary Supplements in Disease Management, Churchill Livingstone, Edinburgh, 2003.

[16] H. Osiecki, The Physicians Handbook of Clinical Nutrition, seventh edn, Eagle Farm: Bioconcepts, 2000.

[17] J.E. Pizzorno, M.T. Murray, H. Joiner-Bey, The Clinicians Handbook of Natural Medicine, second edn, Churchill Livingstone, St Louis,

[18] L. Braun, M. Cohen, Herbs & Natural Supplements: An evidence based guide, second edn, Elsevier, Sydney, 2007.

[19] R. Trickey, Women, Hormones & The Menstrual Cycle, second edn, Allen & Unwin, Sydney, 2003.

[20] R. Berklow, A.J. Fletcher (Eds.), The Merck Manual, sixteenth edn, Merck Research Laboratories, New Jersey, 1992.

[21] A.H. Bittles, C. Bower, R. Hussain, E.J. Glasson (Eds.), The four ages of Down syndrome. European Journal of Public Health 17 (2) (2006) 221–225.

[22] National Institutes of Health Research Plan on Down syndrome. U.S. Department of Health and Human Services, 2007.

[23] M.J. Gawel, D.M. Park, J. Alaghband-Zadeh, F.C. Rose, Exercise and hormonal secretion, Postgraduate Medical Journal 55 (1979) 373–376.

[24] R.G. McMurray, A.G. Hackney, Interactions of Metabolic Hormones, Adipose Tissue and Exercise, Sports Medicine 35 (5) (2005) 393–412.

[25] W.I. Cohen, L. Nadel, M.E. Madnick (Eds.), Down syndrome: visions for the 21st century, Wiley-Liss Inc., New York, 2002.

[26] C.A. Melville, S.A. Cooper, C.W. McGrother, C.F. Thorp, R. Collacott, Obesity in adults with Down syndrome: a case-control study, Journal of Intellectual Disabilities 49 (Pt2) (2005) 125–133.

[27] J. Higdon, An Evidence Based Approach to Vitamins and Minerals, Thieme, New York, 2003.

[28] R.W. Bryner, I.H. Ullrich, J. Sauers, D. Donley, G. Hornsby, M. Kolar, R. Yeater, Effects of Resistance vs. Aerobic Training Combined With an 800 Calorie Liquid Diet on Lean Body Mass and Resting Metabolic Rate, Journal of the American College of Nutrition 18 (1) (1999) 115–121.

[29] R.F. Hurrell, M. Reddy, J.D. Cook, Inhibition of non-haem iron absorption in man by polyphenolic-containing beverages, British Journal of Nutrition 81 (1999) 289–295.

[30] D. Hoffman, The New Holistic Herbal, Rockport: Element Books, 1992.

[31] S. Mills, K. Bone, Principles & Practice of Phytotherapy; Modern Herbal Medicine, Churchill Livingstone, Edinburgh: London, 2000.

[32] British Herbal Medicine Association, British. Herbal Pharmacopoeia, BHMAA, 1983.

[33] H. Osiecki, The Nutrient Bible, seventh edn, BioConcepts Publishing, Eagle Farm, 2008.

[34] S. Mills, K. Bone, The Essential Guide to Herbal Safety, Churchill Livingstone, St Louis, 2005.

[35] K. Bone, Clinical Applications of Chinese and Ayurvedic Herbs: Monographs for the Western Herbal Practitioners, Phytotherapy Press, Warwick, 1996.

[36] M.A. Grieve, Modern Herbal (revised edition), Tiger Books International, London, 1992.

[37] S. Panda, A. Kar, Changes in thyroid hormone concentrations after administration of ashwagandha root extract to adult male mice, Journal of Pharmacy and Pharmacology 50 (9) (1998) 1065–1068.

[38] H.M. Chang, P.P. But, Pharmacology and Applications of Chinese Materia Medica, World Scientific Publishing, Singapore, 1987.

[39] M. Zana, Z. Janka, J. Kalman, Oxidative stress: A bridge between Down's syndrome and Alzheimer's disease, Neurobiology of Aging 28 (5) (2007) 648–676.

[40] A. Kar, S. Panda, S. Bharti, Relative efficacy of three medicinal plant extracts in the alteration of thyroid hormone concentrations in male mice, Journal of Ethnopharmacology 81 (2) (2002) 281–285.

[41] R. Donfrancesco, A. Dell'uomo, Ginkgo biloba in Down syndrome, Phytomedicine 11 (2004) 469.

[42] M. Ziaudidin, N. Phansaklar, P. Patki, S. Diwanay, B. Patwardhan: in L. Davis, G. Kuttan, Immunomodulatory activity of Withania somnifera, Journal of Ethnopharmacology, (2000) 193–200.

[43] M. Layrisse, M.N. Garcia-Casal, L. Solano, M.A. Baron, F. Arguello, D. Llovera, J. Ramırez, et al., Iron Bioavailability in Humans from Breakfasts Enriched with Iron Bis-Glycine Chelate, Phytates and Polyphenols, The Journal of Nutrition 130 (9) (2000) 2195–2199.

[44] D. Casparis, P. Del Carlo, F. Branconi, A. Grossi, D. Merante, L. Gafforio, Effectiveness and tolerability of oral liquid ferrous gluconate in iron-deficiency anemia in pregnancy and in the immediate post-partum period: comparison with other liquid or solid formulations containing bivalent or trivalent iron (article in Italian), Minerva Ginecol 48 (11) (1996) 511–518.

[45] G.M. Cole, G.P. Lim, F. Yang, B. Teter, B. Aynun, Q. Ma, M.E. Harris-White, et al., Prevention of Alzheimer's disease: Omega-3 fatty acid and phenolic anti-oxidant interventions, Neurobiology of Aging 26S (2005) S133–S136.

[46] E. Ciska, H. Kozlowska, The effect of cooking on the glucosinolates content in white cabbage, European Food Research and Technology 212 (5) (2001) 582–587.

[47] M. McMillan, E.A. Spinks, G.R. Fenwick, Preliminary Observations on the Effect of Dietary Brussels Sprouts on Thyroid Function, Human & Experimental Toxicology 5 (1) (1986) 15–19.

[48] C. Harris, The Vicious Circle of Anæmia and Hæmorrhagia, Canadian Medical Association Journal 77 (2) (1957) 98–100.

[49] W. Boyle, A. Saine, Lectures in Naturopathic Hydrotherapy, Eclectic Medical Publications, Oregon, 1988.

[50] D.D. Buchman, The complete book of water healing, Contemporary Books, McGraw-Hill Companies, New York, 2001.

[51] M. Sinclair, Modern Hydrotherapy for the Massage Therapist, Lippincott Williams & Wilkins, Baltimore, 2008.

[52] F. De Lorenzo, M. Mukherjeem, Z. Kadziolaz, R. Sherwood, V.V. Kakkar, Central cooling effects in patients with hypercholesterolaemia, Clinical Science 95 (1998) 213–217.

[53] M. Gillett, Subclinical Thyroid Disease: Scientific Review and Guidelines for Diagnosis and Management, Journal of the American Medical Association 291 (2004) 228–238.

[54] A. Polmear (Ed.), Evidence-Based Diagnosis in Primary Care, Churchill Livingstone Elsevier, 2008, pp. 274–283.

[55] P.E. Sylvester, Nutritional aspects of Down's syndrome with special reference to the nervous system, British Journal of Psychiatry 145 (1984) 115–120.

[56] A. Luke, M. Sutton, D. Schoeller, N. Roizen, Nutrient intake and obesity in prepubescent children with Down syndrome, Journal of the American Dietetic Association 96 (1996) 1262–1267.

[57] R.E. Fleming, B.R. Bacon, Orchestration of iron homeostasis, N Engl J Med 352 (2005) 1741–1744.

[58] J. Yates, E. Logan, R. Stewart, Iron deficiency anaemia in general practice: clinical outcomes over three years and factors influencing diagnostic investigations, Postgrad Med J 80 (2004) 405–410.

[59] H. Hin, G. Bird, P. Fisher, et al., Coeliac disease in primary care: case finding study, BMJ 318 (1999) 164–167.

[60] M. Galloway, W. Smellie, Investigating iron status in microcytic anaemia, BMJ 333 (2006) 791–793.

[61] A.J. Stellon, S.E. Kenwright, Iron deficiency anaemia in general practice: presentations and investigations, Br J Clin Pract 51 (2) (1997) 78–80.

[62] D. Nardone, Usefulness of physical examination in detecting the presence or absence of anaemia, Arch Intern Med 150 (1) (1990) 201–204.

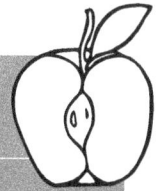

CHAPTER 8

Musculoskeletal system

Rheumatoid arthritis

Case history

Penny Chua, 29, has come to the clinic for help with pain and stiffness in her hands. Over the past 10 weeks Penny has noticed her hands have started to feel stiff, especially in the mornings. She tells you her hands are not sore or swollen, but some of her finger joints are warm to touch and tender when she presses them. The stiffness is there until mid-morning when her hands feel normal again. The stiffness affects both hands and the joint tenderness is not always in the same fingers. Penny also tells you her hands always feel cold.

Penny is a child protection officer and has been finding she is not really enjoying her work as much as she used to. She is wondering whether it is time for a career change but isn't sure what else she would like to do and whether she is willing to go back to study to retrain for another career.

Penny is more tired than she used to be and has lost some weight. She isn't sure why she has lost weight but thinks maybe it has something to do with how she is feeling about work. She thinks this may also be the reason she has been having problems falling asleep.

Penny tells you she feels she eats quite well but concedes her appetite is not what it was. She eats plenty of vegetables with her evening meal and eats chicken two or three times a week, fish once a week and red meat a couple of times a week. Once or twice a week she will have a vegetarian stir-fry or pasta dish. She enjoys fresh fruit and muesli for breakfast with yoghurt and milk and usually has a sandwich with egg, cheese or meat and salad for lunch unless she is out of the office when she will eat whatever is available. Penny loves her morning coffee when she gets to work, and has been drinking more coffee and tea during the day to help with her energy and motivation. She drinks about 500 mL of water each day and has a glass or two of wine with dinner three or four times per week.

Penny tells you she and her partner, Dianne, have been talking about whether or not to have a child together. Both their families are supportive, but they have experienced negative attitudes and behaviour from some people about their relationship, particularly regarding them having a child together. Penny tells you she sometimes feels angry and resentful about the difficulties involved with having a child, particularly when she thinks of some of the family situations she has seen as a child protection officer. She knows she and Dianne could provide a loving and supportive environment for a child and it seems unfair that it should be so much harder for them.

When you ask Penny about her family medical history, she tells you both her mother and her grandmother have arthritis and her grandmother's arthritis has worsened considerably as she has aged.

TABLE 8.1 **COMPLAINT** [1–11]	
Analogy: Skin of the apple	**Complaint:** Define the presenting complaint and symptoms; understand the complaint *Hand pain and stiffness*
AREAS OF INVESTIGATION AND EXAMPLE QUESTIONS	**CLIENT RESPONSES**
Onset *When did you first notice the problem in your hands?*	*About 2½ months ago.*
Timing *Can you feel the pain in your hands all or just some of the time?*	*I feel it pretty well most of the time. They're quite bad in the morning, but get better throughout the day. My hands always feel cold these days.*
Exacerbating factors *Is there anything that makes the pain worse?*	*First thing in the morning.*
Relieving factors *Is there anything that makes the pain better?*	*The pain improves by the middle of the morning.*
Location and radiation *Where do you feel the pain and stiffness?* *Does the pain radiate out from that spot?*	*In my finger joints, but it isn't always the same finger.* *It seems to stay in the same place until it eases off.*
Examination and inspection	Penny looks pale, and has pale palmar creases. There is tenderness of the proximal interphalangeal joints of both hands.

TABLE 8.2 **CONTEXT**	
Analogy: Flesh of the apple	**Context:** Put the presenting complaint into context to understand the disease
AREAS OF INVESTIGATION AND EXAMPLE QUESTIONS	**CLIENT RESPONSES**
Family health *Has anyone else in your family experienced similar symptoms?*	*Yes. My mum and grandmother both have arthritis. Gran's arthritis is really quite bad now.*

▶

▶

Trauma and pre-existing illness *Have you had any trauma to your hands in the past six months?*	No.
Recreational drug use *How much alcohol do you drink each week?* *Do you smoke?* *Do you ever take recreational drugs?*	Not very much, maybe one or two glasses of wine with dinner 3–4 times a week. No. No.
Functional disease *When your hand pain is worse in the mornings do you know if you slept with your arms raised?* (thoracic outlet syndrome)	I'm not sure, I will have to ask my partner if I do that.
Infection and inflammation *Do you have difficulty pinching or grasping bigger objects, opening jar tops or turning door knobs?* (osteoarthritis at base of thumb, rheumatoid arthritis)	When I get a bad flare up, it is hard to do things with my hands without causing pain.
Supplements and side effects of medication *Are you taking any supplements or medicines?*	Not at the moment.
Autoimmune disease *Have you noticed any skin rashes develop when you have your swollen hands?* (systemic lupus erythematosus – SLE)	No, my skin seems to be OK.
Stress and neurological disease *Do you experience nocturnal pain in your hands associated with numbness or pain in wrist, hand or forearm?* (carpal tunnel syndrome) *Have you experienced a sore neck or shoulder with weakness and limitation of movement when you have sore hands and fingers?* (nerve compression)	When my hands are swollen they can hurt during the night but I do not get numbness in my hands. I have been told a massage could be good for my back and neck because I'm really stiff, but my hands can be sore when my back feels OK.
Eating habits and energy *Tell me about your diet.*	Penny's diet consists of 2–3 chicken meals per week, 2 red meat meals, 1 fish meal and 1 vegetarian or pasta meal per week. She eats vegetables with each meal. Breakfast is usually muesli, fresh fruit, yoghurt and milk and lunch is usually a sandwich with some form of protein with salad. Her tea and coffee intake has increased recently and she has about 500 mL water daily.

TABLE 8.3 **CORE**	
Analogy: Core of the apple with the seed of ill health	**Core:** Holistic assessment to understand the client
AREAS OF INVESTIGATION AND EXAMPLE QUESTIONS	**CLIENT RESPONSES**
Emotional health *Do you ever feel sad, anxious or depressed?*	*Yes. Di, my partner, and I are thinking about starting a family. Some people are really negative about us as a couple and about us being parents. That really gets me down sometimes. When I think of the situations I see in my job, it is really unfair that people don't think Di and I would be good parents.*
Daily activities *Tell me about your daily routine.*	*I'm up around 6.30 and get to work usually by 8 or 8.30. Home again by about 6. Bedtime is usually around 10.30. On the weekends we spend time at the markets on Saturday morning and do things around the house in the afternoon. Sunday is usually spent catching up with family and friends.*
Stress release *How do you manage your stress?*	*Sometimes work can get quite stressful and also thinking about whether or not to have a child is making me a bit stressed. I try to talk through what is bothering me and then think about other things to reduce stress.*
Occupation *Do you enjoy your work?*	*I used to, not so much anymore. I'm thinking about going back to uni to do something else.*
Action needed to heal *If you could snap your fingers and have anything you need to help your symptoms improve, what would be your wish list?*	*Tell me what's going on with my hands. Give me some supplements or herbs to help.*
Long-term goals *Where do you see yourself in five years?*	*I'd like to be a parent, maybe also doing another job.*

TABLE 8.4 **PENNY'S SIGNS AND SYMPTOMS** [2, 6–8]	
Pulse	92 bpm
Blood pressure	127/81
Temperature	36.9°C
Respiratory rate	15 resp/min
Body mass index	22
Waist circumference	75.7 cm
Face	Pale and tired looking, pale conjunctiva, pale palmar creases; tenderness over proximal interphalangeal joints on both hands
Urinalysis	No abnormality detected (NAD)

▶

Results of medical investigations

No medical investigations have yet been carried out.

TABLE 8.5 **UNLIKELY DIAGNOSTIC CONSIDERATIONS** [2, 6–8, 10, 11, 13, 65]	
CONDITIONS AND CAUSES	WHY UNLIKELY
TRAUMA AND PRE-EXISTING ILLNESS	
Causal factor: **Trauma/ruptured tendons:** can cause pain in finger joints	Need to determine if Penny has experienced an injury to her hands recently; onset of pain would correlate with an injury and be aggravated by movement; joints would appear very red and swollen
INFECTION AND INFLAMMATION	
Dupuytren's contracture: tenosynovitis of flexors of fingers; fixed flexion contraction on the hand; tender fingers and can occur gradually on both hands	Pain felt in her palm at the base of the third and fourth digits; no visible contracture seen on the palms where the fingers bend towards the hand and cannot be flexed
Bacterial infection – staphylococci, TB, Borrelia **Fungal infection** **Viral infection:** rubella, mumps, hepatitis B All types of infection can cause fatigue and pain in fingers	Can present as mono-, oligo- and polyarthritis; self-limiting and resolves quickly; mild fever present
Septic arthritis: may not present with clear symptoms initially; *Staphylococcus aureus* most common cause	No fever; joint pain will develop over a couple of days; joints will appear very red and swollen
Palindromic rheumatism	Rare and short-lived form of arthritis in joints that become acutely painful, swollen and red and then resolves completely
Osteoarthritis: symptoms may be asymmetrical or symmetrical	Pain eases with rest due to the mechanical nature of the disease; distal interphalangeal joints are usually tender; hands will have a square appearance and there is crepitus on movement of the joint; often occurs in older age groups; stiffness can occur after resting but only for a few minutes and there will be pain on movement
Gout: crystal formation; pain in finger	Usually only affects a single joint; will develop quickly; the joint will appear very swollen and red

▶

Causal factor: **Referred arthritis/bursitis of shoulder:** pain in hand and fingers	No shoulder pain reported
ENDOCRINE/REPRODUCTIVE	
Diabetes: peripheral neuropathy and hand stiffness, lack of circulation, cold hands	Urinalysis NAD
AUTOIMMUNE DISEASE	
Autoimmune chronic hepatitis: Presents more commonly in young and middle-aged women with arthritis in small joints of the hand, low appetite and fatigue	No fever present; no jaundice or yellow sclera of the eyes

Case analysis

TABLE 8.6 **POSSIBLE DIFFERENTIAL DIAGNOSIS**		
Not ruled out by tests/investigations already done [2, 6–11, 64–68]		
CONDITION AND CAUSES	**WHY POSSIBLE**	**WHY UNLIKELY**
CANCER AND HEART DISEASE		
Primary or metastatic tumour	Pain in fingers; pain will be worse at rest	Usually deep boring pain
TRAUMA AND PRE-EXISTING ILLNESS		
Causal factor: **Postviral arthritis:** glandular fever, rheumatic fever, reactive arthritis	Fatigue and pain in fingers, Most often presents as polyarthritis involving more than 5 joints	Mild fever present; will have joint pain that moves to different areas over a period of days
FUNCTIONAL DISEASE		
Carpal tunnel syndrome: pain often in wrist, thumb, index and middle fingers; weakness in abduction of thumb and hypalgesia in the index finger [64, 67]	Pain and stiffness in hand; can occur in later stages of rheumatoid arthritis (RA); common in women; symptoms can occur at night; common to have nocturnal pain, will be felt in wrist and sometimes forearm	Hands will often look normal with no joint swelling; should be no pain experienced on palm of the hand
Raynaud's phenomenon/disease: when this condition appears as an underlying cause of another disease it is called 'phenomenon', otherwise this condition is known as Raynaud's disease	Discolouration of the fingertips due to sluggish blood flow	Extremely painful
Thoracic outlet syndrome	Hand pain worse on waking; numbness in hands	Usually only left hand and after arms are hyperabducted on waking; hands will feel weak
Fibromyalgia	Hands feel cold, stiff and condition is exacerbated by stress; sleep disorders	Will have widespread tender joints on pressure; usually diagnosed if has been present for more than 3 months

Causal factor: **Physiologic fatigue:** caused by depression, caffeine, alcohol, excess sleep, poor sleep due to uncomfortable mattress or pillow, being too hot or cold when trying to sleep, hunger during the night, excess exercise and intense emotions	Common to have delay in falling asleep	Symptoms may present for less than 14 days duration and not usually associated with changes in self-esteem, social difficulties or overall mood; diagnostic studies are within normal limits (this needs to be investigated further)
DEGENERATIVE AND DEFICIENCY		
Anaemia/anaemia of chronic disease: where the inflammatory cytokines seem to mediate a decreased release of iron from the bone marrow to developing red blood cells, causing decreased red cell survival; can be common in RA	Symptoms of anaemia include fatigue, insomnia and depression	
AUTOIMMUNE DISEASE		
Rheumatoid arthritis (RA)	Stiffness in the small joints of the hand, symmetrical presentation, improves with activity; symptoms of hand stiffness present for more than 6 weeks, stiffness is worse in the morning; fatigue and anaemia associated with symptoms; proximal interphalangeal joints tender; joints in hands can be warm and red; stiffness can be migratory and involve several joints; persistent pain; not usual for joints to appear red; symptoms are symmetrical	
Systemic lupus erythematosus (SLE)	Pain in hands not usual for joints to appear red; fatigue; symptoms are symmetrical	Intermittent painful episodes; hands will appear normal, no fever
Causal factor: **Overlap syndrome**	Symptoms of RA and SLE and Raynaud's	
STRESS AND NEUROLOGICAL DISEASE		
Causal factor: **Nerve compression** of the brachial plexus or cervical nerve and ulnar nerve [68]	Pain in hand and fingers	Tingling sensation that is localised to nerve distribution on the ulnar border; will often feel sharp shooting pain
Peripheral neuropathy	Can occur in RA	Weakness in fingers; numbness in fingers

General anxiety disorder (GAD)	Has been present for at least 6 months; anxiety disorder is often associated with loss or potential of a loss; weight loss, lack of sleep; feelings of irritation; person often complains of physical symptoms without thinking there may be a mental disorder; difficulties or delay in falling asleep is common	Ascertain whether Penny has experienced significant weight loss; if tension and stress have been overwhelming for at least 6 months; often associated with diarrhoea, tight chest, difficulty breathing; less common to experience frequent waking and early morning wakefulness as in depression
Mixed anxiety and depressive disorder	Depressive disorder often associated with an experience of loss; symptoms of fatigue, apathy, or intense sadness, insomnia; not enjoying work as much as she used to; angry and resentful about difficulties having a child	Can be associated with numerous physical complaints associated with depression such as restlessness, headaches, shortness of breath, gut or skin disorders; need to define if significant incapacity to continue daily activities for work
Causal factor: **Insomnia: primary**	Difficulty falling asleep, frequent waking during the night	Usually associated with no physical or emotional triggers
Causal factor: **Insomnia: secondary**	Due to chronic pain, anxiety or depression	

TABLE 8.7 **DECISION TABLE FOR REFERRAL** [2, 7–11, 13]		
COMPLAINT	**CONTEXT**	**CORE**
Referral for presenting complaint	Referral for all associated physical, dietary and lifestyle concerns	Referral for contributing emotional, mental, spiritual, metaphysical, lifestyle and constitutional factors
REFERRAL FLAGS	**REFERRAL FLAGS**	**REFERRAL FLAGS**
• Stiffness in hands that is persistent • Family history of arthritis • Common age group for women to develop RA	• Weight loss • Finger joints tender • Delayed sleep	• Anger/resentful over difficulties having a child
ISSUES OF SIGNIFICANCE	**ISSUES OF SIGNIFICANCE**	**ISSUES OF SIGNIFICANCE**
Nil	• Fatigue • Loss of appetite • Limited water intake • Excess coffee and tea intake	• Wanting a career change • Not sure if she wants to study for a new qualification • Employment as a child protection officer exposes Penny to cases of extreme child risk or abuse leading to the risk of burnout and depression/anxiety

REFERRAL DECISION	REFERRAL DECISION	REFERRAL DECISION
• Referral for medical investigation for cause of hand stiffness	• Assess diet and test for anaemia and nutritional imbalance	• Counselling about issues surrounding having a child • Career advisor

TABLE 8.8 **FURTHER INVESTIGATIONS THAT MAY BE NECESSARY** [2, 6, 8–11, 13, 65, 66]	
TEST/INVESTIGATION	**REASON FOR TEST/INVESTIGATION**
FIRST-LINE MEDICAL INVESTIGATIONS:	
Musculoskeletal physical examination	Assess bone, muscle or nerve pain, inflammatory or non-inflammatory arthritis
Tinel sign (tapping on medial nerve) and **phalen test** (flexing the wrist)	Carpal tunnel syndrome
Adson tests	Brachial plexus neuralgia
Cold response test	Raynaud's phenomenon
Nail fold capillary test	Raynaud's phenomenon
Full blood count	*Haemoglobin:* low; main function for red cell is carrying oxygen to tissues and returning CO_2 from tissues to lungs *Platelets:* high; the number of platelets (thrombocytes) gives information about efficiency of blood clotting ***Red cell indices:*** *MCV:* slightly low (indicates size of red blood cell) *MCH:* slightly low (indicates weight of red blood cell) *MCHC:* slightly low (indicates haemoglobin concentration in red blood cell)
Film comments	Film comments: microcytic hypochromic RBC *Microcytic* means the red blood cell is a small weight and generally these cells have less haemoglobin *Hypochromic* means the red blood cell has a deficiency in haemoglobin; the presence of anaemia with microcytosis and hypochromia does not necessarily indicate iron deficiency, although this is the most common cause; the commonest other causes are thalassaemia, sideroblastic anaemia and anaemia of chronic disease
Serum ferritin	*Raised* Can be raised in anaemia of chronic disease and sideroblastic anaemia; normal in thalassaemia

Serum iron levels	*Low* Low in anaemia of chronic disease
Total iron binding capacity	*Low* Low in anaemia of chronic disease, raised in iron deficiency anaemia; normal in sideroblastic anaemia and thalassaemia
ESR/CRP	*Raised* Indicates inflammation and possible infection
Rheumatoid factor	*Positive* Circulating autoantibodies, in inflammatory diseases such as RA and SLE, which have a portion of IgG as their antigen and self-aggregates into immune complexes that cause inflammation and joint damage; the most common reactive IgM molecule is rheumatoid factor
Antinuclear antibodies (ANA)	*Negative* An antibody that reacts against cellular nuclear material and is indicative of an autoimmune abnormality; this is very sensitive in detecting SLE, but not specific to this disease as it can be present in other inflammatory and autoimmune diseases
X-ray on left and right hands	Check if there are any fractures, joint or bone abnormalities, arthritis
Liver function test	Hepatitis
IF NECESSARY:	
MRI of the hands and cervical spine	Arthritis, tumour, bone abnormality, nerve entrapment
Electromyogram (EMG) and nerve conduction velocity test (NCV)	Carpal tunnel syndrome

Confirmed diagnosis

PENNY AND RHEUMATOID ARTHRITIS AND ANAEMIA OF CHRONIC DISEASE

Penny is a 29-year-old woman who presented to the clinic with a 10-week history of morning stiffness presenting in both her hands with tender proximal finger joints. Both her hands feel very cold and she is also experiencing symptoms of fatigue, weight loss, lack of appetite, difficulty falling asleep and she is drinking more coffee and tea to maintain daily energy. Penny is not enjoying her work and is now at a crossroads in her life, trying to decide whether she should change career and if so what she would do. During the consultation Penny expresses anger and resentment that she and her partner, Dianne, are experiencing difficulties in having a child of their own when they know what a wonderful home they could offer, especially when Penny has witnessed firsthand the terrible conditions in which some children grow up.

Because of Penny's persistent symptoms of stiff hands and her family history of arthritis, she was referred for immediate medical assessment. Penny returned with a confirmed diagnosis of **rheumatoid arthritis** and **anaemia of chronic disease**. This diagnosis has helped Penny understand why the stiffness in the small joints of both hands has lasted for more than six weeks. RA usually begins as a progressive peripheral arthritis that slowly develops over a few months. The most commonly affected areas are the small joints of the hand, wrist, feet, elbows, shoulders, knees and ankles. The joints have limitation of movement, are warm and tender and there can be evidence of muscle wasting. Soft tissue thickening around affected joints is common. Overall, morning joint stiffness with joint tenderness and symmetrical joint swelling are common characteristics of RA. Additional symptoms that may be present include fatigue, muscle weakness, anaemia, anorexia and weight loss.

RA is a common, chronic, persistently painful systemic disease producing symmetrical inflammatory polyarthritis and progressive joint damage that can cause severe disability in young people. The cause of the disease is unknown and toxic substances produced during the inflammatory process can lead to the destruction of cartilage. RA is three times more common in women and can begin at any age between the ages of 10 and 70, but most often begins between the ages of 30 and 40. The most likely hypothesis for the chronicity of the inflammatory process is a persistent foreign antigen, perhaps bacteria or virus, which is not destroyed or removed leading to systemic inflammation. Because premenopausal women are more likely to develop the condition than men, there seems to be a hormonal link to the disease.

Family history of RA is an influencing factor to developing the disease. There are several types of RA including short monoarticular attacks lasting up to 48 hours, transient and self-limiting episodes lasting up to 12 months similar to postviral arthritis, a remitting disease over several years or a chronic and persistent presentation that can cause more damage. Occasionally RA progresses rapidly resulting in significant damage within the span of just a few years.

General references used in this diagnosis: 2, 6–11, 65, 66

PRESCRIBED MEDICATION

Penny's doctor has prescribed oral NSAIDs and analgesic medication initially and, if symptoms persist, will consider prescribing other medication and referring Penny to a rheumatologist for assessment. Penny wants to try natural therapies first to see how much they can help before she takes any drugs. She will go back to her doctor for regular medical check-ups.

Anaemia of chronic disease will be treated by addressing the inflammatory process of RA rather than giving iron supplementation.

TABLE 8.9 **DECISION TABLE FOR TREATMENT (ONCE DIAGNOSIS IS CONFIRMED)**		
COMPLAINT	CONTEXT	CORE
Treatment for the presenting complaint and symptoms	Treatment for all associated symptoms	Treatment for mental, emotional, spiritual, constitutional, lifestyle issues and metaphysical considerations

TREATMENT PRIORITY	TREATMENT PRIORITY	TREATMENT PRIORITY
• Reduce requirement for anti-inflammatory medication via lifestyle, dietary, physical therapy, herbal and supplement recommendations • Dietary recommendations to reduce inflammation and prevent joint degeneration • Physical therapy suggestions to improve joint strength, flexibility and function • Recommendation for Penny to exercise regularly to maintain joint functionality • Herbal tea, tonic and tablets with anti-inflammatory, circulatory stimulant, antirheumatic and immunomodulatory action to help reduce inflammation and protect joints • Supplemental nutrients to reduce inflammation and improve symptoms, enhance cartilage synthesis and suppress progression of RA joint pathology **NB:** Penny's condition should be managed in collaboration with her doctor; if she experiences no improvement within 12 weeks or her symptoms worsen she should be encouraged to consider other treatment options; if Penny chooses to take prescribed medication from her GP or rheumatologist her herbal tea, tonic and tablets should be reviewed to ensure there are no negative interactions	• Dietary recommendations to identify and eliminate dietary antigens or aggravating foods • Dietary recommendations to increase intake of antioxidants and essential nutrients • Herbal tonic and tablets with immunomodulatory and antimicrobial action to address potential underlying infection • Herbal tea, tonic and tablets with digestive, silagogue, choleretic and cholagogue action to improve digestive function • Supplemental nutrients to modulate immunity, reduce allergic response, support gastrointestinal mucosa and normalise gastrointestinal permeability	• Recommendation for Penny to deal with her psychological and emotional issues through therapy • Recommendation for Penny to exercise regularly to improve her psychological health and stress response • Herbal tea, tonic and tablets with nervine and adrenal tonic action to support Penny's nervous system and stress response

Treatment aims

- Reduce joint pain, stiffness and inflammation [14, 15, 31, 61].
- Prevent disease progression and joint degeneration [14–16, 61].
- Support joint health and enhance proteoglycan and cartilage synthesis [15, 16, 63].
- Modulate Penny's immune response [14–16, 61].
- Enhance intestinal integrity and support optimal digestive health and function [14–16, 62].
- Identify and manage allergies or sensitivities [14–16].
- Identify and correct nutritional deficiencies [14–16].
- Enhance efficacy of conventional medications, reduce dosage and frequency required and minimise adverse drug side effects [14–16].

- Reduce oxidative stress [14–16, 61].
- Help Penny deal with psychological and emotional issues [15, 17] and support her stress response [17].

Lifestyle alterations/considerations

- Encourage Penny to work through her issues surrounding work and parenthood [15, 17]. A tailored cognitive behavioural therapy program may be beneficial [18].
- Penny will benefit from regular exercise to help improve her psychological health and stress response [20, 21]. Exercise is also likely to improve symptoms and maintain joint functionality [19, 22].

Dietary suggestions

- Identify and remove dietary triggers [14, 15, 31]. Commonly implicated foods are wheat and other gluten-containing grains, corn, dairy and food additives [14, 15, 31]. There is a correlation between food sensitivities and RA [14, 17, 28, 29, 31] and Penny may find particular benefit in avoiding allergenic foods [31].
- Encourage Penny to avoid foods from the solanaceae (nightshade) family: eggplant, capsicum, tomato, capsicum (peppers) and potato [14, 15]. They are implicated in promoting inflammation and pain in rheumatic diseases [30].
- Encourage Penny to increase consumption of foods containing omega-3 fatty acids [14, 15, 32, 33] and monounsaturated fats [32] while reducing consumption of omega-6 fatty acids [32] and saturated fats [14, 15, 16]. Reducing linoleic acid and arachidonic acid while increasing omega-3 and monounsaturated fats [32, 34] can enhance the anti-inflammatory action of omega-3 fatty acids [32, 33].
- Encourage Penny to avoid or reduce consumption of refined carbohydrates, sugar, red meat and animal fats [15, 31].
- Penny may find an uncooked vegan diet containing berries, fruit, vegetables, nuts, sprouts and germinated seeds is beneficial [14, 29]. If she feels a raw vegan diet will be difficult to maintain she should consume a mostly vegetarian antioxidant-rich whole-food diet that is high in fibre, whole grains (avoiding grains to which she is sensitive), legumes, vegetables, fruit, flavanoid-rich berries and cold-water fish [15, 29, 31, 34].
- Encourage Penny to eliminate coffee, tea and alcohol [14, 31, 35] and increase her water intake.
- Encourage Penny to drink fresh vegetable juices once or twice daily [31].

Physical treatment suggestions

- Hydrotherapy: moist heat packs to relieve stiffness and tenderness [15].
- Ice massage/cold packs for five minutes around joint to alleviate pain if Penny experiences an acute flare-up, followed by five-minute massage and repeat cycle for 20 minutes [15].
- For hands, a hot Epsom salt hand bath for 20 minutes will help ease the pain [54]. A heat compress on the hand with a plastic pad on top for 20 minutes is beneficial in cold weather [54, 55].
- Alternating hot (three minutes) and cold (30 seconds) hand bath locally to inflamed or painful joints for four rounds [54].
- Constitutional hydrotherapy [55–58].
- Full-body water-based exercise when the symptoms radiate to other joints in the body [59, 60].

- Penny is likely to benefit from exercises to strengthen muscles, increase range of movement and preserve joint function [15, 19]. High-intensity exercise therapy can improve functionality [15, 22].
- Penny may find massage therapy is beneficial to reduce symptoms and improve her stress response [23–25].
- Acupuncture may be beneficial to Penny [26, 27].

TABLE 8.10 **HERBAL FORMULA (1:2 LIQUID EXTRACTS)**		
HERB	**FORMULA**	**RATIONALE**
Devil's claw *Harpagophytum procumbens*	80 mL	Anti-inflammatory [36, 37]; analgesic [36, 37]; antirheumatic [37]; chondroprotective [36]; digestive bitter [37]; beneficial for degenerative musculoskeletal disorders [36]
Rehmannia *Rehmannia glutinosa*	70 mL	Anti-inflammatory [37, 41]; adrenal trophorestorative [37, 41]; beneficial to reduce inflammation in autoimmune disorders [37, 41]; may help protect against suppressive effects of corticosteroid and chemotherapy [37, 41]
St John's wort *Hypericum perforatum*	50 mL	Anti-inflammatory [36]; antidepressant [36, 37]; anxiolytic [36, 37]; analgesic [36]; antiretroviral [36, 37]; antimicrobial [36, 37]
Supply:	200 mL	Dose: 10 mL twice daily

TABLE 8.11 **HERBAL TABLET ALTERNATIVE**		
Anti-inflammatory herbal tablet to be taken in conjunction with herbal tonic if extra anti-inflammatory support is required; alternative to NSAIDs		
HERB	**DOSE PER TABLET**	**RATIONALE**
Boswellia *Boswellia serrata*	1.9 g	Anti-inflammatory [40, 45]; anti-arthritic [40, 45]; beneficial for RA in combination with turmeric, ginger and withania [46]
Turmeric *Curcuma longa*	2.0 g	Anti-inflammatory [36, 37, 44]; antimicrobial [36, 37]; antioxidant [36, 37]; choleretic [36, 37]; immunomodulator [36]; improves morning stiffness and joint swelling in RA [44]; prevents joint inflammation in RA when taken prior to the onset of joint inflammation [45]
Celery seed *Apium graveolens*	1.0 g	Anti-inflammatory [36, 40]; cholagogue [36]; antirheumatic [36, 40, 43]; sedative [43]
Ginger *Zingiber officinale*	300 mg	Circulatory stimulant [40, 43]; antirheumatic [40, 43]; silagogue [40]
Dose: 1–2 tablets 3 times daily		

TABLE 8.12 HERBAL TEA

Alternative to tea and coffee

HERB	FORMULA	RATIONALE
Passionflower *Passiflora incarnata*	1 part	Anxiolytic [36, 40]; sedative [36, 40]; traditionally used for insomnia [36]; beneficial for anxiety and nervous restlessness [36]
Willowbark *Salix alba*	2 parts	Anti-inflammatory [36, 38, 40]; analgesic [36, 38, 40]; antirheumatic [38, 40]
Prickly ash *Zanthoxylum americanum*	1 part	Circulatory stimulant [38, 40, 43]; antirheumatic [38, 40, 43]; silagogue [38, 40]
Peppermint *Mentha × piperita*	½ part	Mild sedative [36, 37]; antioxidant [36, 37]; enhances cognitive performance [36]; included to improve taste of the tea
Decoction: 1 tsp per cup – 1 cup 3 times daily		

TABLE 8.13 NUTRITIONAL SUPPLEMENTS

SUPPLEMENT AND DOSE	RATIONALE
Omega-3 fish oil 10,000 mg daily in divided doses [14, 36]	Anti-inflammatory [14, 15, 36, 39]; omega-3 supplementation improves clinical status in RA [42, 47] and can reduce the need for antirheumatic medication [47]; omega-3 supplementation reduces tender joints and morning stiffness in RA [32, 33, 42]; benefits of fish oil supplementation in RA are enhanced when an anti-inflammatory diet is followed [33]
1,200 mg **quercetin** and 750 mg **bromelain** daily in divided doses [14, 36]	Quercetin is anti-inflammatory [36, 39]; antioxidant [36, 39]; immunomodulator [36]; quercetin inhibits inflammatory enzymes, prostaglandins and leukotrienes [36], stabilises mast cells [36] and inhibits mast cell release of histamine [39]; Bromelain is an anti-inflammatory [15, 31, 39]; beneficial in auto-immune disease [39]; bromelain reduces inflammation and improves RA symptoms [15, 31, 48]
Glucosamine sulphate 1500 mg daily in divided doses [36]	Anti-inflammatory [36, 52]; chondroprotective [36, 50, 52]; stimulates proteoglycan synthesis and therefore cartilage repair [53]; can provide symptom relief [51] and may suppress progression of joint pathology in RA [52]; enhances health of gastrointestinal mucosa [49]

References

[1] N.J. Talley, S. O'Connor, Pocket Clinical Examination, third edn, Churchill Livingstone Elsevier, Australia, 2009.

[2] P. Kumar, C. Clark, Clinical Medicine, sixth edn, Elsevier Saunders, London, 2005.

[3] J. Silverman, S. Kurtz, J. Draper, Skills for Communicating with Patients, second edn, Radcliff Publishing, Oxford, 2000.

[4] R. Neighbour, The Inner Consultation: how to develop an effective and intuitive consulting style, Radcliff Publishing, Oxon, 2005.

[5] M. Lloyd, R. Bor, Communication Skills For Medicine, third edn, Churchill Livingstone Elsevier, Edinburgh, 2009.

[6] G. Douglas, F. Nicol, C. Robertson, Macleod's Clinical Examination, twelfth edn, Churchill Livingstone Elsevier, Edinburgh, 2009.

[7] J. Jamison, Differential Diagnosis for Primary Care, second edn, Churchill Livingstone Elsevier, London, 2006.

[8] A. Polmear (Ed.), Evidence-Based Diagnosis in Primary Care, Churchill Livingstone Elsevier, Edinburgh, 2008, pp. 274–283.

[9] R. Berkow, A.J. Fletcher, M.H. Beers, The Merck Manual, sixteenth edn, Merck Research Laboratories, Rathway, N.J, 1993 (later edition).

[10] R.H. Seller, Differential Diagnosis of Common Complaints, fifth edn, Saunders Elsevier, Philadelphia, 2007.

[11] R.D. Collins, Differential Diagnosis in Primary Care, fourth edn, Lippincott Williams & Wilkins, Philadelphia, 2008.

[12] K.D. Pagna, T.J. Pagna, Mosby's Diagnostic and Laboratory Test reference, third edn, Mosby, USA, 1997 (later edition).

[13] D. Peters, L. Chaitow, G. Harris, S. Morrison, Integrating Complementary Therapies in Primary Care. Churchill Livingstone, London, (2002)

[14] J. Jamison, Clinical Guide to Nutrition & Dietary Supplements in Disease Management, Churchill Livingstone, Edinburgh, 2003.

[15] J.E. Pizzorno, M.T. Murray, H. Joiner-Bey, The Clinicians Handbook of Natural Medicine, second edn, Churchill Livingstone, St Louis, 2008.

[16] H. Osiecki, The Physicians Handbook of Clinical Nutrition, seventh edn, Bioconcepts, Eagle Farm, 2000.

[17] K.O. Anderson, L.A. Bradley, L.D. Young, L.K. McDaniel, C.M. Wise, Rheumatoid Arthritis: Review of Psychological Factors Related to Etiology, Effects, and Treatment, Psychological Bulletin 98 (2) (1985) 358–387.

[18] A.W. Evers, F.W. Kraaimaat, P.L. van Riel, A.L. de Jong, Tailored cognitive-behavioral therapy in early rheumatoid arthritis for patients at risk: a randomized controlled trial, Pain 100 (2002) 141–153.

[19] T.P. Vliet Vileland, Rehabilitation of people with rheumatoid arthritis, Best Practice & Research Clinical Rheumatology 17 (5) (2003) 847–861.

[20] A.F. Jorm, H. Christensen, K.M. Griffiths, R.A. Parslow, B. Rodgers, K.A. Blewitt, Effectiveness of complementary and self-help treatments for anxiety disorders, Medical Journal of Australia 181 (7) (2004) S29–S46.

[21] A. Byrne, G.D. Byrne, The effect of exercise on depression, anxiety and other mood states: A review, J Psychosom Res 37 (6) (1993) 565–574.

[22] Z. de Jong, M. Munneke, A.H. Zwinderman, H.M. Kroon, A. Jansen, K.H. Ronday, et al., Is a Long-Term High-Intensity Exercise Program Effective and Safe in Patients With Rheumatoid Arthritis? Arthritis & Rheumatism 48 (9) (2003) 2415–2424.

[23] T.F. Field, M. Hernandez-Rief, S. Seligman, J. Krasnegor, W. Sunshine, Juvenile Rheumatoid Arthritis: Benefits from Massage Therapy, Journal of Pediatric Psychology 22 (5) (1997) 607–617.

[24] C.A. Moyer, J. Rounds, J.W. Hannum, A Meta-Analysis of Massage Therapy Research, Psychological Bulletin 130 (1) (2004) 3–18.

[25] T. Field, G. Robinson, F. Scafidi, R. Nawrocki, A. Goncalves, Massage therapy reduces anxiety and enhances EEG pattern of alertness and math computations, International Journal of Neuroscience 86 (1996) 197–205.

[26] J. David, S. Townsend, R. Sathanathan, S. Kriss, C.J. Dore, Effect of acupuncture on patients with rheumatoid arthritis: a randomised, placebo-controlled cross-over study, Rheumatology 38 (1999) 864–869.

[27] X. Liu, L. Sun, J. Xiao, S. Yin, C. Liu, Q. Li, H. Li, et al., Effect of acupuncture and point-injection treatment on immunologic function in rheumatoid arthritis, Journal of Traditional Chinese Medicine 13 (3) (1993) 174–178.

[28] J.A. Jackson, H.D. Riordan, R. Hunninghake, S. Neathery, Joint and Muscle Pain, Various Arthritic Conditions and Food Sensitivities, Journal of Orthomolecular Medicine 13 (3) (1998) 168–172.

[29] L.K. Stamp, M.J. James, L.G. Cleland, Diet and Rheumatoid Arthritis: A Review of the Literature, Seminars in Arthritis and Rheumatism 35 (2005) 77–94.

[30] C.J. Henderson, R.S. Panush, Diets, dietary supplements, and nutritional therapies in rheumatic diseases, in J. Jamison, Clinical Guide to Nutrition & Dietary Supplements in Disease Management, Churchill Livingstone, Edinburgh, 2003.

[31] A.R. Gaby, Alternative Treatments for Rheumatoid Arthritis, Alternative Medicine Review 4 (6) (1999) 392–402.

[32] M.J. James, L.G. Cleland, Dietary n-3 Fatty Acids and Therapy for Rheumatoid Arthritis, Seminars on Arthritis and Rheumatism 27 (1997) 85–97.

[33] O. Adam, C. Beringer, T. Kless, C. Lemmen, A. Adam, M. Wiseman, P. Adam, et al., Anti-inflammatory effects of a low arachidonic acid diet and fish oil in patients with rheumatoid arthritis, Rheumatology International 23 (2003) 27–36.

[34] L. Sköldstam, L. Hagfors, G. Johansson, An experimental study of a Mediterranean diet intervention for patients with rheumatoid arthritis, Annals of Rheumatic Disease 62 (2003) 208–214.

[35] R.H. Martin, The role of nutrition and diet in rheumatoid arthritis, Proceedings of the Nutrition Society 57 (1998) 231–234.

[36] L. Braun, M. Cohen, Herbs & Natural Supplements: An evidence based guide, second edn, Elsevier, Sydney, 2007.

[37] S. Mills, K. Bone, Principles & Practice of Phytotherapy; Modern Herbal Medicine, Churchill Livingstone, Edinburgh, London, 2000.

[38] British Herbal Medicine Association, British Herbal Pharmacopoeia, BHMA, 1983.

[39] H. Osiecki, The Nutrient Bible, seventh edn, BioConcepts Publishing, Eagle Farm, 2008.

[40] S. Mills, K. Bone, The Essential Guide to Herbal Safety, Churchill Livingstone, St Louis, 2005.

[41] K. Bone, Clinical Applications of Chinese and Ayurvedic Herbs: Monographs for the Western Herbal Practitioners, Phytotherapy Press, Warwick, 1996.

[42] D. Volker, P. Fitzgerald, G. Major, M. Garg, Efficacy of fish oil concentrate in the treatment of rheumatoid arthritis, Journal of Rheumatology 27 (10) (2000) 2343–2346.

[43] D. Hoffman, The New Holistic Herbal, Element Books Ltd, Shaftesbury, Dorset, 1990.

[44] N. Chainani-Wu, Safety and Anti-Inflammatory Activity of Curcumin: A Component of Turmeric (Curcuma longa), The J Altern Complement Med 9 (1) (2003) 161–168.

[45] D. Khanna, G. Sethi, K.S. Ahn, M.J. Pandey, A.B. Kunnumakkara, G. Sung, et al., Natural products as a gold mine for arthritis treatment, Current Opinion in Pharmacology 7 (2007) 344–351.

[46] A. Chopra, P. Lavin, B. Patwardhan, D. Chitre, Randomized Double Blind Trial of an Ayurvedic Plant Derived Formulation for Treatment of Rheumatoid Arthritis, The Journal of Rheumatology 27 (6) (2000) 1365–1372.

[47] P. Geusens, C. Wouters, J. Nijs, Y. Jiang, J. Dequeker, Long-term effect of omega-3 fatty acid supplementation in active rheumatoid arthritis, Arthritis and Rheumatism 37 (6) (1994) 824–829.

[48] A.F. Walker, R. Bundy, S.M. Hicks, R.W. Middleton, Bromelain reduces mild acute knee pain and improves well-being in a dose-dependent fashion in an open study of otherwise healthy adults, Phytomedicine 9 (2002) 681–686.

[49] S. Salvatore, R. Heuschkel, S. Tomlin, et al., A pilot study of N-acetylglucosamine, a nutritional substrate for glycosaminoglycan synthesis, in paediatric chronic inflammatory bowel disease, Aliment Pharmacol Ther 14 (2000) 1567–1579.

[50] A.R. Shikman, D. Amiel, D. D'Lima, S.B. Hwang, C. Hu, A. Xu, et al., Chondroprotective activity of N-acetylglucosamine in rabbits with experimental osteoarthritis, Annals of Rheumatic Disease 64 (2005) 89–94.

[51] H. Nakamura, K. Masuko, K. Yudoh, Effects of glucosamine administration on patients with rheumatoid arthritis, Rheumatology International 27 (2007) 213–218.

[52] J. Huan, S. Suguro, S. Hirano, K. Sakamoto, I. Nagaoka, Preventive actions of a high dose of glucosamine on adjuvant arthritis in rats, Inflammation Research 54 (2005) 127–132.

[53] C. Bassleer, L. Rovati, P. Franchimont, Stimulation of proteoglycan production by glucosamine sulfate in chondrocytes isolated from human osteoarthritic articular cartilage in vitro, Osteoarthritis and Cartilage 6 (1998) 427–434.

[54] M. Sinclair, Modern Hydrotherapy for the Massage Therapist, Lippincott Williams & Wilkins, Baltimore, 2008.

[55] L. Chaitow, Hydrotherapy, water therapy for health and beauty, Element, Dorset, 1999.

[56] W. Boyle, A. Saine, Lectures in Naturopathic Hydrotherapy, Eclectic Medical Publications, Oregon, 1988.

[57] J. Geytenbee, Evidence for effective hydrotherapy, Physiotherapy 88 (9) (2002) 514–529.

[58] L.M. Watrous, Constitutional hydrotherapy: from nature cure to advanced naturopathic medicine, Journal of Naturopathic Medicine 7 (2) (1997) 72–79.

[59] D.F. Fernandes de Melo Vitorino, L. Bizari Can de Carvalho, G. Fernandes do Prado, Hydrotherapy and conventional physiotherapy improve total sleep time and quality of life of fibromyalgia patients: Randomized clinical trial, Sleep Medicine 7 (2006) 293–296.

[60] J.P. O'Hare, A. Heywood, L.G. Summerhayes, et al., Observations on the effects of immersion in Bath spa water, British Medical Journal 291 (1985) 1747–1751.

[61] G. Firestein, Evolving concepts of rheumatoid arthritis, Nature 423 (2003) 356–361.

[62] L. Cordain, L. Toohey, M. Smith, M. Hickey, Modulation of immune function by dietary lectins in rheumatoid arthritis, British Journal of Nutrition 83 (2000) 207–217.

[63] S.R. Goldring, Pathogenesis of bone and cartilage destruction in rheumatoid arthritis, Rheumatology 42 (S2) (2003) ii11–ii16.

[64] T. Guidotti, Occupational repetitive strain injury, Am Fam Physician 45 (1992) 585–592.

[65] A. Mies Richie, M. Francis, Diagnostic approach to polyarticular joint pain, Am Fam Physician 68 (6) (2003) 1151–1160.

[66] K.P. Machold, V. Nell, T. Stamm, D. Aletaha, J.S. Smolen, Early Rheumatoid Arthritis, Current Opinion in Rheumatology 18 (3) (2006) 282–288.

[67] C. D'Arcy, S. McGee, Does this patient have carpal tunnel syndrome? JAMA 283 (2000) 3110–3117.

[68] S. Ferry, A. Silman, T. Pritchard, et al., The association between different patterns of hand symptoms and objective evidence of median nerve compression, Arthritis Rheum 41 (1998) 720–724.

Fibromyalgia

Case history

Corrine Devries has come to the clinic to get help for an ongoing problem with muscle aches and fatigue. Corrine is 44 years old and married with three boys in their teens. She recently returned to university to upgrade her nursing qualifications with the aim of returning to the workforce. Before having children Corrine enjoyed working as a nurse and is looking forward to restarting her career. Corrine has dedicated herself to her family for the past 20 years but promised herself she would return to nursing one day. In recent years the burden of parenting has fallen mostly on her – her husband's career as an engineer with a large multinational company can take him away from home for weeks or months at a time.

Corrine loves to be active and is finding her muscle aches mentally and physically debilitating. The muscle pain usually starts as a feeling of stiffness that evolves into a low-grade ache, that can suddenly become acutely painful. The pain moves from place to place, sometimes in her neck and shoulders and then in her lower back and sometimes even in her thighs. When her husband is at home the pain disappears and she feels very well; however, when he leaves again the pain returns and she has problems sleeping. Corrine has also noticed her digestion is affected. She can have symptoms of diarrhoea or constipation and experience significant bloating. The pain leaves her feeling extremely tired and some days she just stays in bed and sleeps all day.

Corinne doesn't think she is stressed; however, when you ask her about her family she tells you that her relationship with her children (all in their mid to late teens) is strained, and she feels they need their father to be around more often.

Corrine has tried massage therapy, which improves the muscle aches temporarily. She has noticed if the massage room is not warm enough she leaves feeling worse than when she arrived.

Corrine recently went to the doctor and had some blood tests in an attempt to find the cause of her pain. All tests came back normal. She is desperate to find out what is causing her pain and to get herself back on track. A fellow nursing student suggested Corrine see a complementary therapist to see if a holistic approach could alleviate her symptoms.

TABLE 8.14 **COMPLAINT** [1–9]	
Analogy: Skin of the apple	**Complaint:** Define the presenting complaint and symptoms; understand the complaint *Muscle pain and fatigue*
AREAS OF INVESTIGATION AND EXAMPLE QUESTIONS	**CLIENT RESPONSES**
Onset *How long have you had these symptoms?*	*Probably for more than a year, on and off. It seems to be getting worse.*
Timing *When do you experience the symptoms?*	*They can come on quite suddenly, always when my husband is away.*
Exacerbating factors *Does anything make it worse?*	*Cold weather seems to, also if I've been very busy and doing a lot of physical work.*

▶

| Relieving factors
Does anything make it better? | *Warmth and rest. Massage helps sometimes. Also my husband being home.* |
| Location
Where do you experience the pain? | *It can occur in a few places, neck and back sometimes my lower back and legs.* |

TABLE 8.15 **CONTEXT**	
Analogy: Flesh of the apple	**Context:** Put the presenting complaint into context to understand the disease
AREAS OF INVESTIGATION AND EXAMPLE QUESTIONS	CLIENT RESPONSES
Recreational drug use *How much alcohol do you drink in a week?* *Do you smoke?*	*Not a lot, just a couple of glasses usually. No.*
Functional disease *Does the muscle ache always move around the body and is most often associated with fatigue?* (fibromyalgia)	*Yes, always this pattern.*
Infection and inflammation *Did you have a virus or influenza before your symptoms started?* *Do you experience early morning stiffness that wears off after a couple of hours of activity?* (inflammatory arthritis)	*I can't remember. Possibly.* *I can be sore in the morning, but it does not tend to wear off with movement.*
Supplements and side effects of medication *Are you taking any supplements or medicines?*	*Just a multivitamin and anti-inflammatories when the pain is bad.*
Endocrine/reproductive *Tell me about your menstrual cycle.*	Corrine describes a regular 28-day cycle with a bleed lasting about 4 days. No pain or discomfort is experienced. Some emotional fragility a couple of days before her period starts.
Stress and neurological disease *Have you developed upper arm, leg and shoulder weakness associated with muscle wasting?* (motor neuron disease)	*I haven't noticed losing weight or muscle on my arms or legs, but I can feel very weak at times and like I have no strength to lift things.*
Eating habits and energy *Tell me about your diet.*	Corrine has a mostly vegetarian diet. She doesn't eat red meat and has a small amount of chicken or fish about 3 times a week. She describes her main weaknesses as chocolate and coffee.

TABLE 8.16 **CORE**	
Analogy: Core of the apple with the seed of ill health	**Core:** Holistic assessment to understand the client
AREAS OF INVESTIGATION AND EXAMPLE QUESTIONS	**CLIENT RESPONSES**
Support systems *Do you get much support when you're on your own?*	*If I really need help I can ask my sister or friends, but I prefer not to.*
Emotional health *Do you ever feel anxious or depressed?*	*Sometimes, particularly when my husband is away.*
Stress release *How do you deal with your stress?*	*If I have the energy and I'm not in too much pain I go to the gym. Otherwise I use chocolate therapy!*
Home life *What are things like for you at home?*	*Up and down. Things can get a little strained with the boys now they're in their teens. It's much harder when my husband is away and I have to deal with them on my own.*
Action needed to heal *What do you feel you need to heal?*	*I'm not sure. Maybe there are some herbs or vitamins that can help.*
Long-term goals *Tell me about your long-term goals.*	*I'm looking forward to getting back into nursing. I think it would be good to be out of the house and be able to focus on something other than my family.*

TABLE 8.17 **CORRINE'S SIGNS AND SYMPTOMS**	
Pulse	86 bpm
Blood pressure	130/75
Temperature	36.7°C
Respiratory rate	17 resp/min
Body mass index	23
Waist circumference	78 cm
Face	Strained look and pale
Urinalysis	No abnormality detected (NAD)

TABLE 8.18 RESULTS OF MEDICAL INVESTIGATIONS [4, 7–10]

TEST/INVESTIGATION	RESULT
Rheumatoid factor (RH factor): in inflammatory diseases such as rheumatoid arthritis; IgG antibodies produced by lymphocytes in membranes act as antigens, which then react with IgG and IgM antibodies to produce immune complexes that cause inflammation and joint damage; the reactive IgM molecule is RH factor	NAD
ESR (erythrocyte sedimentation rate): indicates inflammation in general	NAD
CRP (C-reactive protein): if raised it could be because of infection or inflammation, look to the full blood count to confirm this	NAD
Full blood count Anaemia, infection, inflammation	NAD
Thyroid function test	NAD
Calcium and alkaline phosphatase	NAD
Creatine kinase	NAD

TABLE 8.19 UNLIKELY DIAGNOSTIC CONSIDERATIONS [4, 6–10, 17, 73]

CONDITIONS AND CAUSES	WHY UNLIKELY
FUNCTIONAL DISEASE	
Myopathy: disease of the voluntary muscles	Creatine kinase not raised
Osteomalacia/hypercalcaemia: metabolic bone disease causing generalised aches and pains	Calcium not raised and alkaline phosphatase not raised
DEGENERATIVE AND DEFICIENCY	
Anaemia	Full blood count NAD
INFECTION AND INFLAMMATION	
Bacterial infection: e.g. *Yersinia enterocolitica, Escherichia coli, Shigella, Staphylococcal enterocolitis*, ileocaecal TB; diarrhoea is the main symptom; may cause ulceration and inflammation	Full blood count NAD; usually self-limiting and acute in duration between 1 and 10 days depending on bacterial toxin; violent vomiting can be associated; no bloody diarrhoea reported
Viral infection: retrovirus, hepatitis; diarrhoea, tired, nausea, fatigue, weight loss; generalised aches and pains	Full blood count NAD, no fever present; no history or signs of jaundice; check if stools are pale; no fever
Polymyositis: skeletal muscle inflammation that is more often in women, causing weak proximal muscles, widespread muscle weakness and muscle wasting	Rare disease; creatine kinase and ESR not elevated; full blood count revealed no anaemia, which can be associated with polymyositis
Polymyalgia rheumatica: common to present as stiffness in shoulder and pelvic areas	ESR not raised

▶

▶

Inflammatory bowel syndrome: diarrhoea, often associated with arthritic symptoms of generalised aches and pains	ESR and CRP not raised
Gastroenteritis: abdominal pain, diarrhoea, nausea and vomiting	Associated with vomiting, fever; check if Corrine has experienced generalised crampy abdominal pain; no low-grade fever; acute gastritis usually self-limiting and less than a week
AUTOIMMUNE DISEASE	
Rheumatoid arthritis: autoimmune inflammatory disorder	ESR not raised; full blood count revealed no anaemia, which can be associated with RA
Systemic lupus erythematosus (SLE): widespread aches, inflammatory autoimmune disorder	ESR, CRP not raised indicating no inflammation; full blood count normal indicating no excess antibody reaction in the body
ENDOCRINE/REPRODUCTIVE	
Hypothyroidism: fatigue, general muscle aches and pains, depression, worse for the cold	Thyroid function test NAD

Case analysis

TABLE 8.20 **POSSIBLE DIFFERENTIAL DIAGNOSIS**		
Not ruled out by tests/investigations already done [4, 6–12, 17, 62–76]		
CONDITIONS AND CAUSES	**WHY POSSIBLE**	**WHY UNLIKELY**
ALLERGIES AND IRRITANTS		
Causal factor: **Food intolerance/ allergy** [70]	Fatigue, depression, possible dietary changes when husband is away contributes to feeling fatigued	Need to gain more insight into Corrine's diet when her husband is at home and when he is away
Causal factor: **Lactose intolerance**	Diarrhoea	Corinne has not mentioned symptoms developing after eating particular foods; she has not mentioned significant episodes of abdominal pain
TRAUMA AND PRE-EXISTING ILLNESS		
Causal factor: **Physiological depression: postviral infection**	Depression, fatigue	Need to determine whether Corrine has had viral symptoms in the past 6 months
RECREATIONAL DRUG USE		
Causal factor: **Drug or alcohol abuse**	Digestive disorders, missing husband when he is away, strain with teenage children; not being able to be physically active due to aches and pains, fatigue and sleeping during the day	

▶

FUNCTIONAL DISEASE		
Fibromyalgia: pain in axial skeleton with tender points that has persisted for more than 3 months [70, 71, 74–76]	Pain begins with stiffness, then an ache all over that changes in location, fatigue, irritable bowel symptoms, difficulty sleeping; normal laboratory results rule out organic reasons for symptoms; can be worse from being in cold and with depression	
Chronic fatigue syndrome: fatigue for at least 6 months that has no physical cause, psychoses, bipolar affective disorder, eating disorder or organic brain disease [65–67, 72]	Severe disabling fatigue that affects both mental and physical functioning for at least 6 months; sleeping more, feelings of depression, social withdrawal, crying spells	Need to determine whether Corrine experiences muscular and mental fatigue for at least 24 hours after exertion before some level of recovery occurs; need to determine whether fatigue improves during the day; need to determine if Corrine experiences at least two neurological/cognitive manifestations of chronic fatigue syndrome such as impaired concentration and muscle weakness
Irritable bowel syndrome	Constipation alternating with diarrhoea; stress	Corinne does not mention abdominal pain as a predominant symptom
Causal factor: **Insomnia**	Fibromyalgia sufferers commonly experience difficulty sleeping, which is often attributed to depression	Need to determine if Corrine has difficulty falling asleep, frequent waking during the night and early morning wakefulness
Causal factor: **Physiologic fatigue**	Can be caused by depression, caffeine, alcohol, excess sleep, intense emotions; recent diagnostic studies are within normal limits	Symptoms present for less than 14 days and not usually associated with changes in self-esteem, social difficulties or overall mood
Causal factor: **Functional diarrhoea**	Common in times of stress; usually associated with ongoing fatigue	Need to check if the abdominal pain is associated with diarrhoea; bowel motions are watery and occur first thing in morning with no more passing during the day; bowel motions may only occur after eating food
DEGENERATIVE AND DEFICIENCY		
Causal factor: **Organic fatigue**	Tired, sleep disturbances, no major physical abnormalities	Shorter duration than functional fatigue; need to determine if the feeling of fatigue worsens during the day

INFECTION AND INFLAMMATION		
Osteoarthritis	Pain in many joints, ESR CRP, RH factor can be negative; more common in women	Usually develops in older age groups and shows signs of limited range of movement, bony swellings and instability of joints; not necessarily associated with severe fatigue; need to check Corrine's family history as it can be congenital and begin at an early age
Candidiasis	Diarrhoea, abdominal distension or feeling significant fatigue	No reports of itchy or irritating vaginal discharge
Causal factor: *Helicobacter pylori*	Diarrhoea, bloating; can develop due to increase stress and anxiety	Does not usually have diarrhoea alternating with constipation
SUPPLEMENTS AND SIDE EFFECTS OF MEDICATION		
Causal factor: **Supplement or food additive abuse:** excess vitamin C or magnesium?	Diarrhoea	
STRESS AND NEUROLOGICAL DISEASE		
Type 1: major (clinical) depression – unipolar affective disorder	Can be moderate or severe depression; people often describe symptoms in physical terms; common for fibromyalgia and depression to be linked; misses husband when he is away; sleeps all day when in pain, experiences insomnia and significant fatigue; delayed sleep onset, lack of appetite, can be aggravated by certain conditions and situations that provoke depression; associated symptoms of lack of interest in daily activities, constipation and vague aches and pains are common	Need to determine if Corrine has at least five symptoms of depression for more than 2 weeks and cause considerable incapacity with daily activities; need to define if feel worse in the morning with sense of apprehension; need to determine if Corrine experiences early-morning wakefulness (common); frequent awakening during the night is less common
Type 2: minor depression	Can be mild or moderate depression; common for fibromyalgia and depression to be linked; misses husband when away	Need to show 2–4 symptoms of depression that have lasted at least 2 weeks
Dysthymia: mild depressive illness	Could be experiencing 'double depression' if Corinne has had intermittent periods of depression in the past; symptoms include tiredness, lack of interest in life, low mood; Corrine feels better when her husband is home	Lasts intermittently for 2 years or more; need to determine if Corrine has had a tendency to have episodes of feeling low

Mixed anxiety and depressive disorder: depressive disorder often associated with an experience of loss; symptoms of fatigue, apathy, or intense sadness	Corrine has mentioned significant incapacity to continue daily activities for work and family when symptoms are bad and her husband is away; numerous physical complaints associated with depression such as restlessness, headaches, insomnia, shortness of breath, gut or skin disorders	
Hyperventilation syndrome: functional breathing concern (causes include increased CO_2, fatigue, muscle pain, digestive complaints); habitual patterns of breathing are developed to keep CO_2 levels low that leads to anxiety-provoking consequences	Significant muscle pain or fatigue; shortness of breath, breathing quickly; hyperventilation syndrome can be a consequence of chronic anxiety or irritability	
Causal factor: **Anxiety state**	Family, career and lifestyle stresses; can experience chronic pain that is felt all over the body	Usually pain is widespread in anxiety states alone and not associated with specific tender trigger points; however, anxiety can be concurrently associated with fibromyalgia

Working diagnosis

CORRINE AND PRIMARY FIBROMYALGIA SYNDROME – MYOFASCIAL PAIN SYNDROME

Corrine is a 44-year-old woman who is married with three teenage boys. Recently she has returned to tertiary studies in order to restart her nursing career, something she is very excited about. However, Corrine is experiencing debilitating symptoms that may interfere with her long-term goal of gaining her nursing degree and returning to work. Corrine's husband frequently works away from home for extended periods. During these times Corrine experiences symptoms of muscle aches and pains and extreme fatigue. The pain can move to all areas of the body and can become so debilitating that she has to go to bed and sleep all day. This is most distressing to Corrine as she likes to be physically active. When the whole family is reunited the symptoms disappear and her life feels normal again. Corrine often experiences significant tension with the boys and when her symptoms are aggravated she can experience gastrointestinal disturbances along with her muscular pains.

It is likely that Corrine has developed **primary fibromyalgia syndrome**. This is a functional condition of the voluntary muscles that gives rise to widespread pain stemming from muscles and their insertion points, tendons, ligaments and other white connective tissue. The term 'myalgia' means muscle pain. Fibromyalgia is a widespread chronic musculoskeletal pain of the axial skeleton (cervical, thoracic spine, anterior chest or lower back) that has persisted for more than 3 months. The widespread pain will be felt over all four quadrants of the body and, although it travels, pain is usually experienced consistently in particular locations. The perception of pain allegedly involves sensory, emotional and cognitive processing in the brain. The pain can present as stiffness initially with a frequent ache that comes on gradually and then can become very acute. Two features of fibromyalgia include the sensation of pain not associated with diseased organs and very tender trigger points across the body. For fibromyalgia to be diagnosed more than five and up to 18 tender points need to be confirmed on the body. More recent opinion on diagnosis questions whether fibromyalgia should better be understood as unexplained widespread pain and that the number of tender points indicate the severity rather than the actuality of the condition. Tender points do not refer pain in the typical way a trigger point does and the number of painful points can vary from day to day. The pain is often aggravated by the cold, mechanical trauma, fatigue and emotional stress. Females are more likely to experience this pain, or are more likely to report the symptoms of fibromyalgia than men. People who experience fibromyalgia often do not sleep well and lack non-rapid eye movement sleep. The muscles often affected are occiput, lower back, neck, shoulders, thorax, gluteal region and thighs. The condition is often linked with irritable bowel syndrome and is considered psychogenic in nature. There are studies that suggest that fibromyalgia syndrome has a genetic predisposition associated with the condition, and the syndrome is likely to develop after a traumatic/viral/infection event [12].

General references used in this diagnosis: 4, 6–12, 66, 69–71, 74, 75

TABLE 8.21 **DECISION TABLE FOR TREATMENT PRIOR TO REFERRAL**		
COMPLAINT	**CONTEXT**	**CORE**
Treatment for the presenting complaint and symptoms	Treatment for all associated symptoms	Treatment for mental, emotional, spiritual, constitutional, lifestyle issues and metaphysical considerations
TREATMENT PRIORITY	**TREATMENT PRIORITY**	**TREATMENT PRIORITY**
• Herbal tonic, tablets or tea with anti-inflammatory, analgesic, adaptogenic and tonic actions • Nutritional supplements to help reduce pain and increase energy levels • Physical therapies to help reduce pain levels	• Dietary recommendations to improve digestive health • Dietary recommendations to increase intake of essential nutrients and antioxidants • Nutritional supplements to improve digestive function and energy production	• Herbal tonic, tablets or tea with anxiolytic and adaptogenic action to support nervous system, stress response and reduce anxiety levels • Physical therapy recommendations to help reduce anxiety and stress levels • Physical therapy suggestions to improve sleep

TABLE 8.22 **DECISION TABLE FOR REFERRAL** [4, 7–9, 10, 13]		
COMPLAINT	**CONTEXT**	**CORE**
Referral for presenting complaint	Referral for all associated physical, dietary and lifestyle concerns	Referral for contributing emotional, mental, spiritual, metaphysical, lifestyle and constitutional factors
REFERRAL FLAGS	**REFERRAL FLAGS**	**REFERRAL FLAGS**
• Unexplained and undiagnosed muscle pain • Bed rest provides no pain relief	• Periods of extreme fatigue • Sleep disturbance that impairs daily functions	• Diminished interest/capability to keep up with daily activities when the symptoms are aggravated and her husband is away • Corrine may not feel in control of the choices being made in her lifestyle • Corrine is feeling overwhelmed with life
ISSUES OF SIGNIFICANCE	**ISSUES OF SIGNIFICANCE**	**ISSUES OF SIGNIFICANCE**
Nil	• Bloating, constipation and diarrhoea, indicating impaired digestive function and nutrient absorption • Potential for dietary or environmental allergies or sensitivities to be contributing to Corrine's problems • Impaired energy metabolism	• Strained relationship with teenage children • Emotional stress may affect her goal of completing her studies and gaining a qualification in nursing • Not being as physically active as she would like when the symptoms are acute
REFERRAL DECISION	**REFERRAL DECISION**	**REFERRAL DECISION**
• Refer to a GP for a musculoskeletal examination and trigger-point evaluation	• Medical investigations for diarrhoea • Medical and dietary investigations for food allergies	• Counselling to assess and support Corrine's mental health status due to physical, emotional and environmental stressors • Support to continue her studies and cope with daily activities

TABLE 8.23 **FURTHER INVESTIGATIONS THAT MAY BE NECESSARY** [4, 6, 8–11, 76]	
TEST/INVESTIGATION	**REASON FOR TEST/INVESTIGATION**
FIRST-LINE INVESTIGATIONS:	
Musculoskeletal examination of trigger points: trigger-point test in areas of localised soft-tissue tenderness in the dorsal spine, interscapular region, base of the neck, over both sacroiliac joints, over the elbows and the medial side of the knee	Fibromyalgia
Abdominal examination: guarding, rebound tenderness, palpation, abnormal pulsations (auscultation)	Assess abdominal distension, tenderness, hyperactive bowel sounds

►

▶

Hydrogen breath test: to detect bacterial overgrowth; when bacteria is metabolised by lactose or glucose there is a production of hydrogen; if there is lactose in the small intestine that has not been broken down there will be an early rise in breath hydrogen	*H. pylori*
Stool test	Rule out parasitic infections and occult blood that suggests possible diagnosis of diverticulosis, ulcers, polyps, inflammatory bowel disease, GI tumour, haemorrhoids and *H. pylori*; if acidic stools are passed it indicates lactose intolerance
Counselling/psychiatry consultation: mental health assessment	Emotional assessment and support
Diet diary	Have a more detailed look at the foods Corrine is eating, what times she eats, how she prepares food and the amount of food ingested
Elimination diets	Detect food intolerance
Nijmegen questionnaire	Hyperventilation syndrome
Sleep diary: for one week	Assess patterns of sleep and activities prior to sleep; note time Corrine goes to bed, how long she takes to fall asleep, how many times she wakes during the night, the last time of waking before morning, any dreams or nightmares, need to urinate, and comments from her sleep partner; writing down thoughts before bed and when waking is also helpful
IF NECESSARY:	
Epstein-Barr/Ross River virus blood test	Check for postviral infection
Antinuclear antibodies: a protein antibody that reacts against cellular nuclear material and is indicative of an autoimmune abnormality; it is very sensitive in detecting systemic lupus erythematosus (SLE), but not specific to this disease as it can be present in other inflammatory and autoimmune diseases	Connective tissue disease such as SLE
Oral tolerance lactose test	Determine lactose metabolism
Capnometer/pulmonary gas exchange during orthostatic tests	Hyperventilation syndrome
ROUTINE TESTS DUE TO GENDER AND AGE	
Cervical smear	Cervical cancer, sexually transmitted diseases, *Candida*

Confirmed diagnosis

Primary fibromyalgia syndrome with associated physiological depression

PRESCRIBED MEDICATION

- Selective serotonin reuptake inhibitor (SSRI) antidepressants: Corrine would like to try natural therapies before taking prescribed antidepressant medication

TABLE 8.24 **DECISION TABLE FOR TREATMENT (ONCE DIAGNOSIS IS CONFIRMED)**		
COMPLAINT	**CONTEXT**	**CORE**
Treatment for the presenting complaint and symptoms	Treatment for all associated symptoms	Treatment for mental, emotional, spiritual, constitutional, lifestyle issues and metaphysical considerations
TREATMENT PRIORITY	**TREATMENT PRIORITY**	**TREATMENT PRIORITY**
• Continue with herbal tonic, tablets or tea with anti-inflammatory, analgesic, adaptogenic and tonic actions • Continue with nutritional supplements to help reduce pain and increase energy levels • Continue with physical therapies to help reduce pain **NB:** If Corrine takes the prescribed antidepressant medication her herbal tea/tonic will have to be reformulated to ensure there is no interaction between St John's wort and the prescribed medication	• Continue with dietary recommendations to improve digestive health • Continue with dietary recommendations to increase her intake of essential nutrients and antioxidants • Herbal tonic, tablets or tea to support neurotransmitter function and hypothalamic-pituitary-adrenal (HPA) function • Recommendation to identify and eliminate any dietary or environmental triggers • Nutritional supplements to improve digestive function and energy production	• Continue with herbal tonic, tablets or tea to support the nervous system and stress response, and to reduce anxiety levels • Continue with physical therapy recommendations to help reduce anxiety and stress levels • Continue with stress-management techniques • Recommendation for cognitive behavioural therapy

Treatment aims

- Reduce muscle pain and increase mitochondrial energy production in muscle cells [14, 21, 35].
- Reduce levels of inflammatory mediators [22].
- Support adrenal glands; treat apparent adrenal exhaustion and improve stress response [15, 21, 60].
- Improve quality of sleep [16, 21].
- Balance neurotransmitter production [21, 58], HPA axis [15, 21] and enhance serotonin levels [54, 58].
- Support Corrine's nervous system and help her manage her anxiety and stress levels [15, 61].
- Support and improve digestive function [17, 35, 59, 60] and normalise bowel flora [19, 59, 60, 62].

- Support liver detoxification and reduce endotoxinaemia [18, 57, 60].
- Support normal thyroid function. Inadequate thyroid hormone regulation or cellular resistance to the thyroid hormone are postulated to be involved in the development of fibromyalgia symptoms [21, 60].
- Increase aerobic exercise [4, 8, 12, 42].

Lifestyle alterations/considerations

- Corrine will benefit from stress-management techniques such as meditation, yoga and relaxation training [21, 35, 43, 60].
- Corrine may experience benefit from cognitive behavioural therapy [41].
- Corrine should undertake regular daily exercise. It can help improve her physical symptoms [12, 39, 40, 42] and can help improve stress, anxiety [44, 45] and her sleep patterns [45, 46].

Dietary suggestions

- Whole-food, vegetarian diet. Some fibromyalgia sufferers have experienced mild to moderate improvements following a vegetarian diet [31].
- Corrine may find a low-oxalate diet helpful in controlling her symptoms [32]. If she follows a low-oxalate diet it is essential to maintain her intake of essential nutrients.
- Increase Corrine's dietary intake of antioxidants. Elevated free-radical levels and oxidative stress are associated with fibromyalgia [33, 56].
- Eliminate excitotoxins (glutamate, aspartame, MSG) from the diet. Some fibromyalgia sufferers respond to their elimination [20, 21].
- Ensure sufficient dietary intake of omega-3 fatty acids [33, 35].
- Balance blood-sugar levels using a low GI/GL diet [21, 60]. Dysglycaemia can worsen symptoms of fibromyalgia [21].
- Increase consumption of foods that support liver function; onions, garlic, leeks, cruciferous vegetables and lecithin to assist with cellular detoxification [35, 57].
- Eliminate coffee, which may be aggravating Corrine's digestive symptoms [34].
- Determine whether Corrine has any food allergies or intolerances and manage accordingly [55, 60].

Physical treatment suggestions

- Regular massage may reduce muscle pain, improve sleep and assist with stress management [38, 60, 63, 77].
- Prescribed exercise therapy [12, 40, 42] and exercises to increase flexibility and stretch muscles – yoga may be helpful [39].
- Acupuncture may reduce pain symptoms [41, 60].
- Hydrotherapy: full body underwater exercise and Watsu stretches underwater have been shown to be very beneficial for hydrotherapy when practised over a period of six months [55, 47–49, 60].
- Hot baths and showers [50, 60].
- Constitutional hydrotherapy [51, 60].
- Hot foot bath to raise her core temperature and ease abdominal bloating [52].
- Apply a hot apple cider and water or castor oil compress to the abdomen to ease digestive complaints [50, 52].

TABLE 8.25 HERBAL FORMULA (1:2 LIQUID EXTRACTS)

HERB	FORMULA	RATIONALE
Withania *Withania somnifera*	50 mL	Adaptogen [25, 26]; tonic [25, 26]; immunomodulator [25, 26]; anti-inflammatory [25, 26]; anxiolytic [26]; traditionally used for people who are physically and emotionally exhausted [26]
St John's wort *Hypericum perforatum*	50 mL	Antiretroviral [25]; anxiolytic [25, 26]; antidepressant [25, 26]; traditionally used for muscular rheumatism [25]
Rehmannia *Rehmannia glutinosa*	40 mL	Anti-inflammatory [27]; adrenal trophorestorative [27]
St Mary's thistle *Silybum marianum*	30 mL	Hepatoprotective [25, 26], hepatotrophorestorative [25], antioxidant [25]; choleretic [25]; an aid to improve digestive function and to assist in improving liver function [25]
Siberian ginseng *Eleutherococcus senticosus*	40 mL	Adaptogen [25, 26]; immunomodulator [25, 26]; tonic [25, 26]
Supply:	200 mL	Dose: 5 mL 3 times daily

Chaste tree (*Vitex agnus castus*) 1000 mg daily (either as 2 mL of 1:2 liquid extract or tablet) [23] Improves nocturnal melatonin release [28]; considered beneficial in treating insomnia associated with fibromyalgia; can help correct raised prolactin levels, which are sometimes present in fibromyalgia [23]

Willow bark (*Salix alba*) liquid or tablet providing equivalent of 60 mg salicin 2–4 times daily [24]; anti-inflammatory, analgesic and antirheumatic; traditionally used for muscular pain [29]

TABLE 8.26 HERBAL TEA

Alternative to herbal tonic if Corrine prefers a tea

HERB	FORMULA	RATIONALE
St John's wort *Hypericum perforatum*	2 parts	See above
Willow bark *Salix alba*	2 parts	See above
Valerian root *Valeriana officinalis*	1 part	Hypnotic [29]; sedative [25, 29]; mild anodyne [29]; traditionally used as an anxiolytic and to promote sleep [25, 29]; improves sleep latency and quality [30]; traditionally used for nervous unrest, stress and neuralgia [25]
Ginger root *Zingiber officinale*	½ part	Anti-inflammatory [25, 26]; analgesic [26]; circulatory stimulant [25, 26]; antispasmodic [25, 26]; carminative [25, 26]

Decoction: 1 tsp per cup – 1 cup 3–4 times daily

TABLE 8.27 **NUTRITIONAL SUPPLEMENTS**	
SUPPLEMENT AND DOSE	**RATIONALE**
Omega-3 fish oil 6000 mg daily in divided doses [26, 35, 61]	Anti-inflammatory [26, 61]; suppresses production of proinflammatory prostaglandins and cytokines [26, 61]; beneficial to reduce inflammatory processes associated with fibromyalgia [22]
High-potency practitioner-strength **multivitamin, mineral and antioxidant supplement** providing therapeutic doses of essential micronutrients and antioxidants Dosage: as directed by the manufacturer	To reduce oxidative stress and provide essential vitamins and minerals [33, 56]; high doses of a broad range of essential nutrients and antioxidants are indicated in fibromyalgia [21]
Magnesium and malic acid supplement [36]: providing a daily dose of 1200 mg malic acid and 600 mg elemental magnesium [36]	Supplementation with magnesium and malic acid has been shown to improve fibromyalgia symptoms [36]
Coenzyme Q10 100 mg twice daily [26]	Essential for energy metabolism [26, 61]; antioxidant [26, 61]; reduces oxidative stress [26, 37, 61]; indicated for use in fibromyalgia [37]
High-potency practitioner-strength **probiotic supplement** containing therapeutic levels of human strain *Lactobacilli* and *Bifidobacterium* organisms [33, 59]	Disordered intestinal microflora is common in fibromyalgia [17, 59, 60, 64]; supplementation may help improve digestive function, reduce digestive disturbance [17, 19, 59] and reduce neurological symptoms [62, 64]

References

[1] J. Silverman, S. Kurtz, J. Draper, Skills for Communicating with Patients, second edn, Radcliff Publishing, Oxford, 2000.

[2] R. Neighbour, The Inner Consultation: how to develop an effective and intuitive consulting style, Radcliff Publishing, Oxon, 2005.

[3] M. Lloyd, R. Bor, Communication Skills For Medicine, third edn, Churchill Livingstone Elsevier, Edinburgh, 2009.

[4] P. Kumar, C. Clark, Clinical Medicine, sixth edn, Elsevier Saunders, London, 2005.

[5] N.J. Talley, S. O'Connor, Pocket Clinical Examination, third edn, Churchill Livingstone Elsevier, Australia, 2009.

[6] G. Douglas, F. Nicol, C. Robertson, Macleod's Clinical Examination, twelfth edn, Churchill Livingstone Elsevier, Edinburgh, 2009.

[7] R.H. Seller, Differential Diagnosis of Common Complaints, fifth edn, Saunders Elsevier, Philadelphia, 2007.

[8] A. Polmear, Evidence-Based Diagnosis in Primary Care, Churchill Livingstone Elsevier, Edinburgh, 2008.

[9] R.D. Collins, Differential Diagnosis in Primary Care, fourth edn, Lippincott Williams & Wilkins, Philadelphia, 2008.

[10] J. Jamison, Differential Diagnosis for Primary Care, second edn, Churchill Livingstone Elsevier, London, 2006.

[11] R. Berkow, A.J. Fletcher, M.H. Beers, The Merck Manual, sixteenth edn, Merck Research Laboratories, Rathway, N.J, 1993 (later edition).

[12] L. Chaitow, E. Blake, P. Orrock, M. Wallden, P. Snider, J. Zeff, Natropathic Physical Medicine: Theory and Practice for Manual Therapists and Naturopaths, Churchill Livingstone Elsevier, Philadelphia, 2008.

[13] D. Peters, L. Chaitow, G. Harris, S. Morrison, Integrating Complementary Therapies in Primary Care. Churchill Livingstone, London, (2002).

[14] J.H. Park, K.J. Niermann, N.J. Olsen, Evidence for metabolic abnormalities in the muscles of patients with Fibromyalgia, Current Rheumatology Reports 2 (2) (2000) 131–140.

[15] L.J. Crofford, S.R. Pillemer, K.T. Kalogeras, J.M. Cash, D. Michelson, M.A. Kling, et al., Hypothalamic-pituitary-adrenal axis perturbations in patients with Fibromyalgia, Arthritis and Rheumatism 37 (11) (1994) 1583–1592.

[16] S.M. Harding, Sleep in Fibromyalgia Patients: Subjective and objective findings. American Journal of the Medical Sciences, Fibromyalgia 315 (6) (1998) 367–376.

[17] G. Triadafilopoulos, R.W. Simms, D.L. Goldenberg, Bowel dysfunction in Fibromyalgia syndrome, Digestive Diseases and Sciences 36 (1) (1991) 59–64.

[18] M. Pimentel, D. Wallace, D. Hallegua, E. Chow, Y. Kong, S. Park, et al., A link between irritable bowel syndrome and Fibromyalgia may be related to findings on lactulose breath testing, Annals of Rheumatic Disease 63 (2004) 450–452.

[19] M. Pimentel, E.J. Chow, D. Hellegua, D. Wallace, H.C. Lin, Small intestinal bacterial overgrowth: A possible association with Fibromyalgia, Journal of Musculoskeletal Pain 9 (3) (2001) 105–113.

[20] J.D. Smith, J.M. Terpening, S.O. Schmidt, J.G. Gums, Relief of fibromyalgia symptoms following discontinuation of dietary excitotoxins, The Annals of Pharmacotherapy 35 (6) (2001) 702–706.

[21] J.E. Pizzorno, M.T. Murray, H. Joiner-Bey, The Clinicians Handbook of Natural Medicine, second edn, Churchill Livingstone, St Louis, 2008.

[22] I.E. Blanco, F.J. de Serres, E. Fernández-Bustillo, D. Al Kassam, D. Arbesú, C. Rodríguez, et al., α1-Antitrypsin and fibromyalgia: new data in favour of the inflammatory hypothesis of Fibromyalgia, Medical Hypotheses 64 (4) (2005) 759–769.

[23] K. Bone, B. Burgoyne, New uses for Chaste Tree, A Phytotherapist's Perspective 84 (2005) 1–2.

[24] K. Bone, Bark Willow, A Safe and Effective Alternative to NSAIDs, A Phytotherapist's Perspective 87 (2006) 1–2.

[25] S. Mills, K. Bone, Principles and Practice of Phytotherapy, Modern Herbal Medicine, Churchill Livingstone, Edinburgh: London, 2000.

[26] L. Braun, M. Cohen, Herbs & Natural Supplements: An evidence based guide, second edn, Elsevier, Sydney, 2007.

[27] K. Bone, Clinical Applications of Chinese and Ayurvedic Herbs: Monographs for the Western Herbal Practitioners, Phytotherapy Press, Warwick, 1996.

[28] Dericks-Tan, Schwinn, C. Hildt in K. Bone, B. Burgoyne, New uses for Chaste Tree, A Phytotherapist's Perspective 84 (2005) 1–2.

[29] British Herbal Medicine Association, British Herbal Pharmacopoeia, BHMAA, 1983.

[30] F. Donath, S. Quispe, K. Diefenbach, A. Maruer, I. Fietze, I. Roots, Critical evaluation of the effect of valerian extract on sleep structure and sleep quality, Pharmacopsychiatry 33 (2) (2000) 47–53.

[31] M.S. Donaldson, N. Speight, S. Loomis, Fibromyalgia syndrome improved using a mostly raw vegetarian diet: an observational study, BMC Complementary and Alternative Medicine 1 (2001) 7.

[32] C. Solomons, Effective Treatments, The VP Foundation Newsletter 28 (2007) 10–11. Retrieved 21 August 2009 from http://www.thevpfoundation.org/effective_treatment.htm.

[33] S. Ozgocmen, H. Ozyurt, S. Sogut, O. Akyol, Current concepts in the pathophysiology of fibromyalgia: the potential role of oxidative stress and nitric oxide, Rheumatology International 26 (7) (2006) 585–597.

[34] P.J. Boekema, M. Samsom, G.P. van Berge Henegouwen, M. Smout, Coffee and Gastrointestinal Function: Facts and Fiction: A Review, Scandinavian Journal of Gastroenterology 34 (5) Supp (230) (1999) 35–39.

[35] H. Osiecki, The Physicians Handbook of Clinical Nutrition, seventh edn, Bioconcepts, Eagle Farm, 2000.

[36] G.E. Abraham, J.D. Flechas, Management of Fibromyalgia: Rationale for the use of magnesium and Malic Acid, Journal of Nutritional Medicine 3 (1) (1992) 49–59.

[37] M.D. Cordero, A.M. Moreno-Fernandez, M. deMiguel, P. Bonal, F. Campa, L.M. Jimenez-Jimenez, et al., Coenzyme Q10 distribution in blood is altered in patients with Fibromyalgia, Clinical Biochemistry 42 (7–8) (2009) 732–735.

[38] T. Field, M. Diego, C. Cullen, M. Hernandez-Reif, W. Sunshine, S. Douglas, Fibromyalgia Pain and Substance P Decrease and Sleep Improves After Massage Therapy, Journal of Clinical Rheumatology 8 (2) (2002) 72–76.

[39] G.D. da Silva, G. Lorenzi-Filho, L.V. Lage, Effects of Yoga and the Addition of Tui Na in Patients with Fibromyalgia, The J Altern Complement Med 13 (10) (2007) 1107–1114.

[40] D.L. Goldenberg, C. Burkhardt, C. Crofford, Management of Fibromyalgia Syndrome, Journal of the American Medical Association 292 (2004) 2388–2395.

[41] D.P. Martin, C.D. Sletten, B.A. Williams, I.H. Berger, Improvement in Fibromyalgia Symptoms With Acupuncture: Results of a Randomized Controlled Trial, Mayo Clinic Proceedings 81 (6) (2006) 749–757.

[42] S.C.M. Richards, D.L. Scott, Prescribed exercise in people with fibromyalgia: parallel group randomised controlled trial, British Medical Journal 325 (2002) 185.

[43] A.F. Jorm, H. Christensen, K.M. Griffiths, R.A. Parslow, B. Rodgers, K.A. Blewitt, Effectiveness of complementary and self-help treatments for anxiety disorders, Medical Journal of Australia 181 (7) (2004) S29–S46.

[44] A. Byrne, G.D. Byrne, The effect of exercise on depression, anxiety and other mood states: A review, J Psychosom Res 37 (6) (1993) 565–574.

[45] K. Morgan, Daytime activity and risk factors for late-life insomnia, Journal of Sleep Research 12 (2003) 231–238.

[46] E.J. Stepanski, J.K. Wyatt, Use of sleep hygiene in the treatment of insomnia, Sleep Medicine Reviews 7 (3) (2003) 215–225.

[47] D.F. Fernandes de Melo Vitorino, L. Bizari Can de Carvalho, G. Fernandes do Prado, Hydrotherapy and conventional physiotherapy improve total sleep time and quality of life of fibromyalgia patients: Randomized clinical trial, Sleep Medicine 7 (2006) 293–296.

[48] E. Blake, in: L. Chaitow, E. Blake, P. Orrock, M. Wallden, P. Snider, J. Zeff (Eds.), Naturopathic Physical Medicine, Theory and Practice for Manual Therapists and Naturopaths, Churchill Livingstone Elsevier, Philadelhia, 2008.

[49] J.P. O'Hare, A. Heywood, L.G. Summerhayes, et al., Observations on the effects of immersion in Bath spa water, British Medical Journal 291 (1985) 1747–1751.

[50] M. Sinclair, Modern Hydrotherapy for the Massage Therapist, Lippincott Williams & Wilkins, Baltimore, 2008.

[51] L. Chaitow, Hydrotherapy, water therapy for health and beauty, Element, Dorset, 1999.

[52] D.D. Buchman, The complete book of water healing, Contemporary Books, McGraw-Hill Companies, New York, 2001.

[53] L. Chaitow, in: L. Chaitow, E. Blake, P. Orrock, M. Wallden, P. Snider, J. Zeff (Eds.), Naturopathic Physical Medicine, Theory and Practice for Manual Therapists and Naturopaths, Churchill Livingstone Elsevier, Philadelhia, 2008.

[54] L. Bazzichi, G. Giannaccini, L. Betti, G. Mascia, L. Fabbrini, P. Italiani, et al., Alteration of serotonin transporter density and activity in Fibromyalgia, Arthritis Research & Therapy 8 (2006) R99.

[55] R.B. Loblay, A.R. Swain, The role of food intolerance in chronic fatigue syndrome, the clinical and Scientific basis of myalgic encephalomyelitis/chronic fatigue syndrome, (1992) 521–538. Retrieved 3 March 2010 from http://www.sswahs.nsw.gov.au/rpa/allergy/research/RoleOfFoodIntoleranceInCFS.pdf.

[56] S. Bagis, L. Tamer, G. Sahin, R. Bilgin, H. Guler, B. Ercan, et al., Free radicals and antioxidants in primary fibromyalgia: an oxidative stress disorder? Rheumatology International 25 (2005) 188–190.

[57] M. Percival, Fibromyalgia: Nutritional Support, Clinical Nutrition Insights (1997) 1–4.

[58] L.J. Crofford, M.A. Demitrack, Evidence that abnormalities of central neurohormonal systems are key to understanding fibromyalgia and chronic fatigue syndrome, Rheumatic Disease Clinics of North America 22 (1996) 267–284.

[59] D.J. Wallace, D.S. Hallegua, Fibromyalgia: The Gastrointestinal Link, Current Pain and Headache Reports 8 (2004) 364–368.

[60] L. Chaitow, Fibromyalgia: The Oestopathic Naturopathic Approach, Journal of Bodywork and Movement Therapies 2 (4) (1998) 195–199.

[61] J. Jamison, Clinical Guide to Nutrition & Dietary Supplements in Disease Management, Churchill Livingstone, Edinburgh, 2003.

[62] A. Venket Rao, A. Bested, T. Veaulne, M. Katzman, C. Iorio, et al., A randomized, double-blind, placebo-controlled pilot study of a probiotic in emotional symptoms of chronic fatigue syndrome, Gut Pathogens 1 (2009) 6.

[63] T. Field, J. Delage, M. Hernandez-Reif, Movement and massage therapy reduce fibromyalgia pain, Journal of Bodywork and Movement Therapies 7 (1) (2003) 49–52.

[64] A. Logan, M. Katzman, Major depressive disorder: probiotics may be an adjuvant therapy, Medical Hypotheses 64 (2005) 533–538.

[65] L. Darbishire, L. Ridsdale, P.T. Seed, Distinguishing patients with chronic fatigue from those with chronic fatigue syndrome: a diagnostic study in UK primary care, Br J Gen Pract 53 (2003) 441–445.

[66] G. Whiting, et al., Interventions for the treatment and management of chronic fatigue syndrome, Journal of the American Medical Association 286 (2001) 1360–1368.

[67] S. Wessely, Chronic fatigue symptom and syndrome, Ann Intern Med 134 (2001) 838–843.

[68] G. Ellis, J. Robinson, G. Crawford, When symptoms of disease overlap with symptoms of depression, Aust Fam Physician 35 (2006) 647–649.

[69] W.J. Meggs, Neurogenic switching: a hypothesis for a mechanism for shifting the site of inflammation in allergy and chemical sensitivity, Environmental Health Perspectives 103 (1) (1995) 54–56.

[70] P. Croft, Symptoms without pathology: should we try a little tenderness? Rheumatology 42 (2003) 815–817.

[71] L. Crofford, D. Clauw, Fibromyalgia: where are we a decade after the American College of Rheumatology Classification Criteria were developed? Arthritis Rheum 46 (2002) 1136–1138.

[72] B. Carruthers, A. Jain, K. De Meirleir, et al., Myalgic encephalomyelitis/chronic fatigue syndrome: clinical working case definition, diagnostic and treatment protocols, J Chronic Fatigue Syndr 11 (2003) 7–115.

[73] I. Hickie, T.A. Davenport, D. Wakefield, et al., Post-infective and chronic fatigue syndromes precipitated by viral and non-viral pathogens: prospective cohort study, BMJ 333 (2006) 575–578.

[74] A. Elvin, A.K. Siosteen, A. Nilsson, E. Kosek, Decreased muscle blood flow in fibromyalgia patients during standardised muscle exercise: a contrast media enhanced colour Doppler study, European Journal of Pain 10 (2) (2006) 137–144.

[75] K. Henriksson, Is fibromyalgia a distinct clinical entity? Pain mechanism's in fibromyalgia syndrome. A mycologist's view, Baillieres Clinical Rheumatology 3 (1999) 455–461.

[76] J. Nijs, M. Meeus, K. Meirleria, Chronic musculoskeletal pain in chronic fatigue syndrome, Manual Therapy 11 (2006) 187–191.

[77] L. Barnes, The self-perceived effects of massage in palliative care patients, Honours thesis, Southern Cross University, Australia, 2004.

Systemic lupus erythematosus

Case history

Amira Zandi, 42, has come to the clinic for help and advice regarding pain in her hands. Amira has been experiencing intermittent hand pain for about two years, which is progressively worsening. The pain seems to affect her finger joints the most and Amira's hands feel quite cold and numb first thing in the morning; a hot shower alleviates the sensation of coldness and discomfort. She has noticed the pain seems worse in cold weather, and she has come to dislike winter because the cold affects her hands so much.

Amira tells you she has also noticed a rash that appears on her face across her nose. She thinks it is probably stress-related eczema and keeping it well moisturised seems to keep it under control. Amira has wondered if cortisone cream would help when it gets particularly bad. Amira has noticed that her rash is worse if she is out in the sun so she makes sure she always covers up with a broad-brimmed hat, long-sleeved clothing and sunscreen.

Further questioning reveals that Amira has been feeling quite tired recently and she feels as if she is always on the brink of getting the flu. She has also been having more problems with constipation recently. Amira knows her health is out of balance and wants to find out how she can get back into balance again.

Amira eats red meat three or four times a week, chicken at least three times a week and fish usually once a week. She eats cooked vegetables with her main meal in winter and salads in summer. She usually has cooked porridge or cereal and milk for breakfast and has at least two pieces of fruit each day. Lunch is either leftovers or a sandwich. She drinks four to six glasses of water daily and starts every morning with a strong coffee to help her get started and then drinks another cup or two during the day.

When you ask Amira about her family and social life she shares that she is experiencing great grief at the moment because her 19-year-old son is leaving home to travel overseas. Her husband divorced her three years ago and she has lived life for her children since then. Two years ago her daughter married and now her son is leaving too. Her relationship with her son has been difficult during his teenage years, but she always hoped things would improve. She feels as if everyone she loves and cares for has left her. You notice her wringing her hands as she expresses her emotions. Amira says she keeps mostly to herself and does not usually socialise with friends or colleagues as her focus has been on homemaking for many years. Amira also tells you that recently she has been having more trouble sleeping than usual.

Amira has worked part time as an administrative assistant since her husband left her and is thinking of increasing her hours, particularly now there is nobody at home to care for. She is concerned she will not be able to cope with the additional work because of the pain in her hands.

Amira has a family history of osteoarthritis (OA) and systemic lupus erythematosus (SLE). Because of this history she thinks she should see her family doctor to run some tests, but she has come to the clinic today because she would like your perspective and suggestions before she sees a medical practitioner or specialist.

TABLE 8.28 COMPLAINT [1–11]

Analogy: Skin of the apple	Complaint: Define the presenting complaint and symptoms; understand the complaint *Hand pain*
AREAS OF INVESTIGATION AND EXAMPLE QUESTIONS	**CLIENT RESPONSES**
Onset *When did you first notice the pain in your hands?*	*I have had this for about two years. It is worse now than when it first began.*
Exacerbating factors *What makes the pain worse?*	*It is worse first thing in the morning and if my hands are cold.*
Relieving factors *What makes the pain better?*	*Warmth makes it better.*
Location and radiation *Where exactly do you get the pain?* *Does the pain radiate out from that spot?*	*In the joints of my fingers.* *No, just the fingers.*
Examination and inspection	Amira's fingertips appear discoloured and there is evidence of soft tissue swelling in the fingers. There appear to be mild vascular lesions on her fingertips and nail folds. There is a slight 'butterfly' formation redness across Amira's cheeks and nose.

TABLE 8.29 CONTEXT

Analogy: Flesh of the apple	Context: Put the presenting complaint into context to understand the disease
AREAS OF INVESTIGATION AND EXAMPLE QUESTIONS	**CLIENT RESPONSES**
Family health *Has anyone in your family had similar symptoms?*	*Yes. My aunt has SLE and my mother has OA.*
Trauma and pre-existing illness *Do your fingers feel weak after using them when repeating certain movements like working on the computer?* (repetitive strain injury)	*Yes, I do notice that after working on the computer they are sore.*
Functional disease *Does the pain in your hands become worse with physical activity and improve with rest?* (mechanical causes, OA)	*It does get sore when I am using my hands, but it seems to be sore when I am resting them too.*

▶

Infection and inflammation *Do you feel joint pain in your hands during the night?* (arthritis) *Do you experience any shoulder stiffness or pain with the sore hands and fingers?* (referred arthritis pain)	*When I have a flare up it can hurt all day and all night.* *I do feel pain in my back sometimes but not specifically my shoulders.*
Endocrine/reproductive *Tell me about your menstrual cycle.*	Amira's cycle is between 26 and 30 days, with a bleed of about 4–5 days. She experiences no significant pain or discomfort but does sometimes feel more anxious in the days before her period.
Stress and neurological disease *Do you have weakness in your fingers associated with numbness?* (peripheral neuropathy)	*They do not feel numb, but they can feel weak sometimes.*
Eating habits and energy *Tell me about your diet.* *How are your energy levels?*	Amira's diet contains red meat meals 3–4 times a week, chicken usually 3 times a week and fish usually once a week. She has either cooked vegetables or salad with her main meal and has porridge or cereal and milk for breakfast. She has leftovers or sandwiches for lunch and has about 3 cups of coffee during the day. *I'm quite tired a lot of the time, I think maybe it is because I'm having problems sleeping at night.*

TABLE 8.30 **CORE**	
Analogy: Core of the apple with the seed of ill health	**Core:** Holistic assessment to understand the client.
AREAS OF INVESTIGATION AND EXAMPLE QUESTIONS	**CLIENT RESPONSES**
Emotional health *You mentioned you sometimes feel sad or anxious. Can you tell me more about that?*	*I'm very sad. My husband divorced me 3 years ago and now my son is leaving me too. Things have been difficult between us for the past few years, I was hoping they would get better before he left home.*
Stress release *How do you deal with stress and sadness?*	*I don't know. Sometimes I just cry about it. I tell my mother but I don't think she understands how it feels for your husband to leave you.*
Occupation *Tell me about your work.*	*I work in an office. I like my work and the people are kind and friendly. Maybe I'll increase my hours there since I'm not needed at home anymore.*

Family and friends Do you spend much time with family and friends?	Not really. I see my parents and sister sometimes. Most of the time I'm at home.
Action needed to heal How were you hoping I could help you?	Tell me what to do, give me some herbal medicine to help with my hands and help me feel well again.
Long-term goals What do you think you will be doing in five or 10 years?	I think I will be working full time and living alone. Maybe I will feel happier then.

TABLE 8.31 **AMIRA'S SIGNS AND SYMPTOMS** [2, 6–8]	
Pulse	86bpm
Blood pressure	122/81
Temperature	38.5°C
Respiratory rate	16 resp/min
Body mass index	22
Waist circumference	76.8 cm
Nails and fingers	Mild vascular lesions on fingertips and nail folds; discolouration of finger tips, soft tissue swelling of fingers
Face	Slight redness across nose and cheeks in butterfly formation
Urinalysis	No abnormality detected (NAD)

Results of medical investigations

No investigations have been carried out as yet.

TABLE 8.32 **UNLIKELY DIAGNOSTIC CONSIDERATIONS** [2, 6–11, 13, 70, 72]	
CONDITIONS AND CAUSES	**WHY UNLIKELY**
TRAUMA AND PRE-EXISTING ILLNESS	
Causal factor: **Trauma/ruptured tendons:** can cause pain in the finger joints	Need to determine if Amira has experienced an injury to her hands recently; onset of pain would correlate with an injury and be aggravated by movement; joints would appear very red and swollen
INFECTION AND INFLAMMATION	
Bacterial: staphylococci, TB, *Borrelia* **Fungal infection** **Viral infection:** rubella, mumps, hepatitis B Fatigue and pain in fingers, mild fever present	Can present as mono-, oligo- and polyarthritis; self-limiting and resolves quickly; would have red swollen joints

▶

Causal factor: **Postviral arthritis:** glandular fever, rheumatic fever, reactive arthritis Fatigue and pain in fingers, mild fever present; most often presents as polyarthritis involving more than 5 joints	Will usually resolve after a few weeks
Reiter's syndrome: intermittent arthritis	No conjunctivitis or urethritis
Enteropathic arthritis: from inflammatory bowel syndrome	No bloody diarrhoea or abdominal pain
Osteoarthritis (OA): usually presents as oligoarthritis affecting only 2–4 joints or polyarthritis affecting 5 or more joints; pain in hands and joints, symptoms may be asymmetrical or symmetrical; family history of OA	Distal interphalangeal joints not specifically tender, hands did not appear square looking, Amira is younger than the usual age to develop severe OA, no crepitus movement of the joint; pain eases with rest due to the mechanical nature of disease; stiffness can occur after resting but only for a few minutes and there would be pain on movement
Gout: crystal formation pain in finger	Usually only affects a single joint and is extremely painful; would develop quickly; the joint will appear very swollen and red
Dupuytren's contracture: tenosynovitis of flexors of the fingers; fixed flexion contraction on the hand; tender fingers; can occur gradually on both hands	Pain felt in the palm at the base of the third and fourth digits; no visible contracture seen on the palm where the fingers bend towards the hand and cannot be flexed
Causal factor: **Referred arthritis/bursitis of shoulder:** pain in the hand and fingers	No shoulder pain reported
ENDOCRINE/REPRODUCTIVE	
Diabetes: peripheral neuropathy and hand stiffness, lack of circulation, cold hands	Urinalysis NAD
AUTOIMMUNE DISEASE	
Rheumatoid arthritis (RA): can be polyarthritis presenting as mono- and oligoarthritis; joint pain in the hands, fatigue and stress; can present with arthritis in the fingers and a skin rash	Pain will often be worse on waking; hands are not swollen and warm, proximal interphalangeal joints not specifically tender, no ulnar deviation to the hand; pain is not intermittent pain but more likely to be persistent
Psoriatic arthritis: usually presents as oligoarthritis affecting only 2–4 joints	No psoriatic lesions on the skin that appear salmon pink, silvery or scaling; no pitting of the nail bed or white appearance
Chronic discoid lupus: benign variant of lupus	Usually only affects the skin and has defined plaques that can scar

Case analysis

CONDITION	WHY POSSIBLE	WHY UNLIKELY
TABLE 8.33 POSSIBLE DIFFERENTIAL DIAGNOSIS		
Not ruled out by tests/investigations already done [2, 6–11, 69–73]		
ALLERGIES AND IRRITANTS		
Atopic eczema: the word 'atopy' means to react to common environmental factors; can be caused and aggravated by diet or genetic factors	Lesions worse for anxiety; symmetrical lesions; eating potentially allergic/intolerant foods such as wheat and dairy	Skin rash that causes itching, begins with small vesicles and then spreads to produce thickening of the skin and weeping of pus and blood if scratched too much; associated with a history of asthma; presenting in flexor folds of the knees, behind the ears, hands, scalp, elbows and face; lesions cause irritation and scratching
Primary irritant eczema: degreasing of skin with water loss and dryness, fissuring and cracking; can happen at work and in the home	On areas of body that have close contact with irritants and where chemicals may be applied on skin	Usually asymmetrical lesions in exposed areas and displayed in streaks; determine if there is a skin rash on the palm of her hands
Photosensitive eczema	Typical features of eczema and thickening of the skin; often in individuals with pre-existing eczema (diagnosis can be missed); can be distributed over areas that skin is exposed to sun such as the hands, face and neck; may also spread to areas of the body where the skin is not directly exposed to the sun	Rare type of eczema, usually develops in middle age or in elderly men; can develop photosensitivity to artificial lighting
CANCER AND HEART DISEASE		
Primary or metastatic cancer	Pain in fingers, fatigue, frequently getting sick	Deep boring pain that would be worse at rest
TRAUMA AND PRE-EXISTING ILLNESS		
Causal factor: **Repetitive strain injury**	Typing at work and strains fingers, intermittent pain	
Haemochromotosis	Fatigue, constipation, polyarthritis, eating regular meat and high iron-containing foods	

▶

FUNCTIONAL DISEASE		
Thoracic outlet syndrome	Hand pain worse on waking; common in middle-aged women	Usually only affects left hand and after the arms are hyperabducted on waking; hands would feel weak and numb
Raynaud's phenomenon/disease: when this condition appears as an underlying cause of another disease it is called 'phenomenon', otherwise this condition is known as Raynaud's disease	Discolouration of the fingertips due to sluggish blood flow; can be a complication of SLE and RA; finger pain is worse in cold weather	Extremely painful
Carpal tunnel syndrome: pain often in wrist, thumb, index and middle fingers; weakness in abduction of thumb and hypalgesia in the index finger	Pain and stiffness in hand; can be in later stage of RA; common in women; hands will often look normal with no joint swelling; should be no pain felt on palm of the hand	Common to have nocturnal pain in the wrist; need to ascertain level of stiffness and weakness accompanying hand pain
Causal factor: Functional constipation	Stress; currently Amira is highly emotional; constipation can develop	
INFECTION AND INFLAMMATION		
Buerger's disease: vasculitis of the arteries	Pain and numbness in the fingers; can cause Raynaud's phenomenon symptoms and common between the ages of 20 and 40; can be confused with autoimmune diseases such as SLE	Would also involve feet; criteria includes current or recent history of smoking, lack of circulation in the hands and feet, painful walking; usually more common in men; need to as ascertain if the numbness is a symptom experienced with pain in the fingers
Acne rosacea	Inflammatory disorder common on the face with pustules and papules on the nose, forehead and cheeks; more common in women; has associated symptoms of facial flushing; usually develops in adults aged over 30 rather than adolescents	
SUPPLEMENTS AND SIDE EFFECTS OF MEDICATION		
Causal factor: Oral contraceptive pill	SLE symptoms	Ascertain if Amira has taken the oral contraceptive pill recently
Causal factor: Drug-induced SLE: hydralazine and procainamide most common	Rashes, pain in fingers	Need to establish if any medication has been taken over the past two years

ENDOCRINE/REPRODUCTIVE		
Hypothyroidism/ Hashimoto's disease	Feels the cold, constipation, fatigue, sadness and swelling in joints of the hand	No visible goitre, weight gain, skin and hair changes
AUTOIMMUNE DISEASE		
Systemic lupus erythematosus (SLE): will present with polyarthritis affecting 5 or more joints	Fatigue, joint pain in hands, pain in the morning, Raynaud's phenomenon, skin rash, intermittent and transient arthritis with mild fever; not usual for joints to appear red; symptoms are symmetrical; family history of SLE	
Systemic sclerosis	Skin rash, gastrointestinal disturbance, Raynaud's phenomenon, swelling in joints of the hands, raised antinuclear antibodies and RH factor can be present along with a normochromic normocytic film content; less common than SLE	Skin rash can be extensive and spread all over the body; skin on the face forms a beak-like nose and small mouth; painful ulcers on the fingers can develop; heartburn, hypertension and renal involvement can present
Overlap syndrome	Symptoms of RA and SLE and Raynaud's; not usual for joints to appear red; symptoms are symmetrical	
Causal factor: **Posttraumatic stress disorder (PTSD):** Symptoms often develop within 6 months of the stressful event	Symptoms developed after divorce to husband	Has not mentioned flashbacks to a particular traumatic event
STRESS AND NEUROLOGICAL DISEASE		
Causal factor: **Mixed anxiety and depressive disorder**	Depressive disorder often associated with an experience of loss; symptoms of fatigue, apathy, or intense sadness, insomnia	Can be associated with numerous physical complaints associated with depression such as restlessness, headaches, shortness of breath, gut or skin disorders; need to determine if significant incapacity to continue daily activities for work
Stress	Lack of sleep, constipation, skin rash	

Causal factor: **Functional fatigue, depression**	Tiredness that has lasted for several months; grief from being separated from husband and children; feeling lonely; can be moderate or severe depression; people often describe symptoms in physical terms; has insomnia, change in appetite, fatigue; delayed sleep onset, lack of appetite, can be aggravated by certain conditions and situations that provoke depression	Need to determine if the feeling of fatigue improves during the day; early morning waking is common in depression
Peripheral neuropathy	Numbness in fingers	Weakness in fingers
EATING HABITS AND ENERGY		
Causal factor: **Diet: excess saturated fatty acids**	Increase inflammation; eating a lot of red meat	

TABLE 8.34 **DECISION TABLE FOR REFERRAL** [2, 7–11, 13]		
COMPLAINT	**CONTEXT**	**CORE**
Referral for presenting complaint	Referral for all associated physical, dietary and lifestyle concerns	Referral for contributing emotional, mental, spiritual, metaphysical, lifestyle and constitutional factors
REFERRAL FLAGS	**REFERRAL FLAGS**	**REFERRAL FLAGS**
• Pain in the hands intermittent over 2 years • Family history of SLE and OA • In age group for women to develop symptoms of SLE	• Rash on the face across the nose that is worse with exposure to sunlight	• Significant grief about children leaving home • Grief and loneliness after her divorce 3 years ago • Would like to work more to avoid feeling lonely but the hand pain may prevent this
ISSUES OF SIGNIFICANCE	**ISSUES OF SIGNIFICANCE**	**ISSUES OF SIGNIFICANCE**
• Pain in hands worse in the cold weather	• More saturated fatty acids in diet (red meat and dairy) than essential fatty acids (fish and legumes) • Difficulty sleeping	• Does not socialise with friends • After the divorce has put all her energy into the children
REFERRAL DECISION	**REFERRAL DECISION**	**REFERRAL DECISION**
• Immediate referral for medical investigations regarding chronic intermittent pain in the hands	• Medical assessment of the skin rash • Dietary assessment	• Grief counselling and mental health assessment

TABLE 8.35 **FURTHER INVESTIGATIONS THAT MAY BE NECESSARY** [2, 6, 8–11, 13, 70, 72, 73]	
TEST/INVESTIGATION	**REASON FOR TEST/INVESTIGATION**
FIRST-LINE MEDICAL INVESTIGATIONS:	
Full blood count	Rule out infection, tumour, inflammation, anaemia *White blood cell count:* low; can be low in autoimmune disease *Platelets:* low (haemolytic anaemia) The number of platelets (thrombocytes) gives information about efficiency of blood clotting and destruction of platelets can be secondary to antibodies
Film comments	*Normochromic normocytic* (iron deficiency detected early; normochromic means normal haemoglobin content and colour; normocytic means normal red blood cell size)
ESR (erythrocyte sedimentation rate): inflammation in general	*Raised*
CRP (C-reactive protein): infection, cancer, inflammation	*Normal*
Rheumatoid factor (RH factor)	*Positive:* circulating autoantibodies, in inflammatory diseases such as RA, which have a portion of IgG as their antigen and self-aggregates into immune complexes that cause inflammation and joint damage; the most common reactive IgM molecule is RH factor
Antinuclear antibodies (ANA)	*Positive:* high; antibody that reacts against cellular nuclear material and is indicative of an autoimmune abnormality; this is very sensitive in detecting SLE
Immunoglobulins	IgG and IgM raised
Thyroid function test **TSH, T4, T3**	Rule out thyroid disease *TSH:* high *T4:* low in hypothyroidism
Thyroid antibody blood test: thyroid perioxidase antibody, antithyroglobulin antibody	To rule out Hashimoto's disease
IF NECESSARY:	
X-rays on left and right hands	Check if there are any fractures, joint or bone abnormalities; systemic sclerosis shows deposits of calcium around the fingers in an x-ray
Skin prick testing	Response to immediate contact allergies; test for extrinsic specific allergies
Skin patch tests to particular allergens	Review 2–4 days later for specific delayed contact allergies

Confirmed diagnosis

AMIRA AND SYSTEMIC LUPUS ERYTHEMATOSUS WITH RAYNAUD'S PHENOMENON

Amira is a 42-year-old woman with intermittent hand pain present for more than two years which is worsening. Her fingers feel very cold and the pain is worse in cold weather. Amira has come to the clinic seeking help to reduce her hand pain and to clear a skin rash which has developed on her face. She would also like help to feel less tired and to improve her digestion. During the consultation Amira shares information about her diet and lifestyle. She becomes emotional when explaining that both her children have left home and her husband divorced her three years ago. This has left an enormous gulf in her life, which she currently fills with work. Amira is concerned that the pain in her hands will affect her work capability and leave her with more time alone to think about grief and loneliness.

Amira was referred for an immediate medical assessment and returned with a confirmed diagnosis of **systemic lupus erythematosus** (SLE) with **Raynaud's phenomenon**. This explained the symptoms of fatigue, joint pain in her hands, Raynaud's phenomenon, skin rash, low white cell and platelet count, normochromic normocytic film content.

SLE is a connective tissue disorder with a definitive diagnosis of the presence of antinuclear antibodies. The condition is more common in premenopausal women and those people with a family history of lupus. The typical age of onset of the disease is usually between 20 and 40 years. Medically it is referred to as a 'loss of self-tolerance' because the disease attacks so many parts of the body and there are several immunological factors involved in the disease process. It is a multisystem disease that can present with general symptoms of fever, depression and fatigue along with clinical features of a butterfly skin rash across the face, photosensitive skin rash, chest infections, Raynaud's phenomenon, arthritis in the joints that presents like RA, although the joints appear normal. Heart disease, nervous system disorders, abdominal pain, kidney disease, muscle pain and anaemia, reduced white cells and platelets may also be integrated into the SLE diagnostic picture.

Episodes of SLE symptoms are commonly followed by complete remissions for long periods. In most situations the pattern of episodes becomes apparent in the first few years. In that time if serious complications have not developed, it is less likely they will do so. Arthritis is usually intermittent and the destruction of joints which can occur in RA and OA does not occur. However, some people with SLE may develop an ulnar deviation.

General references used in this diagnosis: 2, 6–11

PRESCRIBED MEDICATION

- NSAIDs for arthralgia symptoms and oral corticosteroids if symptoms persist
- Amira would like to try natural therapies first before resorting to prescribed medication

TABLE 8.36 **DECISION TABLE FOR TREATMENT (ONCE DIAGNOSIS CONFIRMED)**		
COMPLAINT	**CONTEXT**	**CORE**
Treatment for the presenting complaint and symptoms	Treatment for all associated symptoms	Treatment for mental, emotional, spiritual, constitutional, lifestyle issues and metaphysical considerations

▶

TREATMENT PRIORITY	TREATMENT PRIORITY	TREATMENT PRIORITY
• Recommendation to exercise daily to reduce inflammatory response and improve symptoms • Dietary recommendations to identify and avoid aggravating foods and to increase consumption of foods with anti-inflammatory and immune-modulating properties • Physical therapy recommendations to reduce pain, increase range of movement and preserve joint function • Herbal tea, tonic and tablets with anti-inflammatory, analgesic, antirheumatic and immunomodulatory action **NB:** Due to the presence of licorice in Amira's herbal tea, her potassium levels should be monitored if she continues to take it for an extended period of time; it is unlikely there will be any problems at this dose **NB:** If Amira takes prescribed steroid or immunosuppressant medications her herbal tonic, tea and tablet formulas will need to be reviewed to ensure there are no negative interactions • Supplemental nutrients with anti-inflammatory properties **NB:** Amira's serum vitamin levels can be monitored while she takes supplemental nutrients to ensure they stay within normal range; it is essential for Amira's case to be managed collaboratively with her medical practitioners to ensure effective and appropriate treatment	• Lifestyle recommendation to exercise daily to improve health and wellbeing • Dietary recommendations to increase consumption of essential nutrients and antioxidants to reduce oxidative stress and promote general health • Herbal tea and tablets with antioxidant, digestive stimulant, liver tonic and laxative action; also antimicrobial action to address the potential of underlying infection • Supplemental nutrients with anti-inflammatory, kidney-protective and antioxidant properties to reduce oxidative stress and enhance health and wellbeing • Supplemental nutrients to support the health of her gastrointestinal mucosa	• Lifestyle suggestions to improve Amira's physical and mental health • Dietary and supplement recommendations to improve symptoms of depression • Herbal tea and tonic with nervine, sedative, anxiolytic, adaptogenic and antidepressant actions to support Amira's nervous system, psychological health and improve her sleep pattern

Treatment aims

- Reduce systemic inflammation [14–16, 67].
- Modulate Amira's immune response [14, 16].
- Slow down or prevent progression of the disease [41].
- Alleviate pain [41] and support joint health and mobility [14, 16].
- Deal with any underlying viral or bacterial infection if present [16, 36].
- Enhance integrity of the intestinal wall and support optimal digestive health and function [14, 37, 38].
- Identify and manage food allergies or intolerances [14, 16, 23, 39, 41].

- Identify and correct nutritional deficiencies [16, 39, 40].
- Enhance efficacy of conventional medications, reduce dosage and minimise adverse drug side effects [41].
- Reduce oxidative stress [40, 41, 50].
- Support Amira's emotional health, nervous system and stress response [44, 45].
- Improve Amira's sleep pattern.

Lifestyle alterations/considerations

- Encourage Amira to reconnect socially with friends and colleagues. She needs to make a new support network and find effective ways of dealing with her sense of loss [18].
- Encourage Amira to exercise every day. Exercise is beneficial to her psychological wellbeing [19, 20] and graded aerobic exercise programs can be beneficial in SLE [42, 43]. Moderate exercise is associated with lower levels of inflammatory mediators [46].
- Encourage Amira to seek counselling to help her find positive coping strategies as she deals with her issues of grief and rejection [17, 18].

Dietary suggestions

- Identify and remove dietary triggers [14, 39, 41]. There is a correlation between food sensitivities and some immune-related rheumatic disorders [14, 16, 23, 39, 41]; Amira may find avoiding allergenic foods is greatly beneficial [41].
- Encourage Amira to avoid foods from the solanaceae (nightshade) family: eggplant, capsicum, tomato, capsicum (peppers) and potato [14, 16]. They are implicated in promoting inflammation and pain in rheumatic diseases [24].
- Encourage Amira to increase consumption of foods containing omega-3 fatty acids [41, 46] while reducing consumption of omega-6 fatty acids [46] and *trans*-fatty acids [47] and saturated fats [48]. Reducing linoleic acid and arachidonic acid while increasing omega-3 can enhance anti-inflammatory action of omega-3 fatty acids [49].
- Encourage Amira to avoid or reduce consumption of refined carbohydrates, sugar and animal fats while eating an antioxidant-rich whole-food diet that is high in fibre, whole grains, legumes, vegetables, fruit and flavanoid-rich berries [16, 40, 41, 48, 50].
- Encourage Amira to increase consumption of foods rich in vitamins A, E and C [39, 41, 50, 51].
- Encourage Amira to include plenty of turmeric and ginger in her diet. Turmeric has anti-inflammatory [25, 26, 32], antioxidant [25, 26] and immunomodulatory [25] actions. Ginger has anti-inflammatory [25, 26], antioxidant [25], circulatory stimulant [25, 26], immunonodulatory [25] and digestive stimulant [14, 25, 26] actions.
- Amira should replace coffee with green tea [41, 50] or the prescribed herbal tea.

Physical treatment suggestions

- Amira may find massage therapy beneficial to help her relax and reduce stress and anxiety [21, 22]. Massage may also be helpful by relaxing muscles, improving the range of motion of her joints and increasing endorphin production [52].
- Amira may find acupuncture therapy helpful [52, 53].
- Hydrotherapy: for hands, a hot Epsom salt hand bath for 20 minutes will help ease the pain [63]. Apply a heat compress on the hand with a plastic pad on top for 20 minutes – this is beneficial in cold weather [62, 63].
- Alternating hot (three minutes) and cold (30 seconds) hand bath locally to inflamed or painful joints for four rounds [63].

- For constipation place a hot compress on the abdomen, then cover in plastic, with a hot water bottle/heating pad on top for 12 minutes. Follow with cold mitten friction for 30 seconds (repeat process three times) [63].
- Alternating hot and cold showers daily to improve her immune system [64, 66].
- Constitutional hydrotherapy [62, 65].
- Cold water shower on the face daily [67].
- Cold oat sponge on the face to clean and ease the rash [62].
- Amira may benefit from exercises to strengthen her muscles, increase range of movement and preserve joint function [15, 54]. Such exercises are beneficial in RA, a condition with many similarities to SLE.

TABLE 8.37 HERBAL FORMULA (1:2 LIQUID EXTRACTS)		
HERB	**FORMULA**	**RATIONALE**
Rehmannia *Rehmannia glutinosa*	70 mL	Anti-inflammatory [26, 30]; adrenal trophorestorative [26, 30]; beneficial to reduce inflammation in autoimmune disorders [26, 30]; may help protect against suppressive effects of corticosteroid and chemotherapy [26, 30]
St John's wort *Hypericum perforatum*	40 mL	Anti-inflammatory [25]; anti-depressant [25, 26]; anxiolytic [25, 26]; analgesic [25]; antiretroviral [25, 26]; antimicrobial [25, 26]
Bupleurum *Bupleurum falcatum*	45 mL	Anti-inflammatory [29, 30]; hepatoprotective [29, 30]; adaptogenic [56]; mild sedative [56]; beneficial in autoimmune disorders involving the kidneys [30]
Hemidesmus *Hemidesmus indicus*	45 mL	Immunusuppressant [30, 56]; therapeutic benefits in autoimmune conditions [30, 56]
Supply:	200 mL	Dose: 5 mL 3 times daily

TABLE 8.38 HERBAL TABLET ALTERNATIVE		
Anti-inflammatory herbal tablet may be taken in addition to herbal tonic if necessary to reduce pain and inflammation as an alternative to NSAIDs		
HERB	**DOSE PER TABLET**	**RATIONALE**
Boswellia *Boswellia serrata*	1.9 g	Anti-inflammatory [29, 33]; anti-arthritic [29, 33]; beneficial for autoimmune rheumatic conditions [58, 59]
Turmeric *Curcuma longa*	2.0 g	Anti-inflammatory [25, 26, 32]; antimicrobial [25, 26]; antioxidant [25, 26]; choleretic [25, 26]; immunomodulator [25]
Celery seed *Apium graveolens*	1.0 g	Anti-inflammatory [25, 29]; cholagogue [25]; antirheumatic [25, 29, 31]; sedative [31]
Ginger *Zingiber officinale*	300 mg	Anti-inflammatory [25, 26]; antioxidant [25]; circulatory stimulant [25, 26]; immunomodulator [25]; digestive stimulant [14, 25, 26]
Dose: 1 tablet 3 times daily		

TABLE 8.39 HERBAL TEA

Alternative to coffee

HERB	FORMULA	RATIONALE
Lemon balm *Melissa officinalis*	2 parts	Anxiolytic [25, 55]; sedative [25, 29, 55]; anti-inflammatory [25]; analgesic [25]; beneficial for sleeping problems [25, 29, 55]
Willowbark *Salix alba*	2 parts	Anti-inflammatory [25, 27, 29]; analgesic [25, 27, 29]; antirheumatic [29]
Prickly ash *Zanthoxylum americanum*	1 part	Circulatory stimulant [27, 29, 38]; antirheumatic [27, 29, 31]; silagogue [27, 29]
Green tea *Camellia sinensis*	1 part	Antioxidant [25, 41, 50]
Licorice root *Glycyrrhiza glabra*	1 part	Anti-inflammatory [25, 26]; adrenal tonic [25, 26]; antioxidant [25, 26]; antimicrobial [25, 26]; immunomodulator [25]; mild laxative [26]

Decoction: 1 tsp per cup – 1 cup 3 times daily

TABLE 8.40 NUTRITIONAL SUPPLEMENTS

SUPPLEMENT AND DOSE	RATIONALE
Omega-3 fish oil 10,000 mg daily in divided doses [25]	Anti-inflammatory [14, 25, 28, 46]; omega-3 3 supplementation improves clinical status in autoimmune conditions [41, 46] and can reduce the need for antirheumatic medication [46]; omega-3 supplementation decreases inflammatory cytokine levels in autoimmune conditions [46]; EPA favours the formation of immunoinhibitory prostaglandins [39]; helps protect against renal damage in SLE [41] and delays the onset and progression of autoimmune lupus nephritis [57]; beneficial in depression [25, 60, 61]
Supplement providing approx 1000 mg vitamin C, 400 mg quercetin, 100 mg bromelain and 250 IU vitamin E per dose Dose: one dose twice daily [14, 25] **NB**: Combining the above supplements in one product is likely to improve compliance by making it easier for Amira to take all the required supplements in one dose and by reducing the financial cost	Quercetin is an anti-inflammatory [25, 28]; antioxidant [25, 28]; immunomodulator [25]; quercetin inhibits inflammatory enzymes, prostaglandins and leukotrienes [25], stabilises mast cells [25] and inhibits mast cell release of histamine [28] Bromelain is anti-inflammatory [15, 35, 28]; beneficial in autoimmune disease [28]; bromelain reduces inflammation [60]; and may be beneficial in inflammatory autoimmune conditions [34] Vitamin E supplementation can induce remission in SLE [39] Vitamin C supplementation may prevent occurrence of active SLE [51] SLE sufferers have lower serum antioxidant levels [41, 50]

References

[1] N.J. Talley, S. O'Connor, Pocket clinical examination, third edn, Churchill Livingstone Elsevier, Australia, 2009.

[2] P. Kumar, C. Clark, Clinical medicine, sixth edn, Elsevier Saunders, London, 2005.

[3] J. Silverman, S. Kurtz, J. Draper, Skills for Communicating with Patients, second edn, Radcliff Publishing, Oxford, 2000.

[4] R. Neighbour, The Inner Consultation: how to develop an effective and intuitive consulting style, Radcliff Publishing, Oxon, 2005.

[5] M. Lloyd, R. Bor, Communication Skills For Medicine, third edn, Churchill Livingstone Elsevier, Edinburgh, 2009.

[6] G. Douglas, F. Nicol, C. Robertson, Macleod's Clinical Examination, twelfth edn, Churchill Livingstone Elsevier, 2009.

[7] J. Jamison, Differential Diagnosis for Primary Care, second edn, Churchill Livingstone Elsevier, London, 2006.

[8] A. Polmear (Ed.), Evidence-Based Diagnosis in Primary Care, Churchill Livingstone Elsevier, Edinburgh, 2008, pp. 274–283.

[9] R. Berkow, A.J. Fletcher, M.H. Beers, The Merck Manual, sixteenth edn, Merck Research Laboratories, Rathway, N.J, 1993 (later edition).

[10] R.H. Seller, Differential Diagnosis of Common Complaints, fifth edn, Saunders Elsevier, Philadelphia, 2007.

[11] R.D. Collins, Differential Diagnosis in Primary Care, fouth edn, Lippincott Williams & Wilkins, Philadelphia, 2008.

[12] K.D. Pagna, T.J. Pagna, Mosby's Diagnostic and Laboratory Test reference, third edn, Mosby, USA, 1997 (later edition).

[13] D. Peters, L. Chaitow, G. Harris, S. Morrison, Integrating Complementary Therapies in Primary Care, Churchill Livingstone, London 2002.

[14] J. Jamison, Clinical Guide to Nutrition & Dietary Supplements in Disease Management, Churchill Livingstone, Edinburgh, 2003.

[15] J.E. Pizzorno, M.T. Murray, H. Joiner-Bey, The Clinicians Handbook of Natural Medicine, second edn, Churchill Livingstone, St Louis, 2008.

[16] H. Osiecki, The Physicians Handbook of Clinical Nutrition, seventh edn, Bioconcepts, Eagle Farm, 2000.

[17] D. Morawetz, What works in therapy: what Australian clients say, Psychotherapy in Australia 9 (1) (2002) 66–70.

[18] G.A. Bonnano, Loss Trauma and Human Resilience, American Psychologist 59 (1) (2004) 20–28.

[19] A.F. Jorm, H. Christensen, K.M. Griffiths, R.A. Parslow, B. Rodgers, K.A. Blewitt, Effectiveness of complementary and self-help treatments for anxiety disorders, Medical Journal of Australia 181 (7) (2004) S29–S46.

[20] A. Byrne, G.D. Byrne, The effect of exercise on depression, anxiety and other mood states: A review, J Psychosom Res 37 (6) (1993) 565–574.

[21] C.A. Moyer, J. Rounds, J.W. Hannum, A Meta-Analysis of Massage Therapy Research, Psychological Bulletin 130 (1) (2004) 3–18.

[22] T. Field, G. Robinson, F. Scafidi, R. Nawrocki, A. Goncalves, Massage therapy reduces anxiety and enhances EEG pattern of alertness and math computations, International Journal of Neuroscience 86 (1996) 197–205.

[23] J.A. Jackson, H.D. Riordan, R. Hunninghake, S. Neathery, Joint and Muscle Pain, Various Arthritic Conditions and Food Sensitivities, Journal of Orthomolecular Medicine 13 (3) (1998) 168–172.

[24] C.J. Henderson, R.S. Panush, Diets, dietary supplements, and nutritional therapies in rheumatic diseases, in J. Jamison, Clinical Guide to Nutrition & Dietary Supplements in Disease Management, Churchill Livingstone, Edinburgh, 2003.

[25] L. Braun, M. Cohen, Herbs & Natural Supplements: An evidence based guide, second edn, Elsevier, Sydney, 2007.

[26] S. Mills, K. Bone, Principles & Practice of Phytotherapy: Modern Herbal Medicine, Churchill Livingstone, Edinburgh, London, 2000.

[27] British Herbal Medicine Association, British Herbal Pharmacopoeia, BHMAA, 1983.

[28] H. Osiecki, The Nutrient Bible, seventh edn, BioConcepts Publishing, Eagle Farm, 2008.

[29] S. Mills, K. Bone, The Essential Guide to Herbal Safety, Churchill Livingstone, St Louis, 2005.

[30] K. Bone, Clinical Applications of Chinese and Ayurvedic Herbs: Monographs for the Western Herbal Practitioners, Phytotherapy Press, Warwick, 1996.

[31] D. Hoffman, The New Holistic Herbal, Element Books Ltd, Shaftesbury, Dorset, 1990.

[32] N. Chainani-Wu, Safety and Anti-Inflammatory Activity of Curcumin: A Component of Turmeric (Curcuma longa), The J Altern Complement Med 9 (1) (2003) 161–168.

[33] D. Khanna, G. Sethi, K.S. Ahn, M.J. Pandey, A.B. Kunnumakkara, G. Sung, et al., Natural products as a gold mine for arthritis treatment, Current Opinion in Pharmacology 7 (2007) 344–351.

[34] D.J. Fitzhugh, S. Shan, M.W. Dewhirst, L.P. Hale, Bromelain treatment decreases neutrophil migration to sites of inflammation, Clinical Immunology 128 (2008) 66–74.

[35] A.R. Gaby, Alternative Treatments for Rheumatoid Arthritis, Alternative Medicine Review 4 (6) (1999) 392–402.

[36] K.W. Wucherpfennig, Mechanisms for the induction of autoimmunity by infectious agents, Journal of Clinical Investigation 108 (2001) 1097–1104.

[37] W. Luman, K.B. Chua, W.K. Cheong, H.S. Ng, Gastrointestinal Manifestations of Systemic Lupus Erythematosus, Singapore Medical Journal 42 (8) (2001) 380–384.

[38] A. Fasano, T. Shea-Donohue, Mechanisms of Disease: the role of intestinal barrier function in the pathogenesis of gastrointestinal autoimmune diseases, Nature Clinical Practice Gastroenterology & Hepatology 2 (9) (2005) 416–422.

[39] J. Homsy, W.J.W. Morros, J.A. Levy, Nutrition and autoimmunity: a review, Clinical and Experimental Immunology 65 (1986) 473–488.

[40] S.C. Bae, S.J. Kim, M.K. Sung, Impaired antioxidant status and decreased dietary intake of antioxidants in patients with systemic lupus erythematosus, Rheumatology International 22 (2002) 238–243.

[41] T. Patavino, D.M. Brady, Natural Medicine and Nutritional Therapy as an Alternative Treatment in Systemic Lupus Erythematosus, Alternative Medicine Review 6 (5) (2001) 460–471.

[42] C.M. Tench, J. McCarthy, I. McCurdie, P.D. White, D.P. D'Cruz, Fatigue in systemic lupus erythematosus: a randomized controlled trial of exercise, Rheumatology 42 (2003) 1050–1054.

[43] C. Ayan, V. Martin, Systemic lupus erythematosus and exercise, Lupus 16 (2007) 5–9.

[44] B. Zeitz, T. Reber, M. Oertel, T. Gluck, J. Scholmerich, R.H. Straub, Altered function of the hypothalamic stress axes in patients with moderately active systemic lupus erythematosus. II. Dissociation between androstenedione, cortisol, or dehydroepiandrosterone and interleukin 6 or tumor necrosis factor, Journal of Rheumatology 27 (4) (2000) 911–918.

[45] S.G. Adams, P.M. Dammers, T.L. Saia, P.J. Brantley, G.R. Gaydos, Stress, Depression, and Anxiety Predict Average Symptom Severity and Daily Symptom Fluctuation in Systemic Lupus Erythematosus, Journal of Behavioral Medicine 17 (5) (1994) 459–477.

[46] A.P. Simopoulis, Omega-3 Fatty Acids in Inflammation and Autoimmune Diseases, Journal of the American College of Nutrition 21 (6) (2002) 495–505.

[47] D. Mozaffarian, T. Pischon, S.E. Hankinson, N. Rifai, K. Joshiparu, W.C. Willett, et al., Dietary intake of trans fatty acids and systemic inflammation in women, The American Journal of Clinical Nutrition 79 (2004) 606–612.

[48] Y. Ioannou, D.A. Isenberg, Current concepts for the management of systemic lupus erythematosus in adults: a therapeutic challenge, Postgraduate Medical Journal 78 (2002) 599–606.

[49] O. Adam, C. Beringer, T. Kless, C. Lemmen, A. Adam, M. Wiseman, P. Adam, et al., Anti-inflammatory effects of a low arachidonic acid diet and fish oil in patients with rheumatoid arthritis, Rheumatology International 23 (2003) 27–36.

[50] S.G. Sukkar, E. Rossi, Oxidative stress and nutritional prevention in autoimmune rheumatic diseases, Autoimmunity Reviews 3 (2004) 199–206.

[51] Y. Minami, T. Sasaki, Y. Arai, Y. Kurisu, S. Hisamichi, Diet and systemic lupus erythematosus: a 4 year prospective study of Japanese patients, Journal of Rheumatology 30 (4) (2003) 747–754.

[52] S. Shirato, How CAM Helps Systemic Lupus Erythematosus, Holistic Nursing Practice 19 (1) (2005) 36–39.

[53] C.M. Greco, A.H. Kao, K. Maksimowicz-McKinnon, R.M. Glick, M. Houze, S.M. Sereika, et al., Acupuncture for systemic lupus erythematosus: a pilot RCT feasibility and safety study, Lupus 17 (2008) 1108–1116.

[54] T.P. Vliet Vileland, Rehabilitation of people with rheumatoid arthritis, Best Practice & Research Clinical Rheumatology 17 (5) (2003) 847–861.

[55] R.F. Weiss, Weiss' Herbal Medicine Classic Edition, Thieme, Stuttgart, 2001.

[56] B. Burgoyne, M. Morgan, Herbs for autoimmunity, A Phytotherapist's Perspective 29 (2003) 1–2.

[57] B. Chandrasekar, D.A. Troyer, J.T. Venkatraman, G. Fernandes, Dietary Omega-3 Lipids Delay the Onset and Progression of Autoimmune Lupus Nephritis by Inhibiting Transforming Growth Factor β mRNA and Protein Expression, Journal of Autoimmunity 8 (1995) 381–393.

[58] K. Bone, Boswellia effective for Osteoarthritis, Modern Phytotherapist 8 (2) (2004) 27–28.

[59] K. Bone, M. Morgan, Boswellia Serrata-Boswellia, Mediherb Professional Review 69 (1999) 1–5.

[60] B.M. Ross, J. Seguin, L.E. Sieswerda, Omega-3 fatty acids as treatments for mental illness: which disorder and which fatty acid? Lipids in Health and Disease 6 (2007) 21.

[61] B. Nemets, Z. Stahl, R.H. Belmaker, Addition of Omega-3 Fatty Acid to Maintenance Medication Treatment for Recurrent Unipolar Depressive Disorder, American Journal of Psychiatry 159 (2002) 477–479.

[62] L. Chaitow, Hydrotherapy, water therapy for health and beauty, Element, Dorset, 1999.

[63] M. Sinclair, Modern Hydrotherapy for the Massage Therapist, Lippincott Williams & Wilkins, Baltimore, 2008.

[64] E. Blake, in: L. Chaitow, E. Blake, P. Orrock, M. Wallden, P. Snider, J. Zeff (Eds.), Naturopathic Physical Medicine: Theory and Practice for Manual Therapists and Naturopaths, Churchill Livingstone Elsevier, Philadelphia, 2008.

[65] W. Boyle, A. Saine, Lectures in Naturopathic Hydrotherapy, Eclectic Medical Publications, Oregon, 1988.

[66] N. Shevchuk, S. Radoja, Possible stimulation of anti-tumour immunity using repeated cold stress: a hypothesis, Infect Agent-Cancer 2 (2007) 20.

[67] D.D. Buchman, The complete book of water healing, Contemporary Books, McGraw-Hill Companies, New York, 2001.

[68] S. El-Hashemy, Naturopathic Standards of Primary Care, CCNM Press Inc, Toronto, 2007.

[69] T. Guidotti, Occupational repetitive strain injury, Am Fam Physician 45 (1992) 585–592.

[70] A. Mies Richie, M. Francis, Diagnostic approach to polyarticular joint pain, Am Fam Physician 68 (6) (2003) 1151–1160.

[71] C. D'Arcy, S. McGee, Does this patient have carpal tunnel syndrome? JAMA 283 (2000) 3110–3117.

[72] S. Ferry, A. Silman, T. Pritchard, et al., The association between different patterns of hand symptoms and objective evidence of median nerve compression, Arthritis Rheum 41 (1998) 720–724.

[73] D.L. Goldenberg, Septic arthritis, Lancet 351 (1998) 197–202.

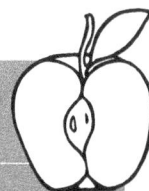

CHAPTER 9

Urinary system

Chronic recurrent cystitis

Case history

Marion Black is 34 years old. She has come to the clinic for help with an ongoing problem of increased nocturnal urination. At times she also experiences increased frequency during the day. Along with the increased urination, Marion experiences a burning and stinging sensation and the urine has an unusual and unpleasant odour that comes on suddenly and usually resolves within two days. She has had this problem before, and it was treated successfully with antibiotics. Marion mentions that sometimes she also experiences pelvic discomfort and an increase in vaginal discharge.

Marion has just entered into a new relationship and she has noticed these symptoms return after sexual intercourse. When she abstains from intercourse for a few weeks she notices great improvement. When she is symptom-free she finds that things seem to be normal for about a month, but then the symptoms return again following sexual intercourse. This is starting to become a major problem in her new relationship and she doesn't want to just keep taking antibiotics when it occurs but to clear the problem up permanently.

Marion says her menstrual cycle has remained the same. She has a regular 28-day cycle with no pain or premenstrual symptoms, and the bleed lasts for three to four days. She is not taking contraceptive drugs at the moment but is considering doing so.

Marion loves her job as a hairdresser, plays several sports, doesn't smoke, drinks alcohol occasionally and enjoys cooking and eating good food. She hopes one day to travel the world. Marion does mention that sometimes her job requires her to stay in the one position for long periods of time and she will 'hold on' rather than pass urine during the day.

TABLE 9.1 **COMPLAINT**	
Analogy: Skin of the apple	**Complaint:** Define the presenting complaint and symptoms; understand the complaint *Recurrent cystitis*
AREAS OF INVESTIGATION AND EXAMPLE QUESTIONS	**CLIENT RESPONSES**
Onset *When did the symptoms start?*	*The symptoms have been happening for the past few months. They go away for a while but come back again.*

►

Exacerbating factors *What do you think makes it worse?*	*The main thing is it keeps coming back after having sex.*
Relieving factors *What makes it better?*	*Antibiotics make it better and sometimes Ural helps too.*

TABLE 9.2 **CONTEXT**	
Analogy: Flesh of the apple	**Context:** Put the presenting complaint into context to understand the disease
AREAS OF INVESTIGATION AND EXAMPLE QUESTIONS	**CLIENT RESPONSES**
Occupational toxins and hazards *What kind of chemicals do you use in your work?*	*Mostly hair colouring and perming solutions. I always wear gloves to protect myself from the chemicals.*
Functional disease *Were you doing any horseback or bike riding when you developed the symptoms of the stinging sensation on urination and vaginal discharge?* (mechanical urethritis)	*No, I am not that fit!*
Infection and inflammation *Is the stinging and burning sensation on urination worse at the end of the urine stream?* (cystitis) *Are the symptoms of burning pain and increased frequency of urination pain better for a hot bath?* (cystitis) *Do you experience any pain or blood during or after sexual intercourse?*(STD, cancer/ infection)	*Yes, definitely.* *Yes, I do like to have a bath when the symptoms are bad, I think it relaxes me too.* *No blood and pain when having sex but I notice the symptoms are bad afterwards.*
Supplements and side effects of medications *Has taking antibiotics led to any problems?*	*I got thrush a couple of times, but I'm OK at the moment.*
Endocrine/reproductive *Can you tell me about your menstrual cycle?* *Tell me about the vaginal discharge and pelvic discomfort.*	Marion reports a 28-day cycle with normal bleed pattern and duration. She is not currently taking the oral contraceptive pill. Marion notices she sometimes gets increased vaginal discharge, particularly after taking antibiotics which she thinks is thrush. The pelvic discomfort usually happens when she has cystitis.

▶

Eating habits and energy *Tell me about your diet and energy levels.*	Marion describes her diet. It is high in refined carbohydrates and she drinks at least 4 cups of coffee daily. Sometimes she misses out on lunch if the salon is very busy. She tries to eat healthy food most nights. She usually has lots of energy, but when she has cystitis she feels tired.

TABLE 9.3 **CORE**	
Analogy: Core of the apple with the seed of ill health	**Core:** Holistic assessment to understand the client
AREAS OF INVESTIGATION AND EXAMPLE QUESTIONS	**CLIENT RESPONSES**
Daily activities *Tell me about your daily routine.*	*I get up at 6.30 am, have breakfast and get to work by 7.30 am. I finish about 5.30 pm or 6 pm and then go home. Dinner is about 7 pm and then I either go out with Sean or we stay home. I usually go to bed by 11 pm.*
Occupation *Do you enjoy your work?*	*I love it, although standing on my feet all day can be tiring.*
Family and friends *Do you have much contact with family and friends?*	*Not as much as I did before I started going out with Sean. I try to see my parents every couple of weeks and sometimes Sean and I go out with friends.*
Education and learning *Do you understand why your cystitis keeps returning?*	*Not really, but I think it must have something to do with sex.*
Action needed to heal *What do you think you need to do to get better?*	*Hopefully not stop having sex! Maybe I need to go to the toilet more during the day and drink more water.*

TABLE 9.4 **MARION'S SIGNS AND SYMPTOMS [1–3, 13]**	
Pulse	85 bpm
Blood pressure	120/80
Temperature	38°C
Respiratory rate	14 resp/min
Body mass index	22
Waist circumference	77 cm
Face	Pale
Urinalysis	Cloudy colour; foul odour; alkaline pH; leukocytes detected; microscopic blood detected; positive nitrites; increased specific gravity

TABLE 9.5 **RESULTS OF MEDICAL INVESTIGATIONS**	
Marion has not been consistent with contraception recently and had these tests	
TEST	**RESULT**
Home urine HGC pregnancy test	Negative
Follow up blood HGC pregnancy test	Negative

TABLE 9.6 **UNLIKELY DIAGNOSTIC CONSIDERATIONS** [3–8]	
CONDITIONS AND CAUSES	**WHY UNLIKELY**
CANCER AND HEART DISEASE	
Congestive heart failure	No protein in Marion's urine; she does not have high blood pressure, extreme tachycardia or shortness of breath
TRAUMA AND PRE-EXISTING ILLNESS	
Renal failure	No protein in Marion's urine
OBSTRUCTION AND FOREIGN BODY	
Renal calculi: primary hyperoxaluria (oxalate stones); hyperuricaemia and hyperuriosuria (uric acid stones); cysteinuria (results in cystine stones)	Usually presents with acidic urine
FUNCTIONAL DISEASE	
Female urethral syndrome: irritative bladder symptoms in absence of urologic findings; pain in the urethra; can be a component of interstitial cystitis; pain on urination, increased frequency, pelvic pain, sexually active [43]	Onset of symptoms occurred more than 2–7 days ago; usually does not present with blood in the urine; no bacteria usually detected by urinalysis; level of urinary urgency not noted yet in Marion's history; usually no fever presents; does not necessarily have nocturia as a symptom
INFECTION AND INFLAMMATION	
Trigonitis: inflammation of the mouth of bladder; increased urination, pelvic pain	Usually normal urinalysis results
Glomerulonephritis (advanced kidney infection)	Would show protein in urine and possible macrocytic blood; low specific gravity
ENDOCRINE/REPRODUCTIVE	
Causal factor: **Ectopic pregnancy**	Blood and urine HGC tests negative
Causal factor: **Pregnancy**	Blood and urine HGC tests negative
Diabetes: nocturia	No glucose in urinalysis

Case analysis

TABLE 9.7 **POSSIBLE DIFFERENTIAL DIAGNOSIS**		
Not ruled out by tests/investigations already done [2–9, 44, 47]		
CONDITIONS AND CAUSES	WHY POSSIBLE	WHY UNLIKELY
CANCER AND HEART DISEASE		
Bladder carcinoma	Blood in urine; pelvic discomfort; increased frequency of urination (need to determine if the volume is decreased)	Pain on urination is not a common symptom
Cervical cancer	Vaginal discharge, symptoms worse with sexual intercourse	Need to determine if pain/blood is experienced on intercourse
TRAUMA AND PRE-EXISTING ILLNESS		
Causal factor: **Mechanical urethritis/ honeymoon cystitis/trauma**	Pain on urination, increased frequency; sexually active	Urine is usually sterile and urinalysis does not indicate the presence of bacteria or other abnormalities
OBSTRUCTION AND FOREIGN BODY		
Renal calculi/kidney stones/bladder obstruction/ stones (hypercalcaemia/ hypercalciuria)	Blood in the urine; pelvic discomfort noted (need to determine whether discomfort occurs at the end of urination); alkaline pH	No back pain (predominant symptom); normal appetite
FUNCTIONAL DISEASE		
Causal factor: **Stress incontinence**	Can be associated with pain on urination, increased frequency of urination and urgency	Usually no nocturia in stress incontinence
Nocturnal polyuria syndrome	Nocturia, increased volume of urine	Usually occurs in the elderly from conditions such as diabetes, heart disease and from certain medications
DEGENERATIVE AND DEFICIENCY		
Osteoporosis (hypercalcaemia)	Alkaline urine, pelvic pain	No family history reported yet; Marion is not in the common age group
Anaemia	Marion's face looks pale	Need more information about Marion's diet and gastrointestinal function

▶

INFECTION AND INFLAMMATION		
Urinary tract infections (UTIs): can affect anywhere along the whole urinary tract **Recurrent cystitis:** lower urinary tract infection/ bladder infection [42, 47]	Increased urination during the day and at night; passing urine is painful, high temperature, urine contains blood, has strong odour and the condition is worsened by sexual intercourse; symptoms develop quickly; recurrence of the same symptoms; urinalysis detected nitrates, leukocytes (pyuria), blood, foul odour and increased pH; pain on urination with pus (pyuria) in urine is diagnostic for cystitis; common in women of this age group	
Pyelonephritis (upper UTI in the kidneys)	White blood cells in urine (pyuria), pelvic pain, raised temperature	No anorexia, severe abdominal pain, back pain, headache, fatigue, chills or vomiting reported
Interstitial cystitis: painful bladder syndrome	Marion is in the age group most commonly affected, recurrent pain on urination, pelvic pain, marked frequency, nocturia	Level of urinary urgency not noted yet in Marion's history; need to determine whether pain is relieved when voiding urine; usually no pus is present (leukocytes in urine)
Reiter's syndrome: can begin with gonorrhoeal urethritis	Pain on urination and increased discharge; urinary symptoms that begin after sexual intercourse; syndrome can be asymptomatic	No conjunctivitis or arthritis or skin lesions reported
ENDOCRINE/REPRODUCTIVE		
Hyperthyroidism/ hyperparathyroidism (hyercalcaemia)	Nocturia, alkaline urine, increased urination	Need more information about thirst, appetite, weight and energy levels
Pelvic inflammatory disease/salpingitis	Pelvic pain, vaginal discharge, fever, sexually active, unsure about contraceptive use	Periods are regular, unsure whether vaginal discharge is purulent and offensive, no significant backache or lower abdominal pain reported; no period pain; unsure at this stage of severity of Marion's pelvic pain
Vaginitis: *Candida albicans*, *Trichomonas*, chemical reaction to vaginal sprays, douches or bubble baths	Vaginal discharge, pain on urination (need to determine if external pain)	No vaginal itching reported; pyuria not commonly detected in urinalysis (leukocytes)

Urethritis: *Chlamydia trachomatis, Mycoplasma,* D streptococci, *Trichomonas, Candida albicans,* gonorrhoeal, herpes urethritis, masturbation, foreign body, horseback or bike riding [48]	Vaginal discharge, Marion is sexually active and has a new partner; the form of contraception Marion and her partner are currently using is unclear; Marion is experiencing pain on urination (need to determine whether it is internal pain)	Less common in women to have blood in urine with urethritis; pyuria not commonly detected in urinalysis (leukocytes)
STRESS AND NEUROLOGICAL DISEASE		
Neurologic disease: multiple sclerosis (MS), spinal cord injury, cauda equina syndrome	Lower urinary tract symptoms; more common in women; increased urination, nocturia	Usually occurs in advanced stages of MS; no significant trauma or injury mentioned in health history so far; no lower back pain reported; no numbness, weakness or tingling in lower limbs

TABLE 9.8 **DECISION TABLE FOR REFERRAL** [1, 3–6, 8, 12]		
COMPLAINT	**CONTEXT**	**CORE**
Referral for presenting complaint	Referral for all associated physical, dietary and lifestyle concerns	Referral for contributing emotional, mental, spiritual, metaphysical, lifestyle and constitutional factors
REFERRAL FLAGS	**REFERRAL FLAGS**	**REFERRAL FLAGS**
• Recurrent UTIs • Marion experiences persistent increase in urinary frequency	• Pelvic pain and vaginal discharge • Dehydration • Return of symptoms following sexual intercourse • Holds on to urine rather than going to the toilet when she needs to while at work • Unclear what form of contraception Marion and her partner are using	• Marion's concerns about her condition affecting her relationship
ISSUES OF SIGNIFICANCE	**ISSUES OF SIGNIFICANCE**	**ISSUES OF SIGNIFICANCE**
Nil	• Recurrent antibiotic therapy	Nil
REFERRAL	**REFERRAL**	**REFERRAL**
• For medical assessment and definitive diagnosis • Second medical opinion on urinalysis result [45]	• Medical investigations to help rule out underlying pathologies (e.g. STD) [48] • Pap (cervical) smear check-up	• Women's health centre or family planning to discuss contraception options and safe sex practice

TABLE 9.9 **FURTHER INVESTIGATIONS THAT MAY BE NECESSARY** [1–8, 42, 45]	
TEST/INVESTIGATION	**REASON FOR TEST/INVESTIGATION**
FIRST-LINE INVESTIGATIONS:	
Urinalysis – repeat test [42, 46, 49–51]	UTI, kidney infection, stones, diabetes, blood
Abdominal examination	Suprapubic tenderness on palpation and percussion
Pelvic examination	Appearance of labia, vulva, entire vagina, cervix, vaginal discharge should be inspected; cervical manipulation for masses or points of tenderness; scabies, contact dermatitis; bulky uterus indicates uterine cancer; vulval inflammation more often in *Candida* than in bacterial vaginosis; vaginal discharge visible with vaginitis
Pap smear (cervical smear) [42, 46]	Check for signs of STIs
Full blood count	Check for infections and/or anaemia
ESR/CRP blood test	Check for inflammation, tumour detection, bacteria and viral detection
Urea, creatinine and **electrolytes** (sodium, potassium, chloride, bicarbonate) **blood test**	Gives an indicator of renal excretory function as urea and blood creatinine is excreted entirely by the kidneys; this will show in renal abnormalities and diabetes
Gram stain and culture of urethral discharge [48]	Chlamydia and gonorrhoea
Potassium hyroxide/saline wet mount	*Candida albicans, Trichomonas*
Urine microscopy	To eliminate the possibility of renal disease; will give information about specific white blood cells (indicates an inflammatory reaction in urinary tract), red blood cells, casts (clumps of materials or cells and can indicate renal disease) and crystals (indicate renal stone formation is imminent)
IF NECESSARY:	
Calcium, phosphate and serum alkaline phosphatase	Metabolic bone disease and renal calculi due to calcium excess, renal infarction; calcium excretion can be monitored
Thyroid function test TSH, T4, T3	TSH (thyroid-stimulating hormone) suppressed in hyperthyroidism; thyroid-specific antibodies, to confirm auto-immune cause of hyperthyroidism (Graves')
Estimated glomerular filtration rate (eGFR)	Kidney function
Renal ultrasound/x-ray	If renal disease is suspected; ultrasound/x-ray will give information about renal size, failure, stones, mass formation, lesions
Pelvic x-ray	Osteoporosis

Cystoscopy: bladder	Direct visualisation of urethra and bladder; check for interstitial cystitis; evaluate blood in urine, bladder cancer, trigonitis
HLA-B27 antigen: human lymphocyte antigen B-27	Reiter's syndrome

Confirmed diagnosis

MARION AND RECURRENT CHRONIC CYSTITIS

Marion is a 34-year-old woman who has recently been experiencing increased urination during the night along with symptoms of burning and stinging on urination, pelvic discomfort, increased vaginal discharge, raised temperature and her urine has an unpleasant odour. Marion has experienced these symptoms in the past and has noticed the symptoms return after sexual intercourse. Marion has only recently entered into a new sexual relationship and is concerned this pattern of symptoms is beginning to have a negative impact on her relationship.

Marion's symptom picture reflects recurrent cystitis that develops as a reinfection in an otherwise functionally normal urinary tract. This is a condition that requires attention as persistent infection may result in further upper UTIs.

Cystitis is a term used for urinary tract infection and is very common in women. Microbial transfer is more likely to happen due to the short urethra to the bladder in women compared with the longer urethra in males. Infection is most often due to the person's own bowel flora and transfer to the urinary tract can be via the bloodstream or lymphatic system. Microbial transfer in women most commonly occurs via the transurethral route between the anus and the vagina. Bacteria can be further carried to the bladder by sexual intercourse. Infrequent and poor bladder emptying can predispose to infection.

It is important to define what kind of cystitis is presenting. There is both **functionally normal urinary tract** (persistent infection rarely results in kidney damage) and **abnormal urinary tract** (from such conditions as urinary stones or diabetes mellitus, which can cause kidney damage and can be made worse by a urinary infection).

Additionally the case history can help ascertain whether the cystitis is due to **relapse** (recurrence of the same bacterial infection within seven days of treatment implying failure to eradicate the infection and indicating kidney stones, scarred kidneys, polycystic disease of the kidneys) or **reinfection** (bacteria is absent after treatment for at least 14 days followed by a reoccurrence of infection with the same or different organism; 80 per cent of recurrent infections are due to this).

General references used in this diagnosis: 3, 5–7, 47

PRESCRIBED MEDICATION

• Antibiotics for the current urinary infection [52]

TABLE 9.10 DECISION TABLE FOR TREATMENT (ONCE DIAGNOSIS IS CONFIRMED)		
COMPLAINT	CONTEXT	CORE
Treatment for the presenting complaint and symptoms	Treatment for all associated symptoms	Treatment for mental, emotional, spiritual, constitutional, lifestyle issues and metaphysical considerations

TREATMENT PRIORITY	TREATMENT PRIORITY	TREATMENT PRIORITY
• Lifestyle recommendations to reduce the frequency and severity of symptoms • Dietary recommendations to improve immune function, inhibit the growth of pathogenic bacteria and reduce the frequency and severity of symptoms • Physical therapy recommendations to reduce frequency and severity of symptoms • Herbal tonic with antimicrobial, diuretic, immune-stimulating and mucous membrane tonic action to help reduce the severity of acute symptoms • Herbal tea with antiseptic, diuretic and demulcent action to help reduce the severity of acute symptoms • Nutritional supplements to improve immunity, inhibit growth of pathogenic bacteria, inhibit adherence of bacteria to the bladder wall and protect the bladder from damage • Lifestyle recommendations to alleviate the discomfort of symptoms of acute cystitis • Physical treatment recommendations to help alleviate the discomfort and severity of symptoms **NB:** Marion's vitamin and mineral levels should be monitored to ensure she stays within normal range. Recommendation to reduce normal dose of vitamin A once symptom improvement has been achieved [16]	• Lifestyle recommendations to help prevent a recurrence of symptoms and improve urinary hygiene • Physical therapy recommendations to help prevent a recurrence of symptoms • Dietary recommendations to improve general health and immunity • Dietary supplements to boost immunity, support bowel flora and prevent a recurrence of cystitis • Herbal tea to help prevent a recurrence of cystitis	• Counselling regarding sexual health • Recommendation for massage to help reduce stress

Treatment aims

- Prevent or reduce frequency of UTIs by reducing urinary stasis [16] and increasing urine flow to aid expulsion of bacteria [14, 16, 18].
- Enhance Marion's immune function [14, 18].
- Improve Marion's urinary hygiene [16, 17].
- Adjust Marion's urinary pH to assist in preventing growth of pathogenic bacteria [14, 15].

- Inhibit adherence of pathogenic bacteria to the urinary bladder wall [14].
- Deal with underlying causative or aggravating factors such as lifestyle and diet [14, 18].

Lifestyle alterations/considerations

- Marion can improve urinary hygiene by emptying her bladder completely before going to bed [16] and by drinking at least 2½ L of water daily [14, 16, 17].
- Encourage Marion to should minimise exposure of the urethra to *E. coli* by ensuring she wipes from front to back when she has a bowel motion and wearing cotton underpants rather than nylon underpants and/or pantyhose [17].
- Encourage Marion to empty her bladder as soon as she feels the urge [17].
- Marion's partner should wear condoms during intercourse [17] and avoid the use of spermicides [16].
- Encourage Marion to urinate after intercourse [14, 17] and can wash her labia and urethra with a strong tea of golden seal (2 tsp/cup) both before and after intercourse [14].
- During acute episodes of cystitis Marion can reduce the sensation of burning and stinging by pouring warm water over her labia and urethral opening while urinating to dilute the urine.
- Weekly vaginal insertion of a pessary containing *Lactobacillus rhamnosus* and *Lactobacillus gasseri* may be helpful to prevent recurrence [16, 28].

Dietary suggestions

- Encourage Marion to drink at least 2½ litres of water each day [14–18].
- Drinking 250 mL of unsweetened cranberry or fresh berry juice [14, 15, 33] and eating a cup of cranberries daily can help prevent recurrence [17, 21, 33].
- Barley water (30 g barley in 1 L of water, reduced by boiling it down to 500 mL) can help alleviate symptoms [16].
- Encourage Marion to avoid refined carbohydrates and simple sugars [14].
- Identify and manage food allergies or intolerances [14].
- Encourage Marion to consume of garlic and onions [14] and eat unsweetened yoghurt with live lactobacilli several times per week [14, 33].
- Encourage Marion to have an antioxidant and flavanoid-rich whole-food diet [30, 31].

Physical treatment suggestions

- Hydrotherapy: a hot shallow bath several times a day or hot foot baths in the acute stage [36]. Apply a hot Epsom salt compress on the bladder, covered with wool and kept warm by a heating pad/hot water bottle [37]. Alternate hot compress with neutral sitz bath [35, 37]. *Note: ice packs or ice compresses are contraindicated over the bladder in cystitis.*
- Myofascial trigger point therapy on pelvic floor trigger points may help alleviate symptoms of urgency and frequency [26].
- Acupuncture may help reduce the severity and frequency of symptoms [27].
- Marion may benefit from massage to help reduce stress [38, 39].

TABLE 9.11 **ACUTE HERBAL FORMULA (1:2 LIQUID EXTRACTS)**		
HERB	**FORMULA**	**RATIONALE**
Bearberry *Arctostaphylos uva-ursi*	60 mL	Urinary antiseptic [19, 23]; astringent [19]; anti-inflammatory [19]; urinary alkaliser [15]; indicated for use in recurrent cystitis [19]; particularly effective against *E. coli* [14]; in combination with other herbs can significantly reduce the recurrence of cystitis [20]

▶

Echinacea root *Echinacea angustifolia/purpurea*	60 mL	Immunostimulant [19, 21]; anti-inflammatory [19, 21]; antioxidant [21]; increases resistance to infection [19]
Golden rod *Solidago virgaurea*	40 mL	Diuretic [21, 22]; anti-inflammatory [21, 22]; antibacterial [21]; the European Scientific Cooperative on Phytotherapy (ESCOP) indicates its use as an adjunctive treatment for bacterial UTIs [21]
Andrographis *Andrographis paniculata*	40 mL	Immunostimulant [19, 21]; antimicrobial [21]
Supply:	200 mL	Dose: 5 mL four times daily
This formula is for short-term use in the management of an active UTI. Bearberry should not be taken continuously for longer than 1 month [23]		
Cranberry *Vaccinium oxycoccus, Vaccinium macrocarpon* Cranberry is bacteriostatic [21]; antioxidant [21]; prevents bacterial adhesion [15, 23, 25] and deodorises urine [16]; an effective adjunctive treatment in UTI [21]. Cranberry may interfere with the action of bearberry [16], so should not be used in conjunction with it [16]; cranberry can be used when Marion is not taking the acute herbal tonic Dose: 10,000 mg capsule or tablet 3–4 times daily [21] or 500 mL unsweetened juice daily [14, 17] in acute cystitis. One 10,000 mg capsule or 250 mL juice daily can be used as a preventative [21]; cranberry may be contraindicated if Marion has a history of oxalate kidney stones [21]		

TABLE 9.12 **HERBAL TEA**

In addition to herbal liquid

HERB	FORMULA	RATIONALE
Buchu leaf *Barosma betulina*	1 part	Urinary tract disinfectant [19, 23]; mild diuretic [19]; traditional therapeutic use for UTIs [19]
Cornsilk *Zea mays*	1 part	Diuretic [22]; urinary demulcent [22]
Dandelion leaf *Taraxacum officinale*	1 part	Diuretic [16, 22, 23]; beneficial to reduce the risk of hypokalaemia and hypertension from long-term use of licorice in herbal tea [40]
Couch grass *Agropyron repens*	1 part	Soothing diuretic [22]; urinary demulcent [22]; indicated for use in cystitis with inflammation or irritation of the urinary tract [24]; may prevent bacterial adhesion [23]
Licorice root powder *Glycyrrhiza glabra*	½ part	Anti-inflammatory [19, 21]; mucoprotective [19, 21]; antibacterial [19, 21]; adrenal tonic [19, 21]; immunomodulator [19, 21]; demulcent [19, 21]; may help prevent bacterial adhesion to the bladder wall [41]
Infusion: 1 cup 3–4 times daily		
This tea can be used during acute episodes of cystitis at a dose of 3–4 cups daily, and can also be consumed at a dose of 1–2 cups daily as a preventative and alternative to tea and coffee; using herbal teas in the management of cystitis provides additional benefits by helping increase fluid intake		

TABLE 9.13 **NUTRITIONAL SUPPLEMENTS**	
SUPPLEMENT AND DOSE	**RATIONALE**
Vitamin C 500 mg every 2 hours during the first day of infection [14, 15] then reduce dose to 500 mg twice daily [34]	4–12 g vitamin C daily acidifies urine and facilitates the formation of reactive nitrogen oxides which are toxic to *E. coli* and other microorganisms [17, 18]; antioxidant [18, 29]; immunostimulant [18, 29]
High-potency practitioner-strength **probiotic supplement** containing *L. acidophilus* [16], *L. rhamnosus* and *L. reuteri* [17] Dosage as recommended by the manufacturer	Probiotic supplementation is helpful in preventing recurrent UTIs in women [16, 17, 21]; immune stimulant [21]; may help prevent disruption to intestinal microflora following antibiotic therapy [21, 32]
High-potency practitioner-strength **multivitamin, mineral and antioxidant supplement** providing therapeutic doses of antioxidants and flavanoids [30, 31] including a daily dose of 30 mg elemental zinc and 10000 IU Vitamin A [16, 21] Dosage as recommended by the manufacturer to achieve recommended doses of specific nutrients Dose should be maintained until there is a consistent improvement in symptoms and then reviewed **NB:** Ensure Marion is using effective contraception while taking vitamin A at this dose. Vitamin A supplementation should be reviewed and reduced to no more than 2500 IU daily [16,21] once her symptoms improve	Supplemental antioxidants and flavanoids may help prevent bladder damage [30, 31]; vitamin A and zinc are important antioxidants, essential for immune function and mucous membrane health [16, 21]; deficiency can result in impaired immunity [16, 21]

References

[1] G. Douglas, F. Nicol, C. Robertson, Macleod's Clinical Examination, twelfth edn, Churchill Livingstone Elsevier, 2009.

[2] N.J. Talley, S. O'Connor, Pocket Clinical Examination, third edn, Churchill Livingstone Elsevier, Australia, 2009.

[3] P. Kumar, C. Clark, Clinical Medicine, sixth edn, Elsevier Saunders, London, 2005 pp. 640–643, 651, 663.

[4] R. Berkow, A.J. Fletcher, M.H. Beers, The Merck Manual, sixteenth edn, Merck Research Laboratories, Rathway, N.J, 1993 (later edition).

[5] J. Jamison, Differential Diagnosis for Primary Care, second edn, Churchill Livingstone Elsevier, London, 2006.

[6] A. Polmear (Ed.), Evidence-Based Diagnosis in Primary Care, Churchill Livingstone Elsevier, 2008.

[7] R.H. Seller, Differential Diagnosis of Common Complaints, fifth edn, Saunders Elsevier, Philadelphia, 2007.

[8] R.D. Collins, Differential Diagnosis in Primary Care, fourth edn, Lippincott Williams & Wilkins, Philadelphia, 2008.

[9] J. Silverman, S. Kurtz, J. Draper, Skills for Communicating with Patients, second edn, Radcliff Publishing, Oxford, 2000.

[10] R. Neighbour, The Inner Consultation; how to develop an effective and intuitive consulting style, Radcliff Publishing, Oxon, 2005.

[11] M. Lloyd, R. Bor, Communication Skills For Medicine, third edn, Churchill Livingstone Elsevier, Edinburgh, 2009.

[12] D. Peters, L. Chaitow, G. Harris, S. Morrison, Integrating Complementary Therapies in Primary Care, Churchill Livingstone, London, 2002.

[13] K.D. Pagna, T.J. Pagna, Mosby's Diagnostic and Laboratory Test reference, third edn, Mosby, USA, 1997 (later edition).

[14] J.E. Pizzorno, M.T. Murray, H. Joiner-Bey, The Clinicians Handbook of Natural Medicine, second edn, Churchill Livingstone, St Louis, 2008.

[15] S. El-Hashemy, Naturopathic Standards of Primary Care, CCNM Press Inc, Toronto, 2007.

[16] J. Jamison, Clinical Guide to Nutrition & Dietary Supplements in Disease Management, Churchill Livingstone, Edinburgh, 2003.

[17] T. Hudson, Treatment and Prevention of Bladder Infections, Alternative and Complementary Therapies 12 (6) (2006) 297–302.

[18] H. Osiecki, The Physicians Handbook of Clinical Nutrition, seventh edn, Bioconcepts, Eagle Farm, 2000.

[19] S. Mills, K. Bone, Principles & Practice of Phytotherapy; Modern Herbal Medicine, Churchill Livingstone, Edinburgh: London, 2000.

[20] B. Larsson, A. Jonasson, S. Fianu, Prophylactic effect of UVA-E in women with recurrent cystitis, in K.Abascal, E.Yarnell, Botanical Medicine for Cystitis, Alternative and Complementary Therapies 14 (2) (2008) 69–77.

[21] L. Braun, M. Cohen, Herbs & Natural Supplements: An evidence based guide, second edn, Elsevier, Sydney, 2007.

[22] S. Mills, K. Bone, The Essential Guide to Herbal Safety, Churchill Livingstone, St Louis, 2005.

[23] K. Abascal, E. Yarnell, Botanical Medicine for Cystitis, Alternative and Complementary Therapies 14 (2) (2008) 69–77.

[24] British Herbal Medicine Association, British Herbal Pharmacopoeia, BHMA, 1983.

[25] S. Ahuja, B. Kaack, J. Roberts, Loss Of Fimbrial Adhesion With The Addition Of Vaccinium Macrocarpon To The Growth Medium Of P-Fimbriated Escherichia Coli, The Journal of Urology 159 (2) (1998) 559–562.

[26] J.M. Weiss, Pelvic Floor Myofascial Trigger Points: Manual Therapy For Interstitial Cystitis And The Urgency-Frequency Syndrome, The Journal of Urology 166 (6) (2001) 2226–2231.

[27] T. Alraek, A. Baerheim, The Effect of Prophylactic Acupuncture Treatment in Women with Recurrent Cystitis: Kidney Patients Fare Better, The J Altern Complement Med 9 (5) (2003) 651–658.

[28] S. Coudeyras, G. Jugie, M. Vermerie, C. Forestier, Adhesion of Human Probiotic Lactobacillus rhamnosus to Cervical and Vaginal Cells and Interaction with Vaginosis-Associated Pathogens, Infectious Diseases in Obstetrics and Gynaecology 2008.

[29] J. Higdon, An Evidence Based Approach to Vitamins and Minerals, Thieme, New York, 2003.

[30] A. Ozcan, A. Korkman, S. Oter, O. Coskun, Contribution of flavonoid antioxidants to the preventive effect of mesna in cyclophosphamide-induced cystitis in rats, Archives of Toxicology 79 (2005) 461–465.

[31] I. Yidrim, A. Korkman, S. Oter, A. Ozcan, E. Oztas, Contribution of antioxidants to preventive effect of mesna in cyclophosphamide-induced hemorrhagic cystitis in rats, Cancer Chemotherapy Pharmacology 54 (2004) 469–473.

[32] J.A. Madden, S.F. Plummer, J. Tang, I. Garaiova, N.T. Plummer, M. Herbison, J.O. Hunter, et al., Effect of probiotics on preventing disruption of the intestinal microflora following antibiotic therapy: A double-blind, placebo-controlled pilot study, International Immunopharmacology 5 (2005) 1091–1097.

[33] T. Kontiokari, J. Laitnen, L. Jarvi, T. Pokka, K. Sundqvist, M. Uhari, Dietary factors protecting women from urinary tract infection, The American Journal of Clinical Nutrition 77 (2003) 600–604.

[34] H. Osiecki, The Nutrient Bible, seventh edn, BioConcepts Publishing, Eagle Farm, 2008.

[35] L. Chaitow, Hydrotherapy, water therapy for health and beauty, Element, Dorset, 1999.

[36] D.D. Buchman, The complete book of water healing, Contemporary Books, McGraw-Hill Companies, New York, 2001.

[37] W. Boyle, A. Saine, Lectures in Naturopathic Hydrotherapy, Eclectic Medical Publications, Oregon, 1988.

[38] T. Field, G. Robinson, F. Scafidi, R. Nawrocki, A. Goncalves, Massage therapy reduces anxiety and enhances EEG pattern of alertness and math computations, International Journal of Neuroscience 86 (1996) 197–205.

[39] C.A. Moyer, J. Rounds, J.W. Hannum, A Meta-Analysis of Massage Therapy Research, Psychological Bulletin 130 (1) (2004) 3–18.

[40] R. Trickey, Women, Hormones & The Menstrual Cycle, second edn, Allen & Unwin, Sydney, 2003.

[41] X. Shen, X. Xiao, C. Liu, Research and application of Radix Glycyrrhizae, Asian Journal of Pharmacodynamics and Pharmacokinetics 7 (3) (2007) 181–200.

[42] J.D. Bremnor, R. Sadovsky, Evaluation of dysuria in adults, Am Fam Physician 65 (2002) 1589–1596.

[43] D.R. Bodner, The urethral syndrome, Urol Clin North Am 15 (1988) 699–703.

[44] R. Maskell, Broadening the concept of urinary tract infection, Br J Urol 76 (1995) 2–8.

[45] S. Bent, B. Nallamothu, D. Simel, et al., Does this woman have an acute uncomplicated urinary tract infection? JAMA 287 (2002) 2701–2710.

[46] P. Little, S. Turner, K. Rumsby, et al., Developing clinical rules to predict urinary tract infection in primary care settings: sensitivity and specificity of near patient tests (dipsticks) and clinical scores, Br J Gen Pract 56 (2006) 606–612.

[47] J. Car, Urinary tract infection in women: diagnosis and management in primary care, BMJ 332 (2006) 94–97.

[48] T. Shapiro, M. Dalton, J. Hammock, et al., The prevalence of urinary tract infections and sexually transmitted disease in women with symptoms of a simple urinary tract infection stratified by low colony count, Acad Emerg Med 12 (2005) 38–44.

[49] D. Medina-Bombardo, M. Segui-Diaz, C. Roca-Fusalba, et al., What is the predictive value of urinary tract infection in women? Fam Pract 20 (2003) 103–107.

[50] B. Bulloch, J. Bausher, W. Pomerantz, et al., Can urine clarity exclude the diagnosis of urinary tract infection? Pediatrics 106 (2000) E60.

[51] L. Deville, J. Yzermans, N. Van Duijn, et al., The urine dipstick test useful to rule out infections. A meta-analysis of the accuracy, BMC Urol 4 (2004) 4.

[52] S.D. Fihn, Acute uncomplicated urinary tract infection in women, N Engl J Med 349 (2003) 259–266.

Kidney stones (renal calculi)

Case history

Max Costas is 60 years old and has come to the clinic for help with backache that has been bothering him for the past couple of weeks. Max describes his pain as dull and intermittent, travelling across his lower back, radiating around to his stomach, down the front of his abdomen and into his groin. The pain has been gradually worsening and in the past three or four days the pain in his lower back has become constant, and he finds himself moving around a lot to ease the discomfort. In the past two days he has experienced sharp pains across his lower back on a few occasions. He tells you the pain was much worse after a long day building a limestone block wall, a task that involved a lot of heavy lifting and physical stress.

Max explains that he owns a landscaping business and this last year has been particularly physically demanding. Over the past few months of summer he has been working long hours to make the most of the daylight, and often forgets to eat and drink properly until he finishes for the day. This is partly because he has so much work to get through but also because he hasn't always been feeling well. Recently his gut has been bloated and he sometimes feels a bit nauseous. He mentions that when he gets home and tries to catch up on his water intake, the pain in his lower back seems to worsen.

When you ask Max about his diet he tells you he loves dairy food even though he doesn't eat as much as he used to. He laughs when he tells you that his apprentice jokes that he thinks Max enjoys a glass of cold milk as much as a beer. Before he was diagnosed with gout four years ago Max used to drink red wine and eat much more red meat and dairy products than he does now. Now he and his wife eat more chicken and fresh fish as well as vegetables and salads. He tells you he particularly enjoys eating spinach and would happily eat it every day. He has also started craving chocolate in the evenings after work. He admits that he isn't always as strict with his new healthier diet as he should be, but since the back pain has started his appetite has gone a bit off, particularly because he feels nauseous so often now. Max is a tea drinker and can consume quite a few cups during the day, particularly if he is working on a residential job and the homeowners offer him cups of tea.

Max and his wife have four children who are now grown up, and four grandchildren with another two on the way. He tells you being a grandfather is the best thing in the world and if he could he'd spend all day every day with the grandkids. He has thought about retiring and travelling around the country with his wife, but the thought of being away from the grandchildren for an extended period of time puts him off doing anything about it. He has been running his landscaping business for the past 25 years and it has become so busy that he has several staff and two apprentices to help him keep up with the workload. While he really enjoys landscaping, Max is aware that his body doesn't cope as well with the physical demands of his work as it did 10 years ago.

Max's doctor prescribed 200 mg Progout daily when he diagnosed Max with gout four years ago, and Max has been taking it consistently each day since then. When he recently saw his doctor to get a repeat prescription for Progout he told his doctor about the back pain and that he wasn't feeling very well. The doctor did some blood tests that revealed Max has kidney stones. Max would now like to learn how he can manage his condition as naturally as possible and prevent this happening again. He thinks a massage may help his back pain and ease his tension.

TABLE 9.14 **COMPLAINT**	
Analogy: Skin of the apple	**Complaint:** Define the presenting complaint and symptoms; understand the complaint *Kidney stones*
AREAS OF INVESTIGATION AND EXAMPLE QUESTIONS	**CLIENT RESPONSES**
Onset	About two weeks.
Understanding the cause (client)	Max knows he has kidney stones because the doctor told him. Because he thinks massage might alleviate the pain, it is apparent he needs further information about his condition and how to manage it.
Exacerbating factors *When does your back pain feel worse?*	*At the end of the day when I get home and drink lots of water.*
Relieving factors *Is there anything that seems to make it better?*	*Not that I can think of. I'm hoping a massage might help a bit.*
Location and radiation	The pain started in Max's lower back and radiates around to his stomach, down the abdomen and into his groin.
Rating scale *On a scale of 1 to 10, with 1 being no pain and 10 being the worst pain you have ever experienced how would you rate your back pain?*	*At the moment it's about a 5, but sometimes it gets worse and it's about an 8. It seems to be getting worse.*

TABLE 9.15 **CONTEXT**	
Analogy: Flesh of the apple	**Context:** Put the presenting complaint into context to understand the disease
AREAS OF INVESTIGATION AND EXAMPLE QUESTIONS	**CLIENT RESPONSES**
Family health *Has anyone in your family ever had back pain or kidney stones?*	*My dad used to suffer from back pain when he was older and my brother has arthritis in his back. I don't think anyone else has kidney stones.*
Surgery and hospitalisation *Have you had surgery or been hospitalised in the last year or so?*	*No.*

▶

Occupational toxins and hazards *Are you exposed to any chemicals in your work? Do you think your work is contributing to your back pain?*	*Not really. I think work does have an effect on my back, I do some pretty heavy lifting although I try and leave most of that type of work to the younger blokes.*
Functional disease *Does lying on your back with rest relieve your back pain?* (acute lumbosacral strain/ mechanical/disc syndrome) *Is the back pain worse by coughing, laughing, passing a bowel motion, sneezing, sitting or bending?* (disc syndrome)	*No. I usually feel very restless and need to move around to ease the pain.* *No. I haven't noticed that.*
Degenerative and deficiency *Did the doctor tell you if they found arthritis in your back when they did the tests?* *Do you experience early-morning stiffness that wears off after a couple of hours of activity?* (inflammatory arthritis) *Is the lower back pain associated with pain in other joints?* (osteoarthritis)	*No, I don't remember them saying anything.* *No. The pain can be there any time of the day.* *No, the pain is just in the back area and radiates to the groin when it's really bad.*
Endocrine/reproductive *Is your back pain associated with burning urination, difficulty urinating or fever?* (prostatitis)	*No urine problems yet, but sometimes I notice the colour is darker than normal.*
Supplements and side effects of medications *Are you taking any supplements or medications such as pain killers at the moment?*	*Yes, the doctor gave me some tablets to take for the pain when I needed them.* Max shows you a pack of paracetamol and codeine tablets.
Stress and neurological disease *Do you experience upper arm, leg, shoulder weakness associated with muscle wasting?* (motor neuron disease)	*No muscle weakness that I've really noticed. I can still lift things at work if this other pain is not irritating me.*

TABLE 9.16 CORE

Analogy: Core of the apple with the seed of ill health	**Core:** Holistic assessment to understand the client
AREAS OF INVESTIGATION AND EXAMPLE QUESTIONS	**CLIENT RESPONSES**
Emotional health *You have been experiencing some physical setbacks recently; how is this affecting your moods?*	*I really like my work, but it's getting harder on my body. I don't usually get stressed, but I've been working really hard lately. I suppose I get a bit grumpy when I get stressed.*

▶

Daily activities *Apart from work, what do you do during the day?*	*At the moment it really is just work. I'm up at about 5.30 and get home about 6. Then it's dinner and bed. I'm working most of the weekends at the moment too. Things should quieten down in the next month and I'll have more time for my wife and family.*
Family and friends *Tell me about your family and social life.*	*I really just live for the grandkids, they're really great. If I could, I'd get out of the business and look after them all the time although the wife might have something to say about that! I haven't spent much time with friends recently since work has been so busy. It usually eases off over winter so I should get some more time then.*
Education and learning *Do you understand how kidney stones can cause a backache?*	*Not really. Will massage make it better?*
Action needed to heal *What do you think will help you get better?*	*I don't really know. The doctor said something about what I eat and to drink more water. He said I might have to have surgery if it doesn't get better, so I'm here for something natural to help.*

TABLE 9.17 **MAX'S SIGNS AND SYMPTOMS** [1–3]	
Pulse	88 bpm
Blood pressure	140/90
Temperature	37.2°C
Respiratory rate	14 resp/min
Body mass index	23
Waist circumference	85.7 cm
Face	Sunburned
Urinalysis	Colour – brown/orange pH – low (acidic urine is associated with xanthine, cysteine, uric acid and calcium oxalate stones; if pH was high it would indicate presence of calcium carbonate, calcium phosphate and magnesium phosphate stones instead) Multiple crystals found in urinary sediment Specific gravity – high Blood present – small amount (microscopic)

TABLE 9.18 **RESULTS OF MEDICAL INVESTIGATIONS** [1–8, 37]	
TEST	**RESULTS**
Abdominal inspection: guarding, rebound tenderness, palpation, abnormal pulsations (auscultation)	No sign of appendicitis, pancreatitis, enlarged liver, bowel obstruction, perforated ulcer; no positive Murphy's sign for inflamed gall bladder; hiatus hernia signs, swallowed air; no middle epigastric tenderness in gastric and peptic ulcer; mild kidney discomfort on percussion
Urine microscopic investigation: define type of urine crystals and red blood cells [38] Radio-opacity of stone	*Result:* calcium oxalate – radio-opaque **All types:** Calcium stones – radio-opaque, cysteine stones radio-opaque, magnesium ammonium phosphate – moderately radio-opaque *Ruled out:* uric acid stones: radiolucent
Urinary calcium, oxalate and uric acid output: two 24-hour samples	High oxalate output
Estimated glomerula filtration rate (eGFR)	Kidney function: NAD
Electrolytes (sodium, potassium, chloride, bicarbonate blood test) urea and creatinine; signal muscle breakdown and tissue damage and gives an indicator for renal excretory function as urea and blood creatinine is excreted entirely by the kidneys; this will show in renal abnormalities	NAD
Full blood count: anaemia, infection	NAD
ESR/CRP: indication of infection, cancer, inflammation	NAD
Fasting blood glucose test: raised in pancreatic cancer, pancreatitis, drug therapy and acute stress response; diabetes; decreased levels, liver disease	NAD
Calcium, phosphate, serum alkaline phosphatase: metabolic bone disease such as osteomalacia, Paget's disease and renal calculi due to calcium excess, renal infarction; calcium excretion can be monitored	NAD
Prostate-specific antigen: raised in prostatic cancer, benign prostatic hypertrophy, prostatitis	NAD
Liver function test: hepatitis, substance abuse	NAD
Plain abdominal x-ray: to rule out appendicitis, intestinal obstruction such as constipation and hiatus hernia; abdominal aneurysm	Detected urinary calculi on x-ray
Stool test: detect ova, parasites, bacteria and fat levels, and occult blood; if acidic stools are passed it indicates lactose intolerance	NAD

TABLE 9.19 **UNLIKELY DIAGNOSTIC CONSIDERATIONS** [2, 4–8]	
CONDITIONS AND CAUSES	**WHY UNLIKELY**
ALLERGIES AND IRRITANTS	
Causal factor: **Lactose intolerance:** abdominal pain, bloating, nausea; possible recurrent abdominal pain with onset of lactose ingestion	Usually significant diarrhoea; no acidic stools
CANCER AND HEART DISEASE	
Prostate cancer: metastases into bone	Prostate specific antigen NAD; CRP within normal range
Neoplasms: kidney, stomach, pancreatic, intestinal, prostate	ESR/CRP not raised, abdominal x-ray did not detect, full blood count NAD
Hypertension	Blood pressure is within normal range, although in the higher range of normal
TRAUMA AND PRE-EXISTING ILLNESS	
Causal factor: **Trauma:** (ruptured spleen, stomach, colon)	Abdominal x-ray did not detect
Abdominal aneurysm: deep pain in lumbosacral region; can cause acute pain if likely to rupture; steady pain; Max is in the age group in which this condition is likely to develop; pain relieved by changing positions	Abdominal x-ray did not detect
Kidney embolism/infarction: abdominal pain, steady aching in flank pain that can radiate to the groin; nausea often associated; microscopic blood in the urine usually present	Usually occurs in the elderly and over 60 years of age; most often protein and white blood cells are present in the urine; no advanced hypertension
Primary renal diseases: medullary sponge kidney, renal tubular acidoses	Electrolytes test NAD, urinalysis revealed no protein
OBSTRUCTION AND FOREIGN BODY	
Renal calculi – **hypercalcaemia:** most common causes are hyperparathyroidism, vitamin D ingestion, sarcoidosis	Unlikely due to urinalysis detecting low pH (acidic reading); no excess serum calcium would usually present with alkaline urine (high pH)
Renal calculi – **hypercalciuria:** most common metabolic abnormality detected in calcium stone-formers; causes can be excess dietary intake of calcium, excess resorption of calcium from the skeleton in prolonged immobilisation, idiopathic reasons where there is an increased absorption of calcium from the gut	Unlikely due to urinalysis detecting low pH (acidic reading); no excess serum calcium would usually present with alkaline urine (high pH)
Hyperuricaemia and hyperuriosuria: uric acid stones comprise 3–5% of all kidney stones; uric acid is the endpoint of purine metabolism and hyperuricaemia can be a primary defect in gout and an end result of increased cell turn over in myeloproliferative disorders; dehydration alone can cause uric acid stones to form; some people with calcium stones also have increased uric acid levels; pH was low on urinalysis (acidic)	Unlikely while taking Progout, which reduces the formation and accumulation of uric acid in the body; uric acid stones are radiolucent

Cystinuria: results in formation of cystine stones, but only 1–2% fall into this category; cystinuria is a defective tubular reabsorption and jejunal absorption of cystine, lysine, ornithine and arginine; pH was low on urinalysis (acidic)	No family history mentioned for cysteine kidney stone formation; tests would have revealed radio-opaque cysteine stones
Polycystic kidney disease: symptoms can include some abdominal and loin pain, blood in urine and can result in kidney stones (often uric acid)	No family history yet revealed for polycystic kidney disease, which is often inherited Tests: no uric acid stones, no protein in urinalysis
DEGENERATIVE AND DEFICIENCY	
Osteoporosis: lower back pain, rapid bone remodelling causing calcium excess	Unlikely due to urinalysis detecting low pH (acidic reading); no excess serum calcium; would usually present with alkaline urine (high pH)
Osteomalacia: buffering of H^+ by Ca^{2+} in bone resulting in depletion of calcium from bone; excess calcium excretion can develop	Unlikely due to urinalysis detecting low pH (acidic reading); no excess serum calcium; would usually present with alkaline urine (high pH)
Paget's disease: rapid bone remodelling causing calcium excess	Unlikely due to urinalysis detecting low pH (acidic reading); no excess serum calcium; would usually present with alkaline urine (high pH)
Peptic ulcer: dull constant pain and sharp pain, referred back pain, nausea, lack of appetite	No vomiting or weight change; pain not only at night; pain location usually located in middle of the abdomen and does not radiate; no abnormality with CRP reading in blood tests; not detected in abdominal x-ray
INFECTION AND INFLAMMATION	
Appendicitis: referred back pain, nausea, lack of appetite	No fever; ESR/CRP not raised; full blood count NAD; abdominal x-ray did not detect; pain usually in midgut
Cholecystitis: referred pain, nausea	No fever; ESR/CRP not raised; full blood count NAD; abdominal x-ray did not detect; pain usually above the navel on the abdomen
Pancreatitis: abdominal pain, nausea, lower back pain	No fever; ESR/CRP not raised; full blood count NAD; abdominal x-ray did not detect; no glucose in urinalysis

▶

Inflammatory bowel disease: Crohn's disease, diverticulitis, ischaemic colitis, regional ileitis, amoebicolitis, autoimmune granulomatous colitis	ESR/CRP not raised; no fever; full blood count NAD; abdominal x-ray did not detect, stool test did not detect blood in stool
Kidney infection: pyelonephritis, perinephric abscess	No fever; ESR/CRP not raised; full blood count NAD
Prostatitis: lower back pain, urinary changes	Prostate-specific antigen NAD
Hepatitis: biliary disease can cause excess oxalate-containing foods	Liver function test NAD
Causal factor: **Intestinal abscess**	No raised ESR/CRP; full blood count NAD; no fever; abdominal x-ray did not detect
Causal factor: **Septic infection causing back pain**	ESR/CRP not raised; no fever; full blood count NAD
Urinary tract infection	No leukocytes or nitrates present in urinalysis or alkaline urine
Phlebitis of iliac veins and inferior vena cava	ESR/CRP not raised; abdominal x-ray did not detect; full blood count NAD
Causal factor: **Inflammatory lower back pain:** osteoarthritis, rheumatoid arthritis, fibromyositis, osteomyelitis, spinal, rectal abscess, myelitis, cystitis, ankylosing spondylitis, tuberculosis of spine	ESR/CRP not raised; full blood count NAD
SUPPLEMENTS AND SIDE EFFECTS MEDICATION AND DRUGS	
Causal factor: **Vitamin D intoxication:** causes excess calcium levels due to producing excess bone resorption	Unlikely due to urinalysis detecting low pH (acidic reading); no excess serum calcium; would usually present with alkaline urine (high pH)
ENDOCRINE/REPRODUCTIVE	
Diabetes	Fasting blood glucose test NAD
Benign prosatatic hyperplasia (enlargement): age, abdominal and loin pain; causes symptoms of urinary obstruction such as loin pain	Urinary stream changes not reported by Max as predominant symptoms in case history; prostate specific-antigen NAD
Primary parahyperthyroidism: caused by single or multiple adenomas or by hyperplasia of the parathyroid gland, or compensatory response due to renal failure or vitamin D deficiency	Unlikely due to urinalysis detecting low pH (acidic reading); would usually present with alkaline urine (high pH)
Hyperthyroidism: endocrine condition that can lead to excess calcium and kidney stones	Urinalysis showed acidic urine, no excess calcium; would usually present with alkaline urine (high pH)

Case analysis

TABLE 9.20 **POSSIBLE FURTHER DIFFERENTIAL DIAGNOSIS**		
Not ruled out by tests/investigations already done [2–8]		
CONDITIONS AND CAUSES	**WHY POSSIBLE**	**WHY UNLIKELY**
ALLERGIES AND IRRITANTS		
Causal facotr: **Food allergy:** typically to cow's milk, egg, soya, peanut, wheat and fish	Abdominal discomfort	Often presents with swelling of the lips and tongue, urticaria skin rash, conjunctivitis, rhinitis, anaphylaxis and difficulty breathing
TRAUMA AND PRE-EXISTING ILLNESS		
Causal factor: **Trauma** (strains, sprains, tear, herniated disc, fracture, disc prolapse)	Work strain and lower back pain	
Causal factor: **Leg length discrepancy**	Low back pain, restlessness	Has not experienced this kind of pain before
Causal factor: **Congenital disorders:** scoliosis	Lower back pain	Has not experienced this kind of pain before
FUNCTIONAL DISEASE		
Irritable bowel syndrome	Bloating and pain	Pain not necessarily relieved by passing a bowel motion
Causal factor: **Faulty posture**	Strain for long periods of time at work	
SUPPLEMENTS AND SIDE EFFECTS OF MEDICATIONS		
Casual factor: **Medication/supplementation: Analgesic abuse:** causes calcified papillae that mimic kidney stones	Salicylate excess may predispose to uric acid stone formation; pH would be acidic in this case	This would be prevented by taking Progout
AUTOIMMUNE DISEASE		
Coeliac disease	Abdominal pain, poor diet, diarrhoea	More often upper abdominal pain with bloating; diarrhoea or constipation usually a prominent symptom
EATING HABITS AND ENERGY		
Dehydration	Working long hours, not drinking enough water causing kidney stones; drinking mostly tea which can be more dehydrating; pH was low on urinalysis (acidic)	More often increases uric acid stones; this would be masked by taking Progout

TABLE 9.21 **CONFIRMED DIAGNOSIS** [1–8, 35]	
CONDITION	**RATIONALE**
Kidney stones	Referred pain in the back that can be dull and constant; pain can be sharp when a kidney stone is dislodged, usually after physical exertion; kidney stones are more likely to develop with dehydration, physical exertion in warm environments, increased intake of calcium, high purine and oxalate-containing foods; small amount of blood present in the urine; reduced appetite; occasional nausea; drinking fluids makes the pain worse
Primary hyperoxaluria: Inherited disorder may cause errors in metabolism of glycoxalate that increase endogenous oxalate biosynthesis; calcium oxalate stones will form, which are the most common type (65%) of kidney stone; a more common cause for **milder hyperoxaluria** is the ingestion of high oxalate-containing foods, too much dietary calcium restriction causing compensatory reabsorption of oxalate, and dehydration	Max is consuming a lot of spinach, chocolate and tea and doesn't drink enough water; he has recently reduced dairy products; pH was low on urinalysis (acidic); calcium oxalate stones can present at any urinary pH, unlike most calcium stones that will present at alkaline pH and uric acid stones will present as acid pH; urine microscopy revealed calcium oxalate stones as radio-opaque; high oxalate output in 24-hour urine samples
Tests: urine microscopy, urinalysis, abdominal x-ray	Uric acid – radiolucent detected with urine microscopic investigation; detected urinary calculi on x-ray; high oxalate output in two 24-hour urine samples

Working diagnosis

MAX AND KIDNEY STONES (RENAL CALCULI) COMMON MILD HYPEROXALURIA

Max is a 60-year-old man who enjoys owning and working in a landscaping business. His work requires him to expend physical energy for long hours, which could lead to strain and wear and tear of the musculoskeletal system. Max has previously been diagnosed with gout for which he is currently being prescribed the medication Progout, along with advice to reduce consumption of meat, dairy products and alcohol. Recently Max has experienced symptoms that mirror the development of kidney stones (renal calculi).

From the information provided in his case history it is most likely that Max has the most common type of kidney stone for men (65 per cent), which is composed of calcium oxalate (hyperoxaluria). Kidney stones develop when there is a chemical composition of urine that favours stone crystallisation, when there is production of concentrated urine and an impairment of inhibitors that prevent crystallisation. The pain of kidney stones can be acute, sharp, dull, wax and wane, or may present as a constant ache in the loin. Kidney stones should be considered when abdominal pain lasts for more than 12 hours, there is a loss of appetite, loin and renal tenderness and there is blood in the urine. Nausea and vomiting with a feeling of restlessness is also a symptom of renal calculi.

It is vital to confirm a diagnosis of renal calculi and the composition of kidney stones before proceeding with treatment. A common cause of mild hyperoxaluria is ingestion of high oxalate-containing foods or excessive dietary calcium restriction causing compensatory reabsorption of oxalate and dehydration [39]. Kidney stones can be a recurring problem with 50 per cent of people forming further stones. Along with alleviating initial acute symptoms of discomfort, preventative guidance is therefore essential.

General references used in this diagnosis: 2, 4–8, 36, 38, 39

TABLE 9.22 **DECISION TABLE FOR TREATMENT PRIOR TO REFERRAL**		
COMPLAINT	**CONTEXT**	**CORE**
Treatment for the presenting complaint and symptoms	Treatment for all associated symptoms	Treatment for mental, emotional, spiritual, constitutional, lifestyle issues and metaphysical considerations
TREATMENT PRIORITY	**TREATMENT PRIORITY**	**TREATMENT PRIORITY**
• Lifestyle recommendations to reduce the formation of kidney stones • Physical therapy recommendations to alleviate acute symptoms • Dietary recommendations to reduce stone formation and the risk of stone recurrence • Herbal tonic or tea to reduce stone formation and provide symptom relief • Nutritional supplements to reduce inflammation and the risk of stone formation	• Dietary recommendations to enhance general health and wellbeing • Lifestyle recommendations to enhance general health and wellbeing • Dietary and lifestyle recommendations to help reduce blood pressure	• Lifestyle recommendations to reduce stress levels

TABLE 9.23 **DECISION TABLE FOR REFERRAL** [2–8, 13]		
COMPLAINT	**CONTEXT**	**CORE**
Referral for presenting complaint	Referral for all associated physical, dietary and lifestyle concerns	Referral for contributing emotional, mental, spiritual, metaphysical, lifestyle and constitutional factors
REFERRAL FLAGS	**REFERRAL FLAGS**	**REFERRAL FLAGS**
• Presence of microscopic blood in urine and acidic urine	• Dehydration risk when working long hours • Blood pressure on the high side of normal range • Physically demanding work	• Working long hours

▶

ISSUES OF SIGNIFICANCE	ISSUES OF SIGNIFICANCE	ISSUES OF SIGNIFICANCE
• History of treatment for gout	• Nausea and bloating • Pain in lower back • Excess intake of dairy products in diet • Consistent intake of high oxalate-containing foods	• Worried about the business if his health suffers • Would like more time with the grandchildren
REFERRAL	**REFERRAL**	**REFERRAL**
• Stones need to be surgically removed [2, 16, 36] • Max's case needs to be managed collaboratively with his GP [35]	• Refer for musculoskeletal examination and exercise therapy program to strengthen Max's lower back • Dietary assessment for allergies or intolerances • Refer for thorough abdominal examination	• Regular massage for musculoskeletal support and stress release

TABLE 9.24 **FURTHER INVESTIGATIONS THAT MAY BE NECESSARY** [1–9]	
TEST/INVESTIGATION	**REASON FOR TEST/INVESTIGATION**
FIRST-LINE INVESTIGATIONS:	
Musculoskeletal examination	Flexion, extension, rotation, straight leg test will reveal physical signs of mechanical or inflammatory, compression or degeneration of spine
Elimination diets	Detect food intolerance
IF NECESSARY:	
Renal helical CT scan/excretion urography/IV urography/retrograde pyelography [36–38]	Definitive diagnosis for renal calculi if there are any doubts; detects any urinary obstructive causes, renal infarction, polycystic kidney disease
Cystoscopy	Direct visualisation of urethra, bladder and prostate
Hydrogen breath test	To detect bacterial overgrowth; when bacteria is metabolised by lactose or glucose there is a production of hydrogen
Antigliadin antibodies	Check if antibodies to gluten are present in the blood
Colonoscopy and biopsy	Rule out bowel cancer, polyps, inflammatory bowel disease, diverticulitis or haemorrhoids
Back x-ray/radiography	Osteoarthritis, osteoporosis, herniated disc, cancer, Paget's disease, bone cancer

Confirmed diagnosis

Kidney stones (renal calculi), common mild hyperoxaluria and faulty posture

PRESCRIBED MEDICATION

- Paracetamol and codeine as required for pain

TABLE 9.25 **DECISION TABLE FOR TREATMENT (ONCE DIAGNOSIS IS CONFIRMED)**		
COMPLAINT	**CONTEXT**	**CORE**
Treatment for the presenting complaint and symptoms	Treatment for all associated symptoms	Treatment for mental, emotional, spiritual, constitutional, lifestyle issues and metaphysical considerations
TREATMENT PRIORITY	**TREATMENT PRIORITY**	**TREATMENT PRIORITY**
• Continue with lifestyle recommendations to reduce the formation of kidney stones • Continue with physical therapy recommendations for the relief of back pain • Continue with dietary recommendations to reduce stone formation and the risk of stone recurrence • Continue with herbal tonic or tea and nutritional supplements **NB**: Max's mineral levels should be monitored to ensure they stay within an acceptable range during supplementation; this should be done as part of the collaborative management of Max's case with his GP	• Physical therapy recommendations to help improve muscle strength in Max's lower back and to improve his posture • Continue with lifestyle and dietary recommendations to enhance general health and wellbeing and to reduce blood pressure • Recommendation to test for heavy metals if symptoms continue despite dietary and lifestyle measures; appropriate detoxification program if necessary	• Continue with lifestyle recommendations to reduce stress • Recommendation for Max to participate in hobbies and other activities for pleasure to improve his work/home/social life balance

Treatment aims

- Eliminate stones and prevent recurrence [16, 17].
- Reduce urinary calcium [15] and oxalate [15, 16].
- Increase Max's urine production to at least 2 L each day to dilute and ensure adequate flow of urine [15, 17].
- Alkalise Max's urine [15, 17].
- Support Max's stress response [15, 28].
- Improve Max's diet [17].

Lifestyle alterations/considerations

- Encourage Max to avoid consuming aluminium compounds and alkalis (antacids) [15, 17].
- Consider testing for heavy metal toxicity if Max continues to experience stones despite treatment. Many heavy metals are toxic to the kidneys, and cadmium exposure in particular can lead to renal tubular failure and is known to increase kidney stone formation. It tends to be concentrated in the kidney tissue [15, 17].

- If Max consistently sleeps on the same side, encourage him to change sleep position. Research has shown the side of the stone is the same as the side on which people sleep in 76 per cent of people studied [29].
- Kidney stone formation is more likely to occur with stress [28], so encourage Max to reduce his stress levels. This may involve delegating more of the physical work to his employees to reduce the physical stress on his body and/or taking on additional staff to reduce his workload, stress-management techniques, etc. Stress management can reduce his blood pressure [15, 16, 30].
- Encourage Max to take up some activities for pleasure rather than financial reward. He needs to get more balance between work and play in his life.

Dietary suggestions

- Encourage Max to should increase water consumption aiming for at least 2½–3 L daily [15, 17, 33].
- Encourage Max to should consume 120 mL of lemon juice in water daily. Lemon juice consumption increases citrate excretion in urolithiasis [17]. Lemon juice can be added to water and included in Max's water intake.
- Encourage Max to increase his intake of fibre, complex carbohydrates and green leafy vegetables [15–17, 33] and reduce consumption of refined carbohydrates, sugar, fat and alcohol [15, 17, 33].
- Encourage Max to minimise his salt intake [15, 17, 33]. A high dietary intake of salt increases calcium excretion [11, 17] and can adversely affect blood pressure [15–17, 31, 32].
- Encourage Max to increase his intake of foods rich in vitamin K [15, 17].
- Encourage Max to reduce consumption of animal protein and particularly purine protein (meat, fish, poultry, yeast) [15, 17, 33] and limit his consumption of dairy foods [15, 17].
- Encourage Max to reduce consumption of foods high in oxalates (black tea, chocolate, carrots, cucumber, grapefruit, kale, peanuts, sweet potato, peppers, spinach, beet leaves, rhubarb, parsley and cranberry) [15, 17, 33].
- Encourage Max to reduce his consumption of caffeine. Caffeine consumption is associated with higher levels of urinary calcium [17]. Max will benefit from replacing black tea with herbal tea [33].
- Encourage Max to increase consumption of foods with a high magnesium-to-calcium ratio (barley, bran, corn, buckwheat, rye, soy, oats, brown rice, avocado, banana, lima beans, potato) [15–17].

Physical treatment suggestions

- Acupuncture may help to relieve pain as part of a holistic treatment program [14].
- Hydrotherapy suggestions: hot trunk wrap [34, 35].
- Constitutional hydrotherapy [34, 36, 37].
- Hot fomentations (5–10 minutes) with vinegar water alternating with cold (1–5 minutes) mitten frictions to abdomen and lower back [36, 37].
- Place a cold compress to the head and immerse the body in a hot half-full bath, massage the lower back while in the water [36].
- A hot towel roll massage; fomentation to the lumbar spine [34].
- Full-immersion warm bath [34].
- Swimming in a warm pool, underwater massage and mud baths are helpful for lower back pain [34].
- Hot sitz Epsom salt bath for lower back pain [35].
- Max is likely to benefit from a prescribed graduated activity exercise therapy program to improve lower back strength and reduce pain [38].

TABLE 9.26 HERBAL FORMULA (1:2 LIQUID EXTRACTS)

Made with ethanolic extract herbal liquids (alcohol removed)

HERB	FORMULA	RATIONALE
Crataeva *Crataeva nurvala*	80 mL	Antilithic [19, 20]; anti-inflammatory [19, 20]
Gravel root *Eupatorium purpureum*	30 mL	Antilithic [18], diuretic [18], antirheumatic [18]; indicated for the treatment of renal calculi [18]
Hydrangea root *Hydrangea arborescens*	30 mL	Contains furanocoumarins that promote smooth muscle relaxation, relaxing the ureter and allowing stones to pass [15]; traditionally used for treating urinary calculi [18]
Bearberry *Arctostaphylos uva-ursi*	60 mL	Urinary system anti-inflammatory [18, 34]; diuretic [18]; indicated for urolithiasis [18]
Supply:	200 mL	Dose: 5 mL 3 times daily

TABLE 9.27 HERBAL TEA

Alternative to herbal liquid if Max prefers to drink a herbal tea rather than a tonic

HERB	FORMULA	RATIONALE
Corn silk *Zea mays*	1 part	Antilithic [18]; diuretic [18]
Gravel root *Eupatorium purpureum*	1 part	See above
Hydrangea *Hydrangea arborescens*	1 part	See above
Decoction: 1 tsp per cup – 1 cup 3 times daily		

TABLE 9.28 NUTRITIONAL SUPPLEMENTS

SUPPLEMENT AND DOSE	RATIONALE
Magnesium citrate supplement Providing 480 mg elemental magnesium [17] and 25 mg vitamin B6 daily [15, 17]	Increases calcium oxalate solubility in the urine [15, 17, 33] and inhibits precipitation of calcium phosphate and calcium oxalate [15, 22]; low urinary magnesium:calcium ratio is a risk factor for development of kidney stones [15]; supplemental magnesium is effective in preventing recurrence of kidney stones [15, 17, 33]; the citrate form of magnesium has been shown to be successful in preventing kidney stone recurrence [17]; combining magnesium with B6 is more effective in prevention of kidney stone recurrence than supplementing with magnesium alone [15, 24]; vitamin B6 reduces endogenous production and excretion of oxalates [15]; supplementation decreases oxalate formation [23, 33]

►

Calcium citrate 500 mg daily [17, 33]	Supplementation with calcium citrate can decrease oxalate absorption [17] and reduce urinary oxalate levels [21]; calcium supplementation is preventative for oxalate stones [16, 33]
Vitamin K 2 mg daily [15, 17]	Necessary for carboxylation of glutamic acid to gamma-carboxyglutamic acid [17]; gamma-carboxyglutamic acid inhibits growth of calcium oxalate monohydrate and therefore stone formation [17, 25]
Omega-3 fish oil 10,000 mg daily in divided doses [17]	Anti-inflammatory [17, 33]; decreases transmembrane oxalate exchange [17]; urinary calcium excretion is positively correlated with plasma arachidonic acid levels [26]; can reduce the risk of stone formation [33]
High-potency practitioner-strength **probiotic** containing human strain lactobacillus and bifidobacterium organisms, and specifically containing *Oxalobacter formigenes* [27] Dosage as per the manufacturer's instructions **NB:** probiotic supplements containing *Oxalobacter formigenes* may be difficult to obtain in some locations	To support normal digestive function and synthesis of vitamin K in the gut [15]; people with low levels of *Oxalobacter formigenes* are more likely to form calcium oxalate stones [27]; supplementation with *Oxalobacter formigenes* may reduce the incidence of calcium oxalate stones [15, 27]

References

[1] K.D. Pagna, T.J. Pagna, Mosby's Diagnostic and Laboratory Test reference, third edn, Mosby, USA, 1997 (later edition).

[2] P. Kumar, C. Clark, Clinical Medicine, sixth edn, Elsevier Saunders, London, 2005.

[3] G. Douglas, F. Nicol, C. Robertson, Macleod's Clinical Examination, twelfth edn, Churchill Livingstone Elsevier, 2009.

[4] R.D. Collins, Differential Diagnosis in Primary Care, fourth edn, Lippincott Williams & Wilkins, Philadelphia, 2008.

[5] R.H. Seller, Differential Diagnosis of Common Complaints, fifth edn, Saunders Elsevier, Philadelphia, 2007.

[6] P. Glasziou, Evidence-Based Diagnosis in Primary Care, Churchill Livingstone Elsevier, 2008.

[7] J. Jamison, Differential Diagnosis for Primary Care, second edn, Churchill Livingstone Elsevier, London, 2006.

[8] R. Berkow, A.J. Fletcher, M.H. Beers, The Merck Manual, sixteenth edn, Merck Research Laboratories, Rathway, N.J, 1993 (later edition).

[9] N.J. Talley, S. O'Connor, Pocket Clinical Examination, third edn, Churchill Livingstone Elsevier, Australia, 2009.

[10] J. Silverman, S. Kurtz, J. Draper, Skills for Communicating with Patients, second edn, Radcliff Publishing, Oxford, 2000.

[11] R. Neighbour, The Inner Consultation; how to develop an effective and intuitive consulting style, Radcliff Publishing, Oxon, 2005.

[12] M. Lloyd, R. Bor, Communication Skills For Medicine, third edn, Churchill Livingstone Elsevier, Edinburgh, 2009.

[13] D. Peters, L. Chaitow, G. Harris, S. Morrison, Integrating Complementary Therapies in Primary Care, Churchill Livingstone, London, 2002.

[14] A. Holdgate, J. Hardcastle, Renal Colic: A Diagnostic and Therapeutic Review, Emergency Medicine 11 (1) (1999) 9–16.

[15] J.E. Pizzorno, M.T. Murray, H. Joiner-Bey, The Clinicians Handbook of Natural Medicine, second edn, Churchill Livingstone, St Louis, 2008.

[16] S. El-Hashemy, Naturopathic Standards of Primary Care, CCNM Press Inc, Toronto, 2007.

[17] R.A. Anderson, A complementary approach to urolithiasis prevention, World Journal of Urology 20 (2002) 294–301.

[18] British Herbal Medicine Association, British Herbal Pharmacopoeia, BHMAA, 1983.

[19] K. Bone, Clinical Applications of Chinese and Ayurvedic Herbs: Monographs for the Western Herbal Practitioners, Phytotherapy Press, Warwick, 1996.

[20] S. Mills, K. Bone, The Essential Guide to Herbal Safety, Elsevier Churchill Livingstone, St Louis, 2005.

[21] B.S. Levine, J.S. Rodman, S. Wienerman, R.S. Bockman, J.M. Lane, D.S. Chapman, Effect of calcium citrate supplementation on urinary calcium oxalate saturation in female stone formers: implications for prevention of osteoporosis, The American Journal of Clinical Nutrition 60 (1994) 592–596.

[22] P.O. Schwille, A. Schmiedel, U. Hermann, J. Fan, D. Gottliev, M. Manoharan, J. Wipplinger, Magnesium, citrate and magnesium-alkali citrate as modulators of calcium oxalate crystallization in urine: observations in patients with recurrent idiopathic calcium urolithiasis, Urological Research 27 (2) (1999) 117–126.

[23] G.C. Curhan, W.C. Willett, F.E. Speizer, M.J. Stampfer, Intakes of Vitamins B6 and C and the Risk of Kidney Stones in Women, Journal of the American Society of Nephrology 10 (1999) 840–845.

[24] V. Rattan, H. Sidhu, S. Vaidyanathan, S.K. Thind, R. Nath, Effect of combined supplementation of magnesium oxide and pyridoxine in calcium oxalate stone formers, Urological Research 22 (3) (1994) 161–165.

[25] Y. Nakagawa, H.C. Margolis, S. Yokoyama, F.C. Kezdys, E.T. Kaiser, F.L. Coe, Purification and Characterization of a Calcium Oxalate Monohydrate Crystal Growth Inhibitor from Human Kidney Tissue Culture Medium, The Journal of Biological Chemistry 256 (8) (1981) 3936–3944.

[26] B. Battio, A. Budakovic, M.A. Nassuato, G. Vezzoli, E. Manzato, G. Luisetto, M. Zaninotto, Plasma phospholipid arachidonic acid content and calcium metabolism in idiopathic calcium nephrolithiasis, Kidney International 58 (2008) 1278–1284.

[27] S.A. Troxel, H. Sidhu, P. Kaul, R.K. Low, Intestinal Oxalobacter formigenes colonization in calcium oxalate stone formers and its relation to urinary oxalate, Journal of Endourology 17 (3) (2003) 173–176.

[28] G.R. Najem, J.J. Seebode, A.J. Samady, M. Feuerman, L. Friedman, Stressful Life Events and Risk of Symptomatic Kidney Stones, International Journal of Epidemiology 26 (5) (1997) 1017–1023.

[29] B. Shekarriz, H.F. Lu, M. Stoller, Correlation Of Unilateral Urolithiasis With Sleep Posture, The Journal of Urology 165 (4) (2001) 1085–1087.

[30] P. Grossman, L. Niemann, S. Schmidt, H. Walach, Mindfulness-based stress reduction and health benefits. A meta-analysis, Journal of Psychomatic Research 57 (2004) 35–43.

[31] H. Osiecki, The Physicians Handbook of Clinical Nutrition, seventh edn, Bioconcepts, Eagle Farm, 2000.

[32] P.K. Whelton, L.J. Appel, M.A. Espeland, W.B. Applegate, W.H. Ettinger, J.B. Kostis, S. Kumanyika, et al., Sodium Reduction and Weight Loss in the Treatment of Hypertension in Older Persons: A Randomized Controlled Trial of Nonpharmacologic Interventions in the Elderly, Journal of the American Medical Association 279 (11) (1998) 839–846.

[33] J. Jamison, Clinical Guide to Nutrition & Dietary Supplements in Disease Management, Churchill Livingstone, Edinburgh, 2003.

[34] S. Mills, K. Bone, Principles & Practice of Phytotherapy; Modern Herbal Medicine, Churchill Livingstone, Edinburgh: London, 2000.

[35] M. Eskelinen, Usefulness of history-taking, physical examination and diagnostic scoring in acute renal colic, European Journal of Urology 34 (1998) 467–473.

[36] A. Portis, C. Sundaram, Diagnosis and initial management of kidney stones, American Family Physician 63 (2001) 1329–1338.

[37] P. Bove, D. Kaplan, N. Dalrymple, et al., Reexamining the value of haematuria testing in patients with acute flank pain, Journal of Urology 162 (1999) 685–687.

[38] G. Bihl, A. Meyers, Recurrent renal stone disease-advancesinpathogenesisandmanagement, Lancet 358 (2001) 651–656.

[39] L. Borghi, et al., Comparison of two diets for the prevention of recurrent stones in idiopathic hypercalcuria, N Engl J Med 346 (2002) 77–84.

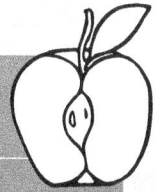

CHAPTER 10

Neurological system

Depression

Case history

Mark Stevens, 48, has come to the clinic because his wife has strongly urged him to.

Mark was laid off work seven months ago when the company he was working for laid off most of its workforce. Mark has worked as a diesel fitter specialising in ore pit vehicles since he finished his apprenticeship many years ago. Since Mark was laid off he has been unable to find other employment and family finances are beginning to become stretched.

Mark and his wife have two teenage children, a 14-year-old boy and a 17-year-old girl, and he is concerned about the example he is setting them. Mark is more tired than he has ever been before although generally his fatigue improves during the day. He sleeps more hours overnight and has started taking a nap during the day because he is so bored. He is spending most of his time at home and the amount of time he spends in front of the television during the day has been causing tension between him and his wife. Mark doesn't feel he can talk to her about how he feels because she seems so anxious about their finances and he feels that is his fault. He hates being on social security benefits and attending the Centrelink office, but he feels there is no other solution at the moment.

Mark tells you he feels old and tired, is drinking about six beers every day, eating lots of junk food and has taken up smoking again. The cost of his cigarettes is another area of friction between him and his wife. Mark also tells you he drinks four to six cups of coffee every day to help give him energy.

Mark has considered retraining and looking for work in another field, but he doesn't know what he would do. Working as a diesel fitter is all he knows and he isn't sure he would enjoy doing anything else. He is also anxious about starting again and not sure how he would feel about retraining alongside a lot of younger people and then competing with them for jobs.

His GP recently did some blood tests and recommended he go on antidepressants. Mark hates popping pills and doesn't believe he is depressed. He didn't understand why the doctor did all the blood tests since he doesn't think he is sick, just bored and unemployed. Mark tells you he did not want his doctor to think he was going crazy but he feels like crying sometimes and is ashamed to do so; at other times he feels numb and doesn't want to talk to anyone. Mark says he used to be a very busy, driven person and he doesn't feel he knows himself anymore.

TABLE 10.1 **COMPLAINT** [3–7, 12–15, 75]	
Analogy: Skin of the apple	**Complaint:** Define the presenting complaint and symptoms; understand the complaint *Depression*
AREAS OF INVESTIGATION AND EXAMPLE QUESTIONS	**CLIENT RESPONSES**
Onset *When did you start experiencing your current symptoms?*	*When I got laid off. It's been getting worse since I can't find another job.*
Understanding the cause (client) *I get the impression you have not been satisfied with the explanations that have been given to you previously for your symptoms, is that correct? What do you think is the cause?*	*Yeah, I get annoyed when my doctor thinks there is something wrong with me, when I know I am just feeling trapped and bored.* *Because I'm at home doing nothing.*
Exacerbating factors *Is there anything that makes them worse?*	*When I argue with my wife or when we have trouble paying bills.*
Relieving factors *Is there anything that makes them better?*	*Not really.*
Examination and inspection	Mark appears passive and withdrawn. His face is inexpressive, his face is red and he has dark rings under his eyes.

TABLE 10.2 **CONTEXT**	
Analogy: Flesh of the apple	**Context:** Put the presenting complaint into context to understand the disease
AREAS OF INVESTIGATION AND EXAMPLE QUESTIONS	**CLIENT RESPONSES**
Family health *Has anyone else in your family ever experienced similar symptoms?*	*I don't think so.*
Obstruction and foreign body *Do you snore during the night and wake up feeling fatigued and unrested?* (sleep apnoea)	*Yeah. I snore a lot but I think it's because I drink too much alcohol at night.*
Recreational drug use *Are you taking any recreational drugs?*	*No. The fact I have taken up smoking again is causing friction at home.*
Occupational toxins and hazards *Could you have been exposed to any potentially toxic chemicals or heavy metals in your previous job?*	*I don't know. I suppose I could have been but nobody ever said anything about it.*

▶

Functional disease *Did the fatigue begin after losing your job or did you feel it before?* (functional origin)	*Yeah, I used to have loads of energy.*
Supplements and side effects of medication *Are you taking any supplements or medication at the moment?*	*No.*
Stress and neurological *Have you experienced any associated symptoms to the tiredness such as decreased libido and vague aches and pains along with disturbed sleep?* (depression) *Have you experienced other symptoms such as headaches, chest pain, palpitations, dizziness, or feelings of nervous foreboding?* (anxiety related)	*All of those things.* *No chest pains or dizziness, I don't feel anything much.*
Eating habits and energy *Tell me about your diet and energy levels.*	Mark tells you he knows his diet isn't particularly good at the moment. He is eating a lot of junk food and drinking too much coffee and beer out of boredom. His wife gives him healthy food but he often doesn't have much appetite for it.

TABLE 10.3 **CORE**	
Analogy: Core of the apple with the seed of ill health	**Core:** Holistic assessment to understand the client
AREAS OF INVESTIGATION AND EXAMPLE QUESTIONS	**CLIENT RESPONSES**
Support systems *Do you have a supportive social or family network?* *Are you aware of the support agencies available to you?*	*If I really needed help I think the family would do something, but don't I like to ask anyone for help.* *Centrelink gave me a list of places, but I haven't gone to any of them.*
Emotional health *Do you think you are depressed?*	*I don't think so, I'm just bored and out of work.*
Daily activities *Tell me about your daily routine.*	Mark tells you he sleeps late, watches TV when he gets up. He might go out to get the paper or shopping with his wife during the day. He is usually in bed by 10 pm.
Stress release *How do you deal with your stress?*	*Smoking and drinking. I know it's not good.*

Home life How are things at home right now?	There is a fair bit of tension with my wife. She says she understands, but I think it's my fault we're having problems paying the bills. I'm washed up and unemployable at 48. Not a good example to set for the kids.
Action needed to heal How do you think I can help you? [76]	I don't know, it was the wife's idea.
Long-term goals Do you have any long-term goals?	To be working again.

TABLE 10.4 MARK' S SIGNS AND SYMPTOMS [1, 6, 7]

Pulse	70 bpm
Blood pressure	125/78
Temperature	36.6°C
Respiratory rate	14 resp/min
Body mass index	29
Waist circumference	97.7 cm
Face	Lack of facial expression, red face, dark rings under the eyes
Urinalysis	No abnormality detected (NAD)

TABLE 10.5 RESULTS OF MEDICAL INVESTIGATIONS [1–5]

TEST/INVESTIGATION	RESULT
Full blood count: To rule out infection, tumour, inflammation, anaemia	All cells appear normal
Epstein-Barr/Ross River virus blood test	Negative for postviral infection
Cholesterol blood test	Within normal range
Thyroid function test	NAD
CRP (C-reactive protein): infection, inflammation, tumour, bacteria	Normal range
Liver function test	NAD
Serum electrolyte blood test	NAD
Serum cortisol blood test	NAD
Toxicology screen	NAD
Lead level	NAD

TABLE 10.6 UNLIKELY DIAGNOSTIC CONSIDERATIONS [1–5, 8–11, 62, 67, 68, 71–73]

CONDITIONS AND CAUSES	WHY UNLIKELY
CANCER AND HEART DISEASE	
Bronchogenic carcinoma	CRP normal
Chronic cardiorespiratory disease	No shortness of breath, hypertension, electrolyte balance normal
RECREATIONAL DRUG USE	
Causal factor: **Liver damage due to alcohol excess**	LFT normal
OCCUPATIONAL TOXINS AND HAZARDS	
Causal factor: **Toxins**	Toxicology screen clear
Causal factor: **Lead toxicity**	Lead levels within normal range
FUNCTIONAL DISEASE	
Electrolyte imbalance (hyponatraemia, hypokalaemia, hypercalcaemia)	Blood test and urinalysis within normal range
DEGENERATION AND DEFICIENCY	
Anaemia	Full blood count normal
Causal factor: **Nutritional deficiency:** Mark is pale	No sign of smooth glossy tongue or cheilosis on sides of mouth
Causal factor: **Organic fatigue:** tired, sleep disturbances, no major physical abnormalities	Shorter duration than functional fatigue; Mark's fatigue does not generally worsen during the day
INFECTION AND INFLAMMATION	
Causal factor: **Current viral infection:** glandular fever, Ross River virus	Full blood count normal, no fever
Causal factor: **Current bacterial infection**	Full blood count normal, no fever
Hepatitis	LFT normal, no sign of jaundice
ENDOCRINE/REPRODUCTIVE	
Hypothyroidism/hyperthryoidism	Thyroid function test normal
Adrenal insufficiency/Cushing's syndrome	No low blood pressure or skin pigmentation, serum cortisol within normal range
Diabetes	Urinalysis NAD
AUTOIMMUNE DISEASE	
Rheumatoid arthritis/systemic lupus erythematosus	CRP normal

▶

STRESS AND NEUROLOGICAL DISEASE	
Causal factor: **Psychological depression:** adjustment disorder, tiredness, hypersomnia, low mood due to a particular life-changing event or psychological cause	Depression does not continue for more than 2 months; not considered major depression
Physiological depression: postviral infection, depression, fatigue [73]	Blood tests reveal no viral illness such as glandular fever during the past 6 months
Type 2 – minor depression: can be mild or moderate depression	Need to show 2–4 symptoms of depression that have lasted at least 2 weeks; Mark shows more than 4 signs of depression currently

TABLE 10.7 **CONFIRMED DIAGNOSIS** [1–3, 10, 11]	
CONDITION	**RATIONALE**
Depression: important differential diagnosis to rule out before exploring other possibilities of mental or organic causes for fatigue symptoms	Tiredness that has lasted several months, feelings of guilt, watching excessive amounts of television, excess coffee, alcohol and junk food, feeling like wanting to cry; anxiety began after the trauma of losing his job; fatigue generally improves during the day
Primary origins: primary depression and endogenous depression are associated with conditions that are regarded as primary disorders, i.e. that do not occur secondarily to other medical or psychiatric disorders; these terms refer to depression that is caused by internal chemical and biological factors rather than external stressors	Type 1: major (clinical) depression; has at least five symptoms of depression for more than 2 weeks and causes considerable incapacity with daily activities; can be moderate or severe depression; people often describe symptoms in physical terms

Case analysis

TABLE 10.8 **POSSIBLE FURTHER DIFFERENTIAL DIAGNOSIS**		
Not ruled out by tests/investigations already done [1–5, 8–11, 16, 62–76]		
CONDITIONS AND CAUSES	**WHY POSSIBLE**	**WHY UNLIKELY**
ALLERGIES AND IRRITANTS		
Food intolerance/allergy	Fatigue, depression, recent dietary change since feeling low; Mark may be eating foods he did not previously eat	Need to gain more insight into Mark's previous and current diet and associated symptoms
OBSTRUCTION AND FOREIGN BODIES		
Obstructive sleep apnoea [63]	Daytime naps, tired; sufferers are often obese and Mark's BMI is 29; can be made worse by drinking alcohol prior to sleeping; Mark wakes up feeling unrefreshed and snores during the night	Do not usually complain of 'sleepiness' but rather fatigue generally

FUNCTIONAL DISEASE		
Chronic fatigue syndrome: fatigue for at least 6 months that has no physical explanation when there is no diagnosis of psychoses, bipolar affective disorder, eating disorder or organic brain disease [65, 72]	Severe disabling fatigue affects both mental and physical functioning for at least 6 months; Mark is sleeping more, has depression, feelings of guilt, social withdrawal and crying spells	Need to determine whether Mark experiences muscular and mental fatigue for at least 24 hours after exertion before some level of recovery; need to determine if fatigue improves during the day; need to determine if Mark experiences at least two neurological/ cognitive manifestations of chronic fatigue syndrome such as impaired concentration and muscle weakness; no significant autonomic, neuroendocrine or immune manifestations of the disorder present for Mark; often due to postviral infection, which Mark has not had
Causal factor: **Seasonal affective disorder**	Secondary to the winter months; symptoms include increased sleep, tiredness, increased appetite, weight gain	Need to determine if Mark has experienced episodes of depression during the winter months in the past
Causal factor: **Physiologic fatigue**	Can be caused by depression, caffeine, alcohol, excess sleep, intense emotions; recent diagnostic studies are within normal limits; could be feeling physiologic fatigue concurrently with functional fatigue from depression	Symptoms present for less than 14 days and are not usually associated with changes in self-esteem, social difficulties or overall mood
Causal factor: **Functional fatigue**	Tiredness that has lasted several months, began after the trauma of losing his job; feeling of fatigue generally improves during the day	
STRESS AND NEUROLOGICAL DISEASE		
Bipolar disorders: mental illness where individual alternates between manic episodes and major depression [66, 74]	May not think he needs help or there is anything out of balance mentally	Need to determine if there are episodes of manic behaviour that may include restlessness, fast speech, weight loss, difficulty sleeping; not sure if there is any family history of mental illness

▶

Dysthymia: mild depressive illness [70]	Mark could be experiencing 'double depression' if he has had intermittent periods of depression in the past; symptoms include tiredness, lack of interest in life, low mood	Lasts intermittently for 2 years or more; need to determine if Mark had episodes of feeling low prior to losing his job
Mixed anxiety and depressive disorder	Depressive disorder often associated with an experience of loss; symptoms of fatigue, apathy or intense sadness; Mark has mentioned a significant incapacity to continue daily activities for work and family	Numerous physical complaints associated with depression such as restlessness, headaches, insomnia, shortness of breath, gut or skin disorders
Posttraumatic stress disorder (PTSD): symptoms often develop within 6 months of the stressful event	Family tension could indicate emotional detachment from his family; Mark's symptoms developed after he was made redundant; Mark has mentioned anxiety about re-training and finding a new job	Has not mentioned flashbacks to a particular traumatic event such as losing job
Causal factor: **Emotional stress**	Tired, concerns about job security, financial difficulties, family strain; longer duration than acute organic origin of tiredness	No irritability or shortness of breath reported
Causal factor: **Suicidal tendencies**	Secondary to anxiety and depression; more common in males over 45 years of age; Mark appears emotionally depressed	Need to determine if Mark has had thoughts of suicide, a history of suicide attempts, long history of alcohol abuse, family history of substance abuse or has experienced any psychotic symptoms

Working diagnosis

MARK AND DEPRESSION

Mark is a 48-year-old man who was laid off work six months ago. Since this time Mark has experienced increased fatigue, sleepiness and a lack of interest in daily activities. Mark has started smoking again and is eating unhealthy food, not exercising, is emotionally detached from his wife and is experiencing feelings of guilt and worthlessness. Mark recently had a series of blood tests that ruled out several organic causes for his current symptoms of depression. His doctor would like him to begin a course of antidepressants but Mark does not believe he is depressed.

Depression is diagnosed when a person has had a shift in their self-esteem and are more self-critical, feel hopeless and helpless, guilty and pessimistic. Other signs of depression include negative physical and cognitive symptoms. Types of depression may be categorised under several terms that include whether the depression is primary, secondary, major, minor, mild, moderate, severe and psychological or physical. Major and minor depression are defined on a rating scale dependent on how many symptoms of depression are present every day for at least two weeks.

Mark's symptoms have now developed into what appears to be a primary major depression with severe symptoms present for more than two weeks. The clinical definition of major depression involves a prominent and persistent depressed or low mood that interferes with daily functioning almost every day for at least two weeks, and normally includes at least four of the following symptoms:

- depressed mood most of the day nearly every day
- diminished interest or pleasure in everyday activities most of the day nearly every day
- insomnia or hypersomnia nearly every day
- significant change in appetite nearly every day with weight loss or gain
- fatigue or loss of energy nearly every day
- psychomotor agitation or retardation such as restlessness or slower movements
- lack ability to think or concentrate nearly every day
- feelings of worthlessness or guilt nearly every day
- recurrent thoughts of death or suicide.

It can be common for a person not to recognise they actually have major (clinical) depression and may only understand their symptoms from the perspective of physical changes rather than psychological. Although Mark may have initially had reactive depression that was a secondary response to a life event, his symptoms have continued and present as a potential chemical and biological imbalance that is difficult to restore to equilibrium.

General references used in this diagnosis: 1–5, 62, 67–69

TABLE 10.9 **DECISION TABLE FOR TREATMENT PRIOR TO REFERRAL**		
COMPLAINT	**CONTEXT**	**CORE**
Treatment for the presenting complaint and symptoms	Treatment for all associated symptoms	Treatment for mental, emotional, spiritual, constitutional, lifestyle issues and metaphysical considerations
TREATMENT PRIORITY	**TREATMENT PRIORITY**	**TREATMENT PRIORITY**
• Lifestyle recommendations to improve symptoms of depression • Physical therapy suggestions to help improve symptoms of depression • Dietary recommendations to increase intake of essential nutrients for optimal production of serotonin and other neurotransmitters • Dietary recommendations to eliminate foods that may be having an adverse effect on Mark's mental health • Herbal tonic, tablets or tea with antidepressant, anxiolytic, tonic and adaptogenic action	• Lifestyle recommendations to eliminate unhelpful habits or behaviours and improve general health and fitness • Dietary recommendations to improve general health and nutrition and avoid consuming food or drinks that may be adversely affecting his mental health • Herbal tonic, tea or tablets with adaptogenic and tonic actions	• Recommendation for Mark to attend counselling • Recommendation for Mark to consult a careers advisor • Prioritising herbal and nutritional supplement recommendations to help with affordability • Emphasise dietary changes and lifestyle modifications that are more affordable

▶

COMPLAINT	CONTEXT	CORE
• Nutritional supplements to improve symptoms of depression **NB:** the use of 5-HTP, l-tryptophan or s-adenosylmethionine (SAMe) must be monitored to ensure there are no adverse reactions; if Mark decides to take l-tryptophan, 5-HTP or SAMe in conjunction with the herbal tonic, tea or tablets, the herbal formula should be reformulated due to the potential for interaction between 5-HTP, l-tryptophan and SAMe with St John's wort	• Nutritional supplements to increase intake of essential nutrients	

TABLE 10.10 **DECISION TABLE FOR REFERRAL** [1–5, 8–11, 16]		
COMPLAINT	CONTEXT	CORE
Referral for presenting complaint	Referral for all associated physical, dietary and lifestyle concerns	Referral for contributing emotional, mental, spiritual, metaphysical, lifestyle and constitutional factors
REFERRAL FLAGS	**REFERRAL FLAGS**	**REFERRAL FLAGS**
• Untreated symptoms of major depression as Mark has not chosen to follow his doctor's advice to take antidepressants • Depressed mood most of the day nearly every day • Diminished interest or pleasure in everyday activities most of the day nearly every day • Hypersomnia nearly every day • Significant change in appetite nearly every day with no weight loss or gain • Fatigue or loss of energy nearly every day • Feelings of worthlessness or guilt nearly every day	• Increased alcohol intake • Taken up smoking again	• Relationship tension with Mark's wife • Doesn't feel he can talk to his wife • Low self-esteem • Financial stress; will affect Mark's ability to afford treatment recommendations • Concerns about employability and retraining options • Unwilling to share the extent of his emotional feelings
ISSUES OF SIGNIFICANCE	**ISSUES OF SIGNIFICANCE**	**ISSUES OF SIGNIFICANCE**
Nil	• Poor diet resulting in inadequate intake of essential nutrients • Lack of physical activity	• Sleeping during the day because he is 'bored' • Watching TV excessively and isolating himself

COMPLAINT	CONTEXT	CORE
REFERRAL DECISION	REFERRAL DECISION	REFERRAL DECISION
• Recommendation for mental health assessment and clear information to be provided to Mark regarding choice of taking antidepressants and working collaboratively with a doctor, psychotherapist and counsellor support symptoms of major depression [69]	• Dietary assessment and evaluation to ensure adequate intake of nutrients for nervous system support	• Counselling and mental health assessment [70] • Family counselling

Confirmed diagnosis

Major clinical depression with functional fatigue

PRESCRIBED MEDICATION

• Antidepressant medication – previously prescribed. Mark has decided not to take the antidepressant medication at this stage and wants to try natural therapies.

TABLE 10.11 FURTHER INVESTIGATIONS THAT MAY BE NECESSARY [1–5, 7, 10, 11, 16]	
TEST/INVESTIGATION	REASON FOR TEST/INVESTIGATION
FIRST-LINE INVESTIGATIONS:	
Referral for counselling	Emotional assessment and support
Referral for mental illness assessment	If it is felt Mark is in danger of hurting himself or someone else; it is important that other health professionals are also aware a client may have suicidal thoughts and tendencies
IF NECESSARY:	
Sleep clinic observation	Sleep apnoea
Anti-nuclear antibody	Autoimmune disorders
Vitamin D [22, 23]	Vitamin D deficiency
Heavy metal toxicity screening: mercury, cadmium, arsenic, nickel, aluminium [8, 9]	Heavy metal toxicity can cause neurological and behavioural changes [24]; lead levels are within normal range, but other heavy metals have not been tested for
Serum test for biotin, folic acid, vitamin B6, B2, B3, B12 and C, calcium, copper, iron, magnesium and potassium	Deficiency can cause depression [8, 9]
Brain scan	Brain tumour

TABLE 10.12 **DECISION TABLE FOR TREATMENT (ONCE DIAGNOSIS IS CONFIRMED)**		
COMPLAINT	**CONTEXT**	**CORE**
Treatment for the presenting complaint and symptoms	Treatment for all associated symptoms	Treatment for mental, emotional, spiritual, constitutional, lifestyle issues and metaphysical considerations
TREATMENT PRIORITY	**TREATMENT PRIORITY**	**TREATMENT PRIORITY**
• Continue with lifestyle recommendations to improve symptoms of depression • Continue with physical therapy suggestions to help improve symptoms of depression • Continue with dietary recommendations • Continue with herbal tonic, tablets or tea • Continue with essential nutritional supplements **NB:** If Mark decides to take prescribed antidepressant medication his herbal formula will need to be reformulated to remove St John's wort; if he is taking l-tryptophan, 5-HTP or SAMe, they will need to be discontinued if he decides to take the prescribed antidepressant; Mark must be monitored collaboratively with his GP to ensure his treatment program is effective and to adjust the program where necessary	• Continue with lifestyle recommendations to eliminate unhelpful habits or behaviours and improve general health and fitness • Continue with dietary recommendations to improve general health and nutrition • Continue with herbal tonic, tea or tablets to support Mark's stress response • Continue with essential nutritional supplements; supplement recommendations may be altered depending on the results of serum and/or hair tissue mineral tests for nutrient deficiencies and heavy metal toxicity	• Recommend Mark continues with counselling • Encourage Mark to continue seeing a career advisor and consider retraining options • Ensure initial and ongoing treatment recommendations are prioritised to ensure affordability • Maintain emphasis on dietary changes and lifestyle modifications to help keep the program affordable

Treatment aims

- Identify and address the factors contributing to Mark's depression [8, 9].
- Balance Mark's neurotransmitter levels [8, 9, 17, 38].
- Improve Mark's stress response and adrenal function [9, 17, 49]. Stress-related adrenal dysfunction can result in depression [9, 49].
- Support normal function of Mark's hypothalamic-pituitary-adrenal axis [9, 17, 49].
- Optimise Mark's nutritional status. Nutritional deficiencies may contribute towards depression [8, 9, 17, 22, 45, 46].
- Direct Mark to therapies that help the development of a positive mental attitude [8, 47] and skills to improve quality of life [9, 47].
- Improve Mark's lifestyle to reduce or eliminate factors such as excessive alcohol consumption, smoking, poor diet and lack of physical activity, which may be contributing towards his depression [8, 9, 21, 35, 47].

Lifestyle alterations/considerations

- Refer Mark for counselling utilising cognitive behavioural therapy that aims to help him develop a positive mental attitude, set realistic goals, avoid negative behavioural patterns and find ways to include laughter and humour into his life [8, 9, 17, 47].
- Regular daily exercise is an effective method of treating depression [8, 9, 17, 47]. Aerobic exercise such as brisk walking, running [21] or weight training [9] has been shown to reduce depression [9, 21].
- Stress-management techniques [49], such as relaxation therapy [9, 47] and yoga breathing exercises [47], might be helpful to Mark.
- Encourage Mark to spend time outside in the fresh air and sunshine to get sufficient sun exposure for adequate vitamin D production. Vitamin D deficiency is associated with depression [22, 23].
- Test Mark for heavy metal toxicity and treat if necessary [9, 24].
- Encourage Mark to live a more healthy lifestyle, incorporating healthy eating, reduced alcohol consumption, quitting smoking and daily physical activity [21, 35, 45, 47].
- Encourage Mark to consult with a careers advisor to help him consider his employment and retraining options.
- Encourage Mark to take up an activity that gives him a purpose and has a positive effect on his family. Planting a vegetable garden may help him to feel he is contributing to the family and may facilitate a greater level of involvement and engagement with his children if they are encouraged to work with him in the garden. Eating home grown vegetables will provide significant nutritional benefits.

Dietary suggestions

- Encourage Mark to follow a Mediterranean-style, nutrient-dense, antioxidant-rich whole-food diet that contains plenty of vegetables, whole grains, legumes, nuts and seeds and cold-water fish [9, 45]. Mediterranean diets have a protective role against depression [45].
- Encourage mark to increase consumption of tryptophan-containing foods such as turkey, salmon, bananas, legumes, fish, whole oats, nuts and seeds, soy and dairy products [8, 9, 17, 40]. Also increase dietary intake of tyrosine from dairy foods, nuts and seeds, oats, whole grains, eggs, fish and soy products [25].
- Encourage mark to increase his dietary intake of omega-3 fatty acids [9, 17, 19, 25, 34].
- Encourage mark to significantly reduce or eliminate refined and processed foods, sugar [9, 17, 19, 46], coffee and other stimulants [9, 17].
- Encourage mark to significantly reduce or eliminate alcohol consumption [9, 35, 56].
- Identify and eliminate foods to which Mark is sensitive or allergic [9, 57].
- Encourage Mark to eat a low GI/GL diet. There is evidence of a link between hypoglycaemia or altered glucose metabolism and depression [19, 20].

Physical treatment suggestions

- Mark may benefit from massage therapy [47, 50, 51]. Massage therapy can reduce anxiety and depression [50, 51]. The use of lavender oil during massage therapy may be particularly helpful [25, 41].
- Electroacupuncture may be of benefit to Mark [42].
- Hydrotherapy: 2–3-minute cold (no less than 55°F/12°C) showers twice a day [18, 52, 55], alternating hot and cold showers with 1–2 minute of hot and 15–30 seconds of cold. Repeat 3–4 times twice a day [18, 54]. Neutral bath from ¼ –1 hour daily for several days [53], full body cold mitten friction [53], constitutional hydrotherapy daily or weekly [53]. Dry skin-brushing prior to bath, followed by wet skin-brushing in the bath with a loofah [54].

TABLE 10.13 **HERBAL FORMULA (1:2 LIQUID EXTRACTS)**		
HERB	**FORMULA**	**RATIONALE**
St John's wort *Hypericum perforatum*	60 mL	Antidepressant [25, 26, 47]; anxiolytic [25, 26]; inhibits synaptic reuptake of serotonin, noradrenalin and dopamine [25, 26]; upregulates serotonin receptors [25, 26]; clinical trials indicate use in treating mild to moderate depression [25, 26] Caution should be exercised if Mark decides to take the prescribed antidepressant medication, his formula should be reformulated to remove St John's wort [25, 26]
Siberian ginseng *Eleutherococcus senticosus*	40 mL	Adaptogenic [25, 28]; tonic [28]; theoretical application in depression is due to the herb's ability to increase serotonin and noradrenalin [29]; clinical indications include stress [25, 28], fatigue [25, 28] and to increase vitality [28]
Damiana *Turnera diffusa*	60 mL	Traditionally used in Western herbal medicine as an antidepressant and anxiolytic [27, 28]; particularly beneficial where there is a sexual factor involved [25]
Rhodiola *Rhodiola rosea*	40 mL	Adaptogenic [31]; tonic [31]; traditionally used to treat fatigue, depression and nervous system disorders [31]; effective in reducing symptoms of depression [32]; effective in reducing symptoms of generalised anxiety disorder [33]
Supply:	200 mL	Dose: 10 mL twice daily

TABLE 10.14 **TABLET ALTERNATIVE TO HERBAL LIQUID: MAY IMPROVE COMPLIANCE**		
HERB	**DOSE PER TABLET**	**RATIONALE**
St John's wort *Hypericum perforatum*	750 mg	See above
Damiana *Turnera diffusa*	675 mg	See above
Schisandra *Schisandra chinensis*	625 mg	Adaptogenic [25, 44]; hepatoprotective [25]; nervine tonic [44]
Skullcap *Scutellaria lateriflora*	500 mg	Nervine tonic [43]; mild sedative [27, 43]; indicated for use in nervous tension [27]
Dose: 2 tablets twice daily		

TABLE 10.15 **HERBAL TEA**

A less expensive option if Mark has concerns about the cost of the herbal tonic or tablet

HERB	FORMULA	RATIONALE
St John's wort *Hypericum perforatum*	2 parts	See above
Damiana *Turnera diffusa*	1 part	See above
Lavender *Lavandula angustifolia*	1 part	Antidepressant [27, 28]; anxiolytic [25, 28]; improves sleep [25], mood [25] and concentration [25]
Oats seed *Avena sativa*	1 part	Antidepressant [27]; nutritive [25]; traditionally used in depressive states and general debility [27]
Vervain *Verbena officinalis*	1 part	Indicated for use in depression and melancholia [27]
Decoction: 1 cup 4 times daily		

TABLE 10.16 **NUTRITIONAL SUPPLEMENTS**

SUPPLEMENT AND DOSE	RATIONALE
Omega-3 fish oil supplement containing 2000 mg EPA daily [36] *An essential and affordable supplement*	Effective in treating depression [8, 9, 17, 25, 34]; supplemental EPA provides significant benefits in treating depression [36, 61]
High-potency practitioner-strength **multivitamin, mineral and antioxidant supplement** containing therapeutic doses of essential micronutrients, particularly B-group vitamins and vitamin D [22, 25, 59, 60] An essential and affordable supplement	Nutritional deficiency can lead to depression [22, 25, 59]; because Mark's current diet is nutrient poor supplementation is advisable B-group vitamins are essential for serotonin production [17, 25, 40]; vitamin D deficiency is associated with depression [22, 60]; because Mark spends most of his time inside he may not be getting sufficient sun exposure to maintain healthy vitamin D levels
Tryptophan supplement providing 400 mg tryptophan daily in divided doses [40] NB: In Australia doses of tryptophan exceeding 100 mg are included in Schedule 4 of the Standard for the Uniform Scheduling of Drugs and Poisons (SUSDP) and require a medical, dental or veterinary prescription [37] or **5-hydroxytryptophan** [5-HTP] 75 mg daily [17] Alternative to herbal treatment; important supplement, but secondary to essential nutritional supplements and dietary recommendations if finances are tight; alternative to herbal formula; the availability and sale of 5-HTP is restricted in many Australian states and territories	Tryptophan deficiency is associated with depression [38, 40]; using contaminated l-tryptophan has been linked to the development of eosinophilia-myalgia syndrome (EMS); caution should be exercised to ensure only high-quality tryptophan products are supplied [9] Immediate serotonin precursor [40]; increases endorphins and catecholamine and is an effective alternative to SSRI medications and tricyclic antidepressants [9]; 5-HTP has a therapeutic use in depression [17, 40];

▶

S-adenosylmethionine (SAMe) 200 mg 3 times daily [40]; an alternative to tryptophan or 5-HTP if difficulties obtaining or prescribing at the recommended dose are experienced; important supplement, but secondary to essential nutritional supplements and dietary recommendations if finances are tight; alternative to herbal treatment	Effective for mild to moderately severe depression [17, 47]; therapeutic use in depression [17, 40, 47]
Magnesium 800 mg elemental magnesium daily in divided doses [37, 40]; important supplement, but secondary to essential nutritional supplements and dietary recommendations if finances are tight	Supplemental magnesium is an effective treatment for depression [25, 37, 39]; magnesium deficiency may be a causative factor in the development of depression [25, 37, 40]

References

[1] P. Kumar, C. Clark, Clinical Medicine, sixth edn, Elsevier Saunders, London, 2005, pp. 1288–1291.

[2] R.D. Collins, Differential Diagnosis in Primary Care, fourth edn, Lippincott Williams & Wilkins, Philadelphia, 2008, pp. 120–121.

[3] A. Polmear, Evidence-Based Diagnosis in Primary Care, Churchill Livingstone Elsevier, Edinburgh, 2008.

[4] R.H. Seller, Differential Diagnosis of Common Complaints, fifth edn, Saunders Elsevier, Philadelphia, 2007, pp. 155–166, 351.

[5] J. Jamison, Differential Diagnosis for Primary Care, second edn, Churchill Livingstone Elsevier, London, 2006, pp. 139–143, 418–420.

[6] N.J. Talley, S. O'Connor, Pocket Clinical Examination, third edn, Churchill Livingstone Elsevier, Australia, 2009.

[7] G. Douglas, F. Nicol, C. Robertson, Macleod's Clinical Examination, twelfth edn, Churchill Livingstone Elsevier, Edinburgh, 2009.

[8] H. Osiecki, The Physicians Handbook of Clinical Nutrition, seventh edn, Bioconcepts, Eagle Farm, 2000.

[9] J.E. Pizzorno, M.T. Murray, H. Joiner-Bey, The Clinicians Handbook of Natural Medicine, second edn, Churchill Livingstone, St Louis, 2008.

[10] R. Berkow, A.J. Fletcher, M.H. Beers, The Merck Manual, sixteenth edn, Merck Research Laboratories, Rathway, N.J, 1993 (later edition).

[11] S. El-Hashemy, Naturopathic Standards of Primary Care, CCNM Press, Toronto, 2008.

[12] J. Silverman, S. Kurtz, J. Draper, Skills for Communicating with Patients, second edn, Radcliff Publishing, Oxford, 2000.

[13] R. Neighbour, The Inner Consultation: how to develop an effective and intuitive consulting style, Radcliff Publishing, Oxon, 2005.

[14] D. Peters, L. Chaitow, G. Harris, S. Morrison, Integrating Complementary Therapies in Primary Care, Churchill Livingstone, London, 2002.

[15] M. Lloyd, R. Bor, Communication Skills For Medicine, third edn, Churchill Livingstone Elsevier, Edinburgh, 2009.

[16] L. Chaitow, E. Blake, P. Orrock, M. Wallden, P. Snider, J. Zeff (Eds.), Natropathic Physical Medicine: Theory and Practice for Manual Therapists and Naturopaths, Churchill Livingstone Elsevier, Philadelphia, 2008.

[17] J. Jamison, Clinical Guide to Nutrition & Dietary Supplements in Disease Management, Churchill Livingstone, Edinburgh, 2003.

[18] N. Shevchuk, S. Radoja, Possible stimulation of anti-tumour immunity using repeated cold stress: a hypothesis, Infect Agent-Cancer 2 (2007) 20.

[19] A.N. Westover, L.B. Marangell, A Cross-National Relationship Between Sugar Consumption And Major Depression? Depression and Anxiety 16 (2002) 118–120.

[20] J.H. Wright, J.J. Jacisin, N.S. Radin, R.A. Bell, Glucose metabolism in unipolar depression, British Journal of Psychiatry 132 (1978) 386–393.

[21] P. Salmon, Effects of physical exercise on anxiety, depression, and sensitivity to stress: A unifying theory, Clinical Psychology Review 21 (1) (2001) 33–61.

[22] M.F. Holick, T.C. Chen, Vitamin D deficiency: a worldwide problem with health consequences, The American Journal of Clinical Nutrition 87 (2008) 1080S–1086S.

[23] M.F. Holick, Vitamin D Deficiency, N Engl J Med 357 (2007) 266–281.

[24] T.W. Clarkson, Metal Toxicity in the Central Nervous System, Environmental Health Perspectives 75 (1987) 59–64.

[25] L. Braun, M. Cohen, Herbs & Natural Supplements: An evidence based guide, second edn, Elsevier, Sydney, 2007.

[26] S. Mills, K. Bone, Principles & Practice of Phytotherapy: Modern Herbal Medicine, Churchill Livingstone, Edinburgh, London, 2000.

[27] British Herbal Medicine Association, British Herbal Pharmacopoeia, BHMAA, 1983.

[28] S. Mills, K. Bone, The Essential Guide to Herbal Safety, Churchill Livingstone, St Louis, 2005.

[29] Z.I. Abramova, Z.K. Cherny, V.P. Natalenko et al. Lek Sredstva Dal'nego Vostoka. 11 (1972) 106–108. in S. Mills, K. Bone. The Essential Guide to Herbal Safety. St Louis, Churchill Livingstone, 2005, pp. 540.

[30] M. Morgan, K. Bone, Rhodiola rosaea – Rhodiola, Mediherb Phytotherapist's Perspective 47 (2005) 1–4.

[31] K. Bone, Rhodiola Effective for Depression, Mediherb Clinical Monitor 19 (2007) 1.

[32] A. Bystritsky, L. Kerwin, J.D. Feusner, A Pilot Study of Rhodiola rosea (Rhodax®) for Generalized Anxiety Disorder (GAD), The J Altern Complement Med 14 (2) (2008) 175–180.

[33] B.M. Ross, J. Seguin, L.E. Sieswerda. Omega-3 fatty acids as treatments for mental illness: which disorder and which fatty acid? Lipids in Health and Disease 6 (21) 2007.

[34] F. Bonnet, K. Irving, J.L. Terra, P. Nony, F. Berthez, P. Moulin, Anxiety and depression are associated with unhealthy lifestyle in patients at risk of cardiovascular disease, Atherosclerosis 178 (2005) 339–344.

[35] B. Nemets, Z. Stahl, R.H. Belmaker, Addition of Omega-3 Fatty Acid to Maintenance Medication Treatment for Recurrent Unipolar Depressive Disorder, American Journal of Psychiatry 159 (2002) 477–479.

[36] Minutes of the twenty-eighth meeting of the Complementary Medicines Evaluation Committee, 27 July 2001. www.tga.gov.au/DOCS/pdf/cmec/cmecmi28.pd.

[37] C. Bell, J. Abrahams, D. Nutt, Tryptophan depletion and its implications for psychiatry, The British Journal of Psychiatry 178 (2001) 399–405.

[38] G.A. Eby, K.L. Eby, Rapid recovery from major depression using magnesium treatment, Medical Hypotheses 67 (2) (2006) 362–370.

[39] H. Osiecki, The Nutrient Bible, seventh edn, BioConcepts Publishing, Eagle Farm, 2008.

[40] S.M. Wilkinson, S.B. Love, A.M. Westcombe, M.A. Gambles, C.C. Burgess, An. Cargill, T. Young, et al., Effectiveness of Aromatherapy Massage in the Management of Anxiety and Depression in Patients With Cancer: A Multicenter Randomized Controlled Trial, Journal of Clinical Oncology 25 (5) (2007) 532–539.

[41] C. Han, X. Li, H. Luo, X. Zhao, X. Li, Clinical study on electro-acupuncture treatment for 30 cases of mental depression, Journal of Traditional Chinese Medicine 24 (3) (2004) 172–176.

[42] R. Awad, J.T. Arnason, V. Trudeau, C. Bergeron, J.W. Budzinski, B.C. Foster, Z. Merali, Phytochemical and biological analysis of Skullcap (Scutellaria lateriflora L.): A medicinal plant with anxiolytic properties, Phytomedicine 10 (8) (2003) 640–649.

[43] K. Bone, Clinical Applications of Chinese and Ayurvedic Herbs: Monographs for the Western Herbal Practitioners, Phytotherapy Press, Warwick, 1996.

[44] A. Sanchez-Villegas, M. Delgado-Rodriguez, A. Alonso, J. Schlatter, F. Lahortiga, L.S. Majem, et al., Association of the Mediterranean dietary pattern with the incidence of depression: the Seguimiento Universidad de Navarra/University of Navarra follow-up (SUN) cohort, Archives of General Psychiatry 66 (10) (2009) 1090–1098.

[45] D. Fishbein, The Contribution of Refined Carbohydrate Consumption to Maladaptive Behaviors, Orthomolecular Psychiatry 11 (1) (1982) 17–25.

[46] A.F. Jorm, H. Christensen, K.M. Griffiths, B. Rodgers, Effectiveness of complementary and self-help treatments for depression, Medical Journal of Australia 176 (2002) S84–S96.

[47] C. Hammen, Stress and Depression, Annual Review of Clinical Psychology 1 (2005) 293–319.

[48] C.M. Pariante, Depression, stress and the adrenal axis, Journal of Neuroendocrinology 15 (8) (2003) 811–812.

[49] C.A. Moyer, J. Rounds, J.W. Hannum, A Meta-Analysis of Massage Research, Psychological Bulletin 130 (1) (2004) 3–18.

[50] T. Field, M. Hernandez-Reif, M. Diego, Cortisol decreases and serotonin and dopamine increase following massage therapy, International Journal of Neuroscience 115 (2005) 1397–1413.

[51] N.A. Shevchuk, Adapted cold shower as a potential treatment for depression, Med Hypotheses, 2007, doi:10.1016/j.mehy.2007.04.052.

[52] W. Boyle, A. Saine, Lectures in Naturopathic Hydrotherapy, Eclectic Medical Publications, Oregon, 1988.

[53] D.D. Buchman, The complete book of water healing, Contemporary Books, McGraw-Hill Companies, New York, 2001.

[54] N. Shevchuk, Hydrotherapy as a possible neuroleptic and sedative treatment, Medical Hypotheses 70 (2) (2008) 23–238.

[55] M.H. Pietraszek, T. Urano, K. Sumioshi, K. Serizawa, S. Takahashi, Y. Takada, et al., Alcohol-Induced Depression: Involvement Of Serotonin, Alcohol & Alcoholism 26 (2) (1991) 155–159.

[56] G. Parker, T. Watkins, Treatment-resistant depression: when antidepressant drug intolerance may indicate food intolerance, Australian & New Zealand Journal of Psychiatry 36 (2) (2002) 263–265.

[57] L. Chaitow, Naturopathic Physical Medicine: Theory and Practice for Manual Therapists and Naturopaths, Churchill Livingstone, London, 2007.

[58] J. Alpert, M. Fava, Nutrition and depression: the role of folate, Nutrition Review 55 (5) (1997) 145–149.

[59] C. Wilkins, Y. Sheline, C. Roe, S. Birge, J. Morris, Vitamin D Deficiency Is Associated With Low Mood and Worse Cognitive Performance in Older Adults, American Journal of Geriatric Psychiatry 14 (12) (2006) 1032–1040.

[60] G. Parker, N. Gibson, H. Brotchie, G. Heruc, A. Rees, D. Hadzi-Pavlovic, Omega-3 Fatty Acids and Mood Disorders, Am J Psychiatry 163 (2006) 969–978.

[61] K. Kendler, C. Gardner, Boundaries of Major Depression: An Evaluation of DSM-IV Criteria, Am J Psychiatry 155 (2) (1998) 172–177.

[62] R.D. Chervin, Sleepiness, fatigue, tiredness, and lack of energy in obstructive sleep apnea, Chest 118 (2000) 372–379.

[63] W.R. Pigeon, M.J. Sateia, R.J. Ferguson, Distinguishing between excessive daytime sleepiness and fatigue: toward improved detection and treatment, J Psychosom Res 54 (2003) 61–69.

[64] S. Wessely, Chronic fatigue symptom and syndrome, Ann Intern Med 134 (2001) 838–843.

[65] A.C. Swann, B. Geller, R.M. Post, L. Altshuler, K.D. Chang, M.P. Delbello, et al., Practical clues to early recognition of bipolar disorder: a primary care approach, Prim Care Companion J Clin Psychiatry 7 (1) (2005) 15–21.

[66] J.M. Thibault, R.W. Steiner, Efficient identification of adults with depression and dementia, Am Fam Physician 70 (6) (2004) 1101–1110.

[67] V. Henkel, R. Mergl, R. Kohnen, et al., Identifying depression in primary care: a comparison of different methods in a prospective cohort study, BMJ 326 (2003) 200–201.

[68] S. Gilbody, A. House, T. Sheldon, Screening and case finding instruments for depression (Cochrane Review). The Cochrane Library, Issue 4, John Wiley, Chichester, 2005.

[69] L. Pezawas, J. Angst, A. Gamma, et al., Recurrent brief depression – past and future, Prog Neuropsychopharmacol Biol Psychiatry 27 (2003) 75–83.

[70] G. Ellis, J. Robinson, G. Crawford, When symptoms of disease overlap with symptoms of depression, Aust Fam Physician 35 (2006) 647–649.

[71] B. Carruthers, A. Jain, K. De Meirleir, et al., Myalgic encephalomyelitis/chronic fatigue syndrome: clinical working case definition, diagnostic and treatment protocols, J Chronic Fatigue Syndr 11 (2003) 7–115.

[72] I. Hickie, T.A. Davenport, D. Wakefield, et al., Post-infective and chronic fatigue syndromes precipitated by viral and non-viral pathogens: prospective cohort study, BMJ 333 (2006) 575–578.

[73] R.H. Belmaker, Bipolar disorders, N Engl J Med 351 (2004) 476–486.

[74] B. Arroll, F. Goodyear-Smith, N. Kerse, et al., Effect of the addition of a 'help' question to two screening questions on specificity for diagnosis of depression in general practice: diagnostic validity study, BMJ 331 (2005) 884–886.

Migraine

Case history

Lexi O'Mara, 25, has come to the clinic for help with headaches. Lexi works as a tour guide leading tours around the city and into country areas as well. Lexi's job involves long hours and she sometimes spends weeks away from home. She likes her job, although not quite as much as she did when she first started working as a tour guide four years ago. The company she is working for was sold about a year ago and the new owners require her to do much more paperwork than she used to. Right now her focus isn't on the job as much as it usually is because she is planning her wedding, which is only three months away.

Lexi started getting bad headaches about six months ago, and recently she seems to have a very bad one about every three weeks. Before then she never really got headaches, at least not such bad headaches. When they come, they last for a couple of days usually starting in the afternoon at the end of a busy day or at the end of a particularly long or stressful tour. Lexi has not been to see her GP as she does not want to take painkillers if possible but rather treat the cause with natural therapies. Lexi tells you her sister sometimes gets migraines and gave Lexi some of her prescribed Panadeine Forte to try to ease her headaches. It did help but she would rather not take them long term.

The pain develops rapidly and starts behind and above her right eye and then radiates into her temple. Before the pain comes on Lexi can experience a temporary loss of vision in her eye and have a series of flashes and spots in her vision. The pain is then usually an intense throbbing pain that intensifies until she needs to avoid noise and light and lie down in a darkened room. Lexi tells you that once she falls asleep the pain seems to go away and she usually wakes up without a headache, although she usually feels washed out for a couple of days afterwards. Sometimes she feels nauseous and vomits when she has a headache, although she has never noticed a particular food or drink making her nauseous and causing the headache.

When you ask Lexi about her general health you discover that she has been having problems with constipation recently. Lexi drinks lots of coffee and tea and knows she should drink more water. Lexi says she tries to eat well but has to eat what is available when she is on tour. She loves red wine, chocolate and cheese and her comfort food is Vegemite on hot buttered toast.

Lexi tells you she is not sure how much longer she wants to work as a tour guide, particularly doing tours that take her away from home. She isn't sure what she would like to do instead but is thinking that maybe she will try for a baby soon and be a mum for a few years. Lexi has been taking the oral contraceptive pill for about three years and sometimes skips her bleed when she is doing a country tour because it is much easier if she doesn't have to deal with a bleed when she is travelling. Before taking the contraceptive pill Lexi had a regular cycle and didn't have any problems with PMS or pain.

Lexi is very excited about her forthcoming wedding. She is having a traditional church wedding with 130 guests. She sometimes gets quite stressed and anxious about it because there is still so much to do and travelling away makes it more difficult for her to organise things. She is finding it a bit difficult to juggle her time between doing the paperwork, preparing for her tours and organising the wedding. Lexi tells you she doesn't want to sound like she is complaining, it's just that there's so much to do at the moment. She tries not to burden her parents or fiancé since they already have enough to do so she tends to keep things to herself.

TABLE 10.17 **COMPLAINT** [1–9, 57, 63, 65]	
Analogy: Skin of the apple	**Complaint:** Define the presenting complaint and symptoms; understand the complaint *Headaches*
AREAS OF INVESTIGATION AND EXAMPLE QUESTIONS	**CLIENT RESPONSES**
Exacerbating factors *Do you know what makes the headaches worse after they come on?*	*I think stress is probably the main trigger, but they do get worse with light and noise.*
Relieving factors *What makes them better?*	*Dark, quiet, rest and painkillers.*

TABLE 10.18 **CONTEXT**	
Analogy: Flesh of the apple	**Context:** Put the presenting complaint into context to understand the disease
AREAS OF INVESTIGATION AND EXAMPLE QUESTIONS	CLIENT RESPONSES
Family health *Does anyone else in your family have problems with headaches?*	*My sister gets headaches, but not as bad as mine.*
Allergies and irritants *Do you ever notice your headaches are any worse after eating chocolate, cheese, Vegemite on toast, bananas or drink red wine?* (amine intolerance)	*I am not sure, but I would not be surprised if it is linked somehow.*
Cancer and heart disease *Have you experienced any changes in smell or taste recently?* (brain tumour)	*No, not really, sometimes I lose my appetite but that is not related to not being able to taste things.*
Recreational drug use *How much alcohol do you usually consume in a week?* *Do you smoke?* *Do you take any other recreational drugs?*	*I'm not a big drinker. I sometimes have a glass of red wine with dinner to help me wind down, but not every day. I usually have 3–4 glasses on the weekend if I go out.* *No, I never have.* *No.*
Functional disease *Do your symptoms of headache improve when you are not working?* *Do you know if you grind your teeth during the night?* (muscle contraction headache) *Does your headache come on after exercise, coughing or having sexual intercourse?* (exertional headache)	*Yes, I did think that, but now that I'm organising my wedding when I'm not working, I notice them coming on any time more frequently.* *My fiancé has not mentioned me doing this and I have not had any suggestions from my dentist about this in the past.* *I can not find a rhyme or reason for why it comes on yet, so I am not really sure.*
Infection and inflammation *Is your headache aggravated by bending down?* (frontal sinusitis, temporal arteritis)	*I do tend to want to lie down when I have a headache, but it hurts any way I am, not only if I bend down.*
Supplements and side effects of medication *Are you taking any supplements or medication?*	*The pill.*
Stress and neurological disease *Do the headaches increase in intensity during the day and lessen in the evening?* (tension headache) *Have you noticed any discharge or swelling from your eye when you have a headache?* (cluster headache) *Do you ever notice redness in one eye, facial sweating and develop the need to move around when you have the headache?* (cluster headache)	*No, they can be any time of day.* *No, I just cannot stand any bright lights.* *No, I need to just lie still and flat when it gets bad, moving would make it worse.*

►

Eating habits and energy *Tell me about your diet.*	Lexi tries to eat a healthy diet, but has to eat whatever is available when she is leading a tour. She knows she should drink more water, and wonders whether this is why she gets constipated at times. Her favourite foods are cheese, chocolate and red wine. Comfort food is Vegemite on hot buttered toast.

TABLE 10.19 **CORE**	
Analogy: Core of the apple with the seed of ill health	**Core:** Holistic assessment to understand the client
AREAS OF INVESTIGATION AND EXAMPLE QUESTIONS	**CLIENT RESPONSES**
Emotional health *Do you ever feel anxious or depressed?*	*I have been getting a bit anxious about the wedding. Not about getting married but just about having to organise so many things when I have to go away so much. It can be hard to get it all done.*
Stress release *How do you deal with stress?*	*I might have a glass of red, or maybe some chocolate (all the things I probably should not have!). If I have the time and opportunity I might go for a bike ride or a run.*
Occupation *Tell me about your job.* *What is it about your job that you are not enjoying as much as you used to?*	*I work as a tour guide taking tours around the city and into the country. I can sometimes be away from home for a couple of weeks at a time.* *The business was sold last year and I have to do a lot more paperwork now. I really hate all the paperwork.*
Action needed to heal *How are you hoping I can help you?*	*Do you have any natural remedies I can take for my headaches instead of painkillers?*
Long-term goals *What do you see yourself doing in five years?*	*Probably with a couple of children, maybe at home or working part time.*

TABLE 10.20 **LEXI'S SIGNS AND SYMPTOMS**	
Pulse	75 bpm
Blood pressure	119/82
Temperature	36.9°C
Respiratory rate	14 resp/min
Body mass index	22
Waist circumference	75.6 cm
Face	Tired looking
Urinalysis	No abnormality detected (NAD)

Results of medical investigations

No medical investigations have been carried out.

TABLE 10.21 **UNLIKELY DIAGNOSTIC CONSIDERATIONS** [1–6, 10, 11, 57, 63, 64]	
CONDITIONS AND CAUSES	WHY UNLIKELY
CANCER AND HEART DISEASE	
Vascular complications: acute aneurysms	Sudden extreme and life-threatening acute presentation; BP history not known; often generalised headache pain or in occiput region
Hypertension: sometimes cause dull headaches	BP in normal range; usually generalised headache pain or in occiput region
Transient ischaemic attack (TIA): often begins with loss of vision in one eye due to emboli travelling through the retinal arteries; can have focal prodromal symptoms similar to a migraine	Headache is unusual in TIAs
Subarachnoid haemorrhage: unilateral red eye, acute headache, photophobia	Usually no visual changes and precipitated by trauma; no altered levels of consciousness
TRAUMA AND PRE-EXISTING ILLNESS	
Kidney disease: headache	BP in normal range; often generalised headache pain; urinalysis NAD
INFECTION AND INFLAMMATION	
Viral meningitis: headaches	No fever or skin rash; usually chronic rather than acute presentation; check if Lexi's neck is stiff on flexion and not on extension or rotation (sign of true nuchal rigidity)
Temporal arteritis: unilateral chronic headache	More common in elderly women, would have a low-grade fever, decreased vision

▶

Causal factor: **Sinus headache:** headache worse on waking in the morning	No upper respiratory symptoms mentioned, no frontal facial pain reported; need to check if the dull ache is aggravated by bending; typically worse in the morning and improves throughout the day
Ethmoid sinusitis: headache and pain in the eye	No nasal discharge, sinus tenderness, upper respiratory tract infection; no blood in nasal discharge
ENDOCRINE/REPRODUCTIVE	
Diabetes: migraine headaches can be precipitated by hypoglycaemia	Urinalysis NAD
STRESS AND NEUROLOGICAL DISEASE	
Ipsilateral Horner's syndrome: in some migraine headaches and cluster headaches, lesion of sympathetic nerve to eye	No classic physical signs of drooping of upper eyelid and slight elevation of lower eyelid; constriction of pupil of affected eye with dilatation lag
EATING HABITS AND ENERGY	
Dehydration: headaches and constipation	Urinalysis NAD, specific gravity in normal range

Case analysis

TABLE 10.22 **POSSIBLE DIFFERENTIAL DIAGNOSIS**		
Not ruled out by tests/investigations already done [1–3, 5, 6, 10, 11, 56–64, 68]		
CONDITIONS AND CAUSES	**WHY POSSIBLE**	**WHY UNLIKELY**
ALLERGIES AND IRRITANTS		
Causal factor: **Food intolerance amine sensitivity** [68]	Chronic headaches; loves drinking red wine, eating chocolate, cheese and Vegemite; usually cause or exacerbate migraine headaches	
Causal factor: **Environmental allergy**	Chronic headaches	No nasal congestion, itchy throat, skin rash
CANCER AND HEART DISEASE		
Brain tumour	Intermittent headaches, throbbing headache rather than dull; symptoms of nausea and vomiting can occur; headache that is progressively getting worse; vomiting associated with the headache	Headache worse on waking; usually symptoms of disturbed speech, vision, smell or taste; can have unusual sensations, lack of concentration and paralysis; usually slow regular pulse rate and high blood pressure; often generalised headache pain; headache will be made worse by coughing or bending and will be worse in the morning; headache will disturb sleep rather than be improved by sleep; no fever or seizures; usually more common over the age of 50

Ocular tumour	Localised to one eye	Often midfacial pain presentation of headache; blurred or double vision is more common
TRAUMA AND PRE-EXISTING ILLNESS		
Causal factor: **Liver disease**	High alcohol intake, increased dairy and fatty foods, dull headaches	Pulse is usually low and regular; no jaundice or yellow sclera
OBSTRUCTION AND FOREIGN BODY		
Causal factor: **Intestinal obstruction** e.g. faecal impaction with overflow	Can cause vomiting	Check if Lexi experiences recurrent abdominal pain after eating meals
RECREATIONAL DRUG USE		
Causal factor: **Substance abuse headaches:** oral or inhaled nitrates, MSG, cocaine, cannabis, alcohol	Duration of the headache can be up to 72 hours after taking substance; if a person is prone to migraines, alcohol can give a delayed hangover headache affect	Onset of headache depends on the type of substance
OCCUPATIONAL TOXINS AND HAZARDS		
Causal factor: **Dental work: leaking amalgam** [50]**, abscess, wisdom teeth**	Chronic headaches	Check if Lexi has had any dental work over the past 6 months and if she has fillings
Causal factor: **Sick building syndrome**	Chronic headache	Headaches are worse after working a few days in a row; no upper respiratory complaints or fatigue reported
FUNCTIONAL DISEASE		
Tension headache	Intensity of headaches increases during the day; can present as pain occurring at the end of a busy work day or work period, emotional and stressful time, not enjoying work as much as she used to; usually due to psychogenic cause; more common in females and begins in the second decade; can have tension type headache and migraine headaches together	Often associated with occipital (base of the head) and can occur on waking in chronic tension headaches; tension headaches can lessen during the evening without needing to sleep, then develop again in the morning; this pattern can persist all day for several days in a row and for months; usually bilateral dull pressing pain rather than throbbing and persistent in intensity that builds up gradually; no prodromes or nausea associated and does not prevent daily activity; family history of headaches is not significant to diagnosis
Glaucoma	Pain in one eye, headaches	Usually older age group; present with a visual halo around objects; headaches more likely to develop in a dark environment rather than be helped by it; will present as a frontal headache

▶

Causal factor: **Exertional headache:** can last from 5 minutes to 48 hours [67]	Headache	Check if the headache also comes on after exercise, coughing or sexual intercourse
Causal factor: **Eye strain**	Recurrent headaches; spending a lot of time reading for work and planning her wedding	Usually dull headaches at the base of the head (occiput area) typical of eye strain; headaches are unusual but may generally occur after a few days in a row of using eyes intensively for close vision
Causal factor: **Functional constipation**	Headache, not drinking enough water, high caffeine intake, not opening up to people about her concerns	Need to check if more than 1 in 4 bowel motions is lumpy and hard, and causes strain, a feeling of incomplete evacuation or blockage; need to check if manual help is needed to facilitate a bowel motion passing; if fewer than 3 evacuations a week
Causal factor: **Postural cause:** cervical pain/arthritis	Chronic headaches, can cause nausea	Check what mattress and pillow Lexi is using; check if neck stiffness is board-like or still supple on flexion (as opposed to meningitis stiffness); usually occurs in older age groups
Causal factor: **TMJ dysfunction**	Chronic headaches, can present in temporal region	Dull headache on waking; no pain mentioned specifically in jaw or ear; check if Lexi grinds her teeth during the night
DEGENERATIVE AND DEFICIENCY		
Causal factor: **Anaemia**	Headaches	Usually more generalised headache pain
SUPPLEMENTS AND SIDE EFFECTS OF MEDICATION		
Causal factor: **Oral contraceptive pill**	Side effect of migraine headaches, particularly if Lexi is taking a low oestrogen pill	
Causal factor: **Probable analgesic overuse:** occurs when person uses pain relief medication for over 15 days per month for at least 3 months	Headache that is worsening; headaches can become worse after initially beginning to withdraw the medication; Panadeine Forte can cause constipation	Usually headache presents several times in a month, is bilateral, pressing and tight nature of pain, moderate intensity; can only confirm diagnosis without taking medication for 2 months
ENDOCRINE/REPRODUCTIVE		
Hypothyroid	Constipation, headaches	No temperature intolerance, skin or hair changes, weight changes reported

▶

STRESS AND NEUROLOGICAL DISEASE		
Cluster headaches: migrainous neuralgia is a condition that causes recurrent bouts of excruciating pain that can wake the person at night and is often focused around one eye; not often associated with family history	Alcohol can precipitate the symptoms; can present in the temporal region; pain presents in one eye and radiates to the face or temporal region; can be precipitated by amine foods such as red wine, chocolate, cheese and Vegemite	Commonly occurs in males aged 40–60 years; headache is severe stabbing and burning pain and of short duration and usually lasts 30–180 minutes; presents with a red eye and can have discharge from the eye; can present with nasal congestion, eyelid oedema, facial sweating, restlessness and wants to move around; can have up to 8 attacks a day; can come back every day for 1–2 months; can recur at the same time every year and at the same time every day; early morning onset is typical; can be associated with peptic ulcer disease
Classic migraine (with aura): severe painful headaches; often unilateral and located in the front and temporal regions of the head; migraines last for 2–8 days	Recurrent headaches that can develop in temporal region and be unilateral; family history of headaches; can experience visual disturbances, nausea, vomiting, better for dark room, sleep and reduced noise stress can exacerbate; headaches usually improve upon waking and after sleep; need to stop moving	Investigate Lexi's symptoms of visual flashes and spots; tingling and numbness in limbs is often associated
Common migraine (without aura)	No prodromal symptoms, may experience vague fatigue or nausea and vomiting before migraine; family history of headaches; can have tension-type headache and migraine headaches together	Not always unilateral headache pain; presents more like a bilateral tension headache; can get fevers, chills, diarrhoea and skin rash; can have motion sickness
Neurologic disease: multiple sclerosis (MS)	More common in women; visual disturbance prior to MS usually unilateral and caused by optic neuritis	Need to establish if Lexi experiences double vision; usually advanced stages of MS; no significant trauma or injury mentioned in health history so far; need to define if visual disturbance comes and goes
Epilepsy	Sensory epilepsy (partial seizures) can present with similar symptoms to a migraine headache	Often there is tingling and weakness felt in limbs
Causal factor: **Stress**	Preparing for her wedding and keeping up with work responsibilities	

Causal factor: **Anxiety**	Headaches and increased stress in her lifestyle	Lexi has not reported lack of sleep, palpitations, tight chest, difficulty breathing, loss of appetite, fast talking
EATING HABITS AND ENERGY		
Causal factor: **Fasting**	Preparing for her wedding may have inspired a dietary and fasting program that can precipitate migraine headaches	Need to ask if she has been dieting or fasting
Causal factor: **Caffeine overload**	Having excess tea and coffee and chocolate	

TABLE 10.23 DECISION TABLE FOR REFERRAL [1–3, 6, 10–12]

COMPLAINT	CONTEXT	CORE
Referral for presenting complaint	Referral for all associated physical, dietary and lifestyle concerns	Referral for contributing emotional, mental, spiritual, metaphysical, lifestyle and constitutional factors
REFERRAL FLAGS	**REFERRAL FLAGS**	**REFERRAL FLAGS**
• Lexi experiences a chronic and reoccurring headache • Headache with nausea and vomiting and eye pain • Headache can persist for more than 24 hours • Does not want to get medical guidance in case she is prescribed medication she does not want to take	• Possible dehydration due to lack of water • Taking sister's prescribed analgesic medication without medical guidance and possibly creating more symptoms if not dosed correctly	Nil
ISSUES OF SIGNIFICANCE	**ISSUES OF SIGNIFICANCE**	**ISSUES OF SIGNIFICANCE**
Nil	• Excessive caffeine intake • Constipation • Oral contraceptive pill may be contributing to symptoms	• Stress with juggling work and organising her wedding • Not as happy in her job as she used to be
REFERRAL DECISION	**REFERRAL DECISION**	**REFERRAL DECISION**
• Medical opinion for what is causing the headaches and education on the orthodox approach to treating them so Lexi can make a treatment/management decision from 'informed consent' [66]	• Lexi needs dietary guidance and cooking/eating/drinking alternatives • Determine whether the oral contraceptive pill is triggering or aggravating Lexi's migraines and recommend alternative contraception methods if necessary [16, 17, 20]	• Emotional and career counselling and/or life coaching may help Lexi with time management and to manage personal and work pressures better

TABLE 10.24 **FURTHER INVESTIGATIONS THAT MAY BE NECESSARY** [1–3, 5, 6, 10, 11, 13, 57, 63, 64]	
TEST/INVESTIGATION	REASON FOR TEST/INVESTIGATION
FIRST-LINE INVESTIGATIONS:	
Eye tests: visual	Looking through a pinhole will improve vision if caused by refractive error and shows that retinal function is good
Snellen chart	Visual acuity
Relative afferent pupillary defect (RAPD)	RAPD positive in optic nerve disease, chronic glaucoma and retinal damage
Neurological assessment	Assess speech, language, facial expression, neck stiffness, orientation, memory, judgement and reasoning, cranial nerves, motor function (reflexes and tone), coordination, sensory function of skin, joints and temperature feeling, general observation of mood and behaviour
Musculoskeletal assessment	Eyes, neck movement or deformity, joint movement/ pain or swelling, muscle wasting or weakness, gait abnormalities, structure of spine and movement, general posture
Abdominal examination: inspection, auscultation, palpation, percussion	Intestinal obstruction
Full blood count	Anaemia, infection
Differential white blood cell count IgE (eosinophils antibody blood test)	Diagnosis for allergic triggers
ESR/CRP	Temporal arteritis/tumour/infection/inflammation
Liver function test	Alcohol and recreational drug abuse
Blood lipids	Carotid atherosclerosis, cardiovascular risk, blood cholesterol
Urea, creatine and electrolytes blood test	This will show in renal abnormalities and diabetes
Fasting blood glucose test	Can differentiate between diabetes, impaired fasting glycaemia (IFG) and impaired glucose tolerance (IGT)
Headache diary	Monitor pattern and precipitating factors for headaches
Diet diary	Monitor food intake and possible triggers for headaches
Skin prick testing	Test for specific extrinsic allergies
IF NECESSARY:	
Thyroid function test	Hypothyroid
Abdominal x-ray	Constipation

▶

Brain CT scan or MRI [64]	To confirm or rule out brain tumour/lesion/TIA, sinusitis
EEG (electroencephalogram)	Shows evidence of abnormal seizure activity to confirm epilepsy
Arteriograms	Vascular abnormalities
TMJ/cervical spine radiograph	Cervical damage and musculoskeletal reason for migraine
Teeth x-ray	Abscess, wisdom teeth
Lumbar puncture	Subarachnoid haemorrhage, bacterial encephalitis, meningitis

Confirmed diagnosis

LEXI AND MIGRAINE

Lexi is hoping complementary therapies can assist with recurrent headaches that began six months ago. Organising her forthcoming wedding has taken up a significant amount of her time and attention in addition to her job as a tour guide, which sometimes requires her to travel away from home. Since the ownership of her workplace changed hands, Lexi is not enjoying her job as much as she used to and she has been forced to do more paperwork. Lexi is on the oral contraceptive pill, is feeling more stressed than usual, loves eating chocolate, cheese, Vegemite and drinking red wine, coffee and tea and feels she is not drinking enough water. Over the past six months she has experienced episodes of severe headaches that begin with visual disturbance, pain in one eye and become so intense that only sleep in a dark room can alleviate the pain.

Confirming a diagnosis of headache pain can be a very difficult challenge and it is important that Lexi was referred for medical assessment because her headache pain is severe, associated with vomiting and nausea and can be disabling.

Lexi has been diagnosed with **classic migraine headaches** and defining features include prodromal symptoms that are usually visual where flashes, jagged lines and patches of light occur and sometimes blindness in one eye is experienced. Tingling, numbness or weakness on one side of the body may also occur. The person often feels nauseated. This prodromal feeling can last from 15 to 60 minutes and then the headache follows. The pain often begins in one spot and then radiates all over the head. The climax of the headache may bring on vomiting and the person needs to lie down in a dark room with no noise. Sleep is usually the only thing that alleviates the pain. The migraine headache will be aggravated by physical activity such as walking.

The cause of the headache is not completely understood but it is believed that the throbbing nature of a migraine headache is due to vasodilatation of blood vessels, with stimulation of nerve endings. Migraines often begin before the age of 20 and genetic factors play a role [69].

Migraines can return at regular intervals but usually have no specific pattern; however, they may present as episodes of pain on the weekend after a busy week. Migraines can be precipitated by vasoactive amine foods in the diet and with increased intake of caffeine. They may also be associated with the menstrual cycle for women and can increase in severity when taking the oral contraceptive pill. Other factors that can precipitate migraines include intense emotions, stress, hypoglycaemia, glare and exertion. Migraines can last up to six hours and occur once a week or less frequently.

Often people who experience migraines will also experience tension-type headaches. This can confuse the diagnosis as the two often have the same pathophysiological process [2] but will be treated differently once diagnosed. Family history is a strong indicator for the final diagnosis of migraine headache.

General references used in this diagnosis: 1–3, 6, 10, 11, 56, 59–61, 63

PRESCRIBED MEDICATION
• Ibuprofen with codeine [59]

TABLE 10.25 **DECISION TABLE FOR TREATMENT (ONCE DIAGNOSIS IS CONFIRMED)**		
COMPLAINT	**CONTEXT**	**CORE**
Treatment for the presenting complaint and symptoms	Treatment for all associated symptoms	Treatment for mental, emotional, spiritual, constitutional, lifestyle issues and metaphysical considerations
TREATMENT PRIORITY	**TREATMENT PRIORITY**	**TREATMENT PRIORITY**
• Lifestyle recommendations to avoid environmental or chemical triggers • Dietary recommendations to identify and avoid triggers • Physical treatment suggestions to reduce frequency and severity of migraines • Herbal tea, tonic or tablets with analgesic and migraine-preventative action • Nutritional supplement recommendations to prevent migraine or reduce its frequency	• Dietary recommendations to reduce inflammation and platelet aggregation • Dietary recommendations to consume important nutrients for migraine prevention • Dietary recommendations to maintain blood-sugar balance • Herbal tea, tonic or tablets to reduce inflammation, vasospasm and platelet aggregation • Herbal tea, tonic or tablets to support digestive function and detoxification • Herbal tonic or tablets with neurotransmitter modulating activity • Nutritional supplements to correct deficiencies that may be contributing to migraines • L-tryptophan or 5-HTP to support serotonin levels	• Lifestyle recommendations to manage stress • Physical treatment recommendations to manage and reduce stress • Herbal tea, tonic or tablets with adaptogenic, anxiolytic and sedative action to support Lexi's nervous system and stress response • Recommendation for Lexi to express her anxiety and ask for help from her family and fiancé

Treatment aims

• Reduce frequency and severity of migraines [25].
• Restore Lexi's biochemical homoeostasis and optimise neurotransmitter production [15–17].
• Dampen inflammatory mediators [15–17].

- Decrease platelet aggregation, prevent the release of vasoactive neurotransmitters and reduce vasospasm [15, 17, 39].
- Identify and eliminate dietary and environmental triggers [14, 15, 17, 39].
- Improve Lexi's digestive function [17, 19, 52], correct intestinal dysbiosis [17–19] and reduce toxic overload [17, 19].
- Identify and correct nutritional deficiencies that may be contributing to the problem [17, 39, 51, 52].
- Improve Lexi's stress response and stress management [14, 15, 17, 25].
- Ensure Lexi's blood-sugar levels remain stable. Missing meals and hypoglycaemia may be contributing to her migraines [16, 17, 21].

Lifestyle alterations/considerations

- Stress-management techniques, such as meditation, yoga and relaxation techniques, can help reduce Lexi's stress [23] and may therefore reduce her migraines [14, 15, 17, 25].
- Thermal biofeedback therapy may be helpful [17, 25].
- Encourage Lexi to exercise regularly to help with stress management and to reduce her anxiety levels [23, 26].
- Encourage Lexi to express her anxieties to her parents and fiancé and seek their help with the wedding arrangements to reduce her stress levels.
- Discuss alternative contraception methods with Lexi. The oral contraceptive pill may be contributing to her migraines [16, 17, 20].
- Encourage Lexi to try to identify and avoid exposure to environmental triggers [16, 25].
- Lexi may benefit from a detoxification program to reduce toxic overload resulting from metabolic waste, food allergy or intolerance reactions and intestinal dysbiosis [17–19].

Dietary suggestions

- Identify food allergies and sensitivities and eliminate those foods [14, 15, 17, 39]. A food diary may help Lexi identify foods that are triggering her migraines. The use of withdrawal and challenge testing may help confirm which foods are migraine triggers. A four-day rotation diet should be used until Lexi has been symptom-free for six months [17].
- Eliminate foods containing vasoactive amines such as red wine, chocolate, aged cheese, yoghurt, Vegemite, citrus, overripe bananas, avocado, red plums, tomatoes and shellfish [15, 17, 39]. Lexi may also need to avoid foods that are fermented during processing such as beer, meat extracts and chicken livers [15].
- Encourage Lexi to increase her water intake and eliminate tea, coffee, cola drinks and alcohol [17].
- Encourage Lexi to reduce her consumption of arachidonic acid from animal fats and fatty foods [17, 41, 53] and increase consumption of omega-3 fatty acids [15, 17, 41, 53].
- Encourage Lexi to increase consumption of nutrient and antioxidant-rich whole foods that are not migraine triggers. Increasing dietary fibre will help improve bowel function and detoxification [17, 55]. Foods high in magnesium and B vitamins will help prevent and reduce symptoms [15, 17, 39, 41].
- Encourage Lexi to eat smaller regular meals of low GI/GL foods to help keep her blood glucose levels stable [16, 17, 21].
- Encourage Lexi to eat ginger, onions, garlic and other foods that can reduce excessive platelet aggregation [16, 17].

Physical treatment suggestions

- Lexi may benefit from acupuncture to help with stress management [23, 24] and prevention of migraine [17, 22, 25, 39].
- Transcutaneous electrical nerve stimulation (TENS) therapy may be beneficial to treat migraine symptoms [17].
- Massage can reduce frequency and severity of migraine symptoms [27]. Including aromatherapy oils in the massage can help reduce Lexi's stress levels [28].
- Topical application of a 10 per cent solution lavender and peppermint essential oils to Lexi's temples and occipital region at the onset of symptoms may be helpful [29, 44].
- Hydrotherapy: as soon as headache begins place the head under cold water or pour cold water over it for three minutes, making sure the nostrils keep out of the water to breathe [45].
- Lexi may find that plunging her feet into very hot water at the first signs of a migraine may help reduce the severity or possibly abort it [46]. This is because the heat of the water dilates blood vessels in the feet and causes more blood to flow to that part of the body, theoretically drawing it away from the head [47]. This is a traditional remedy that has been found helpful by some migraine sufferers. Can add 1 tbsp of mustard powder to a hot foot bath for 20 minutes, while placing an ice pack on the back of the neck and a cold compress on the forehead (changing it every three minutes) [45, 46].
- Neutral body bath [48] or 15-minute hot sitz bath (or half bath) finishing off with cold water over the feet and laying down for 20 minutes [45, 49].
- Alternating hot and cold contrast leg douche shower and cold arm shower prior to a head message can be very beneficial in drawing heat away and helping fatigue [45, 49].

TABLE 10.26 **HERBAL FORMULA (1:2 LIQUID EXTRACTS)**		
HERB	**FORMULA**	**RATIONALE**
Feverfew *Tanacetum parthenium* 1:5 fluid extract	30 mL	Anti-inflammatory [29, 30]; analgesic [29, 30]; inhibits platelet aggregation [29, 30]; decreases vascular smooth muscle spasm [29, 30]; prevents migraine headache [29, 30, 37]
Schisandra *Schisandra chinensis*	55 mL	Anti-inflammatory [29]; adaptogenic [29, 34]; nervine tonic [34]; improves detoxifying capacity of the liver [29, 34]; PAF antagonist [29]
Ginkgo *Ginkgo biloba* 2:1 fluid extract	40 mL	Anti-inflammatory [29, 30]; antioxidant [29, 30, 38]; inhibits vasospasm [30]; modulates neurotransmitters and receptors [29, 38]; anti-PAF properties [30, 38]
Ginger *Zingiber officinale*	15 mL	Anti-inflammatory [29, 30]; antiplatelet [29, 30]; analgesic [29]; antiemetic [29, 30]; can prevent and treat migraine [29]
Skullcap *Scutellaria lateriflora*	30 mL	Nervine tonic [31, 33]; mild sedative [31, 33]; spasmolytic [33]; traditional indications for use include nervous tension and anxiety [31, 33]
Dandelion root *Taraxacum officinale*	30 mL	Choleretic [29, 33]; mild laxative [31, 33]; anti-inflammatory [29]; antioxidant [29]
Supply:	200 mL	Dose: 5 mL 3 times daily

TABLE 10.27 TABLET ALTERNATIVES TO HERBAL LIQUID (IF THERE ARE COMPLIANCE PROBLEMS)

HERB	DOSE PER TABLET	RATIONALE
Feverfew *Tanacetum parthenium*	150 mg	See above

Dose: 1 tablet twice daily

HERB	DOSE PER TABLET	RATIONALE
Brahmi *Bacopa monnieri*	1200 mg	Nervine tonic [34]; mild sedative [34]; anti-inflammatory [34]
Ginkgo *Ginkgo biloba*	1500 mg	See above
Rosemary leaf *Rosmarinus officinalis*	250 mg	Anti-inflammatory [29]; traditionally used for migraine headaches [29, 31, 33]; improves oestrogen metabolism [29, 36]

Dose: 1 tablet 3 times daily

TABLE 10.28 HERBAL TEA

To replace tea and coffee

HERB	FORMULA	RATIONALE
Lavender *Lavandula angustifolia*	2 parts	Anxiolytic [29, 33]; sedative [29]; traditionally combined with valerian in migraine headache [31]
Lemon balm *Melissa officinalis*	2 parts	Anxiolytic [29]; sedative [29, 30]; analgesic [29]; anti-inflammatory [29]
Rosemary leaf *Rosmarinus officinalis*	½ part	See above
Valerian root *Valeriana officinalis*	2 parts	Anxiolytic [29, 30]; mild sedative [30]; smooth muscle relaxant [29, 30]; traditionally combined with lavender for migraine headache [31]

Infusion: 1 tsp per cup – 1 cup 3 times daily

TABLE 10.29 NUTRITIONAL SUPPLEMENTS

SUPPLEMENT AND DOSE	RATIONALE
Magnesium citrate supplement providing 600 mg elemental magnesium daily [15, 29]	Migraine sufferers have lower intracellular magnesium levels [29, 40]; low magnesium levels are linked to migraine headaches [17, 29]; beneficial for migraine prevention [17, 29, 35, 39–41]
B vitamin supplement providing a daily dose of 75 mg B6 [17] and 400 mg B2 [14, 17] combined with a B-vitamin complex [17]	Supplementation with vitamins B6 and B2 can be effective in preventing migraine [15, 17]

►

SUPPLEMENT AND DOSE	RATIONALE
Omega-3 fish oil capsules 5 × 1000 mg capsules 3 times daily providing a daily dose of 2.7 g EPA and 1.8 g DHA [15]	Anti-inflammatory [15, 29, 32]; antiplatelet [17, 29, 32]; omega-3 fatty acids have anti-vasopressor effects [41] and supplementation can reduce migraine frequency, duration and severity [15, 17, 41]
L-tryptophan 500 mg every 6 hours [15, 39] NB: In Australia doses of tryptophan exceeding 100 mg are included in Schedule 4 of the Standard for the Uniform Scheduling of Drugs and Poisons [SUSDP] and require a medical, dental or veterinary prescription [42] or **5-hydroxytryptophan** 400 mg daily [17, 43] The availability and sale of 5-HTP is restricted in many Australian states and territories	Serotonin precursor [17, 32]; serotonin disorders are implicated in the pathogenesis of migraine [15, 17, 32]; l-tryptophan supplementation can reduce reduce migraine frequency [15, 39] The use of contaminated l-tryptophan has been linked to the development of eosinophilia-myalgia syndrome (EMS); caution should be exercised to ensure only high-quality tryptophan products are supplied [17] Immediate precursor to serotonin [17, 32]; 400 mg 5-HTP daily is effective in preventing migraine [17, 43]

References

[1] R.H. Seller, Differential Diagnosis of Common Complaints, fifth edn, Saunders Elsevier, Philadelphia, 2007.

[2] A. Polmear (Ed.), Evidence-Based Diagnosis in Primary Care, Churchill Livingstone Elsevier, 2008, pp. 274–283.

[3] J. Jamison, Differential Diagnosis for Primary Care, second edn, Churchill Livingstone Elsevier, London, 2006.

[4] N.J. Talley, S. O'Connor, Pocket Clinical Examination, third edn, Churchill Livingstone Elsevier, Australia, 2009.

[5] G. Douglas, F. Nicol, C. Robertson, Macleod's Clinical Examination, twelfth edn, Churchill Livingstone Elsevier, 2009.

[6] P. Kumar, C. Clark, Clinical Medicine, sixth edn, Elsevier Saunders, London, 2005.

[7] J. Silverman, S. Kurtz, J. Draper, Skills for Communicating with Patients, second edn, Radcliff Publishing, Oxford, 2000.

[8] R. Neighbour, The Inner Consultation: how to develop an effective and intuitive consulting style, Radcliff Publishing, Oxon, 2005.

[9] M. Lloyd, R. Bor, Communication Skills For Medicine, third edn, Churchill Livingstone Elsevier, Edinburgh, 2009.

[10] R.D. Collins, Differential Diagnosis in Primary Care, fouth edn, Lippincott Williams & Wilkins, Philadelphia, 2008.

[11] R. Berkow, A.J. Fletcher, M.H. Beers, The Merck Manual, sixteenth edn, Merck Research Laboratories, Rathway, N.J, 1993 (later edition).

[12] D. Peters, L. Chaitow, G. Harris, S. Morrison, Integrating Complementary Therapies in Primary Care. London, Churchill Livingstone, 2002.

[13] K.D. Pagna, T.J. Pagna, Mosby's Diagnostic and Laboratory Test reference, third edn, Mosby, USA, 1997 (later edition).

[14] S. El-Hashemy, Naturopathic Standards of Primary Care, CCNM Press Inc, Toronto, 2007.

[15] J. Jamison, Clinical Guide to Nutrition & Dietary Supplements in Disease Management, Churchill Livingstone, Edinburgh, 2003.

[16] H. Osiecki, The Physicians Handbook of Clinical Nutrition, seventh edn, Bioconcepts, Eagle Farm, 2000.

[17] J.E. Pizzorno, M.T. Murray, H. Joiner-Bey, The Clinicians Handbook of Natural Medicine, second edn. St Louis, Churchill Livingstone, 2007.

[18] J.H. Cummings, G.T. Macfarlane, The control and consequences of bacterial fermentation in the human colon, Journal of Applied Bacteriology 70 (1991) 443–459.

[19] L. Galland, Intestinal Toxicity, New approaches to an old problem, Alternative and Complementary Therapies 3 (4) (1997) 288–295.

[20] E.A. MacGregor, Menstruation, Sex Hormones and Migraine, Neurologic Clinics 15 (1) (1997) 125–141.

[21] D.E. Jacome, Hypoglycemia Rebound Migraine, Headache: The Journal of Head and Face Pain 41 (9) (2001) 895–898.

[22] H. Diener, K. Kronfeld, G. Boewing, M. Lungenhausen, C. Maier, A. Molsberger, M. Tegenthoff, Efficacy of acupuncture for the prophylaxis of migraine: a multicentre randomised controlled clinical trial, Lancet Neurology 5 (2006) 310–316.

[23] A.F. Jorm, H. Christensen, K.M. Griffiths, R.A. Parslow, B. Rodgers, K.A. Blewitt, Effectiveness of complementary and self-help treatments for anxiety disorders, Medical Journal of Australia 181 (7) (2004) S29–S46.

[24] D.W. Spence, L. Kayumov, A. Chen, A. Lowe, U. Jain, M.A. Katzman, et al., Acupuncture increases nocturnal melatonin secretion and reduces insomnia and anxiety: A preliminary report, Journal of Neuropsychiatry and Clinical Neurosciences 16 (1) (2004) 19–28.

[25] S.D. Silberstein, Practice parameter: Evidence-based guidelines for migraine headache (an evidence-based review): Report of the Quality Standards Subcommittee of the American Academy of Neurology, Neurology 55 (2000) 754–762.

[26] A. Byrne, G.D. Byrne, The effect of exercise on depression, anxiety and other mood states: A review, J Psychosom Res 37 (6) (1993) 565–574.

[27] M. Hernandez-Reif, J. Dieter, T. Field, B. Swerdlow, M. Diego, Migraine Headaches are Reduced by Massage Therapy, International Journal of Neuroscience 96 (1998) 1–11.

[28] J. Edge, A pilot study addressing the effect of aromatherapy massage on mood, anxiety and relaxation in adult mental health, Complementary Therapies in Nursing & Midwifery 9 (2003) 90–97.

[29] L. Braun, M. Cohen, Herbs & Natural Supplements: An evidence based guide, second edn, Elsevier, Sydney, 2007.

[30] S. Mills, K. Bone, Principles & Practice of Phytotherapy: Modern Herbal Medicine, Churchill Livingstone, Edinburgh, London, 2000.

[31] British Herbal Medicine Association, British Herbal Pharmacopoeia, BHMAA, 1983.

[32] H. Osiecki, The Nutrient Bible, seventh edn, BioConcepts Publishing, Eagle Farm, 2008.

[33] S. Mills, K. Bone, The Essential Guide to Herbal Safety, Churchill Livingstone, St Louis, 2005.

[34] K. Bone, Clinical Applications of Chinese and Ayurvedic Herbs: Monographs for the Western Herbal Practitioners, Phytotherapy Press, Warwick, 1996.

[35] J. Higdon, An Evidence Based Approach to Vitamins and Minerals, Thieme, New York, 2003.

[36] B.T. Zhu, D.P. Loder, M.X. Cai, C.T. Ho, M.T. Huang, A.H. Conney, Dietary administration of an extract from rosemary leaves enhances the liver microsomal metabolism of endogenous estrogens and decreases their uterotropic action in CD-1 mice, Carcinogenesis 19 (1998) 1821–1827.

[37] E. Ernst, M.H. Pittler, The efficacy and safety of feverfew (Tanacetum parthenium L.): an update of a systematic review, Public Health Nutrition 3 (4A) (2000) 509–514.

[38] B.J. Diamond, S.C. Shiflett, N. Feiwel, R.J. Matheis, O. Noskin, J.A. Richards, N.E. Schoenberger, Ginkgo biloba extract: Mechanisms and clinical indications, Archives of Physical Medicine and Rehabilitation 81 (5) (2000) 668–678.

[39] S. Sinclair, Migraine headaches: nutritional, botanical and other alternative approaches, Alternative Medicine Review 4 (2) (1999) 86–95.

[40] J. Thomas, J.M. Millot, S. Sebille, A.M. Delabroise, E. Thomas, M. Manfait, M.J. Arnaud, Free and total magnesium in lymphocytes of migraine patients — effect of magnesium-rich mineral water intake, Clinica Chimica Acta 295 (2000) 63–75.

[41] M.F. McCarty, Magnesium Taurate and Fish Oil for Prevention of Migraine, Medical Hypotheses 47 (1996) 461–466.

[42] Minutes of the twenty-eighth meeting of the Complementary Medicines Evaluation Committee, 27 July 2001. www.tga.gov.au/DOCS/pdf/cmec/cmecmi28.pd.

[43] G. DeBenedittis, R. Massei, 5-HT Precursors in Migraine Prophylaxis: A Double-Blind Cross-Over Study With L-5-Hydroxytryptophan Versus Placebo, The Clinical Journal of Pain 2 (2) (1986) 123–129.

[44] V. Hajhashemi, A. Ghannadi, B. Sharif, Anti-inflammatory and analgesic properties of the leaf extracts and essential oil of Lavandula angustifolia Mill, Journal of Ethnopharmacology 89 (2003) 67–71.

[45] M. Sinclair, Modern Hydrotherapy for the Massage Therapist, Lippincott Williams & Wilkins, Baltimore, 2008.

[46] Y. Saeiki, The effect of foot-bath with or without the essential oil of lavender on the autonomic nervous system: a randomised trial, Complementary Therapies in Medicine 8 (2000) 2–7.

[47] D.D. Buchman, The complete book of water healing, Contemporary Books, McGraw-Hill Companies, New York, 2001.

[48] L. Chaitow, Hydrotherapy, water therapy for health and beauty, Element, Dorset, 1999.

[49] W. Boyle, A. Saine, Lectures in Naturopathic Hydrotherapy, Eclectic Medical Publications, Oregon, 1988.

[50] H. Lichtenberg, Symptoms Before and After Proper Amalgam Removal in Relation to Serum-Globulin Reaction to Metals, Journal of Orthomolecular Medicine 11 (4) (1996) 195–204.

[51] M.S. Seelig, Interrelationship of magnesium and estrogen in cardiovascular and bone disorders, eclampsia, migraine and premenstrual syndrome, Journal of the American College of Nutrition 12 (4) (1993) 442–458.

[52] S.D. Silberstein, P.J. Goadsby, Migraine: preventive treatment, Cephalalgia 22 (2002) 491–512.

[53] Z. Harel, G. Gascon, S. Riggs, R. Vaz, W. Brown, G. Exil, Supplementation With Omega-3 Polyunsaturated Fatty Acids in the Management of Recurrent Migraines in Adolescents, Journal Of Adolescent Health 31 (2002) 154–161.

[54] M.G. Tozzi-Ciancarelli, G. DeMatteis, C. DiMassimo, C. Marini, I. Ciancarelli, A. Carolei, Oxidative stress and platelet responsiveness in migraine, Cephalalgia 17 (5) (1997) 580–584.

[55] C. Cherbut, Inulin and oligofructose in the dietary fibre concept, British Journal of Nutrition 87 (S2) (2002) S159–S162.

[56] S.D. Silberstein, Practice parameter: Evidence-based guidelines for migraine headache (an evidence-based review): Report of the Quality Standards Subcommittee of the American Academy of Neurology, Neurology 55 (2000) 754–762.

[57] C.R. Clinch, Evaluation of acute headaches in adults, Am Fam Physician 63 (2001) 685–692.

[58] H.-C. Diener, V. Limmroth, Medication-overuse headache: a worldwide problem, Lancet Neurol 3 (2004) 475–483.

[59] E.V. De Diego, M. Lanteri-Minet, Recognition and management of migraine in primary care: influence of functional impact measured by the headache impact test (HIT), Cephalalgia 25 (3) (2005) 184–190.

[60] Headache classification committee, The International Classification of Headache Disorders, second edn, Cephalalgia 24 (S1) (2004) 1–60.

[61] S.D. Silberstein, Migraine, Lancet 363 (2004) 381–391.

[62] O. Sjaastad, L. Bakketeig, Cluster headache prevalence. Vaga study of headache epidemiology, Cephalalgia 23 (2003) 528–533.

[63] T. Steiner, M. Fontebasso, Headache, BMJ 325 (2002) 881–886.

[64] M. Detsky, D. McDonald, M. Baerlocher, et al., Does this patient with headache have a migraine or need neuroimaging? JAMA 296 (2006) 1274–1283.

[65] R.A. Purdy, Clinical evaluation of a patient presenting with headache, Med Clin North Am 85 (2001) 847–861.

[66] R.E. Ryan, S.H. Pearlman, Common headaches misdiagnoses, Prim Care Clin Office Pract 31 (2004) 395–405.

[67] M.W. Green, A spectrum of exertional headaches, Med Clin North Am 85 (2001) 1085–1092.

[68] V. Ulrich, M. Russell, R. Jensen, J. Olesen, A comparison of tension-type headache in migraineurs and in non-migraineurs: a population based study, Pain 67 (1996) 501–506.

[69] R.G. Lafreniere, M. Zameel Cader, J.F. Poulin, I. Andres-Engiux, M. Simoneau et al, A dominant-negative mutation in the TRESK potassium channel is linked to familial migraine with aura, Nature Medicine (2010) doi:10.1038/nm.2216.

Insomnia

Case history

Gordon Fryer, 72, lives in a small coastal town. Gordon and his wife Adele moved there 10 years ago when they retired. Adele passed away two years ago and he has lived alone ever since. Gordon still misses Adele and is not interested in having a relationship with anyone else.

Gordon is visiting his son's family in the city at the moment and his daughter-in-law has nagged him into coming to the clinic. She has told him you can give him something natural to help him sleep better. Gordon has had problems sleeping since Adele passed away, and some nights he doesn't fall asleep until 2 am. When he does finally fall asleep his sleep is light and he wakes frequently, which makes him very tired the next day. When he is at home Gordon can take an afternoon nap to catch up on his sleep; however, at the moment the noise and activity in his son and daughter-in-law's house is preventing him from doing so. Consequently he is exhausted and has become impatient and irritable with the grandchildren.

Gordon tells you that when is lying awake in the night he often feels very lonely, although when he is up and moving around during the day he doesn't experience the loneliness in such a profound way as he does during the night. He is feeling very frustrated with his inability to get a good night's sleep.

Gordon loves to fish and freshly caught fish has been a staple of his diet since he retired to the coast. He usually has a bowl of porridge or cereal and a cup of coffee for breakfast and drinks six to eight cups of tea during the day. He relaxes in the evenings with a couple of beers. Gordon still tends Adele's vegetable patch and grows most of the vegetables he eats. He feels close to Adele when he is working in the vegetable patch, so consequently the vegetables are very well tended! Gordon's appetite is not what it used to be and he often prefers to have a light meal such as soup or salad for dinner rather than a larger meal.

Gordon has tried reading books, drinking warm milk and having a warm bath before bed. He doesn't want to take the medication his doctor has offered and is open to any suggestions you can come up with.

TABLE 10.30 **COMPLAINT** [1–6, 61]	
Analogy: Skin of the apple	**Complaint:** Define the presenting complaint and symptoms; understand the complaint *Insomnia*
AREAS OF INVESTIGATION AND EXAMPLE QUESTIONS	**CLIENT RESPONSES**
Onset *When did you first start having problems sleeping?* *Did you ever experienced sleep difficulties before Adele passed away?*	*Two years ago, after my wife died.* *No, I used to sleep really well.*
Exacerbating factors *Is there anything that makes it worse?*	*If I can't get an afternoon nap. At the moment I'm staying with my son and daughter-in-law and it's hard to get a sleep in the afternoon. I know I'm getting to be a grumpy old man around the grandkids, but if I could get more sleep I'd be much better.*
Relieving factors *Is there anything that makes it better?*	*Having a nap in the afternoon. I tried warm milk, reading books and having a bath before bed but none of that made any difference.*

TABLE 10.31 **CONTEXT**	
Analogy: Flesh of the apple	**Context:** Put the presenting complaint into context to understand the disease
AREAS OF INVESTIGATION AND EXAMPLE QUESTIONS	**CLIENT RESPONSES**
Family health *Has anyone else in your family had similar problems?*	*I don't think so.*
Allergies and irritants *Do you ever experience sneezing or nose discharge, or itchy skin that is affecting your sleep patterns?* (allergies)	*No, not really – I don't wake up with a blocked nose if that is what you mean.*

▶

Recreational drug use *How much alcohol do you usually drink in a week?* *Do you smoke?* *Do you take any other drugs?*	*Usually a couple of beers in the evening.* *Not for years.* *No.*
Functional disease *Do you generally experience a delay in falling asleep?* (initial insomnia, prolonged latency, common in anxiety, caffeine and alcohol users and elderly)	*I find it hard to fall asleep. Sometimes I don't get to sleep till after 2 am.*
Infection and inflammation *Do you usually wake up during the night?* (middle insomnia, poor quality sleep, medical conditions such as sleep apnoea, diabetes, prostatism)	*When I finally fall asleep I tend to sleep lightly and wake quite often.*
Supplements and side effects of medication *Are you taking any supplements or medicines?*	*No. The doctor gave me a prescription for sleeping pills but I don't want to use them.*
Stress and neurological disease *Do you experience early-morning wakefulness?* (late insomnia, depression, malnutrition)	*Sometimes, but if I don't get to sleep until early morning hours, I tend to sleep in to catch up – I think it's been harder for me to do this staying with my family so it has changed my rhythm of dealing with lack of sleep.*
Eating habits and energy *Tell me about your diet.*	Gordon's usual diet consists of plenty of home-grown organic vegetables from the vegetable patch his wife planted. He usually has porridge or cereal and coffee for breakfast and eats a light meal such as soup or salad in the evenings. He drinks 6–8 cups of tea during the course of the day.

TABLE 10.32 **CORE**

Analogy: Core of the apple with the seed of ill health	**Core:** Holistic assessment to understand the client
AREAS OF INVESTIGATION AND EXAMPLE QUESTIONS	**CLIENT RESPONSES**
Emotional health *You mentioned you sometimes feel sad. Can you tell me more about that?*	*It's only usually at night when I can't sleep. When I'm up and around during the day it isn't so bad. Sometimes when I'm lying awake at night I can feel quite lonely and sad; I suppose I think about Adele.*
Environmental wellness *Can you tell me about the environment where you live? Are you close to any major traffic routes or industries?* *Tell me about your sleeping environment.*	*I live in a very quiet little place out of the way from everything, which is what Adele and I were looking for when we retired.* *There is the bed and TV in the bedroom. I also have a clock radio and phone.*

▶

Daily activities Can you tell me what you usually do during the day?	I'm up quite early so I start with breakfast and then go into Adele's garden. I'll either do some work or just sit and think there. I might go fishing or head into town for a bit of shopping. I'll usually have a nap after lunch and then read or watch TV until bed.
Action needed to heal How do you hope I can help you?	My daughter-in-law said you might have something natural I could take that would improve my sleep.

TABLE 10.33 GORDON'S SIGNS AND SYMPTOMS [7, 8]

Pulse	90 bpm
Blood pressure	139/88 sitting
Temperature	36.9°C
Respiratory rate	16 resp/min
Body mass index	20
Waist circumference	72 cm
Face	Pale
Urinalysis	No abnormality detected (NAD)

Results of medical investigations

No medical investigations have been conducted.

TABLE 10.34 UNLIKELY DIAGNOSTIC CONSIDERATIONS [4–6, 9, 70]

CONDITIONS AND CAUSES	WHY UNLIKELY
CANCER AND HEART DISEASE	
Congestive heart failure: insomnia can be a symptom	Blood pressure and pulse within normal range
Hypertension	Blood pressure within normal range
Brain tumour: a growth in the brain may affect the hypothalamic centre, preventing sleep	It is rare for sleep disturbance to be the only associated symptom of neurological disorder
FUNCTIONAL DISEASE	
Renal disease: cause of insomnia due to nocturia and the toxic effects of uraemia	Blood pressure, pulse and urinalysis NAD
DEGENERATIVE AND DEFICIENCY	
Cirrhosis of the liver: nocturnal delirium with insomnia	No yellow sclera in eyes or jaundice observed

▶

INFECTION AND INFLAMMATION	
Acute infection	No fever
Peptic oesophagitis: insomnia can be a symptom	No abdominal pain reported or sensation of heartburn
ENDOCRINE AND REPRODUCTIVE	
Hyperthyroid: insomnia a common symptom	Blood pressure and pulse within normal limits, appetite has decreased rather than increased, no common eye symptoms, goitre or muscle wasting suggesting thyroid disease
Addison's disease: adrenal exhaustion, restlessness, inability to rest and sleep	No sign of skin pigmentation or loss of body hair
Non-insulin dependent diabetes mellitus: restlessness, weight loss, anxiety, lack of sleep	Has not reported any increase in thirst or urination; urinalysis NAD
Prostate disorder: insomnia due to waking up frequently during the night; age related	No nocturia or difficulty with urination reported

Case analysis

TABLE 10.35 POSSIBLE DIFFERENTIAL DIAGNOSIS

Not ruled out by tests/investigations already done [4–6, 9–11, 57–71]

CONDITIONS AND CAUSES	WHY POSSIBLE	WHY UNLIKELY
ALLERGIES AND IRRITANTS		
Causal factor: **Food intolerance/allergy**	May be eating foods he did not previously eat when Adele was still alive	Need to gain more insight into Gordon's previous and current diet and associated symptoms
OBSTRUCTION AND FOREIGN BODY		
Causal factor: **Obstructive sleep apnoea:** where breathing recurrently stops during sleep for long enough periods of time to cause lack of oxygen to the brain [58, 63, 64]	Daytime naps, tired; can be made worse with drinking alcohol prior to sleeping; more common in males; frequent waking during the night and poor sleep quality is common; may be more pronounced at this time of life now that he is sleeping on his own, as a long-term sleep partner can help him breathe by moving him gently to take a breath again	Do not usually complain of 'sleepiness' but rather fatigue generally; need to determine if Gordon does not feel well rested in the morning and if he snores during the night; this is usually worse in individuals who are overweight; not as common to have early morning wakefulness as in depression

▶

RECREATIONAL DRUG USE		
Causal factor: **Alcohol withdrawal**	Gordon may drink more alcohol when he is at home than he has been while staying with his son and daughter-in-law; while he is staying in her home, the withdrawal may be causing insomnia; common to have a delay in falling asleep and frequent waking	Need to question Gordon more about his alcohol intake; question him further about stress levels, restlessness, weight loss, missing meals, tachycardia
FUNCTIONAL DISEASE		
Insomnia: primary [57, 60]	Difficulty falling asleep, frequent waking during the night	Usually associated with no physical or emotional triggers; Gordon's insomnia is more likely to be connected to lifestyle change after the death of his wife making it a secondary insomnia
Short-term insomnia: secondary (less than 3 weeks); caused by emotion, excitement, life stress, change, noise, stimulation, pain, grief, anxiety, jet lag, change in working hours	Delayed onset of sleep and frequent waking during the night; staying with family, sleeping in an unfamiliar bed, noise of the grandchildren, recent travel	Gordon's insomnia may have been aggravated by recent events; however, he has experienced sleep disturbance since his wife passed away 2 years ago
Chronic insomnia: age related	Common to present with difficulty falling asleep, then fitful and light sleep for a short period of time; with age the body can function on as little as 4 hours' sleep a night; delayed period of going to sleep and poor sleep quality are common	Requires further investigation due to Gordon's age; often there are associated physical, medical and painful reasons for insomnia in older age groups
Nocturnal asthma	Frequent waking during the night	No breathing difficulty reported
Causal factor: **Restless leg syndrome**	Insomnia; delayed period of going to sleep and poor sleep quality common	Gordon has not reported an uncontrollable urge to move his legs when he wakes during the night
Causal factor: **Physiologic fatigue:** caused by depression, caffeine, alcohol, excess sleep, poor sleep due to an uncomfortable mattress or pillow, being too hot or cold when trying to sleep, hunger during the night, excess exercise and intense emotions	Common to have delay in falling asleep	Symptoms present for less than 14 days and not usually associated with changes in self-esteem, social difficulties or overall mood; diagnostic studies are within normal limits (this needs to be investigated further)

▶

Causal factor: **Organic fatigue**	Tired, sleep disturbances, no major physical abnormalities	Shorter duration than functional fatigue; need to define if the feeling of fatigue worsens during the day
DEGENERATIVE AND DEFICIENCY		
Dementia	Poor sleep, restless during the night; age related	No significant signs of neurological disturbance; needs further investigation; unusual for sleep disturbance to be the first sign of dementia
Anaemia: iron or B12 deficiency	Low iron intake or absorption can contribute to insomnia; loss of appetite	Need to gain more insight into Gordon's previous and current diet and associated symptoms
INFECTION AND INFLAMMATION		
Osteoarthritis	Insomnia; delayed period of going to sleep and poor sleep quality are common; age related	No associated aches and pains reported
SUPPLEMENTS AND SIDE EFFECTS OF MEDICATION		
Causal factor: **Medication/drug reaction:** psychotropics, beta-blockers, bronchodilators, sympathomimetics, diuretics, hypnotics, appetite suppressants, amphetamines, cocaine	Poor sleep quality and delayed onset of sleep are common	
Causal factor: **Sedative misuse**	Gordon may have used sleeping tablets in the past and misused the dose, causing withdrawal and insomnia; restless sleep when in a different environment	
STRESS AND NEUROLOGICAL DISEASE		
Causal factor: **Adjustment disorder – psychological depression**	Insomnia	Aspects of symptoms need to be clarified; usually adjustment disorder depression does not continue for more than 2 months and is not considered major depression; usually a low mood due to a particular life-changing event or psychological cause; need to clarify how depressed Gordon has been feeling since his wife passed away

General anxiety disorder (GAD)	Has been at least 6 months; anxiety disorder is often associated with loss or threat of a loss; weight loss, lack of sleep; feelings of irritation; person often complains of physical symptoms without thinking there may be a mental disorder; delayed period of getting to sleep is common	Ascertain whether Gordon has experienced significant weight loss; if tension and stress have been overwhelming for at least 6 months; often associated with diarrhoea, tight chest, difficulty breathing; less common to experience frequent waking and early-morning wakefulness as in depression
Chronic depression	Chronic insomnia; missing his wife, feeling lonely without her; can be undiagnosed in the elderly population	The fact that Gordon tends to the garden and enjoys fishing are signs that he is active and productive with his daily activities
Type 1 – major (clinical) depression: unipolar affective disorder [62, 68]	Can be moderate or severe depression; people often describe symptoms in physical terms; has insomnia, change in appetite, fatigue; delayed sleep onset, lack of appetite, can be aggravated by certain conditions and situations that provoke depression	Need to determine if at least 5 symptoms of depression have been present for more than 2 weeks have caused considerable incapacity with daily activities; need to determine if Gordon feels worse in the morning and experiences a sense of apprehension; need to define if Gordon experiences early-morning wakefulness (common); frequent awakening during the night (less common); associated symptoms of lack of interest in daily activities, constipation and vague aches and pains are common
Type 2 – minor depression [62, 68]	Can be mild or moderate depression; has insomnia, change in appetite	Need to show 2–4 symptoms of depression that have lasted for at least 2 weeks; early morning waking is common in depression
Dysthymia: mild depressive illness	Could be experiencing 'double depression' if Gordon has had intermittent periods of depression in the past; symptoms include tiredness, lack of interest in life, low mood	Lasts intermittently for 2 years or more; need to determine if Gordon has had the tendency to have episodes of feeling low before his wife passed away; early morning waking is common in depression

Mixed anxiety and depressive disorder [62]	Depressive disorder often associated with an experience of loss; symptoms of fatigue, apathy, or intense sadness, insomnia	Can be associated with numerous physical complaints related to depression such as restlessness, headaches, shortness of breath, gut or skin disorders; need to determine if Gordon experiences significant incapacity to continue daily activities
Posttraumatic stress disorder (PTSD): symptoms often develop within 6 months of the stressful event	Symptoms developed after Gordon's wife passed away	Has not mentioned flashbacks to a particular traumatic event such as the moment his wife died
Causal factor: **Extreme worrier/anxiety**	May present with difficulty falling asleep, loss of appetite	Need to question Gordon more about his level of worry and if a significant feeling of restlessness is experienced; usually does not present with early-morning wakefulness
Causal factor: **Short-term anxiety**	Gordon may be more anxious being out of his comfort zone when staying with his son and his son's family; common to have delay in falling asleep	Often presents with additional symptoms of headache, chest pain, dizziness, palpitations, gastrointestinal upset and nervous temperament
Causal factor: **Functional fatigue/depression**	Tiredness that has lasted several months and began after the trauma of wife's death	Need to determine if his feeling of fatigue improves during the day; early morning waking is common in depression
EATING HABITS AND ENERGY		
Causal factor: **Excess caffeine intake**	Gordon is consuming excessive amounts of tea; common to have a delay in falling asleep if caffeine is consumed prior to going to sleep; for some individuals having caffeine 6 hours before bed can affect sleep	Not as common to have early-morning wakefulnesss (need to define this symptom)
Causal factor: **Nutritional imbalance**	Insomnia can be worse if there is lack of balance with diet, lack of tryptophan and magnesium-rich foods in the evenings	Need to gain more insight into Gordon's previous and current diet and associated symptoms; early-morning wakefulness can be caused by malnutrition

Causal factor: **Jet lag:** air travel can affect the hypothalamic region of diencephalon	Insomnia	Did Gordon travel by plane to see his daughter and how far did he travel?
Causal factor: **Daytime naps**	Although helpful in the short term, if this becomes a continuing routine it can make insomnia worse at night	

Working diagnosis

GORDON AND INSOMNIA

Gordon is a 72-year-old man who is currently staying with his son and daughter-in-law. Gordon's daughter-in-law has encouraged him to see a complementary therapist to help him get a good night's sleep. During the consultation Gordon tells you he lives in a small coastal village and has developed sleep problems since the death of his wife two years ago. Often Gordon experiences difficulty in falling asleep and wakes frequently during the night. Consequently Gordon is feeling tired and irritable, and his fatigue has been exacerbated by in a different environment while on holiday.

Gordon is experiencing **insomnia**, a common condition defined as 'difficulty in sleeping', or having 'disturbed sleep patterns' that cause a feeling of having had no sleep at all. Insomnia can be *primary* (longstanding and with little apparent connection with emotional or physical status) or *secondary* (to acquired pain, anxiety, drug-alcohol withdrawal, depression). *Initial insomnia* is difficulty falling asleep and is often associated with an emotional disturbance such as anxiety. *Middle insomnia* refers to frequent waking during the night and is associated with medical conditions including sleep apnoea. *Early morning waking insomnia* is where a person wakes several hours before normal waking time and either cannot go back to sleep or goes into a restless sleep. This is common in the elderly but can also be associated with depression. *Reversals of sleep rhythm* are usually caused by situational and environmental reasons such as work hours changing or jet lag. It is also possible for a disease of the hypothalamic region in the brain to cause significant sleep disturbance.

The consequences of insomnia on daily living are significant and can be life threatening if it affects skills such as driving where being alert is imperative. It is most important to have the cause of insomnia diagnosed and treated rather than allowing unproductive sleep habits to form or dependence on medication to develop.

General references used in this diagnosis: 4, 5, 10, 57, 59–61

TABLE 10.36 **DECISION TABLE FOR TREATMENT PRIOR TO REFERRAL**		
COMPLAINT	CONTEXT	CORE
Treatment for the presenting complaint and symptoms	Treatment for all associated symptoms	Treatment for mental, emotional, spiritual, constitutional, lifestyle issues and metaphysical considerations

TREATMENT PRIORITY	TREATMENT PRIORITY	TREATMENT PRIORITY
• Lifestyle recommendations to improve sleep hygiene • Dietary recommendations to reduce consumption of stimulants and alcohol • Herbal tea, tonic and tablets to reduce sleep latency and improve sleep maintenance • Supplemental nutrients to help improve sleep • Recommendations for physical therapies to help improve sleep	• Recommendation to exercise daily to improve sleep patterns • Dietary recommendations to increase intake of nutrients essential for production of serotonin and melatonin	• Dietary recommendations to increase intake of nutrients essential for production of serotonin • Supplemental nutrients to assist with insomnia may also be helpful to deal with Gordon's depression

TABLE 10.37 DECISION TABLE FOR REFERRAL [4–6, 11]

COMPLAINT	CONTEXT	CORE
Referral for presenting complaint	Referral for all associated physical, dietary and lifestyle concerns	Referral for contributing emotional, mental, spiritual, metaphysical, lifestyle and constitutional factors
REFERRAL FLAGS	**REFERRAL FLAGS**	**REFERRAL FLAGS**
• Chronically disturbed sleep pattern	• Excessive caffeine intake	• Gordon feels persistent sadness and loneliness after his wife's death 2 years ago
ISSUES OF SIGNIFICANCE	**ISSUES OF SIGNIFICANCE**	**ISSUES OF SIGNIFICANCE**
	• Alcohol intake potentially disturbing sleep pattern • Reduced appetite may lead to malnutrition	• Gordon is feeling exhausted and irritable, particularly when spending time with his son's family
REFERRAL DECISION	**REFERRAL DECISION**	**REFERRAL DECISION**
• Medical opinion on secondary medical and psychiatric causes of insomnia	• Dietary assessment required	• Counselling and mental health assessment to rule out severe depression

TABLE 10.38 FURTHER INVESTIGATIONS THAT MAY BE NECESSARY [4–6, 8–10, 64, 67, 70]

TEST/INVESTIGATION	REASON FOR TEST/INVESTIGATION
FIRST-LINE INVESTIGATIONS:	
Full blood count	Rule out infection, tumour, inflammation, anaemia
Electrolyte imbalance	Renal and heart disease
Liver function test	Signs of drug or alcohol abuse
Thyroid function test TSH, T4, T3	TSH (thyroid-stimulating hormone) suppressed in hyperthyroidism; thyroid-specific antibodies, to confirm auto-immune cause of hyperthyroidism (Graves')

▶

Fasting blood glucose test	Raised levels can indicate diabetes mellitus, Addison's disease
Counselling/psychiatry consultation: mental health assessment	Bereavement, new lifestyle, early onset of dementia
Nijmegen questionnaire	Hyperventilation syndrome
Sleep diary for one week	Assess patterns of sleep and activities prior to sleep; note the time Gordon goes to bed, how long took to fall asleep, how many times he wakes during the night, the last time of waking before morning, any dreams or nightmares that were experienced; writing down thoughts before bed and when waking is also helpful
Diet diary for one week	Have a more detailed look at what foods Gordon is eating, what times he is eating, how he is preparing the food, amounts of food being ingested
IF NECESSARY:	
Sleep centre: polysomnography	Sleep overnight at a sleep centre to be monitored for the cause of the sleep disturbance; rule out sleep apnoea
Capnometer/pulmonary gas exchange during orthostatic tests	Hyperventilation syndrome
Serum cortisol levels	Rule out Addison's disease
ACTH stimulation test	More definitive for Addison's disease; given to stimulate adrenal cortisol production
Brain scan	Brain tumour or obstruction causing insomnia
ROUTINE TESTS DUE TO AGE:	
Cholesterol blood test	Hypercholesterolaemia
Rectal physical examination	Benign prostate feels smooth, soft, from plum size to orange size; prostatitis, prostatic abscess feels large and boggy; cancerous prostate gland feels hard and irregular nodular enlargement
Prostate-specific antigen (if rectal examination shows possible malignant gland)	Raised in prostatic cancer, benign prostatic hypertrophy, prostatitis

Confirmed diagnosis

Age-related insomnia with associated minor depression [59, 70]

PRESCRIBED MEDICATION

- Temazepam
- SSRI antidepressant medication if sleep problems are not resolved with short-term use of temazepam [60]
- Gordon has decided to try natural therapies first before taking prescribed medications

TABLE 10.39 **DECISION TABLE FOR TREATMENT (ONCE DIAGNOSIS IS CONFIRMED)**		
COMPLAINT	**CONTEXT**	**CORE**
Treatment for the presenting complaint and symptoms	Treatment for all associated symptoms	Treatment for mental, emotional, spiritual, constitutional, lifestyle issues and metaphysical considerations
TREATMENT PRIORITY	**TREATMENT PRIORITY**	**TREATMENT PRIORITY**
• Lifestyle and physical therapy recommendations to help improve sleep • Dietary recommendations to improve sleep quality and quantity • Herbal tea tonic or tablets with sedative action **NB:** Herbal tonic or tablets and tea should be reviewed and reformulated if Gordon decides to take temazepam • Supplemental nutrients to help improve sleep quality and quantity • Herbs and supplements should be used until normal sleep pattern has been re-established and then slowly reduced • The long-term aim is for dietary and lifestyle changes to manage insomnia and depression **NB:** Gordon's treatment program should be reviewed within two weeks and managed collaboratively with his GP to ensure Gordon's condition is being managed effectively	• Lifestyle recommendations to improve general health and vitality • Dietary recommendations to reduce consumption of food and drinks that are likely to be aggravating Gordon's symptoms • Dietary recommendations to increase consumption of nutrients essential for production of neurotransmitters to help maintain a better sleeping pattern	• Lifestyle recommendations to improve depression • Recommendation for grief counselling • Dietary recommendations to improve depression • Herbal tea, tonic or tablets with antidepressant action **NB:** Herbal formula or tablet may need to be reformulated to remove St John's wort if Gordon decides to take prescribed antidepressants • Nutritional supplements with antidepressant action **NB:** Nutritional supplements should be reviewed if Gordon decides to take prescribed antidepressants • Massage therapy to help improve depression • By restoring Gordon's sleep pattern his depression is likely to be improved [24]

Treatment aims

• Restore a normal sleep pattern [12–14].
• Identify and correct underlying causes of Gordon's insomnia [12–14].
• Address lifestyle and dietary factors that are disturbing normal sleep patterns [12, 14, 26].
• Improve neurotransmitter balance [12, 14, 24].
• Improve sleep hygiene and create an environment conducive to sleep [12, 27].
• Identify and correct nutritional deficiencies that could be contributing to the problem [12, 14, 42, 46].
• Support normal blood-sugar balance. Hypoglycaemia may be a factor in Gordon's insomnia [14, 35].
• Deal with Gordon's underlying depression [12, 14, 24].

Lifestyle alterations/considerations

- Encourage Gordon to work through his grief and loss. He may find grief counselling helpful as part of a program to help him deal with his depression [14, 22, 23].
- Encourage Gordon to exercise daily. Daily exercise improves sleep [13, 26, 27]. Daily exercise will also help improve his depression [12, 14, 25, 28].
- Encourage Gordon to regularise his bedtime, going to bed and getting up at the same time each day to help strengthen circadian cycling [27].
- Encourage Gordon to not spend excessively long times in bed as this can result in fragmented and shallow sleep [27].
- Encourage Gordon to not try to force sleep. Rather than allowing himself to become tense and frustrated, he should do something else such as reading until he feels tired [27].
- Encourage Gordon to eliminate all sources of light and reduce noise levels in his bedroom [27].
- Encourage Gordon to eliminate the clock from his bedroom [27].
- Encourage Gordon to make sure his bedroom is not excessively warm [27] .
- Encourage Gordon to avoid daytime naps as they reduce nocturnal sleep quality [27].
- Encourage Gordon to ensure his bed is comfortable [27]. If necessary he should get a new one.

Dietary suggestions

- Encourage Gordon to eliminate tea, coffee and other caffeine-containing foods and drinks [12, 14, 27]. Caffeine interferes with sleep latency and sleep maintenance [12, 27]. Caffeine consumption is interfering with Gordon's sleep even if he doesn't think it is [27].
- Encourage Gordon to drink a caffeine-free alternative to black tea.
- Encourage Gordon to stop drinking alcohol. Alcohol causes fragmented sleep and suppresses REM sleep [27, 34] and also interferes with the normal function of GABA and glutamate, which are involved with wake–sleep states [34].
- Ensure Gordon's nocturnal blood-sugar levels remain stable. Altered glucose metabolism is associated with sleep disorders [35, 54].
- Encourage Gordon to eat a low GI/GL diet to keep his blood glucose levels stable [14]. Hypoglycaemia or altered glucose metabolism is associated with depression [36, 37] as well as sleep disturbance [14, 35, 54].
- Encourage Gordon to increase consumption of tryptophan-rich foods such as turkey, salmon, bananas, legumes, fish, whole oats, nuts, seeds, soy and dairy. Tryptophan is beneficial for both depression and insomnia [12, 14, 19].
- Encourage Gordon to increase consumption of foods rich in omega-3 [15, 19, 48, 47].
- Encourage Gordon to consume a light snack containing tryptophan before bed [14, 27]. The snack will help maintain nocturnal blood glucose [27] and the tryptophan will support melatonin synthesis and reduce sleep latency [12, 14, 38, 39].
- Identify and manage food intolerances or sensitivities. Food intolerances can contribute to sleep disorders [13, 55].

Physical treatment suggestions

- In combination with dietary and lifestyle changes, Gordon may find acupuncture very helpful to improve his sleep [29, 30, 44].
- Massage therapy can improve sleep [31] and depression [32]. Massage combined with acupuncture is also beneficial [33].

- Hydrotherapy: daily ¼–1 hour neutral baths over several days [49], hot hydrotherapy shower 2–10 minutes twice a day [50, 53], followed by a cold foot bath and a cold stomach rub or a cold compress to heat the body prior to sleep [49, 51–53]. Hot full body steam bath excluding the head (Russian bath) followed by a short cold shower or cold mitten friction, cover the body and lie down straight away [49].
- Cool or tepid sponge bath prior to sleep [53]. Cold sitz bath brings on a sedative effect [53]. Hot sitz baths can be relaxing and promote sleep [49].

TABLE 10.40 **HERBAL TEA**		
Alternative to black tea		
HERB	**FORMULA**	**RATIONALE**
Oats seed *Avena sativa*	1 part	Antidepressant [18]; traditionally used as a nervous system nutritive and tonic [15] and for general debility [18]
Skullcap *Scutellaria lateriflora*	½ part	Nervine tonic [20, 43]; mild sedative [20, 43]; traditionally used for insomnia [20]
Vervain *Verbena officinalis*	1 part	Antidepressant [18]; sedative [18, 41]; nervine tonic [41]; combines well with oats and skullcap for depression [18, 41]
Infusion: 1 tsp per cup – 1 cup 3–4 times daily		

TABLE 10.41 **HERBAL FORMULA (1:2 LIQUID EXTRACTS)**		
HERB	**FORMULA**	**RATIONALE**
St John's wort *Hypericum perforatum*	50 mL	Antidepressant [15, 17]; nervine [15, 17]
Zizyphus *Zizyphus spinosa*	80 mL	Sedative [20, 21]; hypnotic [20, 21]; indicated for use in insomnia [20, 21]
Valerian *Valeriana officinalis*	40 mL	Anxiolytic [15, 17]; mild sedative [15, 17, 44]; hypnotic [15, 17]; decreases sleep latency and increases sleep quality in poor sleepers [15, 40]; particularly beneficial for insomniacs with depression when combined with St John's wort [17]
Withania *Withania somnifera* 1:1 liquid extract	30 mL	Adaptogen [15, 17]; anxiolytic [15]; antidepressant [15]; mild sedative [17]; traditionally used for insomnia [15, 17]
Supply:	200 mL	Dose: 5 mL at lunchtime, 10 mL in the evening

TABLE 10.42 **TABLET ALTERNATIVES TO HERBAL LIQUID (MAY IMPROVE COMPLIANCE)**		
HERB	**DOSE PER TABLET**	**RATIONALE**
Lavender *Lavandula angustifolia*	400 mg	Sedative [15]; anxiolytic [15, 20]; hypnotic [15, 20]
Withania *Withania somnifera*	1000 mg	See above

▶

▶

Valerian *Valeriana officinalis*	500 mg	See above
St John's wort *Hypericum perforatum*	800 mg	See above

Dose: 1 tablet at lunchtime, two in the evening

Kava kava (*Piper methysticum*) 300 mg tablet before bed [15]

Mild sedative [15, 17, 20, 44]; hypnotic [15, 17, 20, 44]; skeletal muscle relaxant [15, 17, 20, 44]; kava kava may be taken in addition to the herbal tonic or tablet formula to get an initial improvement in sleep

TABLE 10.43 **NUTRITIONAL SUPPLEMENTS**

SUPPLEMENT AND DOSE	RATIONALE
L-tryptophan 1000 mg at bedtime [12] NB: In Australia doses of tryptophan exceeding 100 mg are included in Schedule 4 of the Standard for the Uniform Scheduling of Drugs and Poisons (SUSDP) and require a medical, dental or veterinary prescription [45] **or** **5-hydroxytryptophan** 100 mg daily [14, 44] The availability and sale of 5-HTP is restricted in many Australian states and territories	Serotonin precursor [12, 19]; tryptophan deficiency is associated with depression [42, 43]; 1000 mg dose reduces sleep latency [44] and reduces wakefulness without decreasing REM sleep [12]; the use of contaminated l-tryptophan has been linked to the development of eosinophilia-myalgia syndrome (EMS); caution should be exercised to ensure only high-quality tryptophan products are supplied [14]; immediate precursor to serotonin [12, 19]; beneficial in depression [12, 19] 100 mg 5-HTP daily increases slow wave sleep [44]
Magnesium (amino acid chelate, aspartate or orotate) supplement with 50 mg vitamin B6 [12, 14] Providing 250 mg elemental magnesium 45 minutes before bed [14]	Magnesium and vitamin B6 are required for conversion of tryptophan to serotonin [12, 14]; magnesium deficiency is associated with insomnia [19, 46]; magnesium deficiency is more common in the elderly [16]
Omega-3 fish oil capsules 4 × 1000 mg capsules 3 times daily providing a daily dose of approx. 2000 mg EPA [48]	Fish oil is effective in treating depression [12, 14, 19, 47, 48]; supplemental EPA provides significant benefits in treating depression [48, 56]

References

[1] J. Silverman, S. Kurtz, J. Draper, Skills for Communicating with Patients, second edn, Radcliff Publishing, Oxford, 2000.

[2] R. Neighbour, The Inner Consultation: how to develop an effective and intuitive consulting style, Radcliff Publishing, Oxon, 2005.

[3] M. Lloyd, R. Bor, Communication Skills For Medicine, third edn, Churchill Livingstone Elsevier, Edinburgh, 2009.

[4] R.H. Seller, Differential Diagnosis of Common Complaints, fifth edn, Saunders Elsevier, Philadelphia, 2007.

[5] P. Kumar, C. Clark, Clinical Medicine, sixth edn, Elsevier Saunders, London, 2005.

[6] A. Polmear, Evidence-Based Diagnosis in Primary Care, Churchill Livingstone Elsevier, 2008.

[7] N.J. Talley, S. O'Connor, Pocket Clinical Examination, third edn, Churchill Livingstone Elsevier, Australia, 2009.

[8] G. Douglas, F. Nicol, C. Robertson, Macleod's Clinical Examination, twelfth edn, Churchill Livingstone Elsevier, Edinburgh, 2009.

[9] R.D. Collins, Differential Diagnosis in Primary Care, fourth edn, Lippincott Williams & Wilkins, Philadelphia, 2008.

[10] R. Berkow, A.J. Fletcher, M.H. Beers, The Merck Manual, sixteenth edn, Merck Research Laboratories, Rathway, N.J, 1993 (later edition).

[11] L. Chaitow, E. Blake, P. Orrock, M. Wallden, P. Snider, J. Zeff (Eds.), Natropathic Physical Medicine: Theory and Practice for Manual Therapists and Naturopaths, Churchill Livingstone Elsevier, Philadelphia, 2008.

[12] J. Jamison, Clinical Guide to Nutrition and Dietary Supplements in Disease Management, Churchill Livingstone, Edinburgh, 2003.

[13] H. Osiecki, The Physicians Handbook of Clinical Nutrition, seventh edn, Bioconcepts, Eagle Farm, 2000.

[14] J.E. Pizzorno, M.T. Murray, H. Joiner-Bey, The Clinicians Handbook of Natural Medicine, second edn, St Louis, Churchill Livingstone.

[15] L. Braun, M. Cohen, Herbs & Natural Supplements: An evidence based guide, second edn, Elsevier, Sydney, 2007.

[16] J. Higdon, An Evidence Based Approach to Vitamins and Minerals, Thieme, New York, 2003.

[17] S. Mills, K. Bone, Principles & Practice of Phytotherapy: Modern Herbal Medicine, Churchill Livingstone, Edinburgh, London, 2000.

[18] British Herbal Medicine Association, British Herbal Pharmacopoeia, BHMAA, 1983.

[19] H. Osiecki, The Nutrient Bible, seventh edn, BioConcepts Publishing, Eagle Farm, 2008.

[20] S. Mills, K. Bone, The Essential Guide to Herbal Safety, Churchill Livingstone, St Louis, 2005.

[21] K. Bone, Clinical Applications of Chinese and Ayurvedic Herbs: Monographs for the Western Herbal Practitioners, Phytotherapy Press, Warwick, 1996.

[22] K.Y. Mak, L.K. Ma, K.C.C. Chan, Management Of Grief (Bereavement), Hong Kong Practitioner 19 (1997) 192–198.

[23] D. Morawetz, What works in therapy: what Australian clients say, Psychotherapy in Australia 9 (1) (2002) 66–70.

[24] D. Morawetz, Insomnia and Depression: Which comes first? Sleep Research Online 5 (2) (2003) 77–81.

[25] P. Salmon, Effects of physical exercise on anxiety, depression, and sensitivity to stress: A unifying theory, Clinical Psychology Review 21 (1) (2001) 33–61.

[26] K. Morgan, Daytime activity and risk factors for late-life insomnia, Journal of Sleep Research 12 (2003) 231–238.

[27] E.J. Stepanski, J.K. Wyatt, Use of sleep hygiene in the treatment of insomnia, Sleep Medicine Reviews 7 (3) (2003) 215–225.

[28] S. El-Hashemy, Naturopathic Standards of Primary Care, CCNM Press Inc, Toronto, 2007.

[29] H.Y. Chen, Y. Shi, C.S. Ng, S.M. Chan, K.K.L. Yung, Q.L. Zhang, Auricular Acupuncture Treatment for Insomnia: A Systematic Review, The J Altern Complement Med 13 (6) (2007) 669–676.

[30] D.W. Spence, L. Kayumov, A. Chen, A. Lowe, U. Jain, M.A. Katzman, J. Shen, et al., Acupuncture Increases Nocturnal Melatonin Secretion and Reduces Insomnia and Anxiety: A Preliminary Report, The Journal of Neuropsychiatry and Clinical Neurosciences 16 (2004) 19–28.

[31] A.C. Llanas, H. Hachul, L. Bittencourt, S. Tufik, Physical therapy reduces insomnia symptoms in postmenopausal women, Maturitas 61 (2008) 281–284.

[32] S.M. Wilkinson, S.B. Love, A.M. Westcombe, M.A. Gambles, C.C. Burgess, A. Cargill, T. Young, et al., Effectiveness of Aromatherapy Massage in the Management of Anxiety and Depression in Patients With Cancer: A Multicenter Randomized Controlled Trial, Journal of Clinical Oncology 25 (5) (2007) 532–539.

[33] Z.G. Zhong, H. Cai, X.L. Li, D. Lu, Effect of acupuncture combined with massage of sole on sleeping quality of the patient with insomnia (article in Chinese), Zhonggou Zhen Jiu 28 (6) (2008) 411–413.

[34] T. Roehrs, T. Roth, Sleep, Sleepiness, and Alcohol Use, Alcohol Research and Health 25 (2) (2001) 101–109.

[35] K. Spiegel, K. Knutson, R. Leproult, E. Tasali, E. Van Cauter, Sleep loss: a novel risk factor for insulin resistance and Type 2 diabetes, Journal of Applied Physiology 99 (2005) 2008–2019.

[36] A.N. Westover, L.B. Marangell, A Cross-National Relationship Between Sugar Consumption And Major Depression? Depression and Anxiety 16 (2002) 118–120.

[37] J.H. Wright, J.J. Jacisin, N.S. Radin, R.A. Bell, Glucose metabolism in unipolar depression, British Journal of Psychiatry 132 (1978) 386–393.

[38] E. Hartmann, Effects of L-Tryptophan on Sleepiness and Sleep, Journal of Psychiatric Research 17 (2) (1982–1983) 107–113.

[39] R.J. Wyatt, D.J. Kupfer, A. Sjoerdsma, K. Engelman, D.H. Fram, F. Snyder, Effects Of L-Tryptophan (A Natural Sedative) On Human Sleep, Lancet 296 (7678) (1970) 842–846.

[40] P.D. Leathwood, F. Chauffard, E. Heck, R. Munoz-Box, Aqueous extract of valerian root (Valeriana officinalis L.) improves sleep quality in man, Pharmacology, Biochemistry and Behaviour 17 (1) (1982) 65–71.

[41] D. Hoffman, The New Holistic Herbal, Element Books, Rockport, 1992.

[42] C. Bell, J. Abrahams, D. Nutt, Tryptophan depletion and its implications for psychiatry, The British Journal of Psychiatry 178 (2001) 399–405.

[43] G.A. Eby, K.L. Eby, Rapid recovery from major depression using magnesium treatment, Medical Hypotheses 67 (2) (2006) 362–370.

[44] A.S. Attele, J.T. Xie, C.S. Yuan, Treatment of Insomnia: An Alternative Approach, Alternative Medicine Review 5 (3) (2000) 249–259.

[45] Minutes of the twenty-eighth meeting of the Complementary Medicines Evaluation Committee, 27 July 2001. Retrieved 22 July 2009 from www.tga.gov.au/DOCS/pdf/cmec/cmecmi28.pd.

[46] D.L. Watts, The Nutritional Relationships of Magnesium, Journal of Orthomolecular Medicine 3 (4) (1988) 197–201.

[47] B.M. Ross, J. Seguin, L.E. Sieswerda, Omega-3 fatty acids as treatments for mental illness: which disorder and which fatty acid? Lipids in Health and Disease 6 (2007) 21.

[48] B. Nemets, Z. Stahl, R.H. Belmaker, Addition of Omega-3 Fatty Acid to Maintenance Medication Treatment for Recurrent Unipolar Depressive Disorder, American Journal of Psychiatry 159 (2002) 477–479.

[49] W. Boyle, A. Saine, Lectures in Naturopathic Hydrotherapy, Eclectic Medical Publications, Oregon, 1988.

[50] N. Shevchuk, Hydrotherapy as a possible neuroleptic and sedative treatment, Medical Hypotheses 70 (2) (2008) 230–238.

[51] G.M. Schleinkofer, Lectures on Hydrotherapy according to S.Kneipp, Sebastian Kneipp School, Bad Worishofen, Germany, July 2008.

[52] R. Newman Turner, Naturopathic Medicine Treating the Whole Person: The principles and practice of Naturopathy, HeALL, Herts, 2000.

[53] E. Blake, in: L. Chaitow, E. Blake, P. Orrock, M. Wallden, P. Snider, J. Zeff (Eds.), Naturopathic Physical Medicine, Theory and Practice for Manual Therapists and Naturopaths, Churchill Livingstone Elsevier, Philadelphia, 2008.

[54] L.F. Taub, N.S. Redeker, Sleep Disorders, Glucose Regulation, and Type 2 diabetes, Biological Research for Nursing 9 (3) (2008) 231–243.

[55] G. Arslan, R. Lind, S. Olafsson, E. Florvaag, A. Berstad, Quality of Life in Patients with Subjective Food Hypersensitivity: Applicability of the 10-Item Short Form of the Nepean Dyspepsia Index, Digestive Diseases and Sciences 49 (4) (2004) 680–687.

[56] G. Parker, N. Gibson, H. Brotchie, G. Heruc, A. Rees, D. Hadzi-Pavlovic, Omega-3 Fatty Acids and Mood Disorders, Am J Psychiatry 163 (2006) 969–978.

[57] M.H. Bonnet, D.L. Arand, Diagnosis and treatment of insomnia, Resp Care Clin North Am 5 (1999) 333–348.

[58] S.M. Caples, G.S. Gami, V.K. Somers, Obstructive sleep apnea, Ann Intern Med 142 (2005) 187–198.

[59] O. Almeida, J. Pfaff, Sleep complaints among older general practice patients: association with depression, Br J Gen Pract 55 (2005) 864–866.

[60] M.J. Sateia, P.D. Nowell, Insomnia, Lancet 364 (2004) 1959–1973.

[61] S. Wilson, D. Nutt, Assessment and management of insomnia, Clinical Medicine 5 (2005) 101–110.

[62] K. Kendler, C. Gardner, Boundaries of Major Depression: An Evaluation of DSM-IV Criteria, Am J Psychiatry 155 (2) (1998) 172–177.

[63] R.D. Chervin, Sleepiness, fatigue, tiredness, and lack of energy in obstructive sleep apnea, Chest 118 (2000) 372–379.

[64] W.R. Pigeon, M.J. Sateia, R.J. Ferguson, Distinguishing between excessive daytime sleepiness and fatigue: toward improved detection and treatment, J Psychosom Res 54 (2003) 61–69.

[65] S. Wessely, Chronic fatigue symptom and syndrome, Ann Intern Med 134 (2001) 838–843.

[66] J.M. Thibault, R.W. Steiner, Efficient identification of adults with depression and dementia, Am Fam Physician 70 (6) (2004) 1101–1110.

[67] V. Henkel, R. Mergl, R. Kohnen, et al., Identifying depression in primary care: a comparison of different methods in a prospective cohort study, BMJ 326 (2003) 200–201.

[68] S. Gilbody, A. House, T. Sheldon, Screening and case finding instruments for depression (Cochrane Review). The Cochrane Library, Issue 4, John Wiley, Chichester, 2005.

[69] L. Pezawas, J. Angst, A. Gamma, et al., Recurrent brief depression – past and future, Prog Neuropsychopharmacol Biol Psychiatry 27 (2003) 75–83.

[70] G. Ellis, J. Robinson, G. Crawford, When symptoms of disease overlap with symptoms of depression, Aust Fam Physician 35 (2006) 647–649.

[71] B. Carruthers, A. Jain, K. De Meirleir, et al., Myalgic encephalomyelitis/chronic fatigue syndrome: clinical working case definition, diagnostic and treatment protocols, J Chronic Fatigue Syndr 11 (2003) 7–115.

Anxiety

Case history

Alan Miller is 40 years old, married with two children. He has come to your clinic for some guidance and assistance with restlessness he has begun to experience in several aspects of his life. Alan is a lecturer in Middle Eastern politics, and his work often entails travel to give seminars in the UK, Europe and the US. He tells you he enjoys his work and appreciates the advancement of his career in recent years, which has allowed him to travel and work internationally. He and his wife met in primary school and have been married for 13 years. They have two children: a nine-year-old boy and six-year-old girl. Alan seems uncomfortable during the consultation, shifting position in his chair frequently and constantly moving his hands. He checks his watch frequently and you notice his breathing quickens and his face starts to look quite pale. You get the distinct feeling Alan is becoming irritated during the questioning process. He answers your questions by talking very fast and looking towards one corner of the room.

Alan finally tells you that he has experienced a range of symptoms over the past two years that include an inability to sit still, shortness of breath, chest tightness, problems with sleeping and low libido. At times when he is preparing for a lecture or meeting he sometimes becomes overwhelmed, feeling as if he is having an asthma attack or that he is going to faint. These symptoms are new and started occurring following a series of rejections from book publishers for a book he took several years to write (a historical novel based in the Middle East). He has now put this aside and is trying to focus more on his family and spend less of his time and energy on his work. He confides that he is becoming increasingly concerned his symptoms are a warning that he is heading for a heart attack (his 47-year-old brother recently had one). Alan tells you that he used to really enjoy social interaction and the opportunity to present lectures and seminars; however, he has started to experience these symptoms whenever he attends social gatherings or if people visit him at home.

Alan's appetite hasn't been particularly good recently and he says it doesn't take very long for him to feel full. Recently he has wanted to eat foods high in sugar and has started to crave chocolate. This is a change from his usual diet, which is very healthy with organic vegetables, mostly vegetarian and minimal amounts of red meat and the occasional chicken. He still enjoys eating fresh fish. He expresses concerns about reports of chemicals used in intensively farmed animals and heavy metal contamination in fish. He drinks tea and coffee, but tries to limit his intake to between one and three cups a day. Alan often has lemon in hot water and drinks dandelion root coffee as alternative to real coffee.

Along with his changes in appetite, Alan is experiencing episodes of diarrhoea and has lost a bit of weight. He is aware that he is not particularly large to begin with and is concerned about further weight loss. He used to spend time bike riding and playing sport with his children but hasn't done much exercise recently due to work commitments and difficulties being motivated to go outdoors with them.

Alan hasn't been to the doctor for a couple of years so he doesn't have any current blood tests. He is concerned that if he goes to his doctor with these symptoms he will be prescribed antidepressants. At the urging of his wife, Alan recently went to a counsellor who recommended he see his doctor suggesting he would probably benefit from a course of medication. He has not gone back.

TABLE 10.44 **COMPLAINT** [1, 3–9, 12–14, 66, 67]	
Analogy: Skin of the apple	**Complaint:** Define the presenting complaint and symptoms; understand the complaint *Restlessness*
AREAS OF INVESTIGATION AND EXAMPLE QUESTIONS	**CLIENT RESPONSES**
Onset *When did you first notice the feeling of 'restlessness' develop for you?*	*About two years ago. The feeling of tightness in my chest is more recent, I started having that after the last publisher I tried rejected my book.*

▶

Understanding the cause (client) *Do you have any ideas about why it is happening?*	*I'm wondering if it might be stress related, although my brother had a heart attack recently so I'm concerned it may be my heart.*
Timing *How long does the feeling last?*	*It can be over fairly quickly, but sometimes lasts for hours. I always feel tired and drained afterwards.*
Exacerbating factors *What triggers or aggravates the symptoms the most?*	*Stress, pressure, people.*
Relieving factors *What makes it better?*	*Being at home and resting.*
Your practitioner impression	Alan appears quite worried or anxious. His face is pale and slightly sweaty.

TABLE 10.45 **CONTEXT**	
Analogy: Flesh of the apple	**Context:** Put the presenting complaint into context to understand the disease
AREAS OF INVESTIGATION AND EXAMPLE QUESTIONS	**CLIENT RESPONSES**
Family health *You have mentioned your brother just had a heart attack, do you know if he was experiencing symptoms like yourself prior to this happening?*	*No, he doesn't worry like I do so he lives very hard and is very upbeat. His heart attack seemed to come out of nowhere.*
Recreational drug use *How much alcohol would you drink in a week?* *Do you smoke?* *Do you take any recreational drugs*	*I don't drink a lot. When I'm socialising I might have a couple of drinks and I will have a glass of wine with dinner occasionally.* *No.* *No, never.*
Occupational toxins and hazards *Does your job ever take you to places you would consider hazardous?*	*Not as much as it used to. I know where I can go safely and where I should stay away from. I think there's risk everywhere really. You could be in a car accident going to the shop to get groceries. It's about understanding the risks and minimising them wherever possible.*
Functional disease *If you feel like wanting to faint is it like a feeling of falling* (dizziness) *or is the room spinning?* (vertigo)	*Definitely just feel like falling to the floor if I feel faint, rather than things moving around.*

Supplements and side effects of medication *Have you ever been prescribed medication for anxiety? If so, have you taken yourself off any medication in the past?* (benzodiazepine withdrawal) [66]	*No, I have not taken anything and I do not like to see doctors.*
Endocrine/reproductive *Have you noticed any excess sweating or unusual intolerance to heat or cold recently?* (hyperthyroidism, endocrine disorder) *You have mentioned that one of your symptoms is low libido, how has this affected intimacy in your relationship?*	*I get sweaty palms and forehead when I feel stressed more these days but I have not noticed a big change in how hot or cold I feel.* *I have been having some problems with performance and when I am stressed I tend to not feel like intimacy. My wife is very understanding, but it does concern me.*
Stress and neurological disease *Would you consider yourself a perfectionist?* (possible obsessive-compulsive disorder tendencies)	*Yes, I do have very high standards of myself and that is why having so many book rejections is just so hard to get my head around.*
Eating habits and energy *Tell me about your diet and energy levels.*	Alan describes a very healthy mostly vegetarian diet. He eats mostly organic food, not much red meat and chicken occasionally. He enjoys fresh fish but chooses the type of fish carefully to minimise exposure to mercury. He explains his choices are based on concerns about chemical and heavy metal contamination in food. He has up to 3 hot drinks daily, often choosing dandelion root coffee or hot water and lemon as an alternative to tea and coffee. He goes on to tell you that recently he has been craving sugar and chocolate.

TABLE 10.46 **CORE**	
Analogy: Core of the apple with the seed of ill health	**Core:** Holistic assessment to understand the client
AREAS OF INVESTIGATION AND EXAMPLE QUESTIONS	**CLIENT RESPONSES**
Support system *What kind of support system do you have around you?*	*I have a supportive group of colleagues and my wife and kids are great.*
Emotional health *Do you think you might be anxious or depressed?*	*I think I probably am.*

Environmental wellness *Is a mobile phone or TV or computer switched on near where you sleep?*	*Yes, I sometimes play music on the computer to help me sleep and I use my mobile phone as an alarm to get me up in the morning.*
Daily activities *Tell me about your daily routine.*	*It depends on what I'm doing. At home I'm up at 6 and help get the kids ready for school before going to the office. Sometimes I work at home. I get home around 7 and try to spend some time with the kids before they go to bed. I try and do something with the family on the weekend if I'm not working. When I'm travelling I have no set routine.*
Stress release *How do you manage your stress?*	*Relaxation techniques and exercise.*
Occupation *Do you enjoy your work?*	*Yes, I do. I feel fortunate to be working in a field I enjoy so much and really appreciate the opportunity for travel it gives me.*
Action needed to heal *How do you hope I can help you today?*	*I'm looking for some diet and lifestyle advice and perhaps some herbal supplements.*
Long-term goals *What plans do you have for the future?*	*I would like to keep on with what I'm doing. I sometimes think I should try again to get my book published, or perhaps write another one. I just don't know if I could take all the rejection again.*
Time needed to heal *If you needed to take some time away from work to help you get better, would you be willing to do that?*	*I have thought about that. I think I would, but don't want to find my symptoms come back again later on. I suppose I need to deal with the cause so that doesn't happen.*
Has not been well since *Describe a time in your life when you did not feel the restlessness that is concerning you now.*	*I was happy about 5 years ago before I began this book venture. Things were more in balance then.*

TABLE 10.47 **ALAN'S SIGNS AND SYMPTOMS** [1, 2]	
Pulse	90 bpm
Blood pressure	140/89
Temperature	36.8°C
Respiratory rate	18 resp/min
Body mass index	19
Waist circumference	78.4 cm
Face	Pale with a worried expression; appears to be sweaty
Hands	Cold, clammy and sweaty
Urinalysis	No abnormality detected (NAD)

Results of medical investigations

No investigations have been carried out.

TABLE 10.48 **UNLIKELY DIAGNOSTIC CONSIDERATIONS** [3, 4, 69]	
CONDITIONS AND CAUSES	**WHY UNLIKELY**
CANCER AND HEART DISEASE	
Phaeochromocytoma: (tumours of sympathetic nervous system where 90% occur in the adrenal gland) anxiety, high pulse rate, bordering on hypertension, weight loss, diarrhoea	Very rare; no sign of fever
INFECTION AND INFLAMMATION	
Infectious states affecting brain: tuberculosis, brain abscess, influenza	No fever, nausea or vomiting
Gastritis: diarrhoea, weight loss, tightness in chest, loss of appetite, sense of fullness; travels extensively	No nausea or vomiting or fever reported
ENDOCRINE/REPRODUCTIVE	
Non-insulin-dependent diabetes mellitus: restlessness, weight loss, anxiety, lack of sleep; craving sugar	Has not reported any increase in thirst or urination; no glucose detected in urinalysis
Addison's disease: weight loss, lack of appetite, diarrhoea, restlessness	No sign of skin pigmentation or loss of body hair; no glucose in urinalysis

Case analysis

TABLE 10.49 **POSSIBLE DIFFERENTIAL DIAGNOSIS**		
Not ruled out by tests/investigations already done [3–6, 8, 10–14, 65, 66, 68–82]		
CONDITION	**WHY POSSIBLE**	**WHY POSSIBLE**
ALLERGIES AND IRRITANTS		
Causal factor: **Lactose intolerance**	Diarrhoea, weight loss, appetite loss	Has not mentioned whether symptoms develop after eating particular foods; unclear whether appetite loss may be due to avoiding a food reaction; has not mentioned significant episodes of abdominal pain
Coeliac disease	Diarrhoea, possible anaemia present, where mental and emotional change may be due to B12 deficiency	Has not mentioned significant episodes of abdominal pain; unclear about family genetic history of GIT disorders
CANCER AND HEART DISEASE		
Brain tumour	Increased restlessness, mood changes, difficulty sleeping, appetite changes, weight loss	No sign of memory loss, headaches, lack of coordination
Gastric cancer	Early satiety, weight loss, diarrhoea	No mention of blood or mucus in stools, abdominal distension or pain relieved by food or antacids; no mention of nausea or vomiting
Angina: classical or exertion angina; can be due to **ischaemic heart disease** (myocardial infarction and coronary atheroma)	Tightness in chest, shortness of breath, restlessness	Not clear whether the tightness in the chest is triggered by exertion, being in cold weather, after eating a meal or aggravated by emotions; not clear about the severity and duration of chest pain
Causal factor: **Prehypertension:** mild borderline hypertension	BP reading of 140/89	
OBSTRUCTION AND FOREIGN BODY		
Causal factor: **Intestinal obstruction**	Diarrhoea	Has not mentioned significant episodes of abdominal pain; no vomiting or abdominal distension reported
RECREATIONAL DRUG USE		
Causal factor: **Alcohol withdrawal**	Stress, restlessness, weight loss, missing meals, tachycardia; disappointment with book publication may have influenced alcohol dependence	Need to question Alan more about his alcohol intake

▶

Causal factor: **Drug abuse/induced psychoses:** cocaine use or alcoholism, cannabis [74]	Wakefulness, restlessness, weight loss	Not clear whether Alan has experienced delusions, hallucinations
FUNCTIONAL DISEASE		
Irritable bowel syndrome	Diarrhoea, stress	Does not mention abdominal pain as a predominant symptom; has not reported alternating between constipation and diarrhoea
Gastric ulcer	Weight loss, tightness in chest, loss of appetite, sense of fullness; can develop from chronic anxiety, tension	Has not pointed to a specific point of abdominal pain that is relieved by food or antacids; has not mentioned nocturnal abdominal pain
Peptic oesophagitis/ oesophageal reflux [69]	Tightness in chest, lack of appetite, becomes full quickly	Has not mentioned vomiting or difficulty swallowing
DEGENERATIVE AND DEFICIENCY		
Anaemia: iron or B12 deficiency	Exertion angina, breathlessness, weight loss, loss of appetite, mostly vegetarian diet	
Hypoglycaemia	Breathless, stress, craving sugar; periods of feeling he may faint	
INFECTION AND INFLAMMATION		
Causal factor: ***Helicobacter pylori***	Diarrhoea, weight loss, tightness in chest, loss of appetite, sense of fullness; can develop due to increased stress and anxiety	Has not mentioned any significant abdominal distension
Causal factor: **Intestinal parasites**	Diarrhoea, weight loss; does extensive travel for work	Lack of appetite rather than increase; no reported symptoms of blood or mucus in stools
Asthma [82]	Breathless, feeling of going to faint	Unclear what triggers the feeling of asthma; unclear if triggers include cold air, emotion, irritants in a particular environment, pollution, medication or recent viral infection
SUPPLEMENTS AND SIDE EFFECTS OF MEDICATION		
Causal factor: **Medication withdrawal:** benzodiazepines (prescribed for anxiety) [66]	Restlessness, difficulty sleeping, irritability, shortness of breath	Need to question Alan about previous medication use

▶

►

ENDOCRINE/REPRODUCTIVE		
Hyperthyroidism [70]	Diarrhoea, increased anxiety, weight loss, difficulty sleeping, irritability, prehypertension	Lack of appetite rather that increase; no sign of goitre, eye signs or muscle wasting as in Graves' disease
STRESS AND NEUROLOGICAL DISEASE		
General anxiety disorder (GAD) [65, 71]	Has been at least 6 months of tension and stress about everyday events; anxiety disorder is often associated with threat of a loss; failed book project may have contributed to anxiety developing; diarrhoea, weight loss, lack of sleep, tight chest; talking fast, irritation; person often complains of physical symptoms without thinking there may be a mental disorder	
Mixed anxiety and depressive disorder	Restlessness, difficulty sleeping, disappointment from book not being published, loss of appetite, weight loss, mood changes; depressive disorder often associated with an experience of loss	Has not mentioned ongoing symptoms of fatigue, apathy or intense sadness; has not mentioned significant incapacity to continue daily activities; speech was not slow
Panic disorder [80]	Episodes of intense fear or discomfort; recurrent panic attacks will not be associated with one particular situation or event	Need to determine if Alan experienced unexpected attacks of intense fear where he does not understand the trigger; has not mentioned that he believes he is going to die when feeling overwhelmed with anxiety; strong genetic influence, need to question more about family tendencies towards anxiety or panic attacks
Posttraumatic stress disorder (PTSD): symptoms often develop within 6 months of the stressful event [72]	Difficulty sleeping, restlessness, anxiety	More questioning needed regarding a traumatic event in the past; has not mentioned emotional detachment from family or friends; has not mentioned flashbacks to a particular traumatic event

►

Obsessive-compulsive disorder (OCD) [73]	May try to hide symptoms of OCD; watching clock regularly, appeared to be irritated	Unclear whether Alan checks things or cleans or washes a lot; unclear if there is a genetic tendency towards OCD in the family
Psychiatric disorder: such as schizophrenia, OCD, neurosis [73, 75]	Obvious signs of stress, weight loss, lack of sleep, restlessness; irritability	Unclear whether Alan was distracted during the consultation due to delusions, obsessive thoughts or intense fear; unclear if there is any genetic tendency towards schizophrenia
Manic depression: bipolar disorders alternating between manic episodes and major depression	Episodes of manic behaviour that may include restlessness, fast speech, weight loss, difficulty sleeping	Unclear whether Alan experiences periods of depression
Causal factor: **Extreme worrier** [68]	Restlessness, diarrhoea, difficulty sleeping, loss of appetite	Did not often answer positively to questions in the consultation (as some with extreme worry can do) and symptoms presented as significantly intense
Phobia: intense fear to specific or set of stimuli that are predictable	Has mentioned stress during a specific event of preparing for lecture or meetings; Alan recognises that the emotional response to preparing for lecture or meeting is excessive	Has not mentioned avoidance for a specific object or event; symptoms of anxiety are not restricted to a specific event or object
Causal factor: **Hyperventilation syndrome – functional breathing** concern (causes include increased CO_2, fatigue, muscle pain, digestive complaints) [78, 79, 81]	Shortness of breath, breathing quickly, hyperventilation syndrome can be a consequence of chronic anxiety, irritability; habitual patterns of breathing are developed to keep CO_2 levels low, which can lead to anxiety-provoking consequences	Has not mentioned significant muscle pain or fatigue

TABLE 10.50 **DECISION TABLE FOR REFERRAL** [2–4, 7, 8, 13]		
COMPLAINT	**CONTEXT**	**CORE**
Referral for presenting complaint	Referral for all associated physical, dietary and lifestyle concerns	Referral for contributing emotional, mental, spiritual, metaphysical, lifestyle and constitutional factors

REFERRAL FLAGS	REFERRAL FLAGS	REFERRAL FLAGS
• Significant feeling of restlessness • Inability to sit still • Has not seen a doctor during the 2 years he has experienced worsening symptoms	• Shortness of breath • Tightness in chest • Sensation of asthma attack/fainting • Family history of heart attack • Elevated blood pressure	• Anxiety about daily activities • Series of book publishing rejections has caused significant emotional instability • Experiencing symptoms when in social situations with people
ISSUES OF SIGNIFICANCE	**ISSUES OF SIGNIFICANCE**	**ISSUES OF SIGNIFICANCE**
• Uncomfortable during the consultation • Frequently shifting in the chair • Constantly moving the hands • Frequently checking his watch • Talking fast	• Change in appetite • Sugar cravings • Diarrhoea • Weight loss • Face looks pale • Excess dandelion coffee may be contributing to symptoms of diarrhoea	• Becomes irritated during the consultation • Not spending as much time with his children due to work commitments • Not enjoying social environments with people like he used to
REFERRAL DECISION	**REFERRAL DECISION**	**REFERRAL DECISION**
• Immediate referral for medical investigations to rule out cardiovascular disease or other conditions that may be causing or aggravating his symptoms • Mental health assessment • Rule out phobic, panic and psychiatric causes for the restlessness	• Medical investigations to rule out underlying pathology for change in appetite • Medical investigation to rule out blood-sugar disorder • Medical investigation to rule out organic heart disease • Medical investigation and management • Investigations to rule out physical causes of diarrhoea (e.g. GIT infection, inflammatory bowel disease) • Investigations to rule out underlying pathology as a cause of weight loss	• Referral for mental health assessment and correct diagnosis

TABLE 10.51 FURTHER INVESTIGATIONS THAT MAY BE NECESSARY
[1–4, 8, 10–14, 67, 70]

TEST/INVESTIGATION	REASON FOR TEST/INVESTIGATION
FIRST-LINE INVESTIGATIONS:	
Referral for counselling	Emotional assessment and support
Referral for mental illness assessment	If it is felt that Alan is in danger of hurting himself or someone else; important that other health professionals are also aware of the suicidal thoughts and tendencies
Full blood count	Rule out infection, tumour, inflammation, anaemia

Cholesterol blood test	Risk of heart disease
Fasting blood lipid test	Triglycerides – these are a form of fat transported by VLDLs (very low density lipoproteins) and LDLs (low-density lipoproteins) and act as storage for energy; when in excess they deposit in fatty tissues and cause a risk of coronary and vascular disease; can rise with alcohol ingestion and fatty foods
Liver function test	Signs of drug or alcohol abuse
Thyroid function test TSH, T4, T3	TSH (thyroid-stimulating hormone) suppressed in hyperthyroidism; thyroid-specific antibodies, to confirm auto-immune cause of hyperthyroidism (Graves')
Stool test	Rule out parasitic infections and occult blood that suggests possible diagnosis of diverticulosis, ulcers, polyps, inflammatory bowel disease, and GI tumour, haemorrhoids, *H. pylori*
Capnometer/pulmonary gas exchange during orthostatic tests/Nijmegen questionnaire	Hyperventilation syndrome [15–17]
IF NECESSARY:	
Fasting blood glucose test	Raised levels can indicate diabetes mellitus, Addison's disease
Electrocardiogram (ECG), echocardiography	ST segment depressed in myocardial ischaemia; sinus rhythm will tell if there is cardiac arrhythmia, organic heart disease; can assess ventricular wall involvement and ventricular function
Lactose intolerance test: ingestion of lactose and glucose tolerance test	Lactose intolerance
Antigliadin antibody blood test	Coeliac disease
C-urea breath test	*Helicobacter pylori*
Endoscopy/gastrocopy	Peptic ulcer, gastric tumour, oeosophageal reflux/spasm
CT/MRI scan of abdomen	Show tumours or lesions in adrenal gland
Peak flow rate	Will be reduced in asthma
Urinary metabolites	Phaeochromocytoma; in Addison's disease classically will show low sodium and high potassium and a high urea
ACTH stimulation test	More definitive for Addison's disease; given to stimulate adrenal cortisol production
Serum cortisol levels	Rule out Addison's disease
Allergies, chemical exposure, heavy metals	Can cause anxiety symptoms [37, 38, 45]

Confirmed diagnosis

ALAN AND GENERALISED ANXIETY DISORDER

Alan is a 40-year-old man who has been experiencing restlessness, shortness of breath, tightness in his chest, weight loss, diarrhoea, difficulty sleeping, loss of libido and has developed a craving for sugar. Alan has developed these symptoms over a period of two years, which commenced during a series of book publication rejections. Alan enjoys his work and career advancements generally and is making his family more of a priority recently.

Alan has been diagnosed with **generalised anxiety disorder** (GAD) as he has experienced at least six months of significant tension and worry about everyday activities [65]. It is important to further investigate and determine that there is no panic, phobic, obsessional, hypochondriacal, psychiatric or organic disorders that are influencing the anxiety symptom picture when considering whether a client may have GAD (it is common, however, for a person to present with more than one anxiety disorder). A client presenting with GAD will often look very worried, display restless behaviour and present as pale and sweaty. The person may experience physical symptoms in multiple body systems:

- gastrointestinal – dry mouth, difficulty swallowing, flatulence, diarrhoea
- respiratory – chest constriction, overbreathing, difficult to breathe in
- cardiovascular – palpitations, feeling of pain over heart, missing a beat
- genitourinary – increased frequency, failure of erection, lack of libido
- nervous system – tinnitus, blurred vision, dizziness, headache, sleep disturbance
- psychological – apprehension, fear, irritability, difficult to concentrate, restless, sensitivity to noise, depression, obsessional and depersonalisation.

General references used in this diagnosis: 3, 4, 8, 10–12, 14, 65, 68, 71

PRESCRIBED MEDICATION

- SSRI medication [71]

TABLE 10.52 **DECISION TABLE FOR TREATMENT (ONCE DIAGNOSIS IS CONFIRMED)**		
COMPLAINT	**CONTEXT**	**CORE**
Treatment for the presenting complaint and symptoms	Treatment for all associated symptoms	Treatment for mental, emotional, spiritual, constitutional, lifestyle issues and metaphysical considerations
TREATMENT PRIORITY	**TREATMENT PRIORITY**	**TREATMENT PRIORITY**
• Recommendation to increase exercise to reduce anxiety symptoms • Recommendation to use relaxation therapies • Dietary recommendations to increase consumption of essential nutrients required for production of neurotransmitters with the goal of increasing endogenous neurotransmitter levels	• Recommendation to increase exercise to improve general health and wellbeing • Breathing retraining • Dietary recommendations to improve general health and wellbeing • Recommendation to identify and manage environmental or dietary sensitivities or allergies	• Recommendation for Alan to continue counselling • Recommendation for physical therapies to support Alan's mental health

▶

• Dietary recommendation to reduce consumption of foods or drinks that may aggravate Alan's symptoms • Herbal tonic or tea to relax nervous system **NB:** If Alan takes 5-HTP the herbal tonic may need to be reformulated to avoid a potential interaction between St John's wort and 5-HTP • Nutritional supplements to support nervous system, increase endogenous levels of serotonin and melatonin **NB:** Use of 5-HTP or l-tryptophan must be monitored to ensure there are no adverse reactions; if Alan decides to take prescribed medication he must be monitored collaboratively with his GP to ensure there are no interactions between St John's wort, 5-HTP or l-tryptophan and the prescribed medication	• Recommendation to identify and manage chemical or heavy metal toxicity • Herbal tonic to support adrenal health and stress response • Nutritional supplements to improve Alan's levels of essential nutrients to enhance general health and wellbeing **NB:** Mineral levels should be monitored to ensure Alan stays within acceptable range to avoid adverse reactions • Alan's blood pressure should reduce as anxiety levels reduce, but must be monitored regularly	

Treatment aims

- Relieve Alan's symptoms of anxiety [11, 29].
- Relieve his associated symptoms [11, 20]; restlessness, sleeplessness, low libido, breathlessness, gastrointestinal symptoms, poor appetite, etc.
- Support/normalise Alan's nervous system function [51].
- Support/normalise Alan's adrenal function [44] and restore HPA balance [44, 51].

Lifestyle alterations/considerations

- Encourage Alan to practise relaxation therapies such as meditation, yoga and autogenic (self-relaxation) training [39].
- Encourage Alan to go back to his counsellor to deal with underlying psychological causes of his anxiety [11, 29, 30].
- Breathing rehabilitation therapy has been shown to have significant improvement for anxiety and hyperventilation states when combined with relaxation and physical therapy [49].
- Check for heavy metal toxicity [37], chemical exposure and/or chemical sensitivity [37, 38].
- Determine whether food and/or environmental allergy may be a factor in the development of Alan's symptoms [45].

Dietary suggestions

- Eliminate caffeine [23, 24, 39].
- Avoid alcohol [39, 48], stimulants [3, 25, 39], sugar and refined and processed foods [25, 39, 47].
- Check for food allergies and sensitivities and manage accordingly [25, 50].
- Encourage Alan to eat tryptophan-rich foods to assist his body's production of serotonin [26, 27].

- Encourage Alan to consume foods high in magnesium [28, 29], B-group vitamins, calcium, potassium, vitamins C and E [29, 49]. These nutrients are all essential for normal production of neurotransmitters [29, 49].
- Encourage Alan to consume foods containing the B-group vitamins [29].
- Encourage Alan to eat a healthy diet. There is an association between unhealthy lifestyle and anxiety and depression [47].
- Increase dietary intake of essential fatty acids, particularly omega-3 oil [29, 30].

Physical treatment suggestions

- Daily exercise. Exercise is strongly associated with decreased levels of stress, anxiety and depression [39, 40].
- Acupuncture has been demonstrated to reduce anxiety [39, 41].
- Massage therapy may help reduce Alan's anxiety levels [42, 43].
- Hydrotherapy: hot foot bath [56]. Alternating hot and cold showers daily [34]. Constitutional hydrotherapy [59]. Full body cold mitten friction [56]. Neutral baths [56]. Hot head shower [57]. Hot baths to relax the mind and body [58].

TABLE 10.53 **HERBAL FORMULA (1:2 LIQUID EXTRACTS)**		
HERB	**FORMULA**	**RATIONALE**
St John's wort *Hypericum perforatum*	50 mL	Nervine [18, 32]; antidepressant [18, 32]; indicated for use in anxiety disorders [18, 32]
Damiana *Turnera diffusa*	50 mL	Traditional uses include depression, anxiety, nervous debility, impotence and as an aphrodisiac and invigorator [19, 20]
Withania *Withania somnifera*	70 mL	Adaptogen [18, 32]; tonic [18, 52]; nervine [18, 32]; sedative [18]; anxiolytic [32]; antidepressant [32]; useful for nervous debility due to stress and impotence due to devitalisation [21]
Lavender *Lavandula angustifolia*	30 mL	Anxiolytic [32, 52]; antidepressant [32, 52]; sedative [32]; improves concentration [32]
Supply:	200 mL	Dose: 5 mL 3–4 times daily

TABLE 10.54 **HERBAL TEA**		
Alternative to liquid herbal tonic if Alan prefers a herbal tea		
HERB	**FORMULA**	**RATIONALE**
Skullcap *Scutellaria lateriflora*	1 part	Nervine tonic and mild sedative [22]; indicated for use in nervous tension [19]
Passionflower *Passiflora incarnata*	½ part	Anxiolytic [52]; spasmolytic [52]; mild sedative [19, 52]; indicated for use with nervous tachycardia [19]
Lemon balm *Melissa officinalis*	2 parts	Sedative [19, 32]; indicated for use with neurasthenia, depressive illness and dyspepsia associated with anxiety or depressive states [19]
Lavender *Lavandula angustifolia*	1 part	See above
Infusion: 1 cup 3 times daily		

TABLE 10.55 **NUTRITIONAL SUPPLEMENTS**	
SUPPLEMENT AND DOSE	**RATIONALE**
Omega-3 fish oil 3 × 1000 mg capsules twice daily providing a daily dose of approx. 1000 mg EPA [64]	Reduces plasma catecholamine levels thereby reducing anxiety levels via the HPA axis [31]; an association exists between lowered erythrocyte omega-3 fatty acid concentrations and anxiety [63]; supplemental omega-3 fatty acids can significantly improve symptoms of anxiety [64]
Magnesium supplement providing a daily dose of 300 mg of elemental magnesium in divided doses [32, 33]	Magnesium deficiency can be associated with symptoms of anxiety, depression, insomnia, hypertension and palpitations [32, 33] and supplementation may be helpful in anxiety disorders [14]
B-group vitamin supplement containing at least 100 mg vitamin B3 [29, 33] and 150 mg [29, 33] daily of vitamin B6	Vitamins B3 and B6 supplementation is indicated in anxiety disorders [11, 14, 33]; vitamin B6 facilitates production of serotonin from tryptophan [14, 33, 60]
Tryptophan supplement providing 300 mg tryptophan in divided doses [33] NB: In Australia doses of tryptophan exceeding 100 mg are included in Schedule 4 of the Standard for the Uniform Scheduling of Drugs and Poisons (SUSDP) and require a medical, dental or veterinary prescription [36] or **5-hydroxytryptophan** 200 mg daily [14] Caution with prescribing 5-HTP together with St John's wort [53] The use of tryptophan or 5-HTP may be considered as an alternative to the herbal tea or tonic or prescribed as additional support The availability and sale of 5-HTP is restricted in many Australian states and territories	Tryptophan depletion is associated with depression and panic disorder [35] and deficiency can be associated with anxiety disorders [33, 61]; the use of contaminated l-tryptophan has been linked to the development of eosinophilia-myalgia syndrome (EMS); caution should be exercised to ensure only high-quality tryptophan products are supplied [26)] Precursor to serotonin [54]; 5-HTP is helpful in treating anxiety at doses of between 200 and 900 mg daily [14]
Supplement providing a daily dose of 1500 mg calcium [29, 33, 60] and 3000 mg potassium [29, 33, 60] daily **NB:** Review use of this supplement once Alan is no longer experiencing panic attacks and hyperventilation	Replenishing calcium and potassium levels may be necessary due to anxiety related hyperventilation depleting these minerals [49, 62]

References

[1] N.J. Talley, S. O'Connor, Pocket Clinical Examination, third edn, Churchill Livingstone Elsevier, Australia, 2009.

[2] G. Douglas, F. Nicol, C. Robertson, Macleod's Clinical Examination, twelfth edn, Churchill Livingstone Elsevier, Edinburgh, 2009.

[3] P. Kumar, C. Clark, Clinical Medicine, sixth edn, Elsevier Saunders, London, 2005.

[4] R.D. Collins, Differential Diagnosis in Primary Care, fourth edn, Lippincott Williams and Wilkins, Philadelphia, 2008.

[5] J. Silverman, S. Kurtz, J. Draper, Skills for Communicating with Patients, second edn, Radcliff Publishing, Oxford, 2000.

[6] R. Neighbour, The Inner Consultation: how to develop an effective and intuitive consulting style, Radcliff Publishing, Oxon, 2005.

[7] D. Peters, L. Chaitow, G. Harris, S. Morrison, Integrating Complementary Therapies in Primary Care, Churchill Livingstone, London, 2002.

[8] A. Polmear, Evidence-Based Diagnosis in Primary Care, Churchill Livingstone Elsevier, Edinburgh, 2008.

[9] M. Lloyd, R. Bor, Communication Skills For Medicine, third edn, Churchill Livingstone Elsevier, Edinburgh, 2009.

[10] R. Berkow, A.J. Fletcher, M.H. Beers, The Merck Manual, sixteenth edn, Merck Research Laboratories, Rathway, N.J, 1993 (later edition).

[11] S. El-Hashemy, Naturopathic Standards of Primary Care, CCNM Press Inc, Toronto, 2008.

[12] L. Chaitow, E. Blake, P. Orrock, M. Wallden, P. Snider, J. Zeff (Eds.), Natropathic Physical Medicine: Theory and Practice for Manual Therapists and Naturopaths, Churchill Livingstone Elsevier, Philadelphia, 2008.

[13] R.H. Seller, Differential Diagnosis of Common Complaints, fifth edn, Saunders Elsevier, Philadelphia, 2007.

[14] J. Jamison, Differential Diagnosis for Primary Care, second edn, Churchill Livingstone Elsevier, London, 2006.

[15] L.P. Malmberg, K. Tamminen, A.R.A. Sovijärvi, Orthostatic increase of respiratory gas exchange in hyperventilation syndrome, Thorax 55 (4) (2000) 295–301.

[16] D. Hess, Capnometry and capnography: Technical aspects, physiologic aspects, and clinical applications, Respir Care 35 (1990) 557–573.

[17] D. O'Flaherty, Capnometry, BMJ Publishing Group, London, 1994.

[18] S. Mills, K. Bone, Principles & Practice of Phytotherapy; Modern Herbal Medicine, Churchill Livingstone, Edinburgh, London, 2000.

[19] British Herbal Medicine Association, British Herbal Pharmacopoeia, BHMAA, 1983.

[20] R. Estrada-Reyes, P. Ortiz-Lopez, J. Gutierrez-Ortiz, L. Martinez-Mota, Turnera diffusa Wild (Turneraceae) recovers sexual behavior in sexually exhausted males, Journal of Ethnopharmacology 123 (3) (2009) 423–429.

[21] K. Bone, Clinical Applications of Chinese and Ayurvedic Herbs: Monographs for the Western Herbal Practitioners, Phytotherapy Press, Warwick, 1996.

[22] R. Awad, J.T. Arnason, V. Trudeau, C. Bergeron, J.W. Budzinski, B.C. Foster, Z. Merali, Phytochemical and biological analysis of Skullcap (Scutellaria lateriflora L.): A medicinal plant with anxiolytic properties, Phytomedicine 10 (8) (2003) 640–649.

[23] D. Charney, G. Henninger, P. Jatlow, Increased anxiogenic effects of caffeine in panic disorder, Archives of General Psychiatry 42 (1984) 233–243.

[24] S. Bolton, G. Null, Caffeine, Psychological Effects, use and abuse, Journal of Orthomolecular Psychiatry 10 (1981) 202–211.

[25] H. Osiecki, The Physicians Handbook of Clinical Nutrition, seventh edn, Bioconcepts, Eagle Farm, 2000.

[26] J.E. Pizzorno, M.T. Murray, H. Joiner-Bey, The Clinicians Handbook of Natural Medicine, second edn, Churchill Livingstone, St Louis, 2008.

[27] B. Boman, L-tryptophan: a rational anti-depressant and a natural hypnotic? Aust NZ Psychiatry 22 (1) (1988) 83–97.

[28] G. Grases, J.A. Perez-Castello, P. Sanchis, A. Casero, J. Perello, B. Isern, et al., Anxiety and stress among science students. Study of calcium and magnesium alterations, Magnesium Research 19 (2) (2006) 102–106.

[29] J. Jamison, Clinical Guide to Nutrition & Dietary Supplements in Disease Management, Churchill Livingstone, Edinburgh, 2003.

[30] P. Green, H. Hermesh, A. Monselise, S. Marom, G. Persburger, A. Weizman, Red cell membrane omega-3 fatty acids are decreased in nondepressed patients with social anxiety disorder, European Journal of Neuropsychopharmacology 16 (2) (2006) 107–113.

[31] B.M. Ross, J. Seguin, L.E. Sieswerda, Omega-3 fatty acids as treatments for mental illness: which disorder and which fatty acid? Lipids in Health and Disease 6 (2007) 21.

[32] L. Braun, M. Cohen, Herbs & Natural Supplements: An evidence based guide, second edn, Elsevier, Sydney, 2007.

[33] H. Osiecki, The Nutrient Bible, seventh edn, BioConcepts Publishing, Eagle Farm, 2008.

[34] N. Shevchuk, Hydrotherapy as a possible neuroleptic and sedative treatment, Medical Hypotheses 70 (2) (2008) 230–238.

[35] C. Bell, J. Abrahams, D. Nutt, Tryptophan depletion and its implications for psychiatry, The British Journal of Psychiatry 178 (2001) 399–405.

[36] Minutes of the twenty-eighth meeting of the Complementary Medicines Evaluation Committee, 27 July 2001. www.tga.gov.au/DOCS/pdf/cmec/cmecmi28.pd.

[37] L. Jarup, Hazards of Heavy Metal Contamination, British Medical Bulletin 68 (2003) 167–182.

[38] H. Tonori, Y. Aizawa, M. Ojima, M. Miyata, S. Ishikawa, K. Sakabe, Anxiety and depressive states in multiple chemical sensitivity, Tokohu Journal of Experimental Medicine 193 (2) (2001) 115–126.

[39] A.F. Jorm, H. Christensen, K.M. Griffiths, R.A. Parslow, B. Rodgers, K.A. Blewitt, Effectiveness of complementary and self-help treatments for anxiety disorders, Medical Journal of Australia 181 (7) (2004) S29–S46.

[40] A. Byrne, G.D. Byrne, The effect of exercise on depression, anxiety and other mood states: A review, J Psychosom Res 37 (6) (1993) 565–574.

[41] D.W. Spence, L. Kayumov, A. Chen, A. Lowe, U. Jain, M.A. Katzman, et al., Acupuncture increases nocturnal melatonin secretion and reduces insomnia and anxiety: A preliminary report, Journal of Neuropsychiatry and Clinical Neurosciences 16 (1) (2004) 19–28.

[42] T. Field, G. Robinson, F. Scafidi, R. Nawrocki, A. Goncalves, Massage therapy reduces anxiety and enhances EEG pattern of alertness and math computations, International Journal of Neuroscience 86 (1996) 197–205.

[43] C.A. Moyer, J. Rounds, J.W. Hannum, A Meta-Analysis of Massage Therapy Research, Psychological Bulletin 130 (1) (2004) 3–18.

[44] C. Tsigos, G.P. Chrousos, Hypothalamic–pituitary–adrenal axis, neuroendocrine factors and stress, J Psychosom Res 53 (2002) 865–871.

[45] P.A. Kovalenko, C.W. Hoven, P. Wu, J. Wicks, D.J. Mandell, Q. Tiet, Association between allergy and anxiety disorders in youth, Australian and New Zealand Journal of Psychiatry 35 (6) (2001) 815–821.

[46] G.E. Simon, W.J. Katon, P.J. Sparks, Allergic to life: psychological factors in environmental illness, American Journal of Psychiatry 147 (7) (1990) 901–906.

[47] F. Bonnet, K. Irving, J.L. Terra, P. Nony, F. Berthez, P. Moulin, Anxiety and depression are associated with unhealthy lifestyle in patients at risk of cardiovascular disease, Atherosclerosis 178 (2005) 339–344.

[48] M.G. Kushner, K.J. Sher, B.D. Beitman, The relation between alcohol problems and the anxiety disorders, American Journal of Psychiatry 147 (1990) 685–695.

[49] L. Chaitow, Naturopathic Physical Medicine: Theory and Practice for Manual Therapists and Naturopaths, Churchill Livingstone, London, 2007.

[50] G. Parker, T. Watkins, Treatment-resistant depression: when antidepressant drug intolerance may indicate food intolerance, Australian & New Zealand Journal of Psychiatry 36 (2) (2002) 263–265.

[51] R. Hoehn-Saric, D.R. McLeod, The peripheral sympathetic nervous system. Its role in normal and pathologic anxiety, Psychiatric Clinics of North America 11 (2) (1988) 375–386.

[52] S. Mills, K. Bone, The Essential Guide to Herbal Safety, Churchill Livingstone, St Louis, 2005.

[53] W.E. Muller, Current St John's wort research from mode of action to clinical efficacy, Pharmacology Research 47 (2) (2003) 101–109.

[54] T.C. Birdsall, 5-Hydroxy Tryptophan: A clinically effective serotonin precursor, Alternative Medicine Review 3 (4) (1998) 271–280.

[55] C.A. Moyer, J. Rounds, J.W. Hannum, A Meta-Analysis of Massage Therapy Research, Psychological Bulletin 130 (1) (2004) 3–18.

[56] L. Chaitow, Hydrotherapy, water therapy for health and beauty, Element, Dorset, 1999.

[57] M. Sinclair, Modern Hydrotherapy for the Massage Therapist, Lippincott Williams & Wilkins, Baltimore, 2008.

[58] D.D. Buchman, The complete book of water healing, Contemporary Books, McGraw-Hill Companies, New York, 2001.

[59] W. Boyle, A. Saine, Lectures in Naturopathic Hydrotherapy, Eclectic Medical Publications, Oregon, 1988.

[60] J. Higdon, An Evidence-Based Approach to Vitamins and Minerals, Thieme, New York, 2003.

[61] I.M. Anderson, C. Mortimore, 5-HT and human anxiety, Evidence from studies using acute tryptophan depletion, Adv Ex Med Biol 467 (1999) 43–55.

[62] F. Wilhelm, R. Gevirtz, W. Roth, Respiratory Dysregulation in Anxiety, Functional Cardiac, and Pain Disorders, Behavior Modification 25 (4) (2001) 513–545.

[63] P. Green, H. Hermesh, A. Monselise, S. Marom, G. Presburger, A. Weizman, Red cell membrane omega-3 fatty acids are decreased in nondepressed patients with social anxiety disorder, Adv Exp Med Biol 467 (1999) 43–55.

[64] G. Parker, N. Gibson, H. Brotchie, G. Heruc, A. Rees, D. Hadzi-Pavlovic, Omega-3 Fatty Acids and Mood Disorders, Am J Psychiatry 163 (2006) 969–978.

[65] C. Gale, M. Oakley-Browne, Generalised anxiety disorder, Clin Evid Dec 12 (2004) 1437–1459.

[66] C.P. O'Brien, Benzodiazepine use, abuse, and dependence, Journal of Clinical Psychiatry 66 (Suppl. 2) (2005) 28–33.

[67] J. McQuaid, M. Stein, Use of brief psychiatric screening measures in a primary care sample, Depress Anxiety 12 (2000) 21–29.

[68] A. Ruscio, Delimiting the boundaries of generalised anxiety disorder: differentiating high worriers with and without GAD, Journal of Anxiety Disorder 16 (2002) 377–400.

[69] J.E. Richter, Oesophageal motility disorders, Lancet 358 (2001) 823–828.

[70] D.S. Cooper, Hyperthyroidism, Lancet 362 (2003) 459–468.

[71] G. Fricchione, Generalised anxiety disorders, N Engl J Med 351 (2004) 675–682.

[72] L. Sher, Recognising posttraumatic stress disorder, Quarterly Journal of Medicine 97 (2004) 1–5.

[73] M.A. Jenike, Obsessive-compulsive disorder, N Engl J Med 350 (2004) 259–265.

[74] L. Arsenault, et al., Causal association between cannabis and psychosis: examination of the evidence, British Journal of Psychiatry 184 (2004) 110–117.

[75] R. Freedman, Schizophrenia, N Engl J Med 349 (2003) 1738–1749.

[76] L. Lum, Hyperventilation and anxiety state (editorial), Journal of the Royal Society of Medicine 74 (1981) 1–4.

[77] L. Lum, Hyperventilation syndromes in medicine and psychiatry, Journal of the Royal Society of Medicine 80 (1987) 229–231.

[78] L. Dratcu, Panic, hyperventilation and perpetuation of anxiety, Progress in Neuro-psychopharmacology and Biological Psychiatry 24 (7) (2000) 1069–1089.

[79] M.J. Ford, M.J. Camilleri, R.B. Hanson, Hyperventilation, central autonomic control, and colonic tone in humans, Gut 37 (1995) 499–504.

[80] D. Klein, False suffocation alarms, spontaneous panics, and related conditions, Archives of General Psychiatry 50 (1993) 306–317.

[81] C.J. Warburton, S. Jack, Can you diagnose hyperventilation? Chronic Respiratory Disease 3 (3) (2006) 113–115.

[82] S. Davies, P. Jackson, L. Ramsay, D. Kuiper, M. Thomas, Dysfunctional breathing and asthma, BMJ 323 (7313) (2001) 323–631.

Bulimia nervosa

Case history

Samantha Collier is 28 years old and recently met the love of her life. Samantha and Owen met eight months ago. It was a case of love at first sight when Samantha accidentally bumped into him in a coffee shop and he dropped his briefcase, which broke open and the contents spilled out all over the floor. Owen just looked at her and smiled, and by the time they finished picking up his papers they were in love.

Samantha is very happy about her new love; however, she is anxious about her physical health. She has been partying harder and drinking more than before she met Owen but has been feeling incredibly tired. She tells you that 'weird things' are happening to her body. She is urinating more often, is constipated and she is getting more pimples than ever before. Also, she often feels her heart racing. Over the past 12 months Samantha's cycle has changed. She is getting her period every two to three months. The bleed lasts for around seven days when it does come but is quite light. Samantha does not experience any significant period pain.

You notice Samantha seems to be hiding her hands from you. Later you notice scars on her knuckles. When you ask her about her diet, Samantha talks about several crash diets she has been on recently. She found the low-carbohydrate diet the most difficult to stick to because of how much meat and fat it contained. She skips from one diet to the next and finds her weight is constantly fluctuating. Samantha confesses she is concerned about how Owen perceives her weight and whether he finds her attractive because her skin is breaking out so much. She feels she is much fatter than she was before and hates being constipated and feeling 'toxic', so she is using laxatives to move her bowels. Samantha tells you her throat is very sore at the moment and was wondering whether she was coming down with something. She really doesn't want to get sick because that would stop her going out with Owen. Just as you are wrapping the conversation up, Samantha tells you that she has been vomiting a lot lately, which may be why her throat is so sore. Samantha is obviously making an effort to open up and a positive rapport has been established.

TABLE 10.56 **COMPLAINT** [1–11, 13, 68–70]	
Analogy: Skin of the apple	**Complaint:** Define the presenting complaint and symptoms; understand the complaint *Weight gain, changes to bowel habits, skin and menstrual cycle*
AREAS OF INVESTIGATION AND EXAMPLE QUESTIONS	**CLIENT RESPONSES**
Onset *How long do you feel your weight has been fluctuating?* *How long ago did you begin vomiting?*	*I've always found it difficult to stay slim.* *That started about 5 or 6 months ago.*
Understanding the cause (client) *Do you have any ideas about what might be causing these changes?*	*Not really. I feel like I might be toxic so maybe that's got something to do with it.*
Timing (duration, frequency) *How often does the vomiting occur?* *How long have you felt uncomfortable about your weight?*	*Depends how I am feeling – could be every second day.* *Since I've met Owen I'm more concerned about it because I don't want him to find my body a turn-off.*
Exacerbating factors *Is there anything that makes your constipation worse?* *Is there anything that makes your vomiting worse?* *Is there anything that makes your skin worse?*	*I haven't thought about it.* *It gets worse when I'm stressed or anxious.* *It's worse before my period.*
Relieving factors *Is there anything that makes your constipation better?* *Is there anything that makes your skin better?*	*If I use laxatives.* *After my period.*
Your practitioner impression	Samantha appears anxious and slightly withdrawn at first. As the consultation progresses she becomes more relaxed. She appears to be covering her hands up.
Examination and inspection	Samantha's tongue has signs of erosion. She has bad breath and you notice raised salivary glands. Her teeth are eroded and her throat looks red and swollen.

TABLE 10.57 **CONTEXT**	
Analogy: Flesh of the apple	**Context:** Put the presenting complaint into context to understand the disease
AREAS OF INVESTIGATION AND EXAMPLE QUESTIONS	**CLIENT RESPONSES**
Family health *Is there anyone else in your family with similar symptoms?*	*I don't think so. My mum and sister have problems with weight, so maybe.*
Allergies and irritants *Is vomiting related to meal times or any specific time of the day?*	*Yes, I can vomit often after eating.*
Obstruction and foreign body *Is there any undigested food in the vomit you bring up?* (obstruction near stomach or peptic condition, or self-induced vomiting before food has digested)	*Yes, often; and I guess that means the food is not being absorbed. Is that right?*
Recreational drug use *How much alcohol would you drink in a week?* *Do you smoke?* *Do you ever take recreational drugs?*	*That depends on what I'm doing. I can drink a fair bit when I'm out with Owen, particularly on the weekend.* *No.* *Sometimes.*
Functional disease *Do you pass a bowel motion less than 3 times a week and often need manual manipulation or laxatives to always assist passing?* (functional constipation)	*I have used laxatives for a while now so my pattern of passing a bowel motion naturally is hard to define now.*
Infection and inflammation *Is vomiting linked with nausea or ever occur without warning?*	*No, I do not feel sick really and I usually know when I am going to vomit.*
Supplements and side effects of medication *How often have you been taking laxatives?*	*I take laxatives to help with my constipation maybe 2 or 3 times a week.*
Endocrine/reproductive *Tell me about your menstrual cycle.*	Samantha tells you her period comes every 2–3 months at the moment. Her bleed is quite light and she doesn't have much pain with it. This pattern has been happening for about a year; previously her period came more often and her bleed was heavier.

▶

▶

Stress and neurological disease *On a typical day, how many hours would you think about your appearance?* (BDD, more than one hour considered excessive)	*I think about it all of the time – like a hum in the back of my mind.*
Eating habits and energy *Tell me about your diet and your energy levels.*	Samantha's eating pattern is erratic. Depending on whether she is trying a weight loss program she may be consuming protein shakes twice daily or focusing mostly on protein and reducing carbohydrate intake. She drinks coffee and Diet Coke to help with her energy levels

TABLE 10.58 **CORE**	
Analogy: Core of the apple with the seed of ill health	**Core:** Holistic assessment to understand the client
AREAS OF INVESTIGATION AND EXAMPLE QUESTIONS	**CLIENT RESPONSES**
Emotional health *Do you ever feel anxious or depressed?*	*Sometimes I get quite anxious.*
Daily activities *Describe what you see when you look at yourself in the mirror every day.*	*I just feel really huge and like I am in someone else's body. I do not like my self-image at all.*
Family and friends *Do you spend much time with family and friends?*	*Not as much as I used to before I met Owen. We try and see my family on the weekend and sometimes we go out with friends.*
Action needed to heal *How were you hoping I could help you?*	*I'm looking for a good detox diet so I can feel better and lose weight.*

TABLE 10.59 **SAMANTHA'S SIGNS AND SYMPTOMS** [1, 3]	
Pulse	95 bpm
Blood pressure	150/95
Temperature	37°C
Respiratory rate	14 resp/min
Body mass index	25
Waist circumference	81 cm
Face	Red, shiny
Inspection of tongue	Signs of erosion
Inspection of throat	Bad breath, salivary glands raised, teeth eroded, throat looks red and swollen
Urinalysis	No abnormality detected (NAD)

Results of medical investigations

No investigations have yet been carried out.

TABLE 10.60 **UNLIKELY DIAGNOSTIC CONSIDERATIONS** [1–5, 8, 9]	
CONDITIONS AND CAUSES	**WHY UNLIKELY**
FUNCTIONAL DISEASE	
Renal impairment: low potassium from excess vomiting	Urinalysis NAD
INFECTION AND INFLAMMATION	
Cystitis: increased urination	Urinalysis NAD
Pancreatitis: vomiting, bowel changes	No fever, would experience nausea and diarrhoea
Gallstone/cholecystitis: vomiting, weight change, bowel changes	Would feel nausea when vomiting, not mentioned in case history; can be associated with abdominal pain and fever
ENDOCRINE/REPRODUCTIVE	
Diabetes: increased urination, anovulatory cycles	Urinalysis NAD
Causal factor: **Ovulatory bleed:** feels emotional	Premenstrual symptoms such as ovulation pain (mittelschmerz) and mood changes; usually spotting or light bleed at time of ovulation, regular cycle; check basal body temperature as it will be biphasic and fluctuate indicating ovulation has occurred
Primary dysmenorrhoea: lower abdominal pain, can get worse with menstrual cycle	Period pain usually begins with menarche and is often associated with no pelvic abnormality, nausea vomiting, headache and dizziness
Secondary dysmenorrhoea: acquired due to pathology; period pain begins several years after menarche and is due to a pelvic abnormality	Painless menstruation
Premenstrual syndrome	Would experience premenstrual mood changes, feel teary, bloated and swollen 1–12 days before period; may experience a dull pelvic ache and abdominal bloating
Endometriosis: irregular periods	No bleeding from the bowel; usually brown vaginal discharge with associated significant abdominal and pelvic pain
Cushing's syndrome: cause amenorrhoea, irregular menstrual cycles, hypertension	No moon-shaped face, frontal balding and oedema; no significant depression mentioned; urinalysis NAD and no indication of glucose intolerance or diabetes which can be associated with Cushing's syndrome

Case analysis

TABLE 10.61 **POSSIBLE DIFFERENTIAL DIAGNOSIS**		
Not ruled out by tests/investigations already done [1–5, 8, 9, 14, 64–70]		
CONDITIONS AND CAUSES	**WHY POSSIBLE**	**WHY UNLIKELY**
CANCER AND HEART DISEASE		
Ovarian, pituitary or adrenal tumour	Will affect androgen levels, produce symptoms of irregular cycles, acne, depression, weight gain	No changes in smell or taste, headaches mentioned indicating a brain tumour
Adult onset and congenital adrenal hyperplasia/ adrenal tumour: can cause primary and secondary amenorrhoea; anovulatory cycles	Can present with anovulatory irregular menstrual bleeding, anxiety, skin breaking out in pimples	Usually presents with severe acne and hirsutism; check if rapid development of symptoms, especially severe virilisation such as frontal balding and enlarged clitoris
Hypertension: borderline	Heart beating fast, BP reading of 150/95	Need to take multiple readings to confirm diagnosis
OBSTRUCTION AND FOREIGN BODY		
Causal factor: **Intestinal obstruction** (bowel cancer, adhesions, hernias, faecal impaction with overflow)	Vomiting and constipation	No abdominal pain; Samantha would experience nausea when vomiting, which is not mentioned in case history
RECREATIONAL DRUG USE		
Causal factor: **Alcohol abuse**	Causes vomiting if drinking heavily, fatigue; can affect skin and digestions; cause dehydration	
FUNCTIONAL DISEASE		
Causal factor: **Functional constipation**	Crash dieting, abuse of laxatives causing a lazy bowel, not drinking enough water, resulting in dehydration	Samantha has indicated that because she has used laxatives for so long her pattern of passing bowel motions naturally is difficult to define
Causal factor: **Vomiting/gagging disorder**	Vomiting, heart racing, increased urination, sore throat, eroded teeth, bad breath	
Causal factor: **Physiologic fatigue:** when diagnostic studies are in normal limits	Can be caused by depression, caffeine, alcohol, excess sleep, intense emotions, crash dieting	Symptoms are present for less than 14 days and are not usually associated with changes in self-esteem, social difficulties or overall mood

▶

Causal factor: **Functional fatigue**	Tiredness that has lasted several months	Need to gain an insight into whether the feeling of fatigue generally improves during the day
Causal factor: **Organic fatigue:** no major physical abnormalities	Tired	Shorter duration than functional fatigue; need to check if fatigue generally worsens during the day
DEGENERATIVE AND DEFICIENCY		
Cardiac arrhythmias: due to low potassium levels from vomiting	Heart beating faster, common in eating disorder with vomiting behaviour such as bulimia and anorexia nervosa	
Causal factor: **Dehydration**	From vomiting and laxative use; causes significant fatigue and heart racing	
Anaemia	Heart racing, fatigue, crash dieting may affect nutritional status causing anaemia	
INFECTION AND INFLAMMATION		
Appendicitis/Meckel's diverticulum	Constipation and nausea; Samantha is in the common age group	Usually intermittent lower abdominal pain; if pain becomes acute it could be a possible diagnosis
Oesophagitis: from vomiting	Sore throat, common for oesophageal disorders to develop from eating disorders with vomiting behaviour such as bulimia and anorexia nervosa	
SUPPLEMENTS AND SIDE EFFECTS OF MEDICATION		
Causal factor: **Drugs:** e.g. diet drugs, after the oral contraceptive pill	Can cause primary and secondary amenorrhoea	Need to learn about relevant history of OCP
ENDOCRINE/REPRODUCTIVE		
Causal factor: **Ectopic pregnancy**	Irregular periods; can present with no pain (rare) and can leak slowly over several days; may be a missed diagnosis; increased desire to urinate	Usually associated with severe and acute abdominal pain, abdominal fullness, increased desire to urinate; may have signs of fever and dull headaches
Pregnancy	Irregular periods; missed periods; vomiting, weight fluctuations, new partner, increased urination, constipation, pimples breaking out	Can present with fever; will have signs of breast tenderness; can present with vaginal discharge and pelvic/abdominal pain; need to clarify if Samantha is experiencing nausea

Ovarian disease: premature menopause often due to autoimmune disease	Menses beginning to change; can present with symptoms of menopause and irregular periods	No hot flushes
Hypothyroidism: cause of secondary amenorrhoea due to hyperprolactinaemia and endocrine disorder; anovulatory cycles	Weight gain, irregular periods, constipation, significant fatigue and sore throat	No skin and hair changes mentioned; no temperature intolerance or visible goitre noted; no significant depression mentioned
Polycystic ovarian syndrome (PCOS): extremely common cause of secondary amenorrhoea; anovulatory cycles	Irregular menstrual cycles, hormonal acne, sugar cravings, weight gain	Check for increased facial and body hair (hirsutism), slow and steady development of symptoms; may have thinning of hair on the head (like men do) called androgenic alopecia
Ovarian cyst	Irregular periods	Ovarian cysts rarely cause heavy menstrual bleeding; may experience lower abdominal pain
Causal factor: **Anovulatory bleeding:** irregular bleeding that appears to be menstrual although no ovulation has occurred; can be associated with both short and long cycles	Irregular cycle; no significant premenstrual symptoms reported to show evidence of regular association with menses cycle; bleed is painless; physical findings will often include acne and indicate PCOS	Check if bleed is unexpected; check basal body temperature, if anovulatory it will not fluctuate (monophasic)
Causal factor: **Oestrogen-withdrawal bleeding:** causes intermenstrual bleeding; occurs when the endometrium proliferates and becomes unstable when oestrogen drops below threshold; can happen outside of the secretory phase or in the absence of progesterone	Common cause of irregular periods in the reproductive years, especially if ovulation has not occurred; menstrual bleeding is prolonged and when it does occur the bleed is usually painless	
Causal factor: **Progesterone-withdrawal bleeding:** only occurs when there is an oestrogen-primed endometrium; can occur when oestrogen therapy continued and progesterone stopped; also when progesterone is administered to test endogenous oestrogen	Irregular menstrual bleed; often occurs in conditions such as PCOS	

Causal factor: **Oestrogen-breakthrough bleeding – 1st type:** when oestrogen levels are low but constant causing sections of oendometrium to degenerate	Intermenstrual bleed; common with PCOS	Need to investigate if Samantha experiences any spotting of blood
Causal factor: **Oestrogen-breakthrough bleeding – 2nd type:** oestrogen levels are well above threshold causing endometrium to become hyperplastic and outgrow blood-borne hormone supply	Causes degeneration of endometrium with prolonged and irregular bleeding	More common in oestrogen-based tumours
Causal factor: **New sexual relationship**	Increased likelihood of pregnancy causing irregular periods	Check if Samantha is sexually active and using contraception
STRESS AND NEUROLOGICAL		
Bulimia nervosa [64–66]	Self-induced vomiting, heart racing from low potassium due to vomiting, increased urination, constipation from lazy bowel due to laxative use, irregular periods, crash dieting, bad breath, sore throat, eroded teeth, swollen salivary glands, scars on knuckles from self-induced vomiting, fear of becoming fat, weight fluctuations	Would need a mental health assessment and diagnosis of depression; obsessive-compulsive disorder is commonly associated
Anorexia nervosa [64–66]	Self-induced vomiting, heart racing from low potassium due to vomiting; low self-esteem; eroded teeth from vomiting	Usually presents with low BMI compared with age norms; usually associated with hypotension, slow pulse; would need a mental health assessment and diagnosis of depression; obsessive-compulsive disorder is commonly associated
Mixed anxiety and depressive disorder	Depressive disorder often associated with an experience of or fear of loss; symptoms of fatigue, apathy or intense sadness; numerous physical complaints associated with depression such as restlessness, gut or skin disorders	

Binge eating disorder	Crash dieting, low self-esteem	A term used for those who have episodes of binge eating but do not make an attempt to lose weight through vomiting or laxatives; physical signs on the hands and in mouth reveal otherwise
Causal factor: **Stress**	Constipation, dietary changes, increased sugar cravings, lack of exercise, heart racing	
Causal factor: **Anxiety**	Can lead to eating disorders, heart racing	
Causal factor: **Depression**	Can lead to eating disorders, fatigue, constipation	Check if fatigue improves during the day
Causal factor: **Abuse**	Scars on knuckles from harming self or from being abused	
EATING HABITS AND ENERGY		
Causal factor: **Diet:** crash dieting	Insulin resistance connection with symptoms of PCOS, constipation, increase stress; cause nutritional deficiencies	Need to clarify dietary changes and duration of changes
Causal factor: **Lack of exercise**	Affects insulin resistance, PCOS, weight gain, stress	

TABLE 10.62 **DECISION TABLE FOR REFERRAL** [1–5, 7–9, 12]		
COMPLAINT	**CONTEXT**	**CORE**
Referral for presenting complaint	Referral for all associated physical, dietary and lifestyle concerns	Referral for contributing emotional, mental, spiritual, metaphysical, lifestyle and constitutional factors
REFERRAL FLAGS	**REFERRAL FLAGS**	**REFERRAL FLAGS**
• Vomiting causing sore throat • Eroded teeth	• Scars on knuckles • Constipation requiring regular use of laxatives • Racing heart	• Excessive concerns about body weight and appearance

ISSUES OF SIGNIFICANCE	ISSUES OF SIGNIFICANCE	ISSUES OF SIGNIFICANCE
• Bad breath	• Increased urination • Fatigue • Anxiety • Increasing outbreaks of pimples • Fad dieting • Change to normal pattern of menstrual bleeding • Partying hard and increased alcohol consumption • Fluctuating weight	• Anxieties about health • Concerns about her physical appearance affecting her relationship with Owen • Body image problems
REFERRAL DECISION	**REFERRAL DECISION**	**REFERRAL DECISION**
• Immediate referral for physical and mental health assessment	• Dietary and nutritional assessment • Gastrointestinal health investigations • Menstrual health assessment and investigations • Cardiovascular investigations	• Cognitive behavioural therapy • Counselling for intimate relationship and body issues • Eating disorder assessment

TABLE 10.63 FURTHER INVESTIGATIONS THAT MAY BE NECESSARY [1–9]

TEST/INVESTIGATION	REASON FOR TEST/INVESTIGATION
FIRST-LINE MEDICAL INVESTIGATIONS:	
Pelvic, vaginal, abdominal examination	Check for bulging uterus, ovaries can be palpable in PCOS, abdominal rebound tenderness, overactive bowel sounds, genital deformities, signs of trauma
Human chorionic gonadotropin (HCG) **blood test/radioimmunoassay** (RIA)	Pregnancy, ectopic pregnancy
Plain abdominal x-ray	Reveals gallstones, rules out intestinal obstruction, appendicitis
Full blood count	Rule out infection, tumour, inflammation, anaemia; anorexia nervosa will present with normocytic normochromic anaemia and leucopenia
Urea, creatinine and electrolytes (sodium, potassium, chloride, bicarbonate) blood test	Signals muscle breakdown and tissue damage; electrolyte values can give indication of danger of cardiac arrest and cardiac arrhythmia; anorexia nervosa and bulimia will present with hypokalaemia from vomiting or purging
Fasting blood glucose test	More definitive test for risk of diabetes, indicate pancreatic conditions and kidney conditions

Thyroid function test	Detects hypothyroidism; anorexia nervosa will reveal low free T3 and T4 without elevation of TSH
Liver function test	Alcohol or drug abuse
Progesterone level	Test 7 days before menstruation is due to see if ovulation has occurred; low serum progesterone level in anovulatory cycles
Oestradiol	*Normal:* PCOS, weight loss, excess exercise *Raised:* pregnancy, ovarian tumour, testicular tumour, adrenal tumour *Low:* PCOS, polycystic ovarian disease, ovarian failure, anorexia nervosa, weight loss, excess exercise, hypothyroidism, Cushing's syndrome, adrenal hyperplasia, menopause, Turner's syndrome, failing pregnancy, fetal death
Oestrone	Elevated in PCOS due to peripheral conversion
FSH (follicle-stimulating hormone)	*Normal:* PCOS, pregnancy, anorexia, weight loss, excess exercise *Raised:* ovarian failure, menopause *Low:* polycystic ovarian disease, anorexia, weight loss, excess exercise, hypothyroidism, Cushing's syndrome, adrenal tumour/hyperplasia
LH (luteinising hormone): due to pulsatile action of this hormone it may not be accurately measured on one random sample	*Normal:* pregnancy, anorexia, weight loss, excess exercise *Raised:* PCOS, polycystic ovarian disease, ovarian failure, menopause *Low:* anorexia, weight loss, excess exercise, hypothyroidism, Cushing's syndrome, adrenal tumour/hyperplasia
PRL (prolactin): common in secondary amenorrhoea to be raised	*Normal:* ovarian failure, anorexia, weight loss, excess exercise, adrenal tumour/hyperplasia *Raised:* PCOS (mildly), hypothyroidism, Cushing's syndrome, pregnancy, amenorrhoea *Low:* pituitary destruction from tumour
Testosterone	*Normal:* ovarian failure, anorexia, weight loss, excess exercise, hypothyroidism, pregnancy *Raised:* PCOS, Cushing's syndrome, adrenal tumour/hyperplasia, ovarian tumour *Low:* corticosteriod use
SHBG (sex hormone-binding globulin)	Low SHBG would indicate the presence of elevated levels of free androgens
Cervical smear	Detects cervical cancer

IF NECESSARY:	
Chest x-ray	Pulmonary heart disease, myocardial calcification, coronary arterial calcification
ECG (exercise electrocardiogram) **Echocardiography**	ST segment depressed in myocardial ischaemia; sinus rhythm will tell if there is cardiac arrhythmia, organic heart disease Can assess ventricular wall involvement and ventricular function
Pelvic ultrasound	Most accurate diagnosis of PCOS and ovarian cysts
Endoscopy	Oesophagitis

Confirmed diagnosis

SAMANTHA AND BULIMIA NERVOSA

Samantha has many reasons to be very happy, as she has recently met and fallen in love with Owen. She has come for help with her overall physical health as she wants to stay attractive to Owen. She is particularly concerned with aspects of her health including her weight, feeling 'toxic', constipation and a sore throat. As the consultation continues Samantha courageously shares her history of crash dieting and that she has been vomiting more lately. During the physical examination you notice she has been hiding her hands because there are visible scars on her knuckles.

Samantha was immediately referred to her GP and for counselling as she has a common condition in her age group known as **bulimia nervosa**. This condition refers to uncontrolled excessive eating (binges). A person will experience a preoccupation with food and habits such as self-induced vomiting, laxative abuse or misuse of drugs to avoid the fattening effects of eating. Fluctuations in body weight are common and women may experience irregular periods. Furthermore, depression, drug (recreational and prescribed) and alcohol addiction can be part of the clinical picture. An official diagnosis of bulimia nervosa requires a person to be binge eating at least two times a week (carried out in secret) for at least three months.

Typical physical signs will be normal weight with a repeated history of diarrhoea, vomiting or non-specific gastrointestinal symptoms. A person with bulimia nervosa will be seeking help with weight concerns when they are clearly not overweight. There will often be clear additional physical signs of repeated vomiting and diarrhoea. Bulimia nervosa is diagnosed when an individual has repeated episodes of binge eating, where a large consumption of food is eaten in a short period of time, during which the person feels out of control with their eating. This causes the person to attempt to avoid weight gain by inducing vomiting or purging with laxatives. Physical complications can include lazy bowel, constipation, hypokalaemia, cardiac arrhythmias and oesophageal rupture due to repeated vomiting.

Mental health features of bulimia nervosa include low self-esteem, obsessive-compulsive behaviour, mood changes and preoccupation with weight changes. Therefore it is essential that a collaborative approach to case management is attempted.

General references used in this diagnosis: 1, 3, 5, 8, 9, 64–66

PRESCRIBED TREATMENT
• SSRI medication and referral to a psychologist for cognitive behavioural therapy [64]

TABLE 10.64 **DECISION TABLE FOR TREATMENT (ONCE DIAGNOSIS IS CONFIRMED)**		
COMPLAINT	**CONTEXT**	**CORE**
Treatment for the presenting complaint and symptoms	Treatment for all associated symptoms	Treatment for mental, emotional, spiritual, constitutional, lifestyle issues and metaphysical considerations
TREATMENT PRIORITY	**TREATMENT PRIORITY**	**TREATMENT PRIORITY**
• Recommendation for counselling and group therapy • Lifestyle and physical therapy recommendations to help reduce symptoms by addressing the underlying triggers • Dietary recommendations to increase consumption of whole foods, balance blood-sugars and increase omega-3 fatty acid intake • Herbal tonic and tea to support nervous system, stress response and hormonal balance • Slippery elm bark powder to soothe and heal sore throat and oesophagus • Nutritional supplements to support nervous system and neurotransmitter production • Levels of supplemented nutrients can be monitored to ensure Samantha stays within normal range **NB:** It is essential that Samantha's case is managed using a multidisciplinary approach	• Recommendations to live a healthier lifestyle and to improve general health and wellbeing • Hydrotherapy suggestions to help with reproductive balance • Dietary recommendations to increase consumption of essential nutrients and reduce consumption of alcohol and caffeine • Herbal tonic or tea with adaptogenic and tonic action • Supplemental nutrients to help correct deficiencies • It is anticipated that Samantha's menstrual cycle will normalise as her nutritional status improves [27]	• Psychological counselling to help her address body image issues and anxiety • Suggestion to become involved in group therapy for support • Lifestyle and physical therapy recommendations to reduce anxiety and support mental health • Herbal tonic and tea with nervine and anxiolytic action • Dietary and nutritional supplement recommendations to support mental health

Treatment aims

- Referral to a clinical psychologist or psychiatrist with experience in treating eating disorders. Bulimia nervosa is condition that requires multidisciplinary care [23].
- Help Samantha establish regular eating patterns that do not involve binging and purging. Balancing blood-sugar levels reduces the likelihood of hypoglycaemia, which may trigger bouts of binging and purging [26].
- Enhance endogenous serotonin production. Low serotonin levels can result in eating disorders [24, 25].
- Correct nutritional deficiencies that may be contributing to Samantha's symptoms [27].
- Encourage Samantha to eat a healthy, balanced diet to ensure optimum levels of essential nutrients and balanced bood-sugar levels [26, 27].

- Encourage Samantha to have a more healthy, balanced lifestyle that includes regular exercise [28] and reduced alcohol consumption [55].
- Deal with Samantha's underlying anxiety [29].
- Normalise Samantha's reproductive hormone balance [30].
- Heal mucous membranes in Samantha's oesophagus and mouth, and restore normal digestive function [30].

Lifestyle alterations/considerations

- Psychotherapy is an important part of Samantha's treatment program [1]. Cognitive behavioural therapy can be helpful in treating bulimia nervosa [1, 51].
- Encourage Samantha to take up regular exercise [28]. This will enhance endogenous serotonin production [48], reduce stress levels [49] and improve Samantha's mental wellbeing [50].
- Encourage Samantha to get involved with a support group. Group psychotherapy using cognitive behavioural therapy may be helpful [52].
- Encourage Samantha to reduce the amount of time she spends partying with Owen. Suggest they find other activities that do not involve so many late nights and so much alcohol consumption.

Dietary suggestions

- Encourage Samantha to eat a whole-food diet, reducing consumption of refined carbohydrates and simple sugars and increasing intake of dietary fibre. This will help to ensure her blood-sugar levels are stable [26].
- Encourage Samantha to eat more foods rich in omega-3, such as deep-ocean fish [39]. A low intake of omega-3 fatty acids has been associated with poor body image and depression [39].
- Encourage Samantha to eat nutrient-dense, antioxidant-rich foods to increase her intake of essential vitamins and minerals. Deficiencies of essential nutrients are common in eating disorders [27, 40].
- Encourage Samantha to reduce alcohol consumption [55].
- Encourage Samantha to avoid coffee and other caffeine-containing beverages [54].
- Encourage Samantha to eat mindfully by learning to listen to her body's cues about hunger, fullness and taste satiety [62].

Physical treatment suggestions

- Samantha may benefit from acupuncture therapy to increase her energy and help alleviate her psychological symptoms [37].
- Hydrotherapy: for low energy and depression, a 2–3-minute cold (no less than 55°F/12°C) shower twice a day [20–22], alternating hot and cold showers with 1–2 minutes hot and 15–30 seconds cold and repeated three to four times twice a day [15, 21], neutral bath from ¼ –1 hour over several days [16], full body cold mitten friction [16], constitutional hydrotherapy daily or weekly [16]. Dry skin-brushing prior to bath, followed by wet skin-brushing in the bath with a loofah [17].
- Hydrotherapy for constipation: place a hot compress on the abdomen, then cover in plastic, with a hot water bottle/heating pad on top for 12 minutes, followed by cold mitten friction for 30 seconds (repeat process three times) [17].
- Alternating hot and cold showers to improve immune function and decrease fatigue [15, 19].
- Arm, wrist, ankle cold shower affusions for fatigue [16, 17, 19].

- A cold, shallow sitz bath with the feet in a hot foot bath simultaneously eases pelvic congestion [15]. For reproductive balance have treatment during the month with weekly contrasting treatments with a hot fomentation on the back and abdomen for 15 minutes, followed by 30-second cold mitten friction. Next, apply heat to the pelvic area and back for another 15 minutes, repeat cold mitten friction with the client in the side lying position (repeat alternating procedure three times) then follow with a abdominal massage [17].
- Facial steam treatment to clean the skin, followed by an oatmeal face pack [19]. Spray the face with a cold shower to finish [15].
- Regular massage could help reduce Samantha's stress and anxiety and improve her mood [38].

TABLE 10.65 HERBAL FORMULA (1:2 LIQUID EXTRACTS)

HERB	FORMULA	RATIONALE
Withania *Withania somnifera*	60 mL	Tonic [31, 32]; adaptogen [31, 32]; mild sedative [31, 32]; as an adaptogen withania is thought to have a normalising action on the HPA axis [32], which can be disturbed in bulimia [35]
Valerian *Valeriana officinalis*	40 mL	Anxiolytic [32, 61]; may be beneficial in anxiety related conditions [32]
Rhodiola *Rhodiola rosea*	40 mL	Adaptogenic [58]; tonic [58]; traditionally used to treat fatigue, depression and nervous system disorders [58]; effective in reducing symptoms of depression [59]; effective in reducing symptoms of anxiety [60]
Supply:	200 mL	Dose: 5 mL 3 times daily
Slippery elm bark powder (*Ulmus rubra*) ½ tsp twice daily, mixed with 1 cup of hot water [32] Demulcent [32, 34]; emollient [32, 34]; nutritive [32, 34]; beneficial to help soothe and heal inflamed oral and oesophageal mucosa		

TABLE 10.66 HERBAL TEA

Alternative to tea and coffee

HERB	FORMULA	RATIONALE
Chamomile flower *Matricaria chamomilla*	1 part	Sedative [32, 31]; vulnerary [32, 31]; beneficial in oral inflammation [31]
Lavender *Lavandula angustifolia*	1 part	Anxiolytic [32, 36]; antidepressant [32, 36]; sedative [32]

Passionflower *Passiflora incarnata*	2 parts	Anxiolytic [31, 32]; mild sedative [31, 32]; beneficial in the treatment anxiety [33]
Oats seed *Avena sativa*	2 parts	Antidepressant [34]; traditionally used as a nervous system nutritive [32]
Infusion: 1 tsp per cup – 1 cup 3 times daily		

TABLE 10.67 NUTRITIONAL SUPPLEMENTS

SUPPLEMENT AND DOSE	RATIONALE
High-potency practitioner-strength **multivitamin and mineral supplement** containing therapeutic doses of essential micronutrients Dosage as recommended by the manufacturer	Deficiency of essential nutrients is common in eating disorders [27, 40] and multivitamin supplementation is indicated [40]
Omega-3 fish oil 3 × 1000 mg capsules twice daily providing a daily dose of approx 1000 mg EPA [63]	Reduces plasma catecholamine levels thereby reducing anxiety levels via the HPA axis [56]; low dietary intake of omega-3 fatty acids have been significantly linked with depression and higher levels of body dissatisfaction [39]; supplemental omega-3 fatty acids can significantly improve symptoms of mood disorders [63]
Zinc citrate 50 mg daily [41]	Zinc deficiency is common in eating disorders [27, 47] and may be a sustaining factor for abnormal eating behaviour in some individuals [42]
L-tryptophan 300 mg plus vitamin B6 45 mg 3 times daily [41, 43] NB: In Australia doses of tryptophan exceeding 100 mg are included in Schedule 4 of the Standard for the Uniform Scheduling of Drugs and Poisons (SUSDP) and require a medical, dental or veterinary prescription before it can be supplied [44] or **5-hydroxytryptophan** 100 mg daily [41] The availability and sale of 5-HTP is restricted in many Australian states and territories *If Samantha is **not** taking prescribed SSRI medication*	To support endogenous production of serotonin and melatonin; Samantha is likely to have lowered levels of plasma tryptophan and altered brain 5-HT function [45]; impaired serotonin-mediated satiety signals may contribute to patterns of recurrent binge eating [53] Tryptophan and B6 supplementation is beneficial in bulimia nervosa [43]
Inositol 6 g daily in divided doses [46] *If Samantha is **not** taking prescribed antidepressant medication*	Effective in treating bulimia nervosa and binge eating [46] and obsessive-compulsive disorder [57]; may be beneficial in circumstances where there are difficulties obtaining l-tryptophan or 5-HTP supplements

References

[1] P. Kumar, C. Clark, Clinical Medicine, sixth edn, Elsevier Saunders, London, 2005, pp. 1288–1291.

[2] R.D. Collins, Differential Diagnosis in Primary Care, fourth edn, Lippincott Williams & Wilkins, Philadelphia, 2008, pp. 120–121.

[3] A. Polmear, Evidence-Based Diagnosis in Primary Care, Churchill Livingstone Elsevier, 2008.

[4] R.H. Seller, Differential Diagnosis of Common Complaints, fifth edn, Saunders Elsevier, Philadelphia, 2007, pp. 155–166,351.

[5] J. Jamison, Differential Diagnosis for Primary Care, second edn, Churchill Livingstone Elsevier, London, 2006, pp. 139–143, 418–420.

[6] N.J. Talley, S. O'Connor, Pocket Clinical Examination, third edn, Churchill Livingstone Elsevier, Australia, 2009.

[7] G. Douglas, F. Nicol, C. Robertson, Macleod's Clinical Examination, twelfth edn, Churchill Livingstone Elsevier, Edinburgh, 2009.

[8] R. Berkow, A.J. Fletcher, M.H. Beers, The Merck Manual, sixteenth edn, Merck Research Laboratories, Rathway, N.J, 1993 (later edition).

[9] S. El-Hashemy, Naturopathic Standards of Primary Care, CCNM Press, Toronto, 2008.

[10] J. Silverman, S. Kurtz, J. Draper, Skills for Communicating with Patients, second edn, Radcliff Publishing, Oxford, 2000.

[11] R. Neighbour, The Inner Consultation: how to develop an effective and intuitive consulting style, Radcliff Publishing, Oxon, 2005.

[12] D. Peters, L. Chaitow, G. Harris, S. Morrison, Integrating Complementary Therapies in Primary Care, Churchill Livingstone, London, 2002.

[13] M. Lloyd, R. Bor, Communication Skills For Medicine, third edn, Churchill Livingstone Elsevier, Edinburgh, 2009.

[14] L. Chaitow, E. Blake, P. Orrock, M. Wallden, P. Snider, J. Zeff (Eds.), Naturopathic Physical Medicine: Theory and Practice for Manual Therapists and Naturopaths, Churchill Livingstone Elsevier, Philadelphia, 2008.

[15] D.D. Buchman, The complete book of water healing, Contemporary Books, McGraw-Hill Companies, New York, 2001.

[16] W. Boyle, A. Saine, Lectures in Naturopathic Hydrotherapy, Eclectic Medical Publications, Oregon, 1988.

[17] M. Sinclair, Modern Hydrotherapy for the Massage Therapist, Lippincott Williams & Wilkins, Baltimore, 2008.

[18] E. Blake, in: L. Chaitow, E. Blake, P. Orrock, M. Wallden, P. Snider, J. Zeff (Eds.), Naturopathic Physical Medicine: Theory and Practice for Manual Therapists and Naturopaths, Philadelphia, Churchill Livingstone Elsevier, 2008.

[19] L. Chaitow, Hydrotherapy, water therapy for health and beauty, Element, Dorset, 1999.

[20] N.A. Shevchuk, Adapted cold shower as a potential treatment for depression, Med Hypoteses, 2007, doi:10.1016/j.mehy.2007.04.052.

[21] N. Shevchuk, Hydrotherapy as a possible neuroleptic and sedative treatment, Medical Hypotheses 70 (2) (2008) 230–238.

[22] N. Shevchuk, S. Radoja, Possible stimulation of anti-tumour immunity using repeated cold stress: a hypothesis, Infect Agent-Cancer 2 (2007) 20.

[23] S.D. Pritts, J. Sussman, Diagnosis of Eating Disorders in Primary Care, American Family Physician 67 (2) (2003) 297–304.

[24] H. Osiecki, The Physician's Handbook of Clinical Nutrition, sixth edn, Bioconcepts Publishing, Eagle Farm, 2001.

[25] T.D. Brewerton, Toward a unified theory of serotonin dysregulation in eating and related disorders, Psychoneuroendocrinology 20 (1995) 561–590.

[26] W.G. Johnson, M.P. Jarrell, K.M. Chupurdia, D.A. Williamson, Repeated binge/purge cycles in bulimia nervosa: role of glucose and insulin, International Journal of Eating Disorders 15 (1994) 331–341.

[27] L. Patrick, Eating disorders: a review of the literature with emphasis on medical complications and clinical nutrition, Alternative Medicine Review 7 (3) (2002) 184–202.

[28] J. Sundgot-Borgen, J.H. Rosenvinge, R. Bahr, L.S. Schneider, The effect of exercise, cognitive therapy, and nutritional counseling in treating bulimia nervosa, Medicine & Science in Sports & Exercise 34 (2) (2002) 190–195.

[29] W.H. Kaye, C.M. Bulik, L. Thornton, N. Barbarich, K. Masters, Comorbidity of Anxiety Disorders with Anorexia and Bulimia Nervosa, American Journal of Psychiatry 161 (2004) 2215–2221.

[30] A.S. Kaplan, D.B. Woodside, Biological aspects of Anorexia Nervosa and Bulimia Nervosa, Journal of Consulting and Clinical Psychology 55 (5) (1987) 645–653.

[31] K. Bone, Clinical Applications of Chinese and Ayurvedic Herbs: Monographs for the Western Herbal Practitioners, Phytotherapy Press, Warwick, 1996.

[32] L. Braun, M. Cohen, Herbs & Natural Supplements: An evidence based guide, second edn, Elsevier, Sydney, 2007.

[33] S. Akhondzadeh, H.R. Naghavi, M. Vazirian, A. Shayeganpour, H. Rashidi, M. Khani, Passionflower in the treatment of generalised anxiety: a pilot double-blind randomised controlled trial with oxazepam, Journal of Clinical Pharmacy and Therapeutics 26 (2001) 363–367.

[34] British Herbal Medicine Association, British Herbal Pharmacopoeia, BHMAA, 1983.

[35] J.F. Mortola, D.D. Rasmussen, S.S. Yen, Alterations of the adrenocorticotropin-cortisol axis in normal weight bulimic women: evidence for a central mechanism, Journal of Clinical EndocrinologyandMetabolism68(3)(1989)517–522.

[36] S. Mills, K. Bone, The Essential Guide to Herbal Safety, Elsevier Churchill Livingstone, St Louis, 2005.

[37] L. Sher, The role of the endogenous opioid system in the effects of acupuncture on mood, behaviour, learning and memory, Medical Hypotheses 50 (1998) 475–478.

[38] T. Field, M. Hernandez-Reif, M. Diego, Cortisol decreases and serotonin and dopamine increase following massage therapy, International Journal of Neuroscience 115 (2005) 1397–1413.

[39] K.A. Bruinsma, D.L. Taren, Dieting, Essential Fatty Acid Intake, and Depression, Nutrition Reviews 58 (4) (2009) 98–108.

[40] C.L. Rock, S. Vasantharajan, Vitamin status of eating disorder patients: relationship to clinical indices and effect of treatment, International Journal of Eating Disorders 18 (3) (1995) 257–262.

[41] H. Osiecki, The Nutrient Bible, seventh edn, BioConcepts Publishing, Eagle Farm, 2008.

[42] C.J. McClain, M.A. Stuart, B. Vivian, M. McClain, R. Talwalker, L. Snelling, L. Humphries, Zinc status before and after zinc supplementation of eating disorder patients, Journal of the American College of Nutrition 11 (6) (1992) 694–700.

[43] M. Mira, S. Abraham, L-Tryptophan as an adjunct to treatment of bulimia nervosa, in L. Patrick, Eating Disorders: A Review of the Literature with Emphasis on Medical Complications and Clinical Nutrition, Alternative Medicine Review 7 (3) (2002) 184–202.

[44] Minutes of the twenty-eighth meeting of the Complementary Medicines Evaluation Committee, 27 July 2001. www.tga.gov.au/DOCS/pdf/cmec/cmecmi28.pd.

[45] I.M. Anderson, M. Parry-Billings, E.A. Newsholme, C.G. Fairburn, P.J. Cowen, Dieting reduces plasma tryptophan and alters brain 5-HT function in women, Psychological Medicine 20 (4) (1990) 785–791.

[46] D. Gelber, J. Levine, R.H. Belmaker, Effect of Inositol on Bulimia Nervosa and Binge Eating, International Journal of Eating Disorders 29 (3) (2001) 345–348.

[47] L. Humphries, B. Vivian, M. Stuart, C.J. McClain, Zinc deficiency and eating disorders, Journal of Clinical Psychiatry 50 (1989) 456–459.

[48] S. Dey, Physical exercise as a novel antidepressant agent: Possible role of serotonin receptor subtypes, Physiology and Behaviour 55 (2) (1994) 323–329.

[49] P. Salmon, Effects of Physical Exercise on Anxiety, Depression, and Sensitivity to Stress: A Unifying Theory, Clinical Psychology Review 21 (1) (2001) 33–61.

[50] K.R. Fox, The influence of physical activity on mental well-being, Public Health Nutrition 2 (1999) 411–418.

[51] P.J. Hay, J. Bacaltchuk, Psychotherapy for bulimia nervosa and binging (Cochrane Review), In: The Cochrane Library, Issue 1, Update Software, Oxford, 2003.

[52] L. Nevonen, A.G. Broberg, M. Lindstrom, B. Levin, A sequenced group psychotherapy model for bulimia nervosa patients: a pilot study, European Eating Disorders Review 7 (1) (1999) 17–27.

[53] B.E. Wolfe, E. Metzger, D.C. Jimerson, Research update on serotonin function in bulimia nervosa and anorexia nervosa, Psychopharmacology Bulletin 33 (1997) 345–354.

[54] M. Bruce, N. Scott, P. Shine, M. Lader, Anxiogenic effects of caffeine in patients with anxiety disorders, Archives of General Psychiatry 49 (11) (1992) 867–869.

[55] M.G. Kushner, K.G. Sher, B.D. Beitman, The relation between alcohol problems and the anxiety disorders, American Journal of Psychiatry 147 (1990) 685–695.

[56] B.M. Ross, J. Seguin, L.E. Sieswerda, Omega-3 fatty acids as treatments for mental illness: which disorder and which fatty acid? Lipids in Health and Disease 6 (2007) 21.

[57] J. Levine, Controlled trials of Inositol in psychiatry, European Neuropsychopharmacology 7 (1997) 147–155.

[58] M. Morgan, K. Bone, Rhodiola rosaea – Rhodiola, Mediherb Phytotherapist's Perspective 47 (2005) 1–4.

[59] K. Bone, Rhodiola Effective for Depression, Mediherb Clinical Monitor 19 (2007) 1.

[60] A. Bystritsky, L. Kerwin, J.D. Feusner, A Pilot Study of Rhodiola rosea (Rhodax®) for Generalized Anxiety Disorder (GAD), The J Altern Complement Med 14 (2) (2008) 175–180.

[61] S. Mills, K. Bone, Principles & Practice of Phytotherapy: Modern Herbal Medicine, Churchill Livingstone, Edinburgh, London, 2000.

[62] J. Mathieu, What Should You Know about Mindful and Intuitive Eating? Journal of the American Dietetic Association 109 (12) (2009) 1982–1987.

[63] G. Parker, N. Gibson, H. Brotchie, G. Heruc, A. Rees, D. Hadzi-Pavlovic, Omega-3 Fatty Acids and Mood Disorders, Am J Psychiatry 163 (2006) 969–978.

[64] C.G. Fairburn, P.J. Harrison, Eating disorders, Lancet 361 (2003) 407–417.

[65] P.S. Mehler, Bulimia Nervosa, N Engl J Med 349 (2003) 875–881.

[66] G.T. Wilson, R. Shafran, Eating disorders guidelines from NICE, Lancet 365 (2005) 79–81.

[67] H. Hoek, D. van Hoeken, Review of the prevalenceandincidenceofeatingdisorders,IntJEat Disord 34 (2003) 383–396.

[68] J. Morgan, F. Reid, J. Lacey, The SCOFF questionnaire: assessment of a new screening tool for eating disorders, BMJ 319 (1999) 1467–1468.

[69] A. Luck, J. Morgan, F. Reid, et al., The SCOFF questionnaire and clinical interview for eating disorders in general practice: comparative study, BMJ 325 (2002) 755–756.

[70] K. Freund, S. Graham, L. Lesky, et al., Detection of bulimia in a primary care setting, J Gen Intern Med 8 (1993) 236–242.

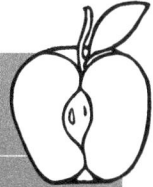

CHAPTER 11

Integumentary system

Eczema

Case history

James Daniels is 17 years old and has come to the clinic for help with an itchy skin rash on his face, hands, behind his ears, on his scalp and in the folds of his knees and elbows. He is considering shaving his head in an effort to relieve the itchiness on his scalp. James has had problems with skin rashes for a few years. Previously he has used a steroid cream prescribed by his doctor, which was usually effective. Right now he is in his final year of high school and has been under a lot of pressure with his studies so he is feeling much more stressed than usual. He has noticed in the last couple of weeks that the rash has started to spread to his feet. His skin is becoming so bad he is trying to cover up as much as possible because he is embarrassed about anyone seeing it. When he was sitting in the clinic waiting room, you noticed he had pulled the sleeves of his jumper down over his hands to cover them up.

James tells you that the rash starts off with tiny red dots that spread and itch and are usually symmetrical on the body. When he scratches the rash it seems to make it spread and then his skin becomes hard and crusted. When the skin is really bad it gets deep cracks and sometimes oozes pus, which he finds so disgusting he always uses the doctor's cream before it gets to that stage.

When you ask James about his diet he tells you he eats just about anything, but he particularly likes bread, things that are cheesy such as cheese toasties from the school canteen and chocolate milk. He also tends to buy a fair bit of junk food from the shops on his way home from school. At home he eats whatever his mum gives him. James hasn't noticed whether any particular food makes his skin worse, although he has never tried to eliminate any foods to see if they make a difference.

James really wants your help for his anxiety and stress levels and is also interested in finding out if there is another way to help control his skin rash apart from using the steroid cream from the doctor. He would like any help you can give him to reduce the itch, which is worse when he washes and also at night when he is in bed.

James has mild asthma, which seems to be worse when he is stressed. He uses a ventolin puffer when necessary and doesn't play much sport because it aggravates his asthma. He prefers to play computer games when he isn't studying.

James' mother tells you that she has allergic rhinitis and had childhood asthma and eczema. She is quite concerned about James at the moment because she has personal experience of how unpleasant and stressful eczema can be.

TABLE 11.1 COMMON AREAS OF INVOLVEMENT AND CAUSES OF ALLERGIC CONTACT DERMATITIS [1–8]

Analogy: Skin of the apple	**Complaint:** Define the presenting complaint and symptoms; understand the complaint *Eczema*
AREAS OF INVESTIGATION AND EXAMPLE QUESTIONS	**CLIENT RESPONSES**
Onset	James says he has always had problems with skin rashes. Recently it has become worse and is spreading to his feet.
Exacerbating factors *What do you think makes it worse?*	*I'm not really sure, but it's much worse since I started to get really stressed about school. It feels worse after I wash and also when I'm in bed at night.*
Relieving factors *What makes it better?*	*The cream the doctor gives me, but that doesn't stop it coming back.*
Location and radiation	James tells you the rash started in the folds of his elbows and knees and then went to his face, hands, behind his ears and scalp. Now it is spreading to his feet.
Examination and inspection *Have you noticed your toe/finger nails have developed ridges?* (eczema)	Erythematous, pruritic, oedematous skin rash with patches of crusted and scaly skin. Signs of possible infection in some lesions. *Some of my toe nails seem to get lines on them.*
Rating scale *On a scale of 1 to 10, with 1 being perfect skin and 10 being the worst you have had, how would you rate your skin at the moment?*	*Probably about 7 or 8 I think. I don't like anyone seeing it because it's so disgusting.*

TABLE 11.2 SKIN DISORDERS

Analogy: Flesh of the apple	**Context:** Put the presenting complaint into context to understand the disease
AREAS OF INVESTIGATION AND EXAMPLE QUESTIONS	**CLIENT RESPONSES**
Family health	James' mother has a history of childhood eczema, hayfever and asthma
Allergies and irritants *Do you know if you are allergic to anything or if there is anything that makes your skin worse?* *Does your rash improve with sunlight?* (atopic eczema, psoriasis, lichen planus) *Has the rash on your feet worsened since wearing leather shoes?* (shoe dermatitis due to chrome in tanning of leather)	*I don't know. Sometimes my skin feels worse after I've had a shower. Mum thinks it is probably soap that makes it worse.* *Yes, I think it is better in the sun so I try not to wear shoes as much.* *Not sure, I don't wear leather shoes much.*

▶

Recreational drug use *Do you ever drink alcohol or any other substances?* This is a difficult question to ask while James' mother is in the room and it may be necessary to ask this without her present.	*No.*
Occupational toxins and hazards *Are you exposed to any chemicals at school, maybe in science or other subjects that might be a problem for your skin?*	*I don't know. I try not to get anything on my skin in science or woodwork.*
Infection and inflammation *Has your skin ever been infected? Do you think there is any infection now?*	*Sometimes in the past I had to have antibiotics. There are couple of spots at the moment that are oozing so maybe they're infected, but I'm not sure.*
Stress and neurological disease *You said your stress levels have gone up recently. Can you tell me about this and whether you think if affects your skin?*	*Yeah, I'm in Year 12 and now they're really piling the work on so I feel pretty stressed. I think stress must make my skin worse since it's worse since my stress increased.*
Eating habits and energy *Tell me about your diet and whether you think what you eat might be affecting your skin.* *What are your energy levels like?*	James tells you he eats anything and has a lot of takeaway and junk food. He hasn't thought about the possibility that what he is eating might be affecting his skin. He thinks his energy levels are pretty good.

TABLE 11.3 **CORE**	
Analogy: Core of the apple with the seed of ill health	**Core:** Holistic assessment to understand the client
AREAS OF INVESTIGATION AND EXAMPLE QUESTIONS	**CLIENT RESPONSES**
Emotional health *Do you have any significant fears or anxieties at the moment?*	*Not really, just stress about school and hoping my marks will be good enough to get me into uni.*
Stress release *What are you doing to deal with your stress?*	*Just having down time when I can. When I'm not studying I probably spend most of my time on the computer.*
Family and friends *How do you get on with your family and friends?*	*Pretty good most of the time though my little sister is really annoying. I see my friends at school and we usually go out on the weekends.*

▶

Home life *How do you feel at home?*	*Good. Sometimes Mum and Dad get on my nerves but they're pretty good really.*
Action needed to heal *What do you feel you need to do to get your skin under control again?*	*I think something to put on it and maybe some medicine. Maybe be less stressed.*

TABLE 11.4 **JAMES' SIGNS AND SYMPTOMS** [1, 2, 9]	
Pulse	75 bpm
Blood pressure	120/75 sitting
Temperature	37.8°C
Respiratory rate	12 resp/min
Body mass index	24
Waist circumference	85.8 cm
Face	Mild erythema on cheeks and around skin line
Inspection of skin on the hands and body	Skin red with signs of secondary thickening and lichenification of the skin; skin trauma (excoriation) from scratching and areas of severe erythema; broken skin in skin folds of knees and elbows and joints of fingers has caused weeping of pus and showing signs of bleeding
Urinalysis	No abnormality detected (NAD)

Results of medical investigations

No medical investigations have been carried out.

TABLE 11.5 **UNLIKELY DIAGNOSTIC CONSIDERATIONS** [2–4, 64, 67]	
CONDITIONS AND CAUSES	**WHY UNLIKELY**
INFECTION AND INFLAMMATION	
Plaque psoriasis vulgaris: onset from 15 years of age is common, can cause plaques of skin on scalp, knees and elbows, can come and go and be worse at times of stress.	Scalp can be involved but usually does not spread past the hair margin; usually dry and does not have vesicles that ooze pus; presents as silvery loose scales with sharp margins; skin rash usually only on extensor surfaces of extremities; not common to have facial skin rash; more common to have arthritic involvement
ENDOCRINE/REPRODUCTIVE	
Diabetes: sometimes children with diabetes will manifest eczema-like skin rashes	Uncommon; urinalysis NAD

Case analysis

TABLE 11.6 **POSSIBLE DIFFERENTIAL DIAGNOSIS**		
Not ruled out by tests/investigations already done [2–5, 9, 10, 59–68]		
CONDITIONS AND CAUSES	**WHY POSSIBLE**	**WHY UNLIKELY**
ALLERGIES AND IRRITANTS		
Endogenous eczema **Atopic eczema:** the word 'atopy' means to react to common environmental factors; can be caused and aggravated by diet, genetic factors, heat, humidity, drying of the skin, contact with woollen clothing, animal saliva touching the skin; house dust mite allergy is thought to be an important factor in facial eczema	Skin rash that causes itching; begins with small vesicles and then spreads to produce thickening of the skin and weeping of pus and blood if scratched excessively; associated with a history of asthma; presenting in flexor folds of the knees, behind the ears, hands, scalp, elbows and face; lesions cause irritation and scratching; lesions worse for anxiety; symmetrical lesions; eating potentially allergic/intolerant foods such as wheat and dairy; maternal link with atopy	
Exogenous eczema **Primary irritant eczema:** degreasing of skin with water loss and dryness, fissuring and cracking; can happen at work and in the home; more commonly occurs in people who use solvents that remove surface skin lipids (fats); cleaning, hairdressing and industrial occupations: musicians, photographers	The rash is on areas of the body that have close contact with irritants and where chemicals may be applied on the skin such as hands, wrists, neck, eyes, hair, knees; can present in adults and children	Usually asymmetrical lesions in exposed areas and displayed in streaks; determine whether James' rash is occurring on the palm of his hands; usually presents with no family history of eczema/atopy
Contact eczema – allergic from repeated exposure to chemicals resulting in the development of an allergic reaction; common allergens include nickel, chromate, latex, perfumes and plants	The rash is on areas of the body that have close contact with irritants and where common contact allergens may be applied on the skin; often occurs with repeated exposure; family history of atopy	

▶

Photosensitive eczema	Typical features of eczema and thickening of the skin; often occurs in individuals with pre-existing eczema (diagnosis can be missed); can be distributed over areas that are exposed to the sun such as the hands, face and neck; may also spread to areas of the body where the skin is not directly exposed to sunlight	Rare type of eczema, usually develops in middle-aged or elderly men; can develop photosensitivity to artificial lighting
Shoe dermatitis: due to chrome in leather tanning	Red scaling of the feet and toes; can occur in adults or children	
Atopic asthma	Comes and goes, associated with eczema, could be associated with foods as well as stress	Unclear if additional triggers include cold air, emotion, irritants in a particular environment, pollution, medication or recent viral infection
Dermatitis herpetiformis	Extremely itchy rash that is symmetrically distributed over extensor surfaces of the body; this condition is usually associated with gluten-sensitive enteropathy, which can be asymptomatic; James is eating a lot of gluten-containing foods; common to present in early adulthood	James has no significant abdominal symptoms of pain, bloating, diarrhoea or constipation associated with his skin rash; usually associated with bullae (fluid filled palpable mass); more common to present on trunk of the body
FUNCTIONAL DISEASE		
Dermatitis artefacta: personality disorder; a person will injure their own skin	High levels of stress and anxiety; skin showing signs of bleeding	Unclear if James is consciously causing his skin lesions and scratching lesions due to stress and has self-destructive tendencies
INFECTION AND INFLAMMATION		
Seborrhoeic dermatitis: affects those areas of the skin where there are sebaceous glands such as the face and scalp and occurs more with times of stress [62]	Occurs on the scalp beyond hair margin; usually undefined margin; can present in small percentage of young male adults in areas of scalp (with dandruff)	Need to determine whether James has yellow greasy scales on his skin; usually occurs in different locations to atopic dermatitis or eczema such as in the centre of the chest, between the nose and lips, eyebrows, navel, groin; develops as 'cradle cap' in young children; more common as an associated symptom of serious illness in adults and the elderly such as Parkinson's disease and HIV

Exfoliative dermatitis: drug therapy, systemic disease, or an idiopathic entity	Scaling of skin; skin rash usually in flexor surfaces	More commonly develops after the age of 40; generalised skin eruption that can cover the whole body
Inverse psoriasis	Will involve flexor skin folds such as the ears; presents as red inflamed areas	Also common areas are axillae, groin, navel, intergluteal crease, penis, lips and webspaces between fingers and toes; does not usually have the white silver scales of typical psoriasis
Dyshidrotic eczema: on the feet	Itching vesicles and rash on feet	Usually presents in older adults; need to determine whether the lesions on James' feet began with feet/toes breaking out in blisters; common to present with coarse pitting of nail beds; check for ridging across the nails
Nummular eczema (discoid eczema)	Scaling plaques on elbows and knees; can present in adults or children; can be anywhere including hands; oozing and itching of lesions is a common symptom	Typically found on extensor surface of extremities, back, buttocks, and hands; coin-shaped lesions
Tinea capitis: fungal infection of the scalp	Lesions often occur on the scalp and it is common in adolescents and adults; can be mild diffuse scaling with no hair loss	More commonly causes patchy hair loss (alopecia); circular scaly patches seen over the entire scalp; in severe conditions pus may form and a crusted 'boggy' scalp will develop; depending on type of fungus it may or may not appear under Wood's light test
Tinea pedis: fungal infection of the feet, between toes	Plaques can appear like nummular eczema; lesions have defined borders; scaling, vesicles and itching	Determine whether the itch is worse in heat; usually red scaly patches with clear centre and redness at the edge; fungal infection of one or more toenails can develop
Scalp bacterial infection	Lesions on the scalp	More common in younger children; need to determine whether there are pustular lesions
Pediculosis on scalp	Widespread itching on scalp	No report of visually seeing white nits on the hair shaft; more common in young children

STRESS AND NEUROLOGICAL DISEASE		
General anxiety disorder (GAD)	Has been at least 6 months of tension and stress about everyday events; anxiety disorder is often associated with threat of a loss (study stresses, fears about losing marks, what to do when he finishes school); craving junk food/sugar	
Hyperventilation syndrome – functional breathing concern (causes include increased CO_2, fatigue, muscle pain and digestive complaints)	Shortness of breath, breathing quickly, hyperventilation syndrome can be a consequence of chronic anxiety, irritability; habitual patterns of breathing are developed to keep CO_2 levels low that leads to anxiety-provoking consequences	James has not mentioned significant muscle pain or fatigue

Working diagnosis

JAMES AND ECZEMA

James is a 17-year-old young man who has come for help with a chronic skin rash on his face, hands, scalp, knees, elbows and behind his ears. He has used a prescribed steroid cream at various times to ease the rash. The cream has improved his symptoms in the short term but has not prevented the rash from returning. James is now in his last year of high school and has been feeling the pressure and stress involved with keeping up with his studies. During this year his skin rash has worsened and he is looking for a more long-term solution to help his symptoms and to reduce his stress levels. James has been eating a lot of bread, cheese and chocolate milk and likes to spend his spare time on the computer rather than doing exercise or sport, which usually aggravates his skin symptoms. He has mild asthma and there is a maternal link to atopy.

James is presenting with symptoms of endogenous eczema – atopic dermatitis, which develops as a skin rash that can worsen with stress, may be caused by dietary factors and is often associated with asthma. The terms 'dermatitis' and 'eczema' are often interchanged in describing this skin condition. The word dermatitis means 'inflammation'. The word eczema means 'flowing over' or 'boiling', linking with the analogy of the skin becoming so hot that pus is like fluid boiling over with heat.

Endogenous eczema is a form of 'atopic dermatitis'. The word 'atopy' means to react to common environmental or food allergic triggers. There are several types of eczema that are usually associated with 'itch' as a predominant symptom. Depending on the type of eczema it can present as acute, subacute or chronic.

Atopic eczema can be caused and aggravated by diet, genetic factors, heat, humidity, drying of the skin, contact with woollen clothing, animal saliva touching the skin and house dust. There is a strong genetic maternal link with atopic eczema and a family history of asthma may be associated. Characteristic features of eczema are red and hot skin usually in the flexures of joints such as the ankles, knees, elbows and around the neck. Swelling is common in acute stages of the rash, with weeping and oozing of fluid to the surface of skin developing after the acute stage. Crusting over of this fluid causes scaling, fissuring and excoriation that can cause intense itching. Chronic scratching can lead to secondary infections and if they are extremely bad over a large area of the body, impaired thermoregulation and increased blood flow can lead to cardiac impairment.

General references used in this diagnosis: 2–4, 59–61, 65, 68

TABLE 11.7 **DECISION TABLE FOR TREATMENT PRIOR TO REFERRAL**		
COMPLAINT	**CONTEXT**	**CORE**
Treatment for the presenting complaint and symptoms	Treatment for all associated symptoms	Treatment for mental, emotional, spiritual, constitutional, lifestyle issues and metaphysical considerations
TREATMENT PRIORITY	**TREATMENT PRIORITY**	**TREATMENT PRIORITY**
• Lifestyle recommendations to reduce the itching and redness of James' skin • Lifestyle recommendations to reduce skin dryness and improve skin quality, thereby reducing irritation and itching • Recommendations to identify and eliminate or limit exposure to allergens that are triggering the eczema • Topical cream or gel to promote skin healing along with reducing inflammation and itching; also with antimicrobial properties to reduce the chance of skin infections • Physical therapy suggestions to reduce symptoms • Herbal tonic and/or tea with depurative and antiallergic properties • Nutritional supplements with anti-inflammatory and antiallergic properties to improve symptoms	• Reduce the reactivity of James' immune system with lifestyle, dietary, herbal and nutritional recommendations • Dietary recommendations to reduce exposure to reactive foods • Dietary recommendations to increase consumption of foods with anti-inflammatory properties • Herbal tonic and/or tea with antioxidant and immunomodulatory properties • Nutritional supplements with antioxidant and immunomodulatory properties and to improve James' nutritional status	• Lifestyle and physical therapy suggestions to help James cope better with his stress • Herbal tonic and/or tea with an adaptogenic and anxiolytic action to help James improve his stress response • Nutritional supplements to provide essential nutrients for health of the nervous system and to improve James' stress response

TABLE 11.8 **DECISION TABLE FOR REFERRAL** [2–5, 10, 11]		
COMPLAINT	**CONTEXT**	**CORE**
Referral for presenting complaint	Referral for all associated physical, dietary and lifestyle concerns	Referral for contributing emotional, mental, spiritual, metaphysical, lifestyle and constitutional factors
REFERRAL FLAGS	**REFERRAL FLAGS**	**REFERRAL FLAGS**
• Worsening skin rash that can ooze pus, making it prone to secondary infection	• Allergies that have not been properly diagnosed or managed	• James may be finding increased stress and anxiety due to an overwhelming study load • Determine if self-harm of skin is occurring – skin showing signs of bleeding
ISSUES OF SIGNIFICANCE	**ISSUES OF SIGNIFICANCE**	**ISSUES OF SIGNIFICANCE**
• Long-term use of corticosteroid cream, which suppresses the condition but does not treat the cause	• James is not providing sufficient nutrients for his needs • Poor quality of James' skin • Stress and anxiety triggering or aggravating his condition • Asthma may be not be optimally managed	• Poor condition of James' skin affecting his self-esteem, which may lead to social isolation
REFERRAL	**REFERRAL**	**REFERRAL**
• Medical check to diagnose the skin rash and review treatment options	• Allergy testing • Dietary assessment • Medical review of his asthma-management program and medication	• Counsellor to assess mental status

TABLE 11.9 **FURTHER INVESTIGATIONS THAT MAY BE NECESSARY** [2, 3, 5, 9, 10]	
TEST/INVESTIGATION	**REASON FOR TEST/INVESTIGATION**
FIRST-LINE INVESTIGATIONS:	
Skin examination by GP/dermatologist	Clinical diagnosis of a skin disorder by sighting the skin lesions; often diagnosis made by seeing the lesion
Chest examination: auscultation, percussion	Signs of asthma, obstruction, infection
Nijmegen questionnaire	Hyperventilation syndrome
Food diary	To help determine any foods that may be triggering or aggravating symptoms
Full blood count	Any fever, bacteria or viral association with the skin rash
ESR/CRP blood test	Indicates level of inflammation; whether bacterial/viral cause

▶

▶

Serum IgE blood test	Atopic eczema and allergic triggers for asthma
Skin prick testing	Response to immediate contact allergies test for extrinsic-specific allergies
Skin patch tests to particular allergens	Review 2–4 days later for specific delayed contact allergies
RAST test (blood)	Test for ingested or inhaled antigens
IF NECESSARY:	
KOH test of skin discharge/lesion (potassium hydroxide)	*Positive:* ringworm, tinea, fungal infections, *Candida* *Negative:* dyshidrotic eczema on feet
Wood's lamp examination (hand-held ultraviolet light shines certain colours for specific conditions)	Fungus: fluorescent
Skin biopsy	Psoriasis, eczema, fungus
Monochromator light-testing	Photosensitive eczema
Antigliadin antibody blood test	Definitive test for gluten allergy
Lung function tests (forced expiratory volume (FEV), peak expiratory flow rate (PEF))	Will be reduced in asthma
Exercise test	Asthma
Capnometer/pulmonary gas exchange during orthostatic tests	Hyperventilation syndrome

Confirmed diagnosis

Atopic eczema with associated atopic asthma

PRESCRIBED MEDICATION

• Topical steroid cream

TABLE 11.10 **DECISION TABLE FOR TREATMENT (ONCE DIAGNOSIS IS CONFIRMED)**		
COMPLAINT	**CONTEXT**	**CORE**
Treatment for the presenting complaint and symptoms	Treatment for all associated symptoms	Treatment for mental, emotional, spiritual, constitutional, lifestyle issues and metaphysical considerations

▶

TREATMENT PRIORITY	TREATMENT PRIORITY	TREATMENT PRIORITY
• Continue with lifestyle recommendations to reduce symptoms and improve the quality of James' skin • Continue to limit exposure to known environmental and dietary triggers • Continue to use topical herbal preparations as necessary to promote skin healing and to reduce redness, irritation, itch and to prevent infection • Continue with physical therapy recommendations as needed to manage symptoms • Continue with herbal tonic and/or tea to manage and prevent symptoms as needed • Continue with nutritional supplements to provide essential nutrients for James' skin and reduce frequency and severity of eczema	• Continue to focus on reducing the reactivity of James' immune system with lifestyle, dietary, herbal and nutritional recommendations • Support and improve James' digestive function with herbal and nutritional supplements • Ongoing dietary changes to improve James' nutritional status • Continue with dietary recommendations to increase consumption of foods with anti-inflammatory properties • Continue with herbal tonic or tea and nutritional supplements to enhance James' antioxidant status and modulate his immune response; review the use of herbal therapy after 2 months based on James' symptoms and compliance to treatment	• Continue with lifestyle and physical therapy suggestions to help James manage his stress, particularly during his final year of high school • Continue with herbal tonic and/or tea and nutritional supplements with adaptogenic and anxiolytic action and essential nutrients to support James' stress response, particularly during his final year of high school; review the use of herbal therapy once James' stress levels have reduced

Treatment aims

- Prevent and relieve the itch [13, 16, 31].
- Reduce the inflammatory response in James' skin [12].
- Promote skin healing and improve the skin quality, hydration and barrier function [14, 17, 31].
- Normalise essential fatty acid and prostaglandin metabolism [12, 13, 46].
- Balance James' immune system, normalise his TH1 and TH2 balance [12–15] and reduce excess histamine release [13].
- Identify and reduce or eliminate exposure to food and environmental allergens [13, 15, 26, 31, 49].
- Identify and reduce or eliminate exposure to other trigger factors [12, 15, 31].
- Identify and correct nutritional deficiencies [13, 14] and improve James' diet.
- Improve James' digestive function, intestinal microflora [14, 47, 48] and support his eliminative process [18].
- Improve James' stress response and reduce stress levels [14, 15, 50].
- Educate James about ways to better manage his condition to improve his quality of life [16, 31, 50].

Lifestyle alterations/considerations

- Encourage James to avoid using soap or soap-based products [13, 20, 30, 31] and use pH-balanced, soap-free alternatives instead [30, 20]. He should apply moisturiser immediately after bathing [12, 20, 31].

- Encourage James to bathe in warm rather than hot water [12, 20, 31].
- James may find soaking in a tepid oatmeal bath soothes his skin and reduces itching [12].
- Encourage James to avoid wearing fabrics that irritate his skin [13, 31]. Clothing should be washed in mild soaps and rinsed thoroughly [13].
- Encourage James to determine the environmental triggers to his eczema and avoid them wherever possible [13, 31, 32]. These may include house dust mites, chemicals, perfumes in personal care products or detergents, climate and airborne allergens [13, 32].
- Testing for food or chemical sensitivities may be helpful [14, 32].
- Encourage James to try to find techniques to help him avoid scratching his skin [13, 14, 30]. Scratching damages the skin, increases the chance of infection and increases lichenification [13].
- James may benefit from stress-management techniques and/or psychotherapy to help him manage the stress-related triggers of his condition [13, 32, 50].
- Encourage James to engage in a form of physical exercise that does not aggravate his eczema. Exercise is strongly associated with decreased levels of stress, anxiety and depression [35, 36].

Dietary suggestions

- Food allergies or intolerances should be identified and managed by removing them from the diet [12–14, 26, 32]. Common allergenic foods include dairy food, wheat, eggs, citrus fruit, peanuts and soya [14, 15, 26, 38].
- Encourage James to increase his intake of omega-3 fatty acids from cold-water fish, almonds, walnuts, pumpkin and flax seed [12, 14, 20, 33]. James should eat oily fish at least three times per week [13, 14]. Omega-3 fatty acids can reduce the severity of eczema and improve skin quality [53, 54].
- Encourage James to ensure he drinks sufficient water to ensure adequate skin hydration [14, 31].
- James needs to improve his diet and increase consumption of antioxidant-rich whole foods providing adequate levels of essential nutrients and antioxidants [49, 51].

Physical treatment suggestions

- James may find massage therapy beneficial for both his symptoms of stress and his anxiety [25, 40] as well as for his eczema [26].
- James may find acupuncture therapy helpful for his anxiety symptoms [27, 28]. Acupuncture also has immune modulating effects, which may also be beneficial [29].
- Hydrotherapy: constitutional hydrotherapy to assist immune function and tone lungs [41, 42, 45]. Oatmeal half-neutral bath 20 minutes twice daily [43, 44]. Alternate hot/cold douche shower direct to thighs and upper chest to tone the body [44]. Cold sponge bath on the body before bed to ease the rash [44].

TABLE 11.11 **HERBAL FORMULA (1:2 LIQUID EXTRACTS)**		
HERB	**FORMULA**	**RATIONALE**
Albizia *Albizia lebbeck*	45 mL	Antiallergic [19, 20]; traditionally used for eczema [19, 20]; stabilises mast cells [19, 20]
Globe artichoke *Cynara scolymus*	40 mL	Antioxidant [20, 21]; hepatoprotective [20, 21]; traditionally used as a depurative for eczema [20, 21]

Rehmannia *Rehmannia glutinosa*	50 mL	Beneficial in inflammatory disorders involving the immune system [19, 21], particularly allergic skin rashes [19]; may help protect against suppressive effects of corticosteroid therapy [19, 21]; traditional therapeutic use for skin rashes [13, 19, 21]
Burdock *Arctium lappa*	20 mL	Depurative [22]; traditionally used for skin disorders, especially eczema [22, 23]
Withania *Withania somnifera*	45 mL	Adaptogen [19, 20]; immunomodulator [19, 20]; anti-inflammatory [19, 20]; antioxidant [20]; tonic [19]; cognitive enhancer [20]; beneficial in stress [19, 20] and anxiety [20]
Supply:	200 mL	Dose: 5 mL 3 times daily

Licorice (*Glycyrrhiza glabra*) applied topically in the form of a gel is effective in reducing redness, swelling and itch in atopic dermatitis [13, 24, 19]
Calendula (*Calendula officinalis*) cream is soothing and healing to the skin [12, 20]

TABLE 11.12 HERBAL TEA

Can be used as an alternative to the herbal tonic or taken in conjunction with the herbal tonic as an alternative to tea and coffee

HERB	FORMULA	RATIONALE
Nettle leaf *Urtica dioica*	3 parts	Anti-inflammatory [20]; antioxidant [20]; depurative [22]; antiallergic [22]; traditionally used in skin conditions such as eczema [20, 22, 23]; specifically indicated for nervous eczema [23]
Licorice root powder *Glycyrrhiza glabra*	2 parts	Anti-inflammatory [20, 19, 13]; antioxidant [20, 19]; adrenal tonic [20, 19]; immunomodulator [20, 19]; antiallergic action [13]
Cleavers *Galium aparine*	2 parts	Depurative [22, 39]; traditionally used for chronic skin disorders such as eczema [22, 39]
Skullcap *Scutellaria lateriflora*	1 part	Nervine tonic [22]; sedative [23]; indicated for use in nervous tension and anxiety [22, 23]

Infusion: 1 tsp per cup – 1 cup 3 times daily

TABLE 11.13 NUTRITIONAL SUPPLEMENTS

SUPPLEMENT AND DOSE	RATIONALE
High-potency practitioner-strength **multivitamin, mineral and antioxidant supplement** containing therapeutic doses of vitamins A, C, D and E, zinc, selenium and B-group vitamins [12–14]	Optimal levels of essential nutrients are associated with reduced symptom severity in eczema [49]; oxidative stress and altered antioxidant function is involved in acute atopic dermatitis [51]; zinc deficiency is common in atopic dermatitis [13]

▶

Omega-3 fish oil 6000 mg daily [20]	Omega-3 fatty acids regulate inflammatory prostaglandin formation [33]; deficiency is associated with dry, itchy, peeling and flaky skin [33]; omega-3 fatty acids have anti-inflammatory and immune-modulating properties that may be beneficial in atopic dermatitis [14, 20]; people with atopic dermatitis have altered essential fatty acid and prostaglandin metabolism [13]; the ratio of omega-3 to omega-6 fatty acids is lower in people with atopic dermatitis [13]; supplementation with 6000 mg of omega-3 oils daily improves clinical symptoms of atopic dermatitis [53, 54]; reduces plasma catecholamine levels thereby reducing anxiety levels via the HPA axis [34]
Quercetin 2000 mg daily in divided doses [20]	Antiallergic [20, 33, 57]; antioxidant [20, 33, 57, 58]; immunomodulator [20, 57]; anti-inflammatory [20, 33, 58]; inhibits inflammatory enzymes, prostaglandins and leukotrienes [20, 57], stabilises mast cells [20, 57] and inhibits histamine release [33, 57]
High-potency practitioner-strength **probiotic supplement** containing therapeutic doses of human strain organisms including *Lactobacillus rhamnosus GG* [20, 48, 52, 56] Dosage as directed by the manufacturer	Moderates inflammatory and immune responses [20, 56]; strengthens intestinal barrier function [20, 56]; supplementation with probiotics may reduce the severity of symptoms in established atopic dermatitis [20, 55, 56]; effective in the primary prevention of eczema [48, 52, 55, 56]

References

[1] N.J. Talley, S. O'Connor, Pocket Clinical Examination, third edn, Churchill Livingstone Elsevier, Australia, 2009.

[2] P. Kumar, C. Clark, Clinical Medicine, sixth edn, Elsevier Saunders, London, 2005.

[3] R.H. Seller, Differential Diagnosis of Common Complaints, fifth edn, Saunders Elsevier, Philadelphia, 2007.

[4] J. Jamison, Differential Diagnosis for Primary Care, second edn., Churchill Livingstone Elsevier, London, 2006.

[5] R.D. Collins, Differential Diagnosis in Primary Care, fourth edn, Lippincott Williams and Wilkins, Philadelphia, 2008.

[6] J. Silverman, S. Kurtz, J. Draper, Skills for Communicating with Patients, second edn, Radcliff Publishing, Oxford, 2000.

[7] R. Neighbour, The Inner Consultation; how to develop an effective and intuitive consulting style, Radcliff Publishing, Oxon, 2005.

[8] M. Lloyd, R. Bor, Communication Skills For Medicine, third edn, Churchill Livingstone Elsevier, Edinburgh, 2009.

[9] G. Douglas, F. Nicol, C. Robertson, Macleod's Clinical Examination, twelfth edn, Churchill Livingstone Elsevier, 2009.

[10] K.D. Pagna, T.J. Pagna, Mosby's Diagnostic and Laboratory Test reference, third edn, Mosby, USA, 1997 (later edition).

[11] D. Peters, L. Chaitow, G. Harris, S. Morrison, Integrating Complementary Therapies in Primary Care, Churchill Livingstone, London, 2002.

[12] J. Jamison, Clinical Guide to Nutrition & Dietary Supplements in Disease Management, Churchill Livingstone, Edinburgh, 2003.

[13] J.E. Pizzorno, M.T. Murray, H. Joiner-Bey, The Clinicians Handbook of Natural Medicine, second edn, Churchill Livingstone, St Louis, 2008.

[14] H. Osiecki, The Physicians Handbook of Clinical Nutrition, seventh edn, Bioconcepts, Eagle Farm, 2000.

[15] D. Wilsmann-Theis, T. Hagemann, J. Jordan, T. Bieber, N. Novak, Facing psoriasis and atopic dermatitis: are there more similarities or more differences? European Journal of Dermatology 18 (2) (2008) 172–180.

[16] J. Schmitt, F. Csötönyi, A. Bauer, M. Meurer, Determinants of treatment goals and satisfaction of patients with atopic eczema, Journal der Deutschen Dermatologischen Gesellchaft 6 (6) (2008) 458–465.

[17] G. Yosipovitch, How to treat that nasty itch, Experimental Dermatology 14 (2005) 478–479.

[18] T. Cook, Effective herbal treatment of allergies, Mediherb Modern Phytotherapist 7 (2) (2003) 1–12.

[19] K. Bone, Clinical Applications of Chinese and Ayurvedic Herbs: Monographs for the Western Herbal Practitioners, Phytotherapy Press, Warwick, 1996.

[20] L. Braun, M. Cohen, Herbs & Natural Supplements: An evidence based guide, second edn, Elsevier, Sydney, 2007.

[21] S. Mills, K. Bone, Principles & Practice of Phytotherapy; Modern Herbal Medicine, Churchill Livingstone, Edinburgh: London, 2000.

[22] S. Mills, K. Bone, The Essential Guide to Herbal Safety, Churchill Livingstone, St Louis, 2005.

[23] British Herbal Medicine Association, British Herbal Pharmacopoeia, BHMAA, 1983.

[24] M. Saedi, S.K. Morteza, M.R. Ghoreishmi, Treatment of atopic dermatitis with licorice gel, The Journal of Dermatological Treatment 14 (3) (2003) 153–157.

[25] T. Field, G. Robinson, F. Scafidi, R. Nawrocki, A. Goncalves, Massage therapy reduces anxiety and enhances EEG pattern of alertness and math computations, International Journal of Neuroscience 86 (1996) 197–205.

[26] J.M. Hanifin, K.D. Cooper, V.C. Ho, S. Kang, B.R. Krafchik, D.J. Margolis, L.A. Schachner, et al., Guidelines of care for atopic dermatitis, Journal of the American Academy of Dermatology 50 (3) (2004) 391–404.

[27] A.F. Jorm, H. Christensen, K.M. Griffiths, R.A. Parslow, B. Rodgers, K.A. Blewitt, Effectiveness of complementary and self-help treatments for anxiety disorders, Medical Journal of Australia 181 (7) (2004) S29–S46.

[28] D.W. Spence, L. Kayumov, A. Chen, A. Lowe, U. Jain, M.A. Katzman, et al., Acupuncture increases nocturnal melatonin secretion and reduces insomnia and anxiety: A preliminary report, Journal of Neuropsychiatry and Clinical Neurosciences 16 (1) (2004) 19–28.

[29] S. Joos, C. Schott, H. Zou, V. Daniel, E. Martin, Immunomodulatory effects of acupuncture in the treatment of allergic asthma: a randomized controlled study, J Altern Complement Med 6 (6) (2000) 519–525.

[30] T. Ruzicka, J. Ring, B. Przybilla, Handbook of atopic eczema, Springer-Verlag, Berlin, 1991, pp. 198–210.

[31] N.H. Cheigh, Managing a common disorder in children: Atopic dermatitis, Journal of Pediatric Healthcare 17 (2) (2003) 84–88.

[32] S.M. Jones, Triggers of atopic dermatitis, Immunology and Allergy Clinics of North America 22 (1) (2002) 55–72.

[33] H. Osiecki, The Nutrient Bible, seventh edn, BioConcepts Publishing, Eagle Farm, 2008.

[34] B.M. Ross, J. Seguin, L.E. Sieswerda, Omega-3 fatty acids as treatments for mental illness: which disorder and which fatty acid? Lipids in Health and Disease 6 (2007) 21.

[35] A.F. Jorm, H. Christensen, K.M. Griffiths, R.A. Parslow, B. Rodgers, K.A. Blewitt, Effectiveness of complementary and self-help treatments for anxiety disorders, Medical Journal of Australia 181 (7) (2004) S29–S46.

[36] A. Byrne, G.D. Byrne, The effect of exercise on depression, anxiety and other mood states: A review, J Psychosom Res 37 (6) (1993) 565–574.

[37] K.J. Kemper, M.R. Lester, Alternative asthma therapies:An evidence-based review, Contemporary Pediatrics 16 (3) (1999) 162–195.

[38] J.C. Baker, J.G. Ayres, Diet and asthma, Respiratory Medicine 94 (2000) 925–934.

[39] M. Morgan, Herbs for the oral treatment of skin conditions, A Phytotherapist's Perspective 65 (2005) 1–2.

[40] J. Edge, A pilot study addressing the effect of aromatherapy massage on mood, anxiety and relaxation in adult mental health, Complementary Therapies in Nursing & Midwifery 9 (2003) 90–97.

[41] W. Boyle, A. Saine, Lectures in Naturopathic Hydrotherapy, Eclectic Medical Publications, Oregon, 1988.

[42] L.M. Watrous, Constitutional hydrotherapy: from nature cure to advanced naturopathic medicine, Journal of Naturopathic Medicine 7 (2) (1997) 72–79.

[43] M. Sinclair, Modern Hydrotherapy for the Massage Therapist, Lippincott Williams & Wilkins, Baltimore, 2008.

[44] D.D. Buchman, The complete book of water healing, Contemporary Books, McGraw-Hill Companies, New York, 2001.

[45] E. Blake, in: L. Chaitow, E. Blake, P. Orrock, M. Wallden, P. Snider, J. Zeff (Eds.), Naturopathic Physical Medicine, Theory and Practice for Manual Therapists and Naturopaths, Churchill Livingstone Elsevier, Philaldelphia, 2008.

[46] D.F. Horrobin, Essential fatty acid metabolism and its modification in atopic eczema, American Journal of Clinical Nutrition 71 (2000) 367S–372S.

[47] K.W. Mah, B. Bjorksten, B.W. Lee, H.P. vanBever, L.P. Shek, T.N. Tan, et al., Distinct pattern of commensal gut microbiota in toddlers with eczema, International Archives of Allergy and Immunology 140 (2) (2006) 157–163.

[48] A.C. Ouwenhand, Antiallergic Effects of Probiotics, Journal of Nutrition 137 (2007) 794S–797S.

[49] P. Ellwood, M.I. Asher, B. Bjorksten, M. Burr, N. Pearce, Diet and asthma, allergic rhinoconjunctivitis and atopic eczema symptom prevalence: an ecological analysis of the International Study of Asthma and Allergies in

Childhood (ISAAC) data, European Respiratory Journal 17 (2001) 436–443.

[50] Y. Chida, A. Steptoe, N. Hirakawa, N. Sudo, C. Kubo, The Effects of Psychological Intervention on Atopic Dermatitis: A Systematic Review and Meta-Analysis, International Archives of Allergy and Immunology 144 (2007) 1–9.

[51] H. Tsukahara, R. Shibatab, Y. Ohshimaa, Y. Todorokia, S. Satoa, S. Ohtaa, et al., Oxidative stress and altered antioxidant defenses in children with acute exacerbation of atopic dermatitis, Life Sciences 72 (2003) 2509–2516.

[52] M. Kalliomäki, S. Salminen, H. Arvilommi, P. Kero, P. Koskinen, E. Isolauri, Probiotics in primary prevention of atopic disease: a randomised placebo-controlled trial, Lancet 357 (2001) 1076–1079.

[53] E. Soyland, J. Funk, G. Rajka, M. Sandberg, P. Thune, L. Rustad, et al., Dietary supplementation with very long-chain n-3 fatty acids in patients with atopic dermatitis. A double-blind, multicentre study, British Journal of Dermatology 130 (6) (1994) 757–764.

[54] A. Bjorneboe, E. Soyland, G.E. Bjorneboe, G. Rajka, C.A. Drevon, Effect of n-3 fatty acid supplement to patients with atopic dermatitis, Journal of Internal Medicine Suppl 731 (1989) 233–236.

[55] G. Caramia, A. Atzei, V. Fanos, Probiotics and the skin, Clinics in Dermatology 26 (2008) 4–11.

[56] J. Lee, D. Seto, L. Bielory, Meta-analysis of clinical trials of probiotics for prevention and treatment of pediatric atopic dermatitis, Journal of Allergy and Clinical Immunology 121 (2008) 116–121.

[57] Y.B. Shaik, M.L. Cateallani, A. Perrella, F. Conti, V. Salini, S. Tete, et al., Role of quercetin (a natural herbal compound) in allergy and inflammation, Journal of Biol Regul Homeost Agents 20 (3–4) (2006) 47–52.

[58] A.W. Boots, G. Haenen, A. Bast, Health effects of quercetin: From antioxidant to nutraceutical, European Journal of Pharmacology 585 (2008) 325–337.

[59] B. Wüthrich, A. Cozzio, A. Roll, G. Senti, T. Kündig, P. Schmid-Grendelmeier, Atopic eczema: genetics or environment? Ann Agric Environ Med 14 (2) (2007) 195–201.

[60] P. Saint-Mezard, A. Rosieres, M. Krasteva, et al., Allergic contact dermatitis, Eur J Dermatol 14 (5) (2004) 284–295.

[61] P.K. Buxton, ABC of dermatology. Eczema and dermatitis, British Medical Journal (Clin Res Ed.) 295 (6605) (1987) 1048–1051.

[62] R.A. Schwartz, C.A. Janusz, C.K. Janniger, Seborrheic dermatitis: an overview, Am Fam Physician 74 (1) (2006) 125–130.

[63] M.L. Heath, R. Sidbury, Cutaneous manifestations of nutritional deficiency, Curr Opin Pediatr 18 (4) (2006) 417–422.

[64] M.W. Greaves, Recent advances in pathophysiology and current management of itch, Ann Acad Med Singap 36 (9) (2007) 788–792.

[65] D.Y.M. Leung, T. Beiber, Atopic Dermatitis, Lancet 361 (2003) 151–160.

[66] R. Twycross, et al., Itch: scratching more than the surface, Quarterly Journal of Medicine 96 (2003) 7–26.

[67] G. Yosipovitch, et al., Itch, Lancet 361 (2003) 690–694.

[68] M. Cork, D. Robinson, Y. Vasilopoulos, et al., New perspectives on epidermal barrier dysfunction in atopic dermatitis: Gene–environment interactions, J Allergy Clin Immunol 118 (2006) 3–21.

Psoriasis

Case history

Margaret Jones is 57 and has recently travelled to Australia from Wales to meet a man she met on the internet. Since arriving in Australia five weeks ago, Margaret's skin has broken out in patches that are progressively worsening. When you inspect Margaret's skin you can see pink lesions on the outside surface of her elbows, knees and hairline of scalp. The lesions are clearly circumscribed and the skin within the lesion has a silvery scaly appearance. Margaret tells you that the patches sometimes feel dry and itchy. Margaret has come to your clinic wanting a natural treatment for her skin.

When you ask Margaret if she has had any skin problems previously she tells you she hasn't experienced this problem before, although she has had problems in the past with some of her toenails. She tells you she is concerned about her toenails as well and is wondering if there is any connection between the toenail problem and the patches on her skin. Margaret confides to you that she is concerned about being intimate with her new man while her skin looks the way it does.

When you ask Margaret about her general health you discover she has been experiencing soreness in her hands, particularly in the finger joints. The soreness doesn't affect every finger, and affects different fingers on each hand. The soreness has caused restriction of movement in her hands, which is preventing her from playing the flute, painting and sculpting. Margaret is passionate about her music and art so she is finding this particularly frustrating at the moment. Margaret goes on to tell you that she has had problems with back pain for many years, which she attributes to long hours of standing in front of her easel or hunched over her sculptures.

Margaret explains that this trip to Australia is very significant for her. She has lived alone happily in her cottage in Wales for eight years but is seriously considering moving to Australia permanently to live with her new man. She admits this is causing her some anxiety because it is such a life-changing decision with major consequences, particularly if things don't work out.

Margaret's mother had rheumatoid arthritis for many years and occasionally her skin would break out into a rash similar to the one Margaret is experiencing now. Margaret doesn't know whether her mother's skin rash was ever properly diagnosed.

Margaret recently had some blood tests to rule out arthritic reasons for her hands being so sore and at the time her skin rash was not very noticeable so a definitive diagnosis was not reached.

TABLE 11.14 **COMPLAINT** [1–8]	
Analogy: Skin of the apple	**Complaint:** Define the presenting complaint and symptoms; understand the complaint *Dry, itchy skin patches*
AREAS OF INVESTIGATION AND EXAMPLE QUESTIONS	**CLIENT RESPONSES**
Location and radiation	Elbows, knees, hairline of scalp.
Account and description *Tell me how the patches have developed and how they feel.*	*There were only a few at first, but then more appeared and they started to get more noticeable. They are now on my scalp and they are flaky and sometimes itchy.*
Examination and inspection	Circumscribed lesions that are pink around the outer edge. Within the lesion the skin has a silvery scaly appearance.

TABLE 11.15 **CONTEXT**	
Analogy: Flesh of the apple	**Context:** Put the presenting complaint into context to understand the disease
AREAS OF INVESTIGATION AND EXAMPLE QUESTIONS	**CLIENT RESPONSES**
Family health	Margaret's mother had rheumatoid arthritis.
Occupational toxins and hazards	Possible chemical exposure from painting and sculpture. Back pain which Margaret attributes to long hours standing at her easel or hunched over sculptures.
Degenerative and deficiency *Has the hand soreness affected your daily activities?*	*It restricts my hand movement and makes it difficult for me to play the flute, paint and sculpt.*
Supplements and side effects of medication and drugs *Do you have a history of taking prescribed lithium, antimalarial or beta-blocker medication?* (can cause and make psoriasis worse)	*No, I try not to take medication for anything, only natural remedies.*
Endocrine/reproductive *Have you noticed a similar rash develop in the genital region?* (psoriasis, Reiter's syndrome) *It would help me make an assessment for how to help you if I could understand more about your sexual relationships. Do you mind me asking you some more personal questions around your sexual history? Have you had a test for HIV before or any investigations for sexually transmitted diseases?* (Reiter's syndrome) You may explain to the client that if she had been intimate in a relationship it could be recommended to have tests for sexually transmitted diseases.	*No, nothing like that.* *No, if it is relevant.* *No, I have never had any tests but I have not been in an intimate relationship for a long while … should I?*
Autoimmune disease *Your blood tests showed a positive result for the HLA-B27 antigen, which can indicate the presence of autoimmune disease. Did your doctor discuss this with you?*	*She did mention this, but I didn't really understand what it meant. I think rheumatoid arthritis is an autoimmune disease and my mother had that.*
Stress and neurological *I imagine recent events in your life such as travelling to Australia from Wales, the new relationship and the possibility of moving to Australia permanently are probably somewhat stressful. How are you feeling about all of this and do you feel stressed?*	*It's wonderfully exciting and exhilarating and at the same time it is stressful and I have times of doubt and anxiety about everything. If I do decide to stay here, there are so many things to consider.*

TABLE 11.16 **CORE**	
Analogy: Core of the apple with the seed of ill health	**Core:** Holistic assessment to understand the client
AREAS OF INVESTIGATION AND EXAMPLE QUESTIONS	**CLIENT RESPONSES**
Support systems *Do you have friends or family nearby?*	*No, I'm here on my own.*
Stress release *How are you managing your stress at the moment?*	*I usually lose myself in my art or music when I'm stressed. At the moment all my gear is back home in Wales and I'm finding it difficult to do much anyway because of the soreness in my hands.*
Family and friends *Tell me about your family and friends in the UK.*	*I have a son and daughter back home, and three grandchildren. They say they will come and visit me if I decide to stay here. I also have some very good friends and we keep in contact through the phone and internet.*
Home life *What is your home life like at the moment?*	*I'm staying in a little flat near Dan's place. It's really very nice and has everything nice and new. I spend most of my time with Dan, but still sleep at my flat.* Margaret confides she and Dan have not yet been intimate.

TABLE 11.17 **MARGARET'S SIGNS AND SYMPTOMS** [1, 2, 9]	
Pulse	80 bpm
Blood pressure	130/80
Temperature	37°C
Respiratory rate	14 resp/min
Body mass index	25
Waist circumference	82.3 cm
Face	Dark under the eyes, tired looking
Skin lesion on elbows and knees	Silvery loose scales with thickening of the skin (lichenification) on extensor surfaces of elbows, knees
Toenails	Appear yellow on three toe nails on left foot (finely pitted); ridging across the nails; onycholysis (lifting of nail bed) and brown stained patches
Urinalysis	No abnormality detected (NAD)

TABLE 11.18 **RESULTS OF MEDICAL INVESTIGATIONS** [2–5, 10]	
Margaret recently had these blood tests to investigate the pain in her hands	
TEST	**RESULTS**
Full blood count	NAD
ESR (erythrocyte sedimentation rate indicates inflammation in general)	NAD
Rheumatoid factor (RH factor): in inflammatory diseases such as rheumatoid arthritis IgG antibodies produced by lymphocytes in membranes act as antigens, which then react with IgG and IgM antibodies to produce immune complexes that cause inflammation and joint damage; the reactive IgM molecule is RH factor	NAD
Antinuclear antibodies: it is a protein antibody that reacts against cellular nuclear material and is indicative of an autoimmune abnormality; this is very sensitive in detecting systemic lupus erythematosus, but not specific to this disease as it can be present in other inflammatory and autoimmune diseases	NAD
HLA-B27 antigen: HLA antigens are under direct genetic control and share a locus on the chromosome; HLA-B27 is found in 90% of people with ankylosing spondylitis and Reiter's syndrome and 70% of people with a similar spinal arthropathy with psoriasis	Detected

TABLE 11.19 **UNLIKELY DIAGNOSTIC CONSIDERATIONS** [2–5, 10, 53, 61]	
CONDITIONS AND CAUSES	**WHY UNLIKELY**
CANCER AND HEART DISEASE	
Solar keratosis: premalignant silvery scaly lesions in sun-exposed areas	Appear as pink macules (flat patches) that are rough like sandpaper; from long term exposure to sun and increases due to age (may not have been as exposed to as much sun in Wales as she is in Australia)
DEGENERATIVE AND DEFICIENCY	
Anaemia: iron deficiency can cause a generalised itch	Full blood count NAD
Anaemia of chronic disease: can develop in rheumatoid arthritis and inflammatory systemic conditions regardless of high dietary levels of iron	Full blood count NAD
INFECTION AND INFLAMMATION	
Atopic dermatitis or eczema: can present with scaling and lichenification (thickening of skin); presenting in folds of knees, elbows, face, hair margin and toe nails; lesions cause some irritation and scratching; lesions worse for anxiety; lesions can be widespread; can present with pitted nail bed in toes and fingers; ridging across the nails	Usually extremely itchy and symmetrical; common to begin in childhood; often family history of allergic rhinitis or asthma; no oozing vesicles; coarse pitted nail bed often associated with weeping skin lesion on toes; skin rash usually in flexor surfaces only; arthritic involvement is not a feature of eczema

▶

Pityriasis rosea: can present like psoriasis with scaling plaques or patches after recurrent scratching; red scales with clear centre and symmetrical; usually resolves within 6 weeks	Usually on trunk and extremities; can be itchy; more common in winter; oval pink patches that are macula (flat discoloured area); usually presents in children and young adults; large solitary herald patch on the trunk develops before generalised lesions
Erythrodermic psoriasis: generalised psoriatic rash that can affect all body sites, including the hands, feet, nails and extremities	Need to clarify if Margaret has ever smoked cigarettes and, if so, how many per day; can also include the face, trunk; pustular psoriasis is common feature and this form can be life threatening; often associated with fever, fatigue and circulation disorders; usually a burning sensation is reported
AUTOIMMUNE DISEASE	
Rheumatoid arthritis: skin rash and inflammatory symptoms, sore hands, fingers and back, genetic link	No RH factor
Systemic lupus disease: facial rash and inflammatory arthritis [53]	No antinuclear antibodies
Ankylosing spondylitis: skin rash and sore back	ESR not raised
Reiter's syndrome: reactive arthritis that is autoimmune in response to another infection in body; pustular dermatitis with inflamed joints; can be sexually transmitted	ESR not raised, no presenting fever, no conjunctivitis or urinary tract inflammation typically associated with inflamed joints

Case analysis

TABLE 11.20 **POSSIBLE DIFFERENTIAL DIAGNOSIS**		
Not ruled out by tests/investigations already done [2–5, 9, 10, 52–62]		
CONDITIONS AND CAUSES	**WHY POSSIBLE**	**WHY UNLIKELY**
ALLERGIES AND IRRITANTS		
Nummular eczema (discoid)	Similar appearance to psoriasis with scaling plaques on the elbows and knees; can present in adults or children; can be anywhere including the hands and especially the limbs; can present in atopic or non-atopic clients; acute/subacute presentations common	Usually oozing of lesions is a common symptom; not clear whether symptoms are the beginning stage of a chronic skin condition or subacute and self-limiting

Contact dermatitis	Present asymmetrically in exposed areas; on areas of the body that have close contact with irritants and where chemicals may be applied on the skin; can present in adults and children; possible reaction to materials used for artwork	No reported oozing vesicles as is common in contact dermatitis; need to determine if the skin rash only developed when having a break from artwork while travelling in Australia
Shoe dermatitis: due to chrome in leather tanning	Red scaling of the feet and toes; can occur in adults or children	
TRAUMA AND PRE-EXISTING ILLNESS		
Trauma (strains, sprains, tear, herniated disc, fracture, disc prolapse)	Work strain and lower back pain	
Congenital disorders: scoliosis	Lower back pain	Need to determine how long the back pain has been experienced
OCCUPATIONAL TOXINS AND HAZARDS		
Faulty posture	Strain for long periods of time while painting and sculpting, playing flute	
Repetitive strain injury (RSI)	Strain for long periods of time while painting and sculpting, playing flute	
INFECTION AND INFLAMMATION		
Plaque psoriasis vulgaris: elbows, knees, hair margin, toenails	Mechanical irritation due to scratching lesions and repetitive actions in art work, stress and anxiety, genetic inheritance of HLA-B27 antigen, pink colour, scaly appearance; rarely on the face; arthritis in distal joints common; often present in adults; usually lesions stop at the hairline; silver scales; yellow pitted nail and lifting of nail bed common on surface of nails for those with psoriasis; brown stained patches on some nail beds; ridging across the nails; can present as red scaly patches with clear centre that weep silvery foam cells; lesions can be widespread and commonly on extensor surfaces Check if Margaret has been prescribed lithium, antimalarials or beta-blockers recently, which can make psoriasis worse	

Psoriatic arthritis: HLA-B27 detected	Pain in the joints of the hands that is not symmetrical, presents like RA but there is no RH factor involved, ESR readings can be normal	
Parapsoriasis: cutaneous disease that resembles psoriasis but does not share pathogenesis; slightly scaly, light salmon-coloured patches that measure less than 5 cm in diameter	Scaling of skin	Usually over the trunk and extremities
Hepatic psoriasis	Psoriasis skin presentation; scaling of skin, thickening of skin on extensor surfaces	Usually develops from chronic long-term hepatic dysfunction; no jaundice observed
Lichen simplex/nodular prurigo (neurodermatitis)	Scaling of skin, thickening of skin on extensor surfaces; more common in females; emotional stress can potentiate this skin disorder	Usually develops due to extremely itchy skin rash that causes intense scratching and rubbing
Seborrhoeic dermatitis: affects those areas of the skin where there are sebaceous glands such as the face and scalp and occurs more with times of stress [52]	Can present like psoriasis with scaling patches; common in adults	May involve scalp but usually beyond hairline; yellow scales; can be orange-red patches; not well-defined borders and greasy scales; more common as associated symptom of serious illness such as Parkinson's disease and HIV in elderly and adults
Dyshidrotic eczema: on feet	Present in adults, itching vesicles; pitting of nails; ridging across the nails	Need to determine if lesions on toes began with feet/toes breaking out in blisters; common to be coarse pitting if present
Osteoporosis	Pain in back	More common to develop in older age group
Osteoarthritis	Distal interphalangeal joints most affected, not asymmetrical; not associated with increase in ESR, RH factor and antinuclear antibodies are negative; more common over 60 years of age	

Tinea unguium: fungal infection of the nails	Nail that is lifting off the nail bed; nails may appear yellow	Nail bed may not be pitted; usually thickening of nail bed with white or brown discolouration; white crumbly material develops under nail bed that can be tested
Tinea pedis: fungal infection of the feet, between toes	Scaling plaques can appear like psoriasis or nummular eczema; lesions have defined border; scaling, vesicles and itching; fungal infection of one or more toe nails can develop	Determine if itch is worse in heat; usually red scaly patches with clear centre and getting red at the edge; not silvery scales
Candida: toe nail	Nail bed disorder on toes	Determine if nail bed is ridged
SUPPLEMENTS AND SIDE EFFECTS OF MEDICATIONS		
Causal factor: **Drug-induced psoriasis:** may be induced by beta-blockers, lithium, antimalarials, terbinafine, calcium channel blockers, captopril, glyburide, granulocyte colony-stimulating factor, interleukens, interferons and lipid-lowering drugs	Lithium, antimalarials, beta-blockers most common and cause psoriasis-like rash	Margaret has not mentioned prescribed medication in initial history taking
STRESS AND NEUROLOGICAL DISEASE		
Causal factor: **Neurotic excoriations**	Thickening of skin and excoriation on extensor surface of knees and elbows	Nervous habit of scratching causes lesions; can develop in childhood

Working diagnosis

MARGARET AND PSORIASIS

Margaret is a 57-year-old woman who recently travelled to Australia from Wales to begin a new relationship with a man she met on the internet. This experience has contributed to Margaret's feelings of excitement and anxiety and is associated with a skin rash. In Wales Margaret lived comfortably on her own creating artwork and playing music. She has experienced pain in her hands and finger joints along with chronic back pain, which she attributes to long hours of artistic work. Margaret would like a professional opinion regarding her symptoms, as her mother had rheumatoid arthritis and developed similar symptoms. Margaret is particularly anxious to have the skin rash cleared up quickly as she is concerned about its impact on her intimate relationship with her new man. The worst affected areas are on the outside of her elbows, her knees and scalp.

Margaret is presenting with symptoms of **psoriasis**, a chronic skin condition where the skin becomes inflamed and there is an increase in cell turnover to produce thickening of the skin layer. Psoriasis lesions are commonly well demarcated and present with silvery scales on red plaques over extensor surfaces such as knees and elbows.

Often coin-like lesions or plaques are found on the scalp, trunk of body and limbs. The nails can present as pitted with yellow discolouring before the appearance of and along with the skin rash. This skin condition has a strong genetic link, is less common in pigmented skin and will usually present between the ages of 16–22 and 55–60. It is not clearly understood why the skin lesion recurs, but environmental factors such as infection, drugs, ultraviolet light, alcohol abuse and stress are known to be involved in symptom aggravation. Emotional and mechanical trauma can trigger psoriasis, while specific medications are known to induce it.

General references used in this diagnosis: 2–4, 55, 56, 58, 60–62

TABLE 11.21 **DECISION TABLE FOR TREATMENT PRIOR TO REFERRAL**		
COMPLAINT	**CONTEXT**	**CORE**
Treatment for the presenting complaint and symptoms	Treatment for all associated symptoms	Treatment for mental, emotional, spiritual, constitutional, lifestyle issues and metaphysical considerations
TREATMENT PRIORITY	**TREATMENT PRIORITY**	**TREATMENT PRIORITY**
• Lifestyle recommendations to reduce skin dryness and improve skin quality • Topical herbal preparations to reduce inflammation, soften lesions and improve skin quality • Physical treatment and lifestyle suggestions to reduce symptoms and improve skin quality • Physical treatment and lifestyle suggestions to reduce trigger factors such as stress and exposure to environmental factors • Physical treatment suggestions to help reduce hand pain and stiffness • Herbal tonic and tea to improve skin function and reduce symptoms of psoriasis • Nutritional supplements to improve skin quality and reduce symptoms of psoriasis	• Recommendations to identify and manage dietary and/or environmental sensitivities or allergies • Dietary recommendations to improve general health, liver and bowel function • Dietary recommendation to include foods with anti-inflammatory, antioxidant and immune-modulating properties • Herbal tonic and tea containing herbs to support liver and bowel function and modulate immune response • Nutritional supplements to improve general health, improve bowel health, reduce inflammation and improve skin quality	• Lifestyle and physical therapy recommendations to help manage and reduce stress • Herbal tonic containing nervine and adaptogenic herbs to help support Margaret's nervous system and stress response

TABLE 11.22 DECISION TABLE FOR REFERRAL [2–5, 10, 11]

COMPLAINT	CONTEXT	CORE
Referral for presenting complaint	Referral for all associated physical, dietary and lifestyle concerns	Referral for contributing emotional, mental, spiritual, metaphysical, lifestyle and constitutional factors
REFERRAL FLAGS	**REFERRAL FLAGS**	**REFERRAL FLAGS**
• Recent appearance of the skin rash, which is not healing • Onset of new rash following international travel and new intimate relationship	• Toenails pitted and lifting, possibly associated with skin lesions • History of back pain • Pain and stiffness in Margaret's hands • Mother's history of rheumatoid arthritis and skin rash	Nil
ISSUES OF SIGNIFICANCE	**ISSUES OF SIGNIFICANCE**	**ISSUES OF SIGNIFICANCE**
Nil	• Onset of skin rash following a life change	• Hand pain restricting Margaret's ability to indulge in her passions of music and art • Stress and anxiety about how the skin rash may affect her relationship with her new man • Significant anxiety about making a life-changing decision
REFERRAL	**REFERRAL**	**REFERRAL**
• Medical opinion for definitive diagnosis of skin rash • Assessment for risk of infection or contagious implications of skin rash	• Diagnosis for the cause of the back and joint pain • Assessment of the toenails and risk of secondary infection	• Depending on severity of anxiety Margaret may want to talk through her concerns with a counsellor

TABLE 11.23 FURTHER INVESTIGATIONS THAT MAY BE NECESSARY [2, 3, 5, 9, 10]

TEST/INVESTIGATION	REASON FOR TEST/INVESTIGATION
FIRST-LINE INVESTIGATIONS:	
Skin examination by GP/dermatologist	Clinical diagnosis of skin disorder by sighting skin lesions; often diagnosis made by sight of lesion
Full blood count	Infectious disease
Serum IgE levels	Allergic disease, atopic eczema

▶

IF NECESSARY:	
Potassium hydroxide (KOH) test	*Positive:* ringworm, tinea, fungal infections, *Candida* *Negative:* dyshidrotic eczema on feet
Wood's lamp examination (hand-held ultra violet light shines certain colours for specific conditions)	Fungus: fluorescent
Skin biopsy	Psoriasis
Microscopy/fungal culture of skin lesion	Fungus
Skin patch tests to particular allergens	Review 2–4 days later for specific delayed contact allergies
Skin prick tests to particular allergens	Response to immediate contact allergies
Antinuclear antibody	Collagen disease, autoimmune disease
Liver function test	Hepatitis or hepatic disorder
X-ray on left and right hands	Rule out fractures, joint or bone abnormalities, osteoporosis, osteoarthritis
X-ray of spine	Osteoporosis
Bone densitometry (DEXA scanning)	Define diagnosis for osteoporosis

Confirmed diagnosis

MARGARET AND PLAQUE PSORIASIS VULGARIS WITH ASSOCIATED PSORIATIC ARTHRITIS

A small percentage of people with psoriasis also have arthropathy where HLA markers are recognised. HLA-B27 is present in up to 70 per cent of people who develop a similar spinal and general arthritis associated with psoriasis. Therefore careful differential diagnosis may be necessary to determine the cause of associated symptoms of inflammation in large or small joints. Commonly psoriatic arthritis will present with joint inflammation of the distal interphalangeal joints with pitted nails. Inflammation of the lower back and similar polyarthritic symptoms to rheumatoid arthritis may also develop.

General references used in this diagnosis: 2–5

PRESCRIBED MEDICATION

NSAIDs and topical steroid cream as necessary. Margaret would prefer to use natural treatments before resorting to prescribed medications.

TABLE 11.24 **DECISION TABLE FOR TREATMENT (ONCE DIAGNOSIS IS CONFIRMED)**		
COMPLAINT	**CONTEXT**	**CORE**
Treatment for the presenting complaint and symptoms	Treatment for all associated symptoms	Treatment for mental, emotional, spiritual, constitutional, lifestyle issues and metaphysical considerations

TREATMENT PRIORITY	TREATMENT PRIORITY	TREATMENT PRIORITY
• Continue to use topical herbal preparations as necessary • Continue with lifestyle recommendations to improve skin quality and reduce dryness • Continue with physical treatment and lifestyle suggestions to reduce exposure to trigger factors and skin quality • Continue with physical treatment suggestions to help reduce hand pain and stiffness • Continue with herbal tonic and tea to reduce psoriasis symptoms and improve skin function • Continue with nutritional supplements to reduce psoriasis symptoms and improve skin **NB:** Margaret's vitamin and mineral levels should be monitored to ensure they stay within acceptable limits; collaborative management of Margaret's condition with her GP is important to ensure her treatment is appropriate and effective	• Continue with recommendations to identify and manage dietary and environmental sensitivities • Continue with dietary recommendations to include anti-inflammatory, antioxidant and immune-modulating foods • Continue with dietary recommendations to improve general health, liver and bowel function • Continue with herbal tonic and tea to support liver and bowel function and modulate immune response • Continue with nutritional supplements to improve general health, improve bowel health, reduce inflammation and improve skin quality	• Continue with lifestyle and physical therapy recommendations to help manage stress • Continue with herbal tonic containing nervine and adaptogenic herbs to help support Margaret's nervous system and stress response

Treatment aims

- Decrease abnormal cell proliferation within the skin with the aim of normalising skin function [12, 41, 49], reducing dryness and improving skin quality [33].
- Reduce inflammatory processes within the skin [12, 41].
- Modulate the immune response. Psoriasis is a TH1-dominant condition [15].
- Enhance function of liver and bowel. Impaired liver function, bile deficiencies and bowel toxaemia are implicated in the development of psoriasis [12]. Altered bowel mucosa and inflammation are associated with psoriasis [50, 51].
- Improve protein digestion. Polyamines produced when breakdown of protein is inadequate are increased in psoriatics [12, 17]. Lowered skin and urinary levels of polyamines are associated with a clinical improvement in psoriasis [17].
- Support and protect Margaret's cardiovascular system. Psoriatics have an increased risk of atherosclerosis [13, 41, 48].
- Support Margaret's stress response. Stress can be a predisposing factor in psoriasis [14, 41].

- Where possible identify and remove dietary and environmental antigens, which may trigger or aggravate the condition [12, 15].
- Determine whether Margaret has a gluten intolerance and manage accordingly [12, 16].

Lifestyle alterations/considerations

- Stress-reduction techniques (e.g. meditation, tai chi, yoga) can be helpful by reducing the impact of stress on Margaret's psoriasis [12, 14].
- The regular use of emollient creams or lotions can help keep Margaret's skin supple and reduce dryness and itching [33].
- Margaret should avoid exposure to cigarette smoke [34].
- Margaret may benefit from exposure to sunlight [35].
- Margaret may benefit from counselling to help her deal with the stress of making a significant life change along with the stress her psoriasis is causing [28].

Dietary suggestions

- Reduce consumption of refined carbohydrates along with sugar, meat, saturated fat and alcohol and follow a low GI/GL diet to ensure her blood glucose levels are stable and stay within normal range [12, 42]. There is an association between psoriasis and abnormal blood-sugar levels [42].
- Margaret's diet should be high in antioxidant-rich, nutrient-dense whole foods. Ensuring a high intake of antioxidants and essential nutrients is very important in psoriasis [12, 16, 48]. High consumption of fruit and vegetables is associated with a lower risk of psoriasis [14].
- Increase consumption of dietary fibre, particularly soluble fibre such as rice bran, oat bran, psyllium and linseeds. Soluble fibre can improve bowel flora and function [26].
- Increase consumption of foods containing omega-3 fatty acids [12, 16, 27]. Margaret may benefit from a period of fasting followed by a vegetarian diet [16].
- Include ½–1 tsp of turmeric in food each day [19]. Turmeric is anti-inflammatory, antioxidant, immunomodulator, hepatoprotective and a cholagogue [18, 19].
- Encourage Margaret to include ginger in her diet. Ginger is anti-inflammatory [19, 40] and an antioxidant [18, 19] and immunomodulator [18, 19].
- Margaret may find a gluten-free diet is helpful [16].

Physical treatment suggestions

- Acupuncture treatment may be beneficial. It may help improve the psoriasis [36] and reduce stress and anxiety [37].
- Hydrotherapy: brief full body baths in apple cider vinegar and salt baths can be beneficial for psoriasis [43]. Oatmeal baths for 20 minutes once or twice daily [44].
- Constitutional hydrotherapy [45, 46].
- Warm Epsom salt bath for 20 minutes to ease pain or tension [44].
- Neutral baths [46].
- Hot foot bath to alleviate stress [47].
- Massage therapy may be beneficial in reducing Margaret's anxiety and stress levels [39].

TABLE 11.25 TOPICAL HERBAL APPLICATIONS

HERB	RATIONALE
Turmeric *Curcuma longa* ½ cup of powdered turmeric plus 1 tsp of bicarbonate of soda mixed with hot water to form a paste; spread cooled paste onto gauze and apply to affected areas [19]	Topical application of turmeric can reduce the severity of active, untreated psoriasis [19]
Chickweed *Stellaria media* Topical application in the form of a cream or ointment can help reduce and soothe itch and soften lesions Chickweed cream may be used as an alternative or in conjunction with topical turmeric application	Antirheumatic [21]; topical antipruritic [21]; vulnerary [21]; emollient [21]; traditionally used as a cooling topical demulcent in eczema and psoriasis [22]

TABLE 11.26 HERBAL FORMULA (1:2 LIQUID EXTRACTS)

HERB	FORMULA	RATIONALE
Turmeric *Curcuma longa*	60 mL	Anti-inflammatory [18, 19]; immunomodulator [19]; depurative [18]; hepatoprotective [19]; antioxidant [18, 19]; cholagogue [18, 19]; improving liver function greatly benefits psoriasis [12]
Withania *Withania somnifera* 1:1 liquid extract	40 mL	Adaptogen [18, 19]; mild sedative [18, 19]; anti-inflammatory [18, 19]; immunomodulator [18, 19]; traditionally used for improving stress adaptation [19]; traditional therapeutic use for psoriasis [18]
Rehmannia *Rehmannia glutinosah*	70 mL	Anti-inflammatory [18, 23]; adrenal trophorestorative [18, 23]; uncured rehmannia is indicated for use in inflammatory disorders of the immune system, particularly skin and autoimmune disorders [23]
Passionflower *Passiflora incarnata*	30 mL	Anxiolytic [21, 19]; sedative [21, 19]; effective in anxiety and nervous restlessness [19, 24]

Supply dose: 200 mL 5 mL 3–4 times daily

TABLE 11.27 HERBAL TEA

Alternative to tea and coffee

HERB	FORMULA	RATIONALE
Oregon grape root *Berberis aquifolium*	½ part	Antipsoriatic [21, 22]; anti-inflammatory [22]; depurative [22]; mild cholagogue [21, 22]; antimicrobial [22]; laxative [21]
Cleavers leaf/stem *Galium aparine*	2 parts	Depurative [21 22]; traditionally used for psoriasis [21, 22]

►

▶

Sarsaparilla root *Smilax officinalis*	1 part	Alterative [20]; antirheumatic [20]; antiseptic [20]; antipruritic [21]; specific for psoriasis [21]
Burdock root *Arctium lappa*	2 parts	Depurative [21, 221]; mild laxative [21, 22]; indicated for use in psoriasis [21]
Decoction: 1 tsp per cup – 1 cup 3 times daily		

TABLE 11.28 **NUTRITIONAL SUPPLEMENTS**	
SUPPLEMENT AND DOSE	**RATIONALE**
Omega-3 fish oil Providing 10, 000–12,000 mg EPA daily for at least 6 weeks [27], decreasing the dose to 6000 mg daily thereafter [19]	Anti-inflammatory [16, 19, 25]; increases adhesion of probiotic bacteria to intestinal wall [25]; fish oil supplementation can reduce inflammatory processes associated with psoriasis [16]; supplementation of up to 10,000–12,000 mg EPA daily can significantly improve psoriasis [27]
Vitamin A 10,000 IU daily for 1–2 weeks until improvement is noticed [19, 25]; thereafter 2500 IU daily [19, 25]	Vitamin A deficiency is common in psoriasis [29]
Zinc supplement providing 50 mg elemental zinc daily [29] 2 mg daily of copper should be included if zinc supplement is taken for more than 1 month [41]	Psoriatics can have increased serum copper:zinc ratio [30] Plasma zinc levels are lower in psoriatics than the general population [31]; psoriatics with extensive surface involvement have lower zinc levels than those with minimal involvement [31]
Supplement providing approx 800 IU **Vitamin E** [19, 25] and 200 mcg **selenium** [19, 25] daily in divided doses	Blood glutathione levels are lower in psoriatics [38] and supplementation with selenium and vitamin E can improve glutathione levels [38]; selenium deficiency is commonly found in psoriasis [32]
High-potency practitioner-strength **multivitamin and mineral formula** providing therapeutic doses of essential micronutrients and antioxidants [12, 16]	To provide broad-spectrum supplemental nutrients and antioxidants; people with psoriasis have increased oxidative stress and decreased antioxidant capacity [16, 48]; nutritional deficiencies are associated with psoriasis and supplemental nutrients and antioxidants may be beneficial [12, 16]

References

[1] N.J. Talley, S. O'Connor, Pocket Clinical Examination, third edn, Churchill Livingstone Elsevier, Australia, 2009.

[2] P. Kumar, C. Clark, Clinical Medicine, sixth edn, Elsevier Saunders, London, 2005.

[3] R.H. Seller, Differential Diagnosis of Common Complaints, fifth edn, Saunders Elsevier, Philadelphia, 2007.

[4] J. Jamison, Differential Diagnosis for Primary Care, second edn, Churchill Livingstone Elsevier, London, 2006.

[5] R.D. Collins, Differential Diagnosis in Primary Care, fourth edn, Lippincott Williams & Wilkins, Philadelphia, 2008.

[6] J. Silverman, S. Kurtz, J. Draper, Skills for Communicating with Patients, second edn, Radcliff Publishing, Oxford, 2000.

[7] R. Neighbour, The Inner Consultation; how to develop an effective and intuitive consulting style, Radcliff Publishing, Oxon, 2005.

[8] M. Lloyd, R. Bor, Communication Skills For Medicine, third edn, Churchill Livingstone Elsevier, Edinburgh, 2009.

[9] G. Douglas, F. Nicol, C. Robertson, Macleod's Clinical Examination, twelfth edn, Churchill Livingstone Elsevier, Edinburgh, 2009.

[10] K.D. Pagna, T.J. Pagna, Mosby's Diagnostic and Laboratory Test reference, third edn., Mosby, USA, 1997 (later edition).

[11] D. Peters, L. Chaitow, G. Harris, S. Morrison, Integrating Complementary Therapies in Primary Care, Churchill Livingstone, London, 2002.

[12] J.E. Pizzorno, M.T. Murray, H. Joiner-Bey, The Clinicians Handbook of Natural Medicine, second edn, Churchill Livingstone, St Louis, 2008.

[13] B.V. Kural, A. Orem, G. Cimsit, Y.E. Yandi, M. Calapogula, Evaluation of the atherogenic tendency of lipids and lipoprotein content and their relationships with oxidant–antioxidant system in patients with psoriasis, Clinica Chimica Acta 328 (2003) 71–82.

[14] J.P. Ortonne, Aetiology and Pathogenesis of Psoriasis, British Journal of Dermatology 135 (Suppl. 49) (1996) 1–5.

[15] D. Wilsmann-Theis, T. Hagemann, J. Jordan, T. Bieber, N. Novak, Facing psoriasis and atopic dermatitis: are there more similarities or more differences? European Journal of Dermatology 18 (2) (2008) 172–180.

[16] M. Wolters, Diet and psoriasis: experimental data and clinical evidence, British Journal of Dermatology 153 (2005) 706–714.

[17] M.S. Proctor, D.I. Wilkinson, E.K. Orenberg, E.M. Farber, Lowered Cutaneous and Urinary Levels of Polyamines With Clinical Improvement in Treated Psoriasis, Archives of Dermatology 115 (8) (1979) 945–949.

[18] S. Mills, K. Bone, Principles & Practice of Phytotherapy; Modern Herbal Medicine, Churchill Livingstone, Edinburgh: London, 2000.

[19] L. Braun, M. Cohen, Herbs & Natural Supplements: An evidence based guide, second edn, Elsevier, Sydney, 2007.

[20] D. Hoffman, The New Holistic Herbal, second edn, Element Books Limited, Shaftesbury, 1996.

[21] British Herbal Medicine Association, British Herbal Pharmacopoeia, BHMA, 1983.

[22] S. Mills, K. Bone, The Essential Guide to Herbal Safety, Elsevier Churchill Livingstone, St Louis, 2004.

[23] K. Bone, Clinical Applications of Chinese and Ayurvedic Herbs: Monographs for the Western Herbal Practitioners, Phytotherapy Press, Warwick 1996.

[24] S. Akhondzadeh, H.R. Naghavi, M. Vazirian, A. Shayeganpour, H. Rashidi, M. Khani, Passionflower in the treatment of generalized anxiety: a pilot double-blind randomized controlled trial with oxazepam, Journal of Clinical Pharmacy and Therapeutics 26 (2001) 363–367.

[25] H. Osiecki, The Nutrient Bible, seventh edn, BioConcepts Publishing, Eagle Farm, 2008.

[26] J.H. Cummings, Constipation, dietary fibre and the control of large bowel function, Postgraduate Medical Journal 60 (1984) 811–819.

[27] P.D. Maurice, B.R. Allen, A. Barkley, S.R. Cockbill, J. Stammers, P.C. Bather, The effects of dietary supplementation with fish oil in patients with psoriasis, British Journal of Dermatology 117 (5) (1988) 599–606.

[28] D.G. Fortune, H.L. Richards, B. Kirby, S. Bowcock, C.J. Main, C.E. Griffiths, A cognitive-behavioural symptom management program as an adjunct in psoriasis therapy, British Journal of Dermatology 146 (3) (2002) 458–465.

[29] S. Majewski, P. Janik, A. Langner, M. Glinska-Ferrenz, B. Swietochowska, I. Sawicki, Decreased levels of vitamin A in serum of patients with psoriasis, Archives of Dermatological Research 280 (1989) 499–501.

[30] A. Donadini, A. Pazzaglia, G. Desirello, C. Minoia, M. Colli, Plasma levels of Zn Cu and Ni in healthy controls and psoriatic patients (author's translation). Acta Vitamin Enzymol 1 (1980) 9–16. Article in Italian.

[31] E.M. McMillan, D. Rowe, Plasma zinc in psoriasis: relation to surface area involvement, British Journal of Dermatology 108 (3) (2003) 301–305.

[32] G. Michaelsson, B. Berne, B. Carlmark, A. Strand, Selenium in whole blood and plasma is decreased in patients with moderate and severe psoriasis, Acta Derm Venerol 69 (1) (1989) 29–34.

[33] A.O. Moden, Role of Topical Emollients and Moisturizers in the Treatment of Dry Skin Barrier Disorders, American Journal of Clinical Dermatology 4 (11) (2003) 771–788.

[34] K. Poikolainen, T. Reunala, J. Karvonen, Smoking, alcohol and life events related to psoriasis among women, British Journal of Dermatology 130 (4) (1994) 473–477.

[35] T. Horio, Skin Disorders that Improve by Exposure to Sunlight, Clinics in Dermatology 16 (1998) 59–65.

[36] S.J. Liao, T.A. Liao, Acupuncture treatment for psoriasis: a retrospective case report, Acupuncture and Electrotherapeutics Research 17 (3) (1992) 195–208.

[37] A. Fassoulaki, A. Paraskeva, K. Patris, T. Pourgiezi, G. Kostopanagiotou, Pressure Applied on the Extra 1 Acupuncture Point Reduces Bispectral Index Values and Stress in Volunteers, Anaesthesia & Analgesia 96 (2003) 885–889.

[38] L. Juhlin, L.E. Edqvist, L.G. Ekman, K. Luinghall, M. Olsson, Blood glutathione-peroxidase levels in skin diseases: effect of selenium and vitamin E treatment, Acta Derm Venerol 62 (3) (1982) 211–214.

[39] C.A. Moyer, J. Rounds, J.W. Hannum, A Meta-Analysis of Massage Therapy Research, Psychological Bulletin 130 (1) (2004) 3–18.

[40] R. Grzanna, L. Lindmark, C.G. Frondoza, Ginger—An Herbal Medicinal Product with Broad Anti-Inflammatory Actions, Journal of Medicinal Food 8 (2) (2005) 125–132.

[41] J. Jamison, Clinical Guide to Nutrition & Dietary Supplements in Disease Management, Churchill Livingstone, Edinburgh, 2003.

[42] P.J. Lynch, Psoriasis and Blood-sugar Levels, Archives of Dermatology 95 (3) (1967) 255–258.

[43] D.D. Buchman, The complete book of water healing, Contemporary Books, McGraw-Hill Companies, New York, 2001.

[44] M. Sinclair, Modern Hydrotherapy for the Massage Therapist, Lippincott Williams & Wilkins, Baltimore, 2008.

[45] W. Boyle, A. Saine, Lectures in Naturopathic Hydrotherapy, Eclectic Medical Publications, Oregon, 1988.

[46] L. Chaitow, Hydrotherapy, water therapy for health and beauty, Element, Dorset, 1999.

[47] Y. Saeiki, The effect of foot-bath with or without the essential oil of lavender on the autonomic nervous system: a randomised trail, Complementary Therapies in Medicine 8 (2000) 2–7.

[48] B. Banizor, A. Orem, G. Cimsit, Y.E. Yandi, M. Calapoglu, Evaluation of the atherogenic tendency of lipids and lipoprotein content and their relationships with oxidant–antioxidant system in patients with psoriasis, Clinica Chimica Acta 328 (2003) 71–82.

[49] P. Moller, L.E. Knudsen, G. Frentz, M. Dybdahl, H. Wallin, B. Nexo, Seasonal variation of DNA damage and repair in patients with non-melanoma skin cancer and referents with and without psoriasis, Mutation Research 407 (1998) 25–34.

[50] R. Scarpa, F. Manguso, A. D'Arienzo, F. D'Armiento, C. Astarita, G. Mazzacca, et al., Microscopic inflammatory changes in colon of patients with both active psoriasis and psoriatic arthritis without bowel symptoms, Journal of Rheumatology 27 (5) (2000) 1241–1246.

[51] C. Ritchlin, Psoriatic disease – from skin to bone, Nat Clin Pract Rheumatol 3 (12) (2007) 698–706.

[52] R.A. Schwartz, C.A. Janusz, C.K. Janniger, Seborrheic dermatitis: an overview, Am Fam Physician 74 (1) (2006) 125–130.

[53] R. Eming, M. Hertl, Autoimmune bullous disorders, Clin Chem Lab Med 44 (2) (2006) 144–149.

[54] D. Roosterman, T. Goerge, S.W. Schneider, N.W. Bunnett, M. Steinhoff, Neuronal control of skin function: the skin as a neuroimmunoendocrine organ, Physiol Rev 86 (4) (2006) 1309–1379.

[55] C.K. Svensson, E.W. Cowen, A.A. Gaspari, Cutaneous drug reactions, Pharmacol Rev 53 (3) (2001) 357–379.

[56] A. Slominski, J. Wortsman, Neuroendocrinology of the skin, Endocr Rev 21 (5) (2000) 457–487.

[57] W.H. McLean, Genetic disorders of palm skin and nail, J Anat 202 (1) (2003) 133–141.

[58] M. Jafferany, Psychodermatology: a guide to understanding common psychocutaneous disorders, Prim Care Companion J Clin Psychiatry 79 (3) (2007) 203–213.

[59] P.R. Cyr, G.K. Dreher, Neurotic excoriations, Am Fam Physician 64 (12) (2001) 1981–1984.

[60] R.S. Fawcett, S. Linford, D.L. Stulberg, Nail abnormalities: clues to systemic disease, Am Fam Physician 69 (6) (2004) 1417–1424.

[61] J. Cahill, R. Sinclair, Cutaneous manifestations of systemic disease, Aust Fam Physician 34 (5) (2005) 335–340.

[62] W. Schon, W.H. Boehncke, Psoriasis, N Engl J Med 352 (2005) 1899–1912.

Acne

Case history

Elias Bagnabol has come to the clinic with his parents, Dorota and Henry. Elias is 16 and still at high school. He is concerned about his acne, which has been worsening over the past 12 months. Elias tells you he started getting pimples when he was 14 and his acne has been slowly getting worse. He started with pimples on his face, now they are all over his face, and also on his back, chest and shoulders. Some of the pimples get quite large and red and can be tender. Elias has blackheads and whiteheads, inflammatory papules and pustules. The skin is greasy and there is obvious facial scarring developing.

Dorota took Elias to their family doctor who prescribed antibiotics. She expressed concern about Elias taking antibiotics long term so the doctor suggested they could try dietary and lifestyle measures to see whether that helped before resorting to antibiotic therapy.

When you ask Elias about his diet he tells you he has either a can of energy drink or toast and coffee for breakfast. He usually buys his morning tea and lunch at the school canteen and has either a sausage roll or a pizza roll at recess and a burger or hot dog for lunch. He drinks either soft drink or fruit juice. Four days per week after school Elias works part time at a fast-food outlet. He usually eats something at work when he starts his shift and usually also eats something there for his evening meal as well. When he is at home Elias likes to have instant noodles or toasted cheese sandwiches. At least three nights per week Elias eats with his family but does not like eating vegetables so usually only has a small amount at the insistence of his mother. Further questioning reveals that Elias eats no fruit or whole grains, usually has one or two energy drinks daily and doesn't drink any water.

Dorota explains that Elias has been feeling episodes of fatigue for the past 12 months and, because he likes to keep up his school and work commitments, he drinks energy drinks and coffee to boost his energy.

When you question Elias about his bowel habits he is quite embarrassed and mumbles that he goes a couple of times a week.

Dorota is hoping you can help with Elias' acne, and perhaps help him to see he needs to eat better. Elias just wants his skin to get better but thinks he might be willing to try your suggestions. Dorota explains that Elias has been suffering from self-esteem issues since developing acne.

TABLE 11.29 **COMPLAINT** [1–10]	
Analogy: Skin of the apple	**Complaint:** Define the presenting complaint and symptoms; understand the complaint *Acne*
AREAS OF INVESTIGATION AND EXAMPLE QUESTIONS	**CLIENT RESPONSES**
Understanding the cause (client) *What do you think is causing your acne? How do you compare your acne today to how it is in general?*	*Puberty, I guess. It is pretty bad today; it can get better than this.*
Location and radiation *Where did the pimples first appear and how and where have they spread?*	Pimples first appeared on Elias' face and have spread to his back, chest and shoulders.
Your practitioner impression	Elias has come with his mother who is seeking a natural treatment to his problem. Your impression is that Elias just wants his skin to clear up and does not care whether that is achieved through natural or conventional medical treatment.
Examination and inspection	Greasy skin, blackheads, whiteheads, inflammatory papules and pustules. Elias' skin has obvious areas of infection, redness, inflammatory papules and pustules. Facial scarring is developing.

TABLE 11.30 **CONTEXT**	
Analogy: Flesh of the apple	**Context:** Put the presenting complaint into context to understand the disease
AREAS OF INVESTIGATION AND EXAMPLE QUESTIONS	**CLIENT RESPONSES**
Family health *Is there a family history of acne?*	*Dad says he used to get it bad when he was growing up.*
Recreational drug use *Do you ever drink alcohol or any other substances?* This is a difficult question to ask while Elias' mother is in the room and it may be necessary to ask this without her present.	*No.*
Functional disease *How often do you have a bowel motion?*	Elias finds this question embarrassing and mumbles. *A couple of times a week.*
Stress and neurological	Elias works part time and is also in Year 11. He is under stress because he wants to maintain school and work commitments. This has resulted in fatigue over the past 12 months.
Eating habits, energy and exercise	Elias has a poor diet with a high level of consumption of fast food and energy drinks, with little or no fruit, whole grains or water. Elias eats only small amounts of vegetables at the insistence of his mother.

TABLE 11.31 **CORE**	
Analogy: Core of the apple with the seed of ill health	**Core:** Holistic assessment to understand the client
AREAS OF INVESTIGATION AND EXAMPLE QUESTIONS	**CLIENT RESPONSES**
Emotional health *Do you have any significant fears or anxieties at the moment?*	*I'm stressed about my skin. Also it is getting harder to keep up with my school and work commitments.*
Environmental wellness *How much time do you spend watching TV, on the computer or on your mobile phone?*	*A lot, I suppose, when I'm not studying or working. I talk to my friends on Facebook or MSN.*
Stress release *How do you manage your stress?*	*I don't know, I suppose I talk to my friends and go out when I can.*

▶

Family and friends *Do you spend much time with family and friends?*	*When I'm not at work I see my friends at school or when we go out. I see my family when I'm at home.*
Action needed to heal *What do you think you need to do to help improve your skin?*	*I don't know, eat better and drink water I suppose. Maybe take some medicine too.*

TABLE 11.32 **ELIAS' SIGNS AND SYMPTOMS** [2, 6, 9, 10]	
Pulse	68 bpm
Blood pressure	120/80
Temperature	37°C
Respiratory rate	14 resp/min
Face	Open and closed comedones present over the whole face, upper back, neck and shoulders; evidence of cyst formation and some scarring; some comedones are red and inflamed
Body mass index	21 – not often recorded as relevant because Elias is aged under 18 years
Urinalysis	No abnormality detected (NAD)

Results of medical investigations

Diagnosis made on physical examination and no medical investigations have been carried out at this stage.

TABLE 11.33 **UNLIKELY DIAGNOSTIC CONSIDERATIONS** [2, 7, 9, 10, 21, 51, 52]	
CONDITIONS AND CAUSES	**WHY UNLIKELY**
INFECTION AND INFLAMMATION	
Seborrhoeic dermatitis: affects those areas of the skin where there are sebaceous glands such as the face and scalp and occurs more with times of stress	Yellow scales; can be orange-red patches; borders are not well defined and have greasy scales; usually occurs in different typical locations such as centre of the chest, between the nose and lips, eyebrows, navel and groin; more common as an associated symptom of serious illness
Gram-negative folliculitis: characteristic bacterial infection with pustules and cysts on the face	Severe form of acne that is rare and can develop after long-term antibiotic use for acne vulgaris
Nodulocystic acne	Cysts that are inflammatory nodules and very severe
Acne rosacea: inflammatory disorder common on the face with pustules and papules on the nose, forehead and cheeks	More common in women; has associated symptoms of facial flushing; develops often in adult years over the age of 30 rather than in adolescence; rosacea has no comedones

ENDOCRINE/REPRODUCTIVE/SEXUAL HEALTH	
Acne conglobata: most severe form of acne, which is an inflammatory disease with blackheads, papules and abscesses; can be caused by steroid use or tumour-producing androgens; associated with testosterone and occurs mainly in men; appears on the face, neck and chest	Lesions fill with pus, crust over and fill again and can spread and remain a long time; sinus symptoms can be present; usually begins between 18 and 40 years of age; can cause severe scarring
Cushing's syndrome: cause of acne	More common on the back and shoulders; no moon-shaped face, obesity, oedema, hypertension; urinalysis NAD
Diabetes: acne symptoms in insulin resistance	Urinalysis NAD
AUTOIMMUNE DISEASE	
Acne fulminans: immune disease with elevated testosterone levels most common in young adolescent males; fatigue can be a common symptom	Rare; would be associated with fever, muscle and bone pain; lack of appetite; begins with bone pain; will be severe acne that is nodulocystic; onset is abrupt
Dermatitis herpetiformis: usually associated with bullae (fluid filled palpable mass); this condition is usually associated with gluten sensitive enteropathy, which can be asymptomatic Elias is consuming considerable amounts of gluten-containing foods; commonly occurs in early adulthood; more common to present on trunk of body	Extremely itchy rash that is symmetrically distributed over extensor surfaces of the body; no significant abdominal symptoms of pain, bloating, diarrhoea or constipation associated with skin rash

TABLE 11.34 **CONFIRMED DIAGNOSIS**	
CONDITION	**RATIONALE**
Acne vulgaris	Common skin condition of this age group in adolescent males; comedones (black and white heads), papules, pustules and nodules; greasy skin, inflammation and scarring; areas of skin most affected with sebaceous glands

Case analysis

TABLE 11.35 **POSSIBLE DIFFERENTIAL DIAGNOSIS**		
Not ruled out by tests/investigations already done [2, 9–11, 21, 24, 50–52]		
CONDITIONS AND CAUSES	**WHY POSSIBLE**	**WHY UNLIKELY**
FAMILY HEALTH		
Causal factor: **Genetics:** increase family history of acne	Acne – father has a history of acne	
ALLERGIES AND IRRITANTS		
Causal factor: **Food intolerances/allergies**	Fatigue, skin break outs, constipation	Need to assess dietary habits more clearly

RECREATIONAL DRUG USE		
Causal factor: **Drugs:** amphetamines, cannabis, cigarette smoking, alcohol	Acne, constipation, episodes of fatigue, spending a lot of time out of the family home	Eyes are not red, no signs of restlessness, still active with everyday routine; need to ascertain if Elias uses recreational drugs
OBSTRUCTION		
Causal factor: **Intestinal obstruction:** e.g. faecal impaction	Constipation	No abdominal pain, diarrhoea, vomiting reported
FUNCTIONAL DISEASE		
Causal factor: **Functional constipation**	Acne and bowel motion only a couple of times a week; not drinking enough water, high caffeine intake; stress	Need to check if more than 1 in 4 bowel motions is lumpy and hard, and causes strain, a feeling of incomplete evacuation or blockage; need to check if manual help is needed to facilitate a bowel motion passing; if Elias has fewer than 3 evacuations a week
DEGENERATIVE AND DEFICIENCY		
Causal factor: **Organic fatigue:** no major physical abnormalities	Tired, sleep disturbances	Shorter duration than functional fatigue; need to determine if the feeling of fatigue worsens during the day
Anaemia	Fatigue; diet may be low in nutrients	Assess iron and B12-rich food intake
Sunlight	Can exacerbate acne	Can help acne [9]; UVB and UVA phototherapy have been used to treat inflammation of acne [2]
INFECTION AND INFLAMMATION		
Causal factor: **Hygiene**	Excess oil and grease can clog pores	Studies are inconclusive that excess washing helps acne and it may exacerbate in some circumstances [15, 16]
SUPPLEMENTS AND SIDE EFFECTS OF MEDICATION OR DRUGS		
Causal factor: **Medications:** lithium, androgens, corticosteroid therapy	Acne	Corticosteroid-induced acne lesions will often be on the back and shoulders (rather than the face); lesions are usually pustules at the same stage of development with no comedones present; no Cushing's symptoms present
ENDOCRINE/REPRODUCTIVE		
Causal factor: **Hormonal balance:** increase androgens in adolescence	Elias is of the gender and age group that most commonly has acne	

STRESS AND NEUROLOGICAL DISEASE		
Depression	Many adolescents with acne show signs of depression and low self-esteem [2]	Need to explore the level of fatigue and intensity of emotions, interest in daily activities and social network
Causal factor: **Physiologic fatigue:** diagnostic studies within normal limits; symptoms present for less than 14 days and not usually associated with changes in self-esteem, social difficulties or overall mood	Can be caused by depression, caffeine, alcohol, excess sleep or intense emotions	Need to question Elias more on self-perception and duration of fatigue
Causal factor: **Functional fatigue – (depression):** tiredness that lasts several months	May be eating junk food as comfort food during depression	Need to determine if the feeling of fatigue improves during the day
Anxiety	Excess sympathetic nervous system response may affect stress and skin lwevels [22]	Speech not fast, no fast pulse rate or no significant weight loss mentioned; lack of sleep not mentioned, not restless or fidgety, no sweating
Causal factor: **Emotional stress:** affects androgen levels [22]	Acne [15, 16]	
EATING HABITS AND ENERGY		
Causal factor: **Dietary factors:** increased carbohydrates and refined sugars increase insulin and then insulin-like growth factor (IGF-1)	Acne, constipation; excess sugar may increase androgen production by influencing SHBG [11–14, 44]	Studies have shown inconclusive evidence that dietary factors affect acne [15, 16]
Causal factor: **Dairy foods:** due to insulin-like growth factor (IGF-1) in dairy cows (journals below)	Acne, constipation [11, 44]	
Causal factor: **Exercise**	Lack of exercise can exacerbate acne if extreme	Exercise can reduce insulin resistance [45] and stress hormones [46] to improve acne
Causal factor: **Dehydration**	Lack of water, constipation, fatigue	

TABLE 11.36 DECISION TABLE FOR TREATMENT PRIOR TO REFERRAL		
COMPLAINT	CONTEXT	CORE
Treatment for the presenting complaint and symptoms	Treatment for all associated symptoms	Treatment for mental, emotional, spiritual, constitutional, lifestyle issues and metaphysical considerations

TREATMENT PRIORITY	TREATMENT PRIORITY	TREATMENT PRIORITY
• Lifestyle recommendations for skin care and topical application of essential oils to improve skin condition and reduce lesions **NB:** Caution should be exercised to ensure Elias does not sensitise to tea tree oil • Dietary recommendations to reduce excessive sebum production • Herbal skin wash with anti-inflammatory, antibacterial and skin healing action to improve condition of the skin and reduce scarring • Herbal tea with depurative and lymphatic action to help improve skin condition • Herbal tablet formulation containing herbs traditionally used for skin disorders with antiseptic, lymphatic, depurative and anti-inflammatory action to improve skin health and quality • Supplemental nutrients with specific indications for acne treatment that support normal skin function, reduce inflammation, support normal hormonal production, improve skin condition and reduce scarring	• Dietary recommendations to improve diet and intake of essential nutrients specific for skin health as well as for general good health • Dietary recommendations to cut out refined carbohydrates, energy drinks, soft drinks, and processed, fried and fatty foods • Recommendation to identify food allergies or sensitivities and manage accordingly • Skin care recommendations to gently cleanse skin and drain comedones and avoid applying topical preparations, which may clog pores and aggravate acne • Recommendation for Elias to give his skin limited exposure to sunlight **NB:** Caution should be exercised that sun exposure is not excessive • Recommendation for Elias to exercise regularly to help improve glycaemic control and reduce the action of insulin on sebum production • Herbal tea with cholagogue, detoxifying and mild laxative action to improve bowel function and detoxification • Supplemental nutrients to improve status of essential nutrients resulting from Elias' poor diet	• Lifestyle recommendations for Elias to reduce stress levels • Physical therapy suggestion to help reduce stress levels • The focus of topical, dietary and herbal and nutritional treatment is to improve Elias' skin; this will support and improve his psychological health

TABLE 11.37 DECISION TABLE FOR REFERRAL

COMPLAINT	CONTEXT	CORE
Referral for presenting complaint	Referral for all associated physical, dietary and lifestyle concerns	Referral for contributing emotional, mental, spiritual, metaphysical, lifestyle and constitutional factors
REFERRAL FLAGS	**REFERRAL FLAGS**	**REFERRAL FLAGS**
• Unclear if decision not to take antibiotics for acne is Elias' or Dorota's decision	• Episodes of fatigue • Inadequate water intake	• Acne causing self-esteem issues

ISSUES OF SIGNIFICANCE	ISSUES OF SIGNIFICANCE	ISSUES OF SIGNIFICANCE
Nil	• Ingestion of high-caffeine foods for energy • Diet high in refined carbohydrates and saturated fatty acids • Lack of vegetables and fruit in diet • Infrequent bowel motions	• Unclear if Elias is committed to changing diet and lifestyle habits • Spending a lot of time away from the family home
REFERRAL	**REFERRAL**	**REFERRAL**
• Options to be explained clearly to Elias so he can make an informed decision about the benefits and side effects of orthodox treatment and natural therapies • Dermatologist to rule out organic causes for acne	• Guidance with dietary options that would suit Elias to try	• Family counselling • Skin-care counselling

TABLE 11.38 FURTHER INVESTIGATIONS THAT MAY BE NECESSARY [2, 6, 9, 10]	
TEST/INVESTIGATION	**REASON FOR TEST/INVESTIGATION**
FIRST-LINE MEDICAL INVESTIGATIONS:	
Full blood count	Anaemia, inflammation, allergies
Fasting blood glucose test	Diabetes or insulin sensitivity
Blood electrolytes	Dehydration
Skin examination and assessment	Specialist dermatology assessment for severity of acne, dehydration
Abdominal inspection: guarding, rebound tenderness, palpation, abnormal pulsations (auscultation)	Constipation or obstruction
Diet diary	Assess food intake over a period of time
Skin diary	Assess any changes in acne over a period of time or patterns/triggers
IF NECESSARY:	
Serum cortisol	Cushing's syndrome, adrenal response
Abdominal x-ray	Constipation

Confirmed diagnosis

ELIAS AND ACNE VULGARIS WITH PHYSIOLOGIC FATIGUE

Elias is a young man of 16 who has come to the clinic with his parents, Dorota and Henry, for help to clear acne on his face, back and chest. Elias has experienced acne since he was 14 and the condition is worsening. Recently he was diagnosed with acne during a routine visit to his medical practitioner and was offered antibiotic treatment. Dorota wanted to try alternative treatment approaches such as diet and lifestyle changes before the prescribed medication. Their doctor referred Elias to the complementary medicine clinic to collaboratively assist clearing the condition.

Many issues with Elias' diet became evident during the consultation including excessive intake of refined carbohydrates, caffeine and fatty foods. There was an obvious lack of vegetables, wholegrains, fibre and fruit in his diet. Elias works four days a week after school in a takeaway food venue and eats with his family only three nights a week. It was difficult to gain information from Elias himself during the consultation, as he was quite closed and seemed uncomfortable; however, he did share that he only usually has two bowel motions a week. Dorota shares that Elias' acne has had a negative impact on his self-esteem.

Elias has been diagnosed with **acne vulgaris**, which is the most common facial skin condition in adolescent years and can continue into mid-adult life. There are several potential causes for the development of acne and some debate exists regarding lifestyle triggers. Generally it is accepted that androgens in puberty mixed with a genetic susceptibility play a major role in the development of acne. Acne presents on areas of the skin that have an increased numer of sebaceous glands such as the face, back and trunk. Three main features include greasy skin along with open comedones (blackheads), closed comedones (whiteheads), papules and pustules. Additional triggers that may have an aggravating impact on acne include the role of high-carbohydrate diets, excessive consumption of saturated fatty acids, insulin resistance, hygiene and emotional stress. There is still considerable debate about the significance of these factors on the development and severity of acne.

Acne is not a trivial condition, and because it develops during the hormonally charged time of adolescence, it can lead to significant issues of low self-esteem, increased depression and even suicide risk.

General references used in this diagnosis: 2, 6, 9, 10, 53

PRESCRIBED MEDICATION [21, 53]

If diet and lifestyle changes are not helping:
First-line medical therapy
• Antibiotic, keratolytics or retinoid topical agents
Second-line medical therapy
• Low-dose oral antibiotic therapy for at least four months
Third-line therapy
• Oral retinoid drug

TABLE 11.39 **DECISION TABLE FOR TREATMENT (ONCE DIAGNOSIS IS CONFIRMED)**		
COMPLAINT	**CONTEXT**	**CORE**
Treatment for the presenting complaint and symptoms	Treatment for all associated symptoms	Treatment for mental, emotional, spiritual, constitutional, lifestyle issues and metaphysical considerations

▶

TREATMENT PRIORITY	TREATMENT PRIORITY	TREATMENT PRIORITY
• Continue with dietary recommendations to reduce excessive sebum production • Continue with lifestyle recommendations for skin care and topical application of essential oils • Continue with herbal skin wash • Continue with herbal tea and tablet • Continue with supplemental nutrients **NB:** Elias' serum vitamin A levels should be monitored to avoid toxicity; vitamin A supplement should be stopped if Elias takes prescribed retinoid medication • Zinc levels should also be monitored to ensure they stay within normal range • Elias' treatment should be reviewed	• Continue with dietary recommendations to improve intake of essential nutrients and eliminate refined carbohydrates, fried and fatty foods, processed foods, energy drinks and sugar • Manage food allergies or sensitivities • Continue with skin care recommendations and limited sunlight exposure • Continue with exercise for general health and glycaemic control • Continue with herbal tea to improve bowel function and detoxification • Continue with supplemental nutrients at least until Elias' diet improves enough to be providing sufficient levels of essential nutrients	• Continue with lifestyle and physical therapy recommendations for stress management

Treatment aims

- Unblock sebaceous glands [18–20].
- Decrease sebaceous gland activity [18–20].
- Reduce bacterial activity within sebum [18, 20] and support skin response against bacterial infection.
- Reduce inflammation and prevent further scarring and cyst formation [18, 19].
- Improve Elias' diet and nutritional status [18–20].
- Improve bowel function and detoxification [19, 20].
- Enhance clearance of dihydrotestosterone to reduce its effects on the skin [19, 20].
- Identify and manage food sensitivities [18, 20].
- Support Elias' stress response and psychological health [22].

Lifestyle alterations/considerations

- Encourage Elias to wash his skin with a mild cleanser no more than twice daily [18, 20].
- Encourage Elias to avoid scrubbing, picking or squeezing his pimples [18]. Squeezing can increase inflammation and scarring of surrounding tissue [18].
- Elias may drain comedones with a comedo extractor [19, 21] but should exercise care not to damage or force sebum into surrounding tissue [18].
- Encourage Elias to avoid applying oil-based creams or topical preparations that may clog pores and aggravate his acne [18].
- Topical application of lavender [18] or tea tree oil [18, 19, 21] directly onto blemishes can reduce bacterial levels and minimise inflammation. A 5 per cent tea tree oil gel is effective in improving skin condition and reducing lesions in acne [43].
- Elias may find washing his skin with oatmeal and/or using a facial mask made with oats, avocado, aloe vera and Manuka honey may improve his skin quality [17].

- Topical application of vitamin E oil [18] and calendula cream [32, 34] may help heal lesions and reduce scarring.
- Elias may benefit from stress-management techniques such as relaxation therapies, yoga, tai-chi or meditation [21–23].
- Elias may benefit from limited exposure to sunlight [17, 18].
- Elias may benefit from regular exercise to improve glycaemic control [45] and help manage his stress [46].

Dietary suggestions

- Encourage Elias to eliminate refined carbohydrates, processed foods, saturated and *trans* fats [18, 19, 20].
- A low GI diet is beneficial in acne [24, 26, 27]. Hyperinsulinaemia may promote production of excessive sebum via androgenic action [24, 26, 27].
- Encourage Elias to significantly increase consumption of whole and unrefined foods, dietary fibre, fruit and vegetables [18, 20, 26]. Encourage him to make healthier food choices from his school canteen and workplace by choosing whole grains, fresh fruit and vegetables and avoid processed meats, fried and fatty foods [18, 20, 26].
- Encourage Elias to increase consumption of foods high in omega-3 fatty acids [20, 26].
- Elias may benefit from reducing or eliminating dairy food [11].
- Encourage Elias to avoid soft drinks and energy drinks [20, 24, 26, 27] and start drinking water instead.
- Encourage Elias to increase dietary intake of zinc, vitamin A and B vitamins, which are all essential nutrients for skin health and are indicated for use in acne [18, 19, 20, 25].

Physical treatment suggestions

- Hydrotherapy: a facial steam treatment to clean the skin followed by an oatmeal sponge. Apply a face pack [47]. A cold shower on the face to finish [48].
- Constitutional hydrotherapy for general detoxing [49].
- Arm, wrist, ankle affusions for fatigue [48].
- Short cold head shower for fatigue [44].
- Neutral oatmeal baths for skin on whole body when the skin is flaring up [47, 48].
- Alternating hot/cold showers daily for immune health and circulation [48].
- Elias may experience benefit from massage therapy to help manage stress [28, 29].

TABLE 11.40 **HERBAL SKIN WASH (1:2 LIQUID EXTRACTS)**		
HERB	**FORMULA**	**RATIONALE**
Echinacea root *Echinacea purpurea*	33 mL	Antimicrobial [30,31]; topical application traditionally used for inflammatory skin conditions [30, 31]
Calendula *Calendula officinalis*	33 mL	Lymphatic [32, 34]; anti-inflammatory [32, 34]; antimicrobial [32, 34]; traditionally used for inflammatory skin lesions and sebaceous cysts [32, 34]; topical application of calendula is beneficial as an antiseptic to reduce inflammation and promote skin healing [30, 32]
Witch hazel *Hamamelis virginiana*	33 mL	Astringent [32, 36]; anti-inflammatory [32]; beneficial as a topical application to inflamed swellings [32, 36]
Supply:	100 mL	Dose: 2½ mL of solution diluted in 60 mL warm water; gently wash skin with solution twice daily

TABLE 11.41 HERBAL FORMULA IN TABLET FORM TO IMPROVE COMPLIANCE

HERB	DOSE PER TABLET	RATIONALE
Cleavers *Galium aparine*	360 mg	Depurative [34, 36]; anti-inflammatory [36]; traditionally used for skin disorders [34, 37]
Sarsaparilla *Smilax ornata*	360 mg	Antiseptic [32]; depurative [37]; traditionally used for skin disorders [32, 37]
Oregon grape *Berberis aquifolium*	360 mg	Depurative [34]; anti-inflammatory [34, 38]; mild cholagogue [32, 34]; laxative [32]; antimicrobial [34, 38]; traditionally used for skin disorders [34, 37]; anticomedogenic [38]
Burdock *Arctium lappa*	270 mg	Depurative [34, 36]; mild laxative [34]; traditionally used for skin conditions [36]
Yellow dock *Rumex crispus*	270 mg	Depurative [34, 37]; cholagogue [32, 34]; mild laxative [32, 34]; traditionally used for skin complaints associated with constipation [32, 36]

Dose: 1 tablet 3 times daily

Myrrh (*Commiphora molmol*) tablet containing 25 mg guggulsterone twice daily [30]
Antiseptic [30]; anti-inflammatory [30, 38]; increases glucose tolerance [38]; anticomedogenic [38]; myrrh supplement containing 25 mg guggulsterone twice daily is effective in improving acne [39, 40]

TABLE 11.42 HERBAL TEA

Alternative to coffee

HERB	FORMULA	RATIONALE
Dandelion root *Taraxacum officinale*	2 parts	Choleretic [30, 33]; enhances liver detoxification [30]; anti-inflammatory [30]; mild laxative effect [30, 33]; traditionally used for skin conditions associated with disordered digestive function [34]
Peppermint leaves *Mentha × piperita*	1 part	Cholagogue [30, 31]; antimicrobial [30, 31]; included in tea formula to improve taste and compliance [31]
Echinacea root *Echinacea purpurea*	2 parts	Antimicrobial [30, 31]; immunostimulant [30, 31]; lymphatic [31]; antioxidant [30, 31]; traditionally used to treat acne [31]
Calendula *Calendula officinalis*	1 part	See above

Decoction: 1 tsp per cup – 1 cup 3 times daily

TABLE 11.43 NUTRITIONAL SUPPLEMENTS

SUPPLEMENT AND DOSE	RATIONALE
Zinc gluconate supplement providing 50 mg elemental zinc daily [30]	Required for production of hormones and retinol-binding protein [19, 25]; essential for normal skin function [19, 25, 33]; low levels of epidermal zinc are associated with acne [42]; supplementation may be beneficial in inflammatory acne [25, 41]
Vitamin A 10,000 IU [18]	Necessary for maintenance of epithelial tissue [18, 33]; reduces sebum production [19] and hyperkeratinisation [18, 19]; low skin and serum levels of vitamin A are associated with acne [18]
Supplement providing a daily dose of **vitamin E** 400 IU and **selenium** 200 µg [18]	Can reduce inflammatory skin lesions in acne [18]; supplemental vitamin E and selenium can improve acne [19]
High-potency practitioner-strength **multivitamin, mineral and antioxidant supplement** providing therapeutic doses of B-group vitamins and chromium [18, 20]	To improve Elias' nutritional and antioxidant status due to his poor diet; supplemental vitamin B2 and B6 is beneficial in acne [30]; chromium improves glucose control [18, 33, 35] and is therefore helpful in reducing hyperinsulinaemia, which can increase sebum production [24, 26, 27]

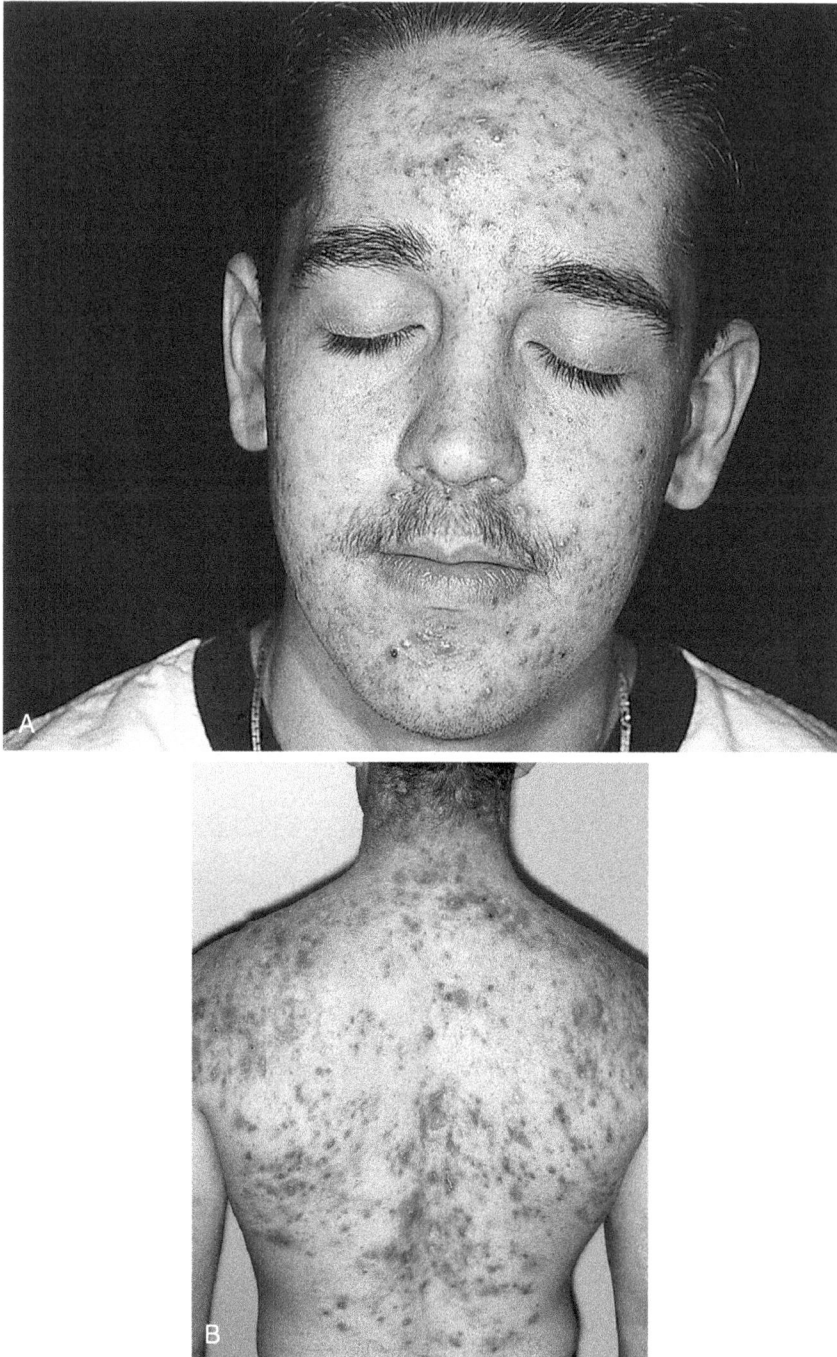

Figure 11.1 Acne vulgaris. A [54]; B [55]

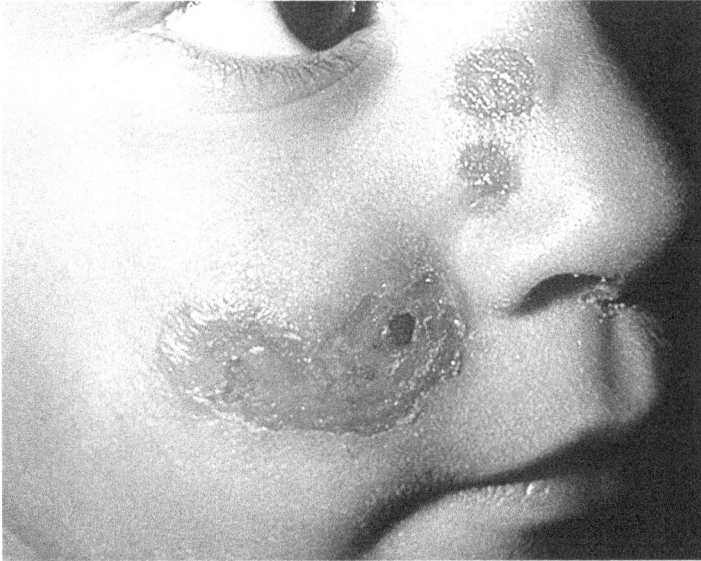

Figure 11.2 *Impetigo.* [55]

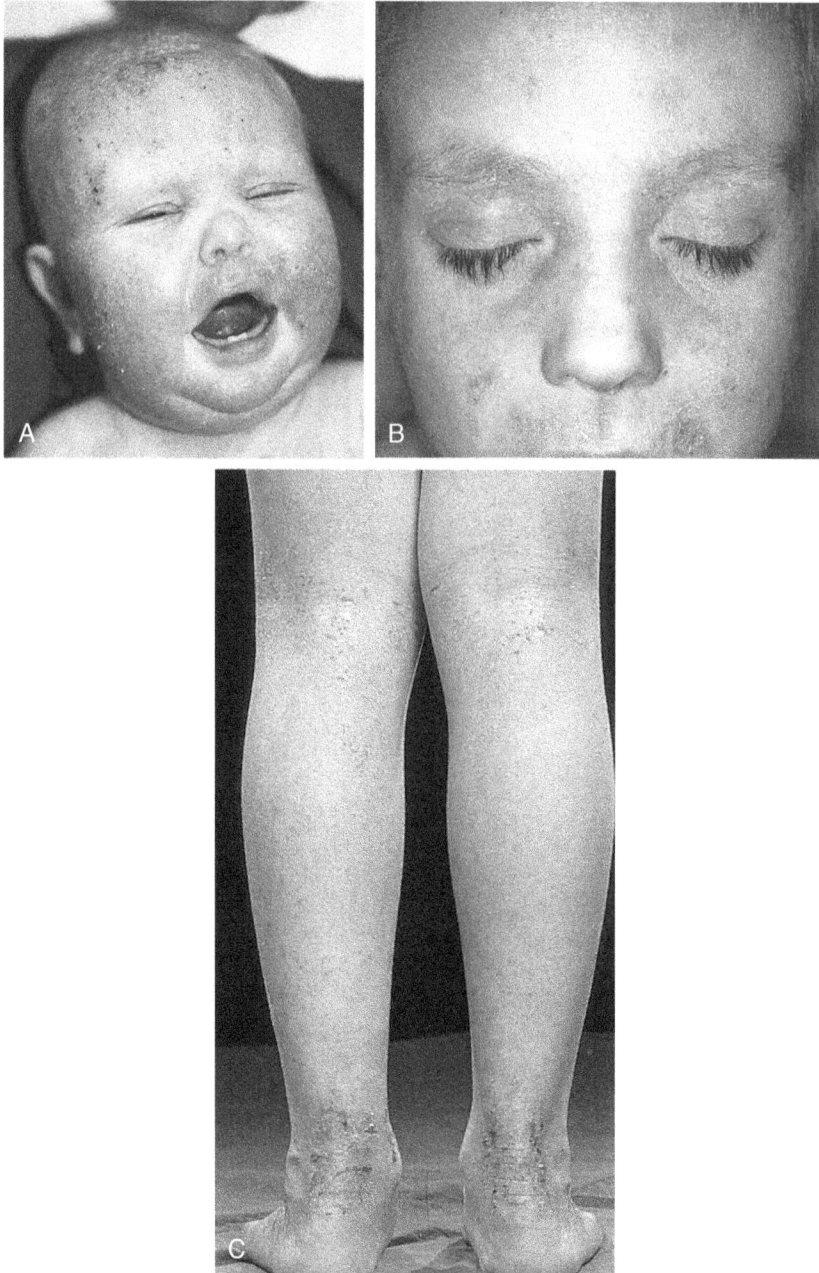

Figure 11.3 Atopic dermatitis. A, B [57]; C [59]

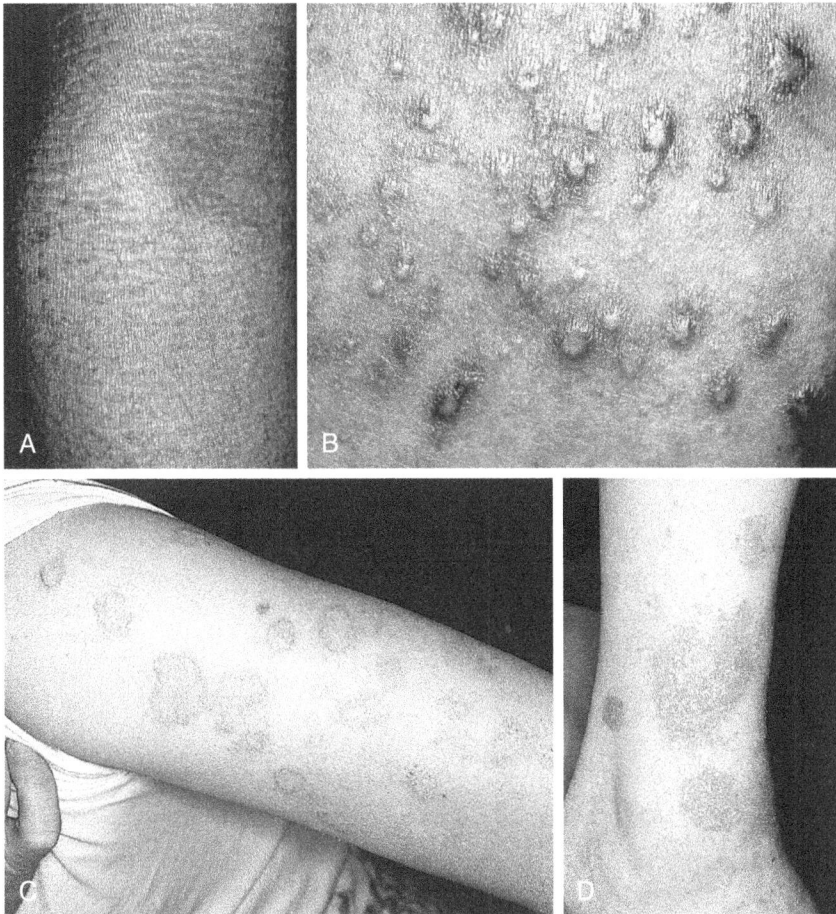

Figure 11.4 *Dermatitis. A: Lichenification and thickening, antecubital fossa [55]; B: Prurigo-like papules in adult atopic dermatitis [55]; C: Nummular eczema on the arm [54]; D: Nummular eczema on the ankle [54]*

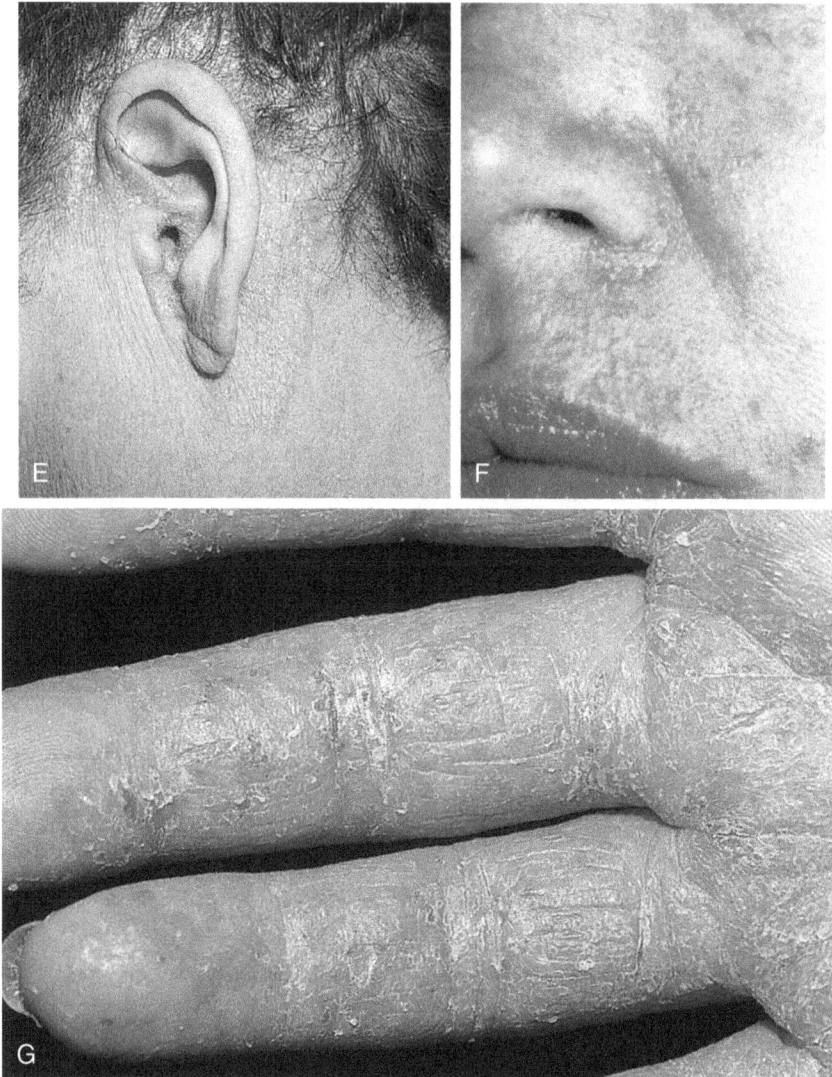

Figure 11.4, cont'd

E: Seborrhoeic dermatitis of the postauricular region [54]; F: Seborrhoeic dermatitis of the nasolabial region [58]; G: Irritant contact dermatitis [58]

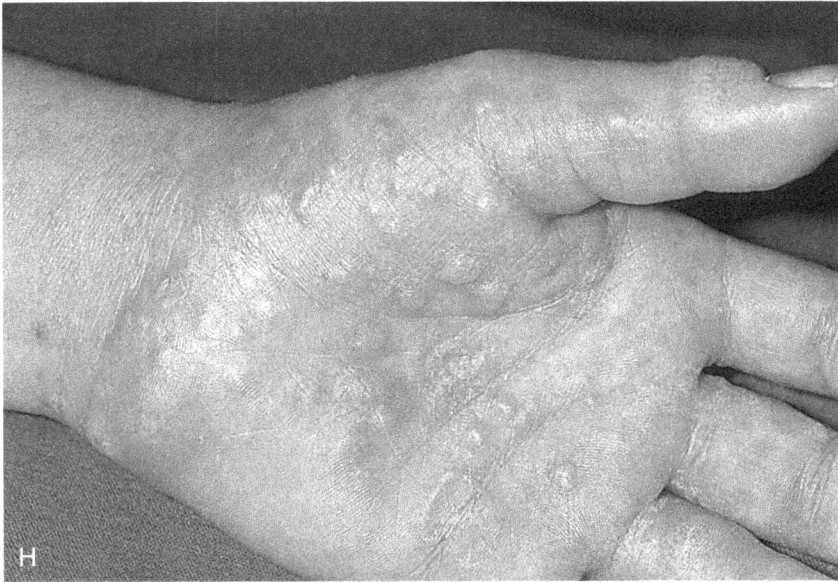

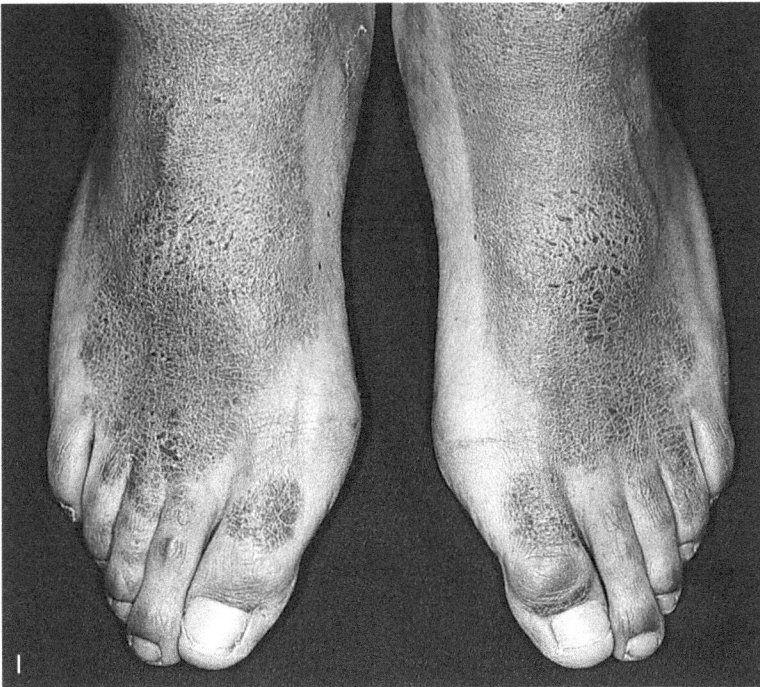

Figure 11.4, cont'd

H: Dyshidrotic eczema (pompholyx) [58]; I: Contact dermatitis of the foot (shoe dermatitis) [54]

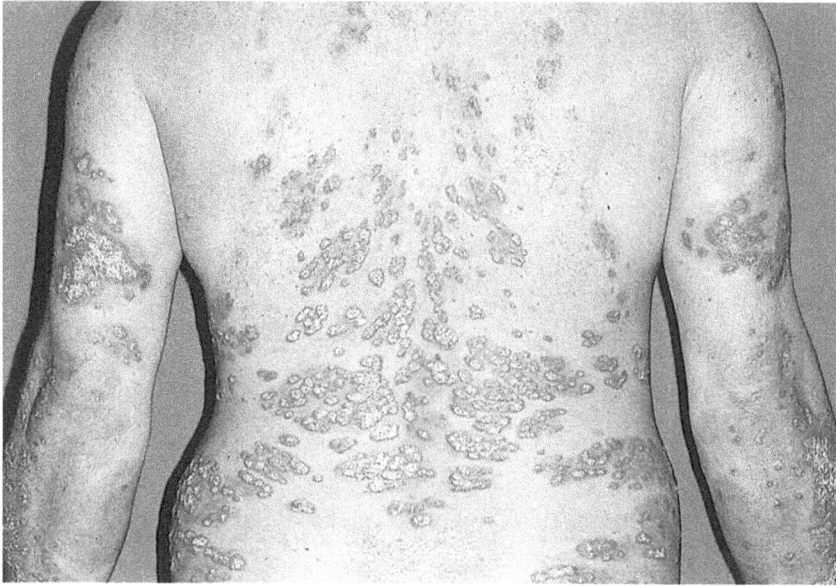

Figure 11.5 *Psoriasis vulgaris. [54]*

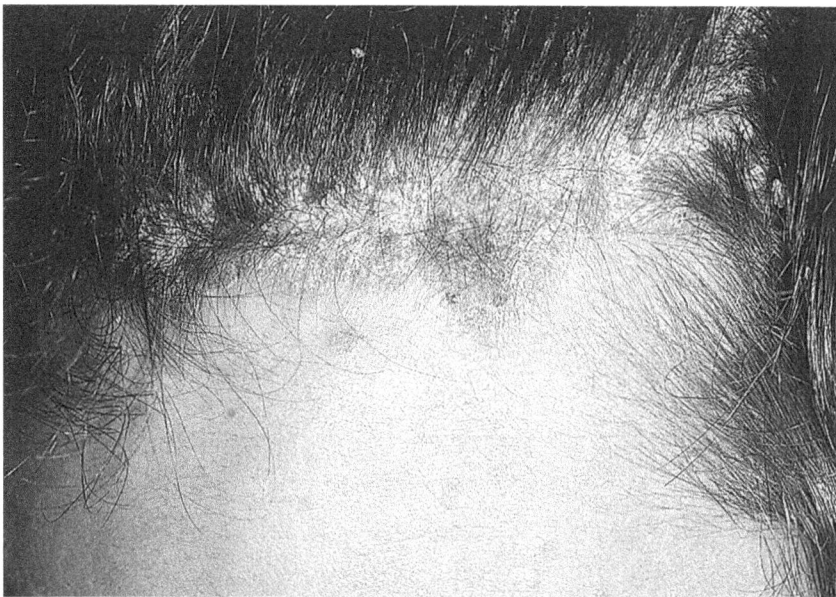

Figure 11.6 *Psoriasis vulgaris of the scalp. [54]*

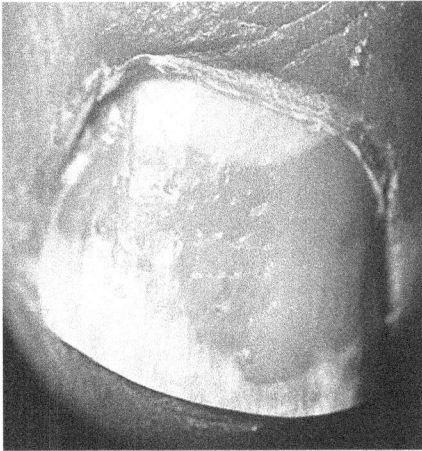

Figure 11.7 Psoriasis vulgaris on nails. [55]

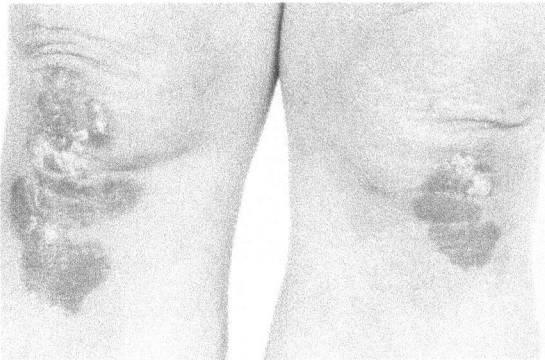

Figure 11.8 Psoriasis on knees. [60]

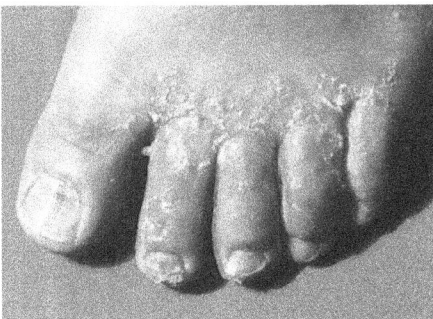

Figure 11.9 Fungal infection on feet/toes. [61]

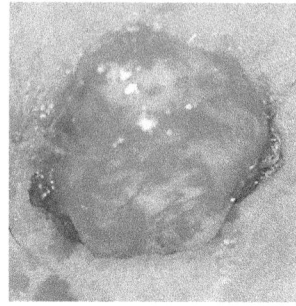

Figure 11.10 Squamous cell cancer. [62]

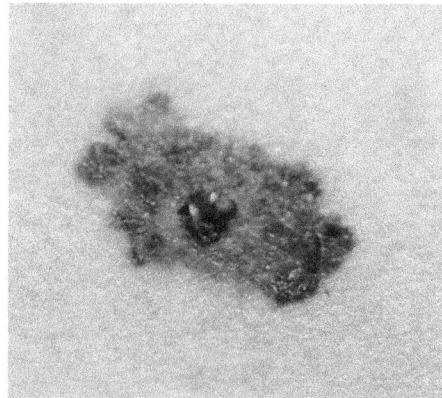

Figure 11.11 Malignant melanoma. [63]

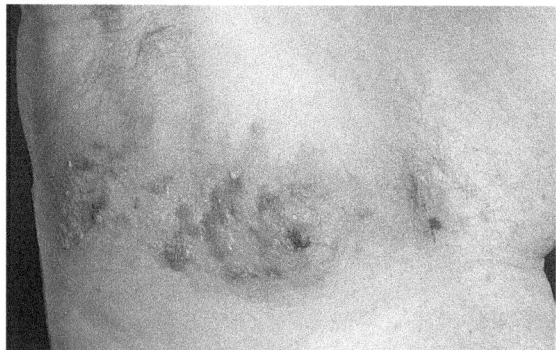

Figure 11.12 Shingles. [64]

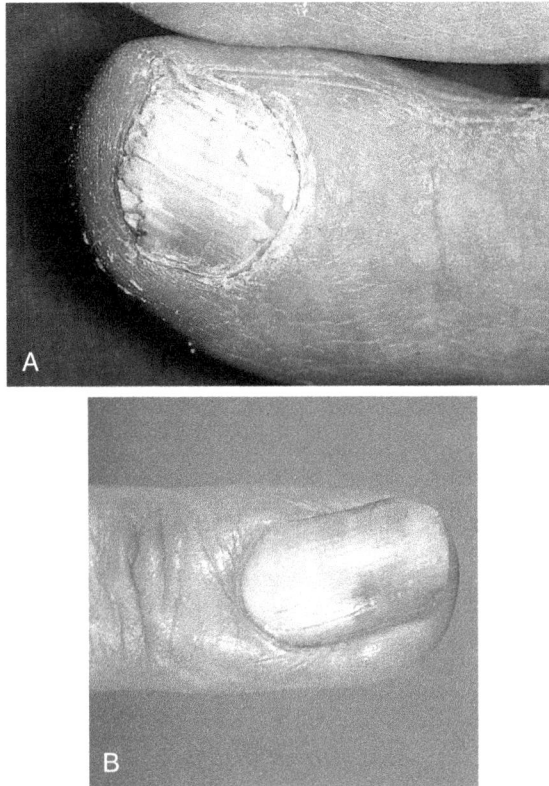

Figure 11.13 A: *Tinea infection of the nail [56]; Psoriasis of the nail [65].*

References

[1] N.J. Talley, S. O'Connor, Pocket Clinical Examination, third edn, Churchill Livingstone Elsevier, Australia, 2009.

[2] P. Kumar, C. Clark, Clinical Medicine, sixth edn, Elsevier Saunders, London, 2005.

[3] J. Silverman, S. Kurtz, J. Draper, Skills for Communicating with Patients, second edn, Radcliff Publishing, Oxford, 2000.

[4] R. Neighbour, The Inner Consultation; how to develop an effective and intuitive consulting style, Radcliff Publishing, Oxon, 2005.

[5] M. Lloyd, R. Bor, Communication skills for medicine, third edn, Churchill Livingstone Elsevier, Edinburgh, 2009.

[6] G. Douglas, F. Nicol, C. Robertson, Macleod's Clinical Examination, twelfth edn., Churchill Livingstone Elsevier, 2009.

[7] J. Jamison, Differential Diagnosis for Primary Care, second edn, Churchill Livingstone Elsevier, London, 2006.

[8] A. Polmear (Ed.), Evidence-Based Diagnosis in Primary Care, Churchill Livingstone Elsevier, 2008, pp. 274–283.

[9] R. Berkow, A.J. Fletcher, M.H. Beers, The Merck Manual. sixteenth edn. Rathway, N.J: Merck Research Laboratories, 1993 (later edition).

[10] R.H. Seller, Differential Diagnosis of Common Complaints, fiftth ed., Saunders, Elsevier Philadelphia, 2007 .

[11] C.A. Adebamowo, D. Spiegelman, F.W. Danby, A.L. Frazier, W.C. Willett, M.D. Holmes, High school dietary dairy intake and teenage acne, Journal of the American Academy of Dermatology 52 (2005) 207–214.

[12] C. Adebamowo, D. Spiegelman, C. Berkey, F. Danby, M. Rockett, H. Colditz, G. Willett, W. Holmes. Milk consumption and acne in teenaged boys, Journal of the American Academy of Dermatology 58 (5) (2005) 787–793.

[13] R. Smith, N. Mann, H. Mäkeläinen, J. Roper, A. Braue, G. Varigos, A pilot study to determine the short-term effects of a low glycemic load diet on hormonal markers of acne: a nonrandomized, parallel, controlled feeding trial, Mol Nutr Food Res 52 (6) (2008) 718–726.

[14] D.M. Selva, K.N. Hogeveen, S.M. Innis, G.L. Hammond, Monosaccharide-induced lipogenesis regulates the human hepatic sex hormone binding globulin gene, J Clin Invest 117 (12) (2007) 3979–3987.

[15] R.N. Smith, N.J. Mann, A. Braue, H. Mäkeläinen, G.A. Varigos, The effect of a high-protein, low glycemic-load diet versus a conventional, high glycemic-load diet on biochemical parameters associated with acne vulgaris: A randomized, investigator-masked, controlled trial, J Am Acad Dermatol 57 (2) (2007) 247–256.

[16] G.F. Webster, Acne Vulgaris. Clinical review, British Medical Journal 325 (2002) 475–479.

[17] P. Magin, D. Pond, W. Smith, A. Watson, A systematic review of the evidence for 'myths and misconceptions' in acne management: diet, face-washing and sunlight, Family Practice 22 (2005) 62–70.

[18] J. Jamison, Clinical Guide to Nutrition and Dietary Supplements in Disease Management, Churchill Livingstone, Edinburgh, 2003.

[19] J.E. Pizzorno, M.T. Murray, H. Joiner-Bey, The Clinicians Handbook of Natural Medicine, second edn, Churchill Livingstone, St Louis, 2008.

[20] H. Osiecki, The Physicians Handbook of Clinical Nutrition, seventh edn, Bioconcepts, Eagle Farm, 2000.

[21] J.S. Strauss, D.P. Krowchuck, J.J. Leyden, A.W. Lucky, A.R. Shalita, E.C. Siegfried, D.M. Thiboutot, et al., Guidelines of care for acne vulgaris management, Journal of the American Academy of Dermatology 56 (2007) 651–663.

[22] A. Chiu, S.Y. Chon, A.B. Kimball, The Response of Skin Disease to Stress; Changes in the severity of Acne Vulgaris as Affected by Examination Stress, Archives of Dermatology 139 (2003) 897–900.

[23] H. Hughes, B.W. Brown, G.F. Lawlis, J.E. Fulton, Treatment of acne vulgaris by biofeedback relaxation and cognitive imagery, J Psychosom Res 27 (3) (1983) 185–191.

[24] R.N. Smith, N.J. Mann, A. Braue, H. Makelainen, G.A. Varigos, The effect of a high-protein, low glycaemic load diet versus a conventional, high glycaemic load diet on biochemical parameters associated with acne vulgaris: A randomized, investigator-masked, controlled trial, Journal of the American Academy of Dermatology 57 (2007) 247–256.

[25] Y.B. Nitzan, A.B. Cohen, Zinc in skin pathology and care, Journal of Dermatological Treatment 17 (2006) 205–210.

[26] L. Cordain, Implications for the Role of Diet in Acne, Seminars in Cutaneous Medicine and Surgery 24 (2005) 84–91.

[27] R. Wolf, H. Matz, E. Orion, Acne and Diet, Clinics in Dermatology 22 (2004) 387–393.

[28] C.A. Moyer, J. Rounds, J.W. Hannum, A Meta-Analysis of Massage Therapy Research, Psychological Bulletin 130 (1) (2004) 3–18.

[29] T. Field, G. Robinson, F. Scafidi, R. Nawrocki, A. Goncalves, Massage therapy reduces anxiety and enhances EEG pattern of alertness and math computations, International Journal of Neuroscience 86 (1996) 197–205.

[30] L. Braun, M. Cohen, Herbs & Natural Supplements: An evidence based guide, second edn, Elsevier, Sydney, 2007.

[31] S. Mills, K. Bone, Principles & Practice of Phytotherapy; Modern Herbal Medicine, Churchill Livingstone, Edinburgh: London, 2000.

[32] British Herbal Medicine Association, British Herbal Pharmacopoeia, BHMA, 1983.

[33] H. Osiecki, The Nutrient Bible, seventh edn, BioConcepts Publishing, Eagle Farm, 2008.

[34] S. Mills, K. Bone, The Essential Guide to Herbal Safety, Churchill Livingstone, St Louis, 2005.

[35] J. Higdon, An Evidence Based Approach to Vitamins and Minerals, Thieme, New York, 2003.

[36] D. Hoffman, The New Holistic Herbal, Element Books Ltd, Shaftesbury, Dorset, 1990.

[37] M. Morgan, Herbs for the oral treatment of skin conditions, A Phytotherapist's Perspective 65 (2005) 1–2.

[38] E. Yarnell, K. Abascai, Herbal Medicine for Acne Vulgaris, J Altern Complement Med 12 (6) (2006) 303–309.

[39] J. Dogra, N. Aneja, V.N. Saxena, Oral gugulipid in acne vulgaris management. Indian Journal of Dermatology, Venerology and Leprology 56 (5) (1990) 381–383.

[40] D.M. Thappa, J. Dogra, Nodulocystic acne: oral gugulipid versus tetracycline, Journal of Dermatology 21 (10) (1994) 729–731.

[41] B. Dreno, P. Foulc, A. Reynaud, D. Moyse, H. Habert, H. Richet, Effect of zinc gluconate on propionibacterium acnes resistance to erythromycin in patients with inflammatory acne: in vitro and in vivo study, European Journal of Dermatology 15 (3) (2005) 152–155.

[42] G. Michaelsson, K. Ljunghall, Patients with dermatitis herpetiformis, acne, psoriasis and Darier's disease have low epidermal zinc concentrations, Acta Derm Venerol 70 (4) (1990) 304–308.

[43] I.B. Bassett, D.L. Pannowitz, R.S. Barnetson, A comparative study of tea-tree oil versus benzoylperoxide in the treatment of acne, Medical Journal of Australia 153 (8) (1990) 455–458.

[44] M. Sinclair, Modern Hydrotherapy for the Massage Therapist, Lippincott Williams & Wilkins, Baltimore, 2008.

[45] A. Maiorana, G. O'Driscoll, C. Goodman, R. Taylor, D. Green, Combined aerobic and resistance exercise improves glycemic control and fitness in type 2 diabetes, Diabetes Research and Clinical Practice 56 (2002) 115–123.

[46] A. Byrne, G.D. Byrne, The effect of exercise on depression, anxiety and other mood states: A review, J Psychosom Res 37 (6) (1993) 565–574.

[47] L. Chaitow, Hydrotherapy, water therapy for health and beauty, Element, Dorset, 1999.

[48] D.D. Buchman, The complete book of water healing, Contemporary Books, McGraw-Hill Companies, New York, 2001.

[49] W. Boyle, A. Saine, Lectures in Naturopathic Hydrotherapy, Eclectic Medical Publications, Oregon, 1988.

[50] S. Feldman, R.E. Careccia, K.L. Barham, J. Hancox, Diagnosis and treatment of acne, Am Fam Physician 69 (9) (2004) 2123–2130.

[51] Y.M. Mengesha, M.L. Bennett, Pustular skin disorders: diagnosis and treatment, Am J Clin Dermatol 3 (6) (2002) 389–400.

[52] K.F. Carter, L.T. Dufour, C.N. Ballard, Identifying primary skin lesions, Nursing 33 (2003) 68–69.

[53] W.D. James, Acne, N Engl J Med 352 (2005) 1463–1472.

[54] J.P. Callen, K.E. Greer, A.S. Paller, L.J. Swinyer, Color Atlas of Dermatology 2e, Saunders, Philadelphia, 1999.

[55] W. James, T. Berger, D. Elston, Andrews' Diseases of the Skin 10e, Saunders, Philadelphia, 2005.

[56] P. Kumar, C. Clark, Clinical Medicine, 6th edn., Elsevier Saunders, London, 2005 Fig. 23.7 p. 1323.

[57] A.S. Paller, A.J. Mancini, Hurwitz Clinical Pediatric Dermatology 3e, Saunders, Philadelphia, 2006.

[58] G.M. White, N.H. Cox, Diseases of the Skin: A Color Atlas and Text 2e, Mosby, , 2006.

[59] G. Douglas, F. Nicol, C. Robertson, Macleod's Clinical Examination, 12th edn, Elsevier, Churchill Livingstone, 2009 Figure 4.3 p. 75.

[60] G. Douglas, F. Nicol, C. Robertson, Macleod's Clinical Examination, 12th edn, Elsevier, Churchill Livingstone, 2009 Figure 4.4 p. 75.

[61] G. Douglas, F. Nicol, C. Robertson, Macleod's Clinical Examination, 12th edn, Elsevier, Churchill Livingstone, 2009 Fig. 4.8 p. 77.

[62] G. Douglas, F. Nicol, C. Robertson, Macleod's Clinical Examination, 12th edn, Elsevier, Churchill Livingstone, 2009 Fig. 4.10 p. 79.

[63] G. Douglas, F. Nicol, C. Robertson, Macleod's Clinical Examination, 12th edn, Elsevier, Churchill Livingstone, 2009 Fig. 4.20 p. 84.

[64] G. Douglas, F. Nicol, C. Robertson, Macleod's Clinical Examination, 12th edn, Elsevier, Churchill Livingstone, 2009 Fig. 4.9 p. 77.

[65] P. Kumar, C. Clark, Clinical medicine, 6th edn, Elsevier Saunders, London, 2005 Fig. 23.17 p. 1333.

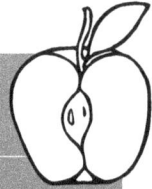

Generic clinical questions

Mnemonic key

SKIN OF THE APPLE	FLESH OF THE APPLE	SEED OF THE APPLE
COMPLAINT	CONTEXT	CORE
Understand the complaint	Understand the disease	Understand the client
'Outer layer' **O**nset **U**nderstanding the cause (client) **T**iming (duration, frequency) **E**xacerbating factors **R**elieving factors **L**ocation and radiation **A**ccount and description **Y**our practitioner impression **E**xamination and inspection **R**ating scale	**'Factors of disease'** **F**amily health **A**llergies and irritants **C**ancer and heart disease **T**rauma and pre-existing illness **O**bstruction and foreign body **R**ecreational drug use **S**urgery and hospitilisation **O**ccupational toxins and hazards **F**unctional disease **D**egenerative and deficiency **I**nfection and inflammation **S**upplements and side effects of medication and drugs **E**ndocrine/reproductive **A**utoimmune disease **S**tress and neurological **E**ating habits and energy	**'Seeds of health'** **S**upport systems **E**motional health **E**nvironmental wellness **D**aily activities **S**tress release **O**ccupation **F**amily and friends **H**ome life **E**ducation and learning **A**ction needed to heal **L**ong-term goals **T**ime to heal **H**as not been well since

Example questions

Demographic information

Name, age, date of birth, sex, height, weight, title, number of children/dependants, occupation, contact details, contact details of GP and/or other health professionals they are currently receiving treatment from.

Complaint questions

Define the presenting complaint and symptoms. Location, timing, character, pattern and modalities [1, 5, 8–14].

INTRODUCTION
Introduce yourself and what to expect from consultation. *Hello, I am [insert name]. Come in and take a seat. I am your CAM practitioner today and my role is to…* *Can I confirm your correct name? What would you prefer I call you?* [1, 7] *So, you are [insert name]. Did I pronounce and spell that correctly?* [7] *You mentioned you are from [insert country]. I'm not familiar with your culture. Do you have a preference for the way I greet you?* [1, 7]
INTRODUCE CAM
Have you been to a CAM therapist before? *Can you tell me what you understand about CAM therapy?*
INTRODUCE THE CLIENT'S PRESENTING COMPLAINT [1]
I would like to spend [insert amount of time] to discuss the reason you are visiting today. Is that alright with you? *Can you tell me what health concerns brought you to have a consultation today?* [7] *How can I help you today?* *What would you like to talk about today?*

DEFINING THE COMPLAINT
Analogy: Skin of the apple Using the mnemonic 'OUTER LAYER'
ONSET
When did you first notice [the complaint]?
UNDERSTANDING THE CAUSE (CLIENT)
So, I understand you have been experiencing [insert symptoms]. Did I get that right? [1] *Can I check I have understood your symptoms correctly … Let me know if I have missed anything …* [1]
TIMING (DURATION, FREQUENCY)
Have you ever noticed this particular complaint before? *How long does [the complaint] last and how often does it occur?*
EXACERBATING FACTORS
Describe what makes [the complaint] worse. *Does [the complaint] prevent you from doing anything in your daily life?*
RELIEVING FACTORS
Describe what makes [the complaint] better.
LOCATION AND RADIATION
Where do you feel [the complaint]? *Can you point to where you feel [the complaint]?* *Does [the complaint] stay in the same area or does it radiate?*

▶

▶
ACCOUNT AND DESCRIPTION
What does [the complaint] feel like generally? *How does it feel now?* *Has [the complaint] changed character since it first began?*

YOUR PRACTITIONER IMPRESSION
What do you notice about the client?

EXAMINATION AND INSPECTION
I can see you have quite a few health concerns. I would like to ask you some general questions and perhaps examine you before we discuss which health concern to begin looking into first. Is that alright with you? [1]

RATING SCALE
On a scale of 1 to 10 how would you rate the complaint?

CHILDREN IN PAIN
Questions directed to the child: Use questioning that involves a favourite toy if it helps the child to share information: *How about we look at your toy's ear* (or relevant body part) *and ask him where it really hurts?* *How does your ear* (or relevant body part) *feel when it hurts?* *How does your toy's ear* (or relevant body part) *feel when it hurts?* *What do you think your toy would need to feel better?* *Does the pain stop you from doing any favourite things or playing with friends?*
Questions for parents: *Can you describe when the pain occurs?* *How long does the pain last?* *Is there anything that makes the pain better or worse?* *To help me understand how much pain your child is in when they are experiencing an acute episode, can you tell me if they are reassured by a hug or being talked to or is there nothing that can comfort him?* *Can your child lie quietly when s/he has the pain or is s/he restless, irritable and tense?* *Does your child's facial expression have a frown? Do they seem withdrawn or disinterested?* *When your child has pain will their chin quiver and jaw clench?* *Does your child's pain stop you from doing anything from day to day?*

Context questions

These questions are to be used as a guide to provide a framework to put the presenting complaint into context and define the cause of the symptoms. It is likely that new symptoms will present following this *context* questioning process where it becomes necessary to ask *complaint* questions for each new symptom picture [1, 2, 4–15].

CONTEXT
Put the presenting complaint into context to *understand the disease*. Common contributing physical, dietary and lifestyle factors that may trigger the presenting complaint and differential diagnosis considerations. **Analogy:** The flesh of the apple Using the mnemonic 'FACTORS OF DISEASE'

▶

FAMILY HEALTH

Describe your family health history.
Describe your mother's/father's/siblings' health.
Can you tell me any information about your birth?
Do you know your biological parents?
Where were you born?

ALLERGIES AND IRRITANTS

Do you have any allergies?

Cough and breathing

Does the cough become worse in the late afternoon or early evening? (asthma, coming home from work in the evening to high pollen area if they have seasonal allergies)
Is your cough worse at night with no sign of shortness of breath? (allergic origin)
Does your cough reoccur at certain times of the year? (seasonal allergies)
Do you experience sneezing or nasal discharge, conjunctivitis and itching on the roof of the mouth with the cough? (allergies)

Eye

Is the red eye associated with discharge, itchy eyes or roof of the mouth, burning of the eyes, sneezing, runny nose or is worse at particular times of the year? (perennial allergic conjunctivitis, seasonal allergic conjunctivitis, vernal keratoconjunctivitis in males aged 3–20 years, contact ophthalmic conjunctivitis)
Do you experience mild pain in the eyes when they are red? (conjunctivitis, allergies)
Do the symptoms of allergic conjunctivitis become worse with forced-air heaters? (dust mites)
Does the generalised red eye(s) have discharge that is scanty, stringy and white? (allergic conjunctivitis)

Nose

Are your nasal symptoms worse in spring or summer? (tree, grass or weed allergies)
Are your nasal symptoms worse after making the bed or doing the house cleaning? (dust mite allergy)
Are your nasal symptoms worse after contact with animals? (allergy to animal dander)

Integumentary

Has the rash on your feet worsened since wearing leather shoes? (shoe dermatitis due to the chrome used in leather tanning)
Is the itching associated with a significant red rash within 24 hours of eating any particular food? (allergy)
Is the itchy skin associated with weeping vesicles? (allergic dermatitis)
Do your itchy skin lesions occur on only one side of your body? (asymmetrical contact dermatitis)
Do your itchy skin lesions occur more often on both sides of your body? (symmetrical atopic dermatitis)
Is the itch associated with wheals or papules? (contact allergy, insect bites)
Is the itching associated with cosmetics or chemicals? (allergic contact dermatitis)

CANCER AND HEART DISEASE

CANCER

Digestive system

Is the indigestion continuous, made worse by food, and associated with symptoms of decreased appetite, nausea and weight loss? (gastric cancer)

Urinary system

Is the increased urination at night associated with decreased urine volume? (renal failure, bladder cancer)
Do you experience blood in the urine along with backache? (prostate cancer)
Do you experience blood in your urine but have no pain with it? (bladder cancer)

Respiratory system

Have you noticed blood in the sputum when you cough? (carcinoma possibility)
Is the sputum associated with your cough profuse and watery? (alveolar cell carcinoma)

Throat

Have you experienced a change in your voice over a period of time? (laryngeal origin)
Have you experienced a change in your voice, hoarseness, difficulty swallowing or breathing? (thyroid tumour)
Have you noticed a nodule or lump around your Adam's apple, with raised lymph nodes around your neck? (thyroid tumour)

Integumentary

Is the dry, scaly skin associated with a thickening of the palm and soles? (Hodgkin's disease)
Is the itchy bottom associated with a thick discharge and persistent lump? (anal cancer or wart)
Does the itchy skin have no sign of a lesion and appear pale, and is it made worse by having a hot shower, or when you have alcohol? (leukaemia)
Is the itchy skin worse and appear red after having a hot shower or when you have alcohol? (polycythemia vera)
Is the itchy skin worse when you have a hot shower or when you have alcohol, and is it associated with night sweats? (lymphoma)

Musculoskeletal

Have you had symptoms of herpes (Zoster) associated with back pain? (consider cancer)
Is the shoulder-tip pain associated with difficult breathing or increased sweating? (bronchogenic carcinoma)
Is the muscle weakness associated with unexplained weight loss? (malignant myopathy)

HEART DISEASE
Cough

Is your cough worse at night and associated with shortness of breath? (paroxysmal nocturnal dyspnoea, congestive heart failure)

Palpitations

Do the palpitations feel like your heart misses a beat, jumps or flutters (150 beats per minute)? (ventricular or atrial extrasystoles)
Do the palpitations feel like your heart is jumping about or racing and associated with breathlessness? (atrial fibrillation)
Do the palpitations feel like your heart is racing or fluttering and are they associated with increased urination (160 beats per minute)? (supraventricular tachycardia)
Do you feel like your heart is racing or fluttering, and also feel breathless and that you might faint? (ventricular tachycardia)
Do the palpitations begin in late afternoon and early evening and occur several hours after eating? (reactive hypoglycaemia)
Do you feel palpitations after exercise, intense emotion or stress? (hyperdynamic circulation)
Do you pass a large amount of urine after experiencing heart palpitations? (T1–T5 lesion in spine, drug induced with smoking and alcohol, anxiety induced)

Breathing

Have you ever woken up in the middle of the night short of breath? (nocturnal dyspnoea)
Is the fatigue associated with shortness of breath and swelling of the ankles? (congestive heart failure)

Pain

Do you experience indigestion that is connected with physical activity? (angina)
Have you experienced pain in your calves when you walk? (claudication)
Do your fingers ever become painful, turn white, then blue and red in the cold? (Raynaud's phenomenon)
Do you experience pain and lack of circulation in the hands and feet, pain on walking and have a history of cigarette smoking? (Buerger's disease)

Headache

Do you wake with a dull headache that worsens during the day and lessens towards evening? (hypertension, tension headache, sinus headaches, intracranial pressure)
Does your headache come from the back of one eye, radiate to the front of the face and is extremely severe but passes quickly? (cluster headache)
Do you experience severe headache pain with swelling and redness in one eye, and pain, facial sweating and wanting to move around? (cluster headache)
Have your headaches and eye pain come on suddenly and disappeared within two hours, then return every day for up to two months at a time? (cluster headaches)
Does your headache return at the same time every year and the same time every day for up to two months? (cluster headache)

Eyes

Do you experience blurry near vision? (retinal circulatory disturbance or macular degeneration should be considered in the elderly, older age group)
Does the visual blurring come and go in episodes? (glaucoma, multiple sclerosis or transient ischaemic attacks, atherosclerotic emboli, carotid insufficiency/amaurosis fugax)
Is the visual loss transient (sometimes progressive) and associated with visual field changes and nocturnal headache? (temporal arteritis, twice as common in elderly women)
Do you experience no pain in the eyes although they are red? (subconjunctival haemorrhage)

Ear

Is the sound in your ears pulsating in character? (vascular disorder)

Musculoskeletal

Does the shoulder-tip pain disappear within 20 minutes? (angina pectoris)

TRAUMA AND PRE-EXISTING ILLNESS

Because we have not met before, it will help if I can get an idea of your medical history. Are you happy for us to do this now? [1]
I understand you have been experiencing [insert symptoms]. Is there anything else bothering you? [1]
You seem concerned that your symptoms may be very serious. Do you have any theories about what might be causing them? [1, 7]
It seems to me that you aren't satisfied with previous explanations for your symptoms. Is that correct? [1]
I realise you may have already explained your symptoms to many other practitioners, but it would be very helpful for me to hear more about your concerns, what treatment you have been having and how you have been coping [7].
You have obviously given your health a great deal of thought and I would appreciate knowing what you believe has been happening for you [1, 7].
What is the worst possible? [1, 7]
Can you tell me if you have had any accidents or injured yourself in the past? [7]
Have you had all childhood vaccinations?

Eyes

Is the red eye only on one side? (foreign body, trauma)

▶

Ears

Has your ear pain developed after plane travel or scuba diving? (otitic barotraumas)
Has your ear pain developed after swimming, cleaning or picking your ear? (otitis externa)
Have you experienced any trauma to your ear recently? (traumatic perforation of ear drum)

Musculoskeletal

Does lying on your back and resting relieve your back pain? (acute lumbosacral strain/ mechanical/disc syndrome)
Is the lower back pain relieved when you are walking or lying on your side with your legs in the fetal position? (disc syndrome)
Do you experience sharp lower back pain that comes on suddenly when turning, lifting, twisting or doing general physical activity? (acute lumbosacral strain)
Is the back pain dull, persistent and accompanied by stiffness? (musculoskeletal strain and postural backache)
Did your back feel like it 'gave way'? (postural backache in the lower lumbar region)
Does the pain radiate across the lower back and into the buttocks? (musculoskeletal strain and faulty posture)
Does the back pain have a sudden onset, radiate to your buttock, and down the leg to the foot? (herniated disc syndrome)
Is the back pain worse by when you cough, laugh, pass a bowel motion, sneeze, sit or bend? (disc syndrome)
Do you feel pain in your shoulder when raising your arm 0–15 degrees? (fracture, dislocation, painful passive movements)
Do you feel pain in your shoulder when raising your straight arm away from your body (abduction) 60–120 degrees and feel tenderness on the shoulder tip? (supraspinatus tendonitis/partial tear)
Do you feel pain in your shoulder when raising your arm 160–180 degrees? (acromioclavicular joint problem)
Do you feel shoulder-tip pain? (brachial neuralgia, cervical dysfunction, myocardial infarction, angina pectoris, pneumothorax, bronchogenic carcinoma, peptic ulceration, cholecystitis)
When you raise your arm does it become weak in the overhead position? (recurrent dislocation)
Do you feel fatigue in your fingers when repeating certain movements like working on the computer? (repetitive strain injury)

Integumentary

Is the itchy bottom associated with a discharge and pain on passing a bowel motion? (fissure)

OBSTRUCTION AND FOREIGN BODY

Digestive system

Is the vomit that comes after the abdominal pain light in colour? (digestive juices and bile – gastritis, cholecystitis obstruction)
Is the itchy skin associated with mucus in your stools but no visible rash? (cholestatic jaundice)
Is there any undigested food in the vomit? (obstruction near the stomach or peptic condition, self-induced vomiting before food has digested)
Is the vomit brown in colour and does it smell like faecal matter? (bowel obstruction)
Have you experienced severe constipation with no gas or wind? (intestinal obstruction)
Is your abdominal pain unaffected by movement and associated with an inability to be still/ restlessness? (obstruction of gallbladder, biliary tree or ureter from stones)
Does abdominal discomfort become worse by bending over or wearing tight clothes and relieved when you pass wind? (gas entrapment, hepatic or splenic flexure syndrome)
Is the blood on the toilet paper bright red and is it there after passing a bowel motion? (haemorrhoids, anal fissure)

▶

▶

Urinary system

Have you experienced reduced urine flow? (kidney stones, prostate conditions)
Do you experience back pain that radiates to the penile tip? (bladder stones)
Is the pain you feel worse at the end of urination? (bladder stone)

Respiratory system

Is there a loud breathing sound associated with the cough? (foreign body or infection in larynx, upper trachea or subglottic area)

Eyes

Do you experience difficulty driving at night because of glare from other headlights or in the day due to bright sunlight? (cataracts)
Do you see glare, a halo, have blurred vision and/or double vision in one eye? (cataracts)
Do you experience blurry distance vision? (cataracts most common in the elderly)

Nose

Do you fall asleep unexpectedly during the day and have a history of snoring? (sleep apnoea)

Throat

Do you frequently need to clear your throat? (PND, obstruction)

Fatigue

Do you snore during the night and wake up feeling unrested and fatigued? (sleep apnoea)

Musculoskeletal

Did the back pain begin gradually on the back and radiate to the groin? (renal colic)

Integumentary

Is the itchy bottom associated with a thick discharge and prolapsed lump? (haemorrhoid)

RECREATIONAL DRUG USE

I would like to ask you about your drinking habits. Do you drink alcohol? [7]
Do you or have you ever used recreational drugs?
Do you smoke? How much do you smoke?
Have you ever smoked in the past?

SURGERY AND HOSPITILISATION

Have you experienced any trauma, injury, surgery or been in hospital?

OCCUPATIONAL TOXINS AND HAZARDS

Are there particular days in the week when your asthma is worse and breathing is more difficult? (allergic, occupational, psychogenic asthma)

FUNCTIONAL DISEASE

Digestive system

Do you have indigestion that has no relation to physical activity? (heart burn, oesophageal reflux)
Does the heartburn pain radiate into the neck, arms, back or jaw? (oesophageal spasm)
Do you feel the heartburn after meals, when lying down or bending over? (oesophageal reflux)
Is the heartburn relieved by taking antacids? (oesophageal reflux)
Is the burning and indigestion made worse by foods such as spices, spearmint, peppermint, garlic, onions, chocolate, fatty foods, alcohol or carbonated beverages? (reduced lower oesophageal pressure and stimulated gastric acidity, oesophageal reflux)

▶

Is the burning and indigestion made worse by cigarette smoking? (reduced lower oesophageal pressure and stimulated gastric acidity, oesophageal reflux)
Is your indigestion made worse by consuming orange juice, tomato juice or spicy foods? (oesophageal reflux)
Do you experience heartburn associated with acid regurgitation and salivation (waterbrash) *at least once a week?* (reflux-dyspepsia)
Do you chew gum or smoke frequently, drink carbonated drinks or wear loose dentures? (aerophagia – swallowing too much air)
Do you have a regular time of day when you pass a bowel motion? (diarrhoea first thing in morning is more often a colon disorder and a functional disorder)
Do you strain to pass at least one in four bowel motions and are left with the feeling of an incomplete evacuation or obstruction? (functional constipation)
Do you experience lumpy or hard stools more frequently than one in four bowel motions? (functional constipation)
Do you pass a bowel motion fewer than three times a week and ever need manual manipulation to assist? (functional constipation)
Is your abdominal pain continuous and has no association with eating, passing a bowel motion or having menses? (functional abdominal pain syndrome)

Urinary system

Do you experience incontinence when you feel the urge to void, have a full bladder or change position? (detrusor muscle instability)
Is the incontinence/passing of urine delayed or gradual? (detrusor muscle instability)
Do you pass large amounts of urine with the incontinence and have a sensation that the bladder is full? (overactive bladder with detrusor muscle instability)
Do you pass large amounts of urine with incontinence without any sensation of abdominal pressure or from the desire to void due to pain? (involuntary destrusor muscle contractions)

Respiratory system

Is the cough worse after eating chocolate, onions, drinking caffeinated coffee or tea? (gastro-oesophageal reflux)
Do you experience a sour taste in the mouth and heartburn with the cough? (gastro-oesophageal reflux)
Have you experienced faster or difficult breathing? (hyperventilation syndrome)

Headache

Does your headache come on after exercise, coughing or having sexual intercourse? (exertional headache)
Do you get headaches associated with grinding your teeth during the night? (muscle contraction headache)

Fatigue

Have you been experience fatigue for a long time? (functional origin)
Do you experience fatigue in the morning? Is it worse in the morning? (functional origin)
Did the fatigue begin at a time of emotional trauma or major life change? (functional origin)
Do you experience a delay in falling asleep? (initial insomnia, prolonged latency, common in anxiety, caffeine and alcohol users and the elderly)
How noisy or warm is your sleeping environment? (environmental reasons for insomnia)
How many daytime naps would you have during the week to catch up on lost sleep?
Do you perform any strenuous exercise in the evenings prior to sleep?
Do you experience severe itching of the skin at night that interferes with sleep?
Do you drink tea or coffee, cola drinks or eat chocolate prior to going to sleep at night? (caffeine induced insomnia)

Musculoskeletal

Has your pain been persistent for more than three months, moves around the body and is it associated with fatigue? (fibromyalgia)
Is your fatigue aggravated by effort? (fibromyalgia, organic fatigue)
Is your back pain relieved by passing a bowel motion? (irritable colon)
When you experience hand pains in the mornings, do you know if you have been sleeping with your arms raised? (thoracic outlet syndrome)

Integumentary

Is the tickling/crawling feeling worse when you are stressed? (psychogenic)
Is the itchy skin associated with dry, scaled skin when you are exposed to cold air? (winter itch)
Is the itchy skin associated with vesicles when you are in humid environments? (prickly heat)
Is the itchy bottom associated with hot weather and wearing nylon underwear? (excessive sweating)

DEGENERATIVE AND DEFICIENCY DISEASES

Digestive system

Can you clearly see any blood in the vomit? (peptic ulcer)
Is your indigestion, upper abdominal pain and burning in the chest relieved by vomiting? (peptic ulcer)
Is the indigestion and burning sensation associated with nausea, sense of fullness and loss of appetite but better after eating? (peptic ulcer)
Is your abdominal pain associated with indigestion/chest pain? (peptic ulcer)
Do your symptoms of indigestion become worse when you are hungry or before eating meals? (peptic ulcer)
Is your abdominal pain better after taking antacids or when sitting up? (peptic conditions)
Is the abdominal pain worse after eating or drinking alcohol? (peptic conditions)
Is the shoulder-tip pain associated with abdominal pain and heartburn? (peptic ulcer)

Urinary

Is the itchy skin associated with no visible rash and do you experience restless legs? (renal failure)

Eyes

Did the blurred vision come on suddenly and without pain? (senile macular degeneration, very common over the age of 55 years)
Do you experience blurred vision, central vision defects and trouble reading? (age-related macular degeneration in older age group)
Did you experience a sudden onset of blurred vision in both eyes? (changes in blood-sugar levels)
Do you experience double vision with blurring that comes and goes and is associated with flashes, stars or dizziness? (vertebrobasilar insufficiency)
Do you experience light flashes in your vision? (usually in the temporal field when a person is in the dark, caused by vitreous shrinking away from the retina)
Do you experience floaters, stars or light flashes in your vision? (contraction of vitreous, common in the older age group, diplopia, unilateral photopsia, posterior vitreous detachment – PVD, retinal detachment and visual blurring)
Do you experience black or grey spots in the vision when looking at a bright background? (vitreous flashes produced when vitreous pulls away from the retina)
Do you experience visual changes in your peripheral field associated with light flashes or a shower of floaters? (retinal detachment)
Do you see the image of halos around lights? (glaucoma)
Do you experience visual field loss? (glaucoma)
Is blurred vision associated with halos around lights, pain in the eye, headache, red eye or nausea? (glaucoma, acute narrow-angle glaucoma)

▶

Ears

Do you experience the ringing sound in both ears? (presbyacusis, NIHL)
Is the ringing in your ears continuous? (otosclerosis, NIHL, presbyacusis, acoustic neuroma)

Respiratory

Is the fatigue associated with shortness of breath, loss of appetite, weight loss and pale skin? (anaemia)
Is the fatigue associated with shortness of breath, weight changes and numbness in the legs? (pernicious anaemia)

Fatigue

Do you have poor-quality sleep? (deficiency of deep and REM sleep)
Do you frequently wake up during the night? (middle insomnia, poor-quality sleep, medical conditions such as sleep apnoea, diabetes, prostatism)
Do you experience early-morning wakefulness? (late insomnia, depression, malnutrition)
Does your fatigue only last a short while and occur after exertion? (organic origin)
Is the fatigue not present in the morning? (organic origin)
Is the fatigue worse as the day progresses and relieved by rest? (organic origin)
Has the fatigue been gradually progressing rather than fluctuating? (organic origin)
Is the fatigue associated with periods of prolonged physical or mental activity, inadequate rest, poor sleep, dieting, a sedentary lifestyle, pregnancy or mental stress? (physiologic fatigue)

Musculoskeletal

Do you feel shoulder-tip pain with restricted movement of the neck? (cervical dysfunction)
Do you have difficulty pinching or grasping bigger objects, opening jar tops or turning door knobs? (osteoarthritis at the base of the thumb)

Integumentary

Is the itchy skin associated with pale skin and no visible sign of a rash? (iron-deficiency anaemia)

INFECTION AND INFLAMMATION

Have you experienced any significant fever or illness?

Digestive system

Is your abdominal pain alleviated by lying down or remaining still? (inflammation)
Is the heartburn relieved by bismuth salts and/or antibiotics? (Helicobacter pylori)
Has the diarrhoea been abrupt, lasted less than a week and is associated with fever, nausea or vomiting? (acute diarrhoea that most often is bacterial, parasitic or viral)
Do you need to get up in the night to pass diarrhoea or loose stools? (organic cause)
Is the abdominal pain relieved by vomiting or passing diarrhoea? (gastroenteritis)
Is the abdominal pain associated with dark urine and light stools? (cholecystitis)
Has the upper abdominal pain, nausea and vomiting been associated with a recent alcohol binge? (acute pancreatitis)
Does the pain occur in your upper abdominal region, radiate to your back, and is it partially relieved by sitting forward? (pancreatitis)
Is there any blood or mucus in your bowel motion? (inflammation, pancreatic disorder)

Urinary system

Do you feel relief from urinary symptoms when you have voided urine? (interstitial cystitis)
Did the incontinence come on suddenly or is it associated with stress? (most often due to infection)
When you experience pain/burning on urination does the discomfort feel internal? (cystitis)
When you experience pain/burning on urination does the discomfort feel external, after the urine has flowed over the external vaginal area? (vaginitis)

▶

▶ *Do you experience pain on urination but not increased frequency?* (vaginitis)
Do you experience burning/pain on urination with increased frequency? (bacterial cystitis)
Did the symptoms of pain and frequency of urination come on over 2–7 days? (female urethral syndrome)
Did the symptoms of pain and frequency of urination come on and resolve quickly? (cystitis)
Is the pain in the abdomen relieved by urination? (cystitis)
Do you avoid urination because the pain is worse on urination? (cystitis)
Are the symptoms of burning pain on urination, increased frequency and abdominal pain better after a hot bath? (cystitis)
Did the symptom of pain on urination come on suddenly accompanied by blood in the urine? (bacterial infection)
Is the pain/blood on urination worse at the end of the urine stream? (cystitis)
Is the pain/blood on urination worse at the beginning of the urine stream? (urethritis)
Is pain on urination and increased frequency associated with high fever, chills, nausea, vomiting and backache? (pyelonephritis)
Have you noticed any pus in your urine? (female urethral syndrome, cystitis)

Respiratory system

Is the cough associated with a sound on inspiration? (whooping cough, viral illness)
Is the cough associated with a shortness of breath/wheeze on expiration? (asthma)
Do you experience shortness of breath with the cough? (asthma)
Is the cough worse during the night? (paroxysmal nocturnal dyspnoea, congestive heart failure, sinusitis, rhinitis)
Is the cough noisy, not very productive and worse at night? (viral, asthma)
Is coughing worse at night, associated with headache, pain when bending the head down, bad breath, coloured nasal discharge and a short burst of coughing? (sinusitis)
Is your cough worse in the morning? (PND, smokers cough, chronic bronchitis)
Have you experienced fever, chills, headache, abdominal pain, conjunctivitis or chest pain with the cough? (bacterial or mycoplasmal origin)
Did the cough begin over a period of days and is it productive with thick yellow mucus? (bacterial, mycoplasmal infection)
Is there a loud 'whoop' sound on inspiration with scanty mucus production? (whooping cough)
Have you had fever, night sweats, and weight loss since you have had the cough? (tuberculosis)
Do you experience sudden and brief episodes of coughing associated with nasal discharge and nasal blockage? (chronic rhinitis)
Do you have muscle pain with the cough? (viral pneumonia)
Does the cough produce scanty mucoid sputum with substernal pain? (acute bronchitis)
Does the cough produce a clear, thick mucus or no mucus at all? (asthma)
Is the mucus from your cough persistent and associated with shortness of breath? (asthma)
Does the cough produce a thick yellow mucus? (bacterial infection)
Does your cough last for a very long time? Is it very productive, loose, moist and is there occasionally blood in the mucus? (bronchiectasis)
Have you noticed if the mucus associated with the cough is purulent and foul smelling? (lung abscess)
Do you experience a productive cough and mucus in your bowel motions? (cystic fibrosis sign)
Have you ever experienced asthma or difficulty breathing during the night? (insomnia due to nocturnal asthma)

▶

Eyes

Do you experience visual changes with pain in the eye? (iritis, acute glaucoma)
Do you experience red eye with pain in the eye? (iritis, acute glaucoma, periorbital cellulitis, corneal abrasion)
Do you often experience red eye(s)? (subconjunctival haemorrhage, episcleritis, scleritis, pterygium, glaucoma, superficial keratitis, uveitis, conjunctivitis)
Did you experience red eye(s) with watery discharge associated with upper respiratory infection? (viral conjunctivitis)
Did the infection begin in one eye and quickly spread to the other? (viral conjunctivitis)
Is the red eye associated with increased discharge that is thick, white/yellow, causes closure of eyelids and worse on waking? (bacterial conjunctivitis)
Do the red eye(s) have discharge that is watery and yellow? (viral conjunctivitis)
Do the red eye(s) have discharge that is green/yellow and thick? (bacterial conjunctivitis)
Is the eyelid swelling associated with discharge? (dacryocystitis)
Does the eyelid have a pustule on it? (stye)
Does the eyelid feel like it is burning and have dry scales? (staphylococcal blepharitis)
Does the eyelid feel like it is burning and have greasy scales? (seborrheic blepharitis)

Ears

Is your pain always in one ear only? (otitis media, serous otitis media, eustachitis)
Do you experience difficulty hearing, crackling noises or tinnitus, but no significant ear pain? (serous otitis media, eustachitis)
Is the throbbing earache you experience aggravated by swallowing? (acute otitis media)
Is it painful to touch behind the ear when you have ear pain? (mastoiditis)
Is it painful to move or touch the ear lobe when you have ear pain? (otitis externa)
Have you experienced any discharge from the ear? (otitis externa, ruptured tympanic membrane from acute otitis media, mastoiditis, trauma to the ear)
Does your child have hearing difficulties, speech delay and ear discomfort that is better when chewing? (serous otitis media)
Is the earache aggravated by swallowing or burping when acute? (otitis media)

Nose

Do you feel pain when you sneeze? (sinusitis)
Do you swallow a lot of mucus? (postnasal drip – PND)
Do you experience sinus pain and scanty mucus with the cough? (PND)

Headache

Is your dull headache aggravated by bending over? (frontal sinusitis, temporal arteritis)

Fatigue

Have you experienced a viral or bacterial infection accompanying your increasing tiredness? (acute fatigue, heart failure, anaemia)

Musculoskeletal

Is the aching/throbbing pain relieved by exercise? (spondyloarthropathy)
Is the aching pain and morning stiffness relieved by resting or lying down? (osteoarthrosis/spondylosis)
Did the back pain develop gradually and is not triggered by physical activity? (degenerative back disease, arthritis)
Does the back pain radiate to the knee, calf or lower leg? (uncommon in degeneration of lumbosacral region)
Is the lower back pain associated with pain in other joints? (osteoarthritis)
Does your lower back pain lessen when you lie on the floor or on a firm mattress? (osteoarthritis)
Is your shoulder pain associated with tenderness over your upper arm (deltoid)? (subacromial bursitis)
When you have the shoulder pain do you also feel sick after eating fatty foods? (cholecystitis)

▶| *Do you experience early-morning stiffness that wears off after a couple of hours of activity?* (inflammatory arthritis)
Do you experience stiffness that is worse with rest and reduces quickly on movement (although there may be pain with movement)? (mechanical arthritis)
Do you have difficulty rising out of a chair or walking up stairs due to your leg muscles feeling so weak? (polymyositis)

Integumentary

Is the skin rash on the palm of your hands? (contact dermatitis, palmo-pustular psoriasis)
Is the skin rash on the inside of the skin folds of your elbows and knees? (eczema)
Is the skin rash on the outside of the skin surfaces such as on the elbows and knees? (psoriasis)
Has the scaly skin rash spread to the genital region? (psoriasis)
Does your skin rash improve with sunlight? (atopic eczema, psoriasis, lichen planus)
Is the itching associated with marked excoriation and is it in hair regions? (nits, pubic lice)
Is the skin itch worse at night and is it associated with a rash? (scabies, lice)
Is the general itching associated with lines of nodules and vesicles with a red base? (scabies)
Is the itchy bottom intense and worse in the morning? (pinworm infestation)
Is the itchy bottom associated with taking medication or antibiotics and is there excoriation associated with loose stools? (Candida)
Is the itching of skin associated with red, scaly patches? (Candida, psoriasis)
Is the itching of skin associated with scaly margin and well-defined borders? (tinea, psoriasis)
Have you noticed your toe/finger nails pitting? (psoriasis, tinea)
Have you noticed your toe/finger nails have developed ridges? (eczema)

SUPPLEMENTS AND SIDE EFFECTS, MEDICATION/DRUGS

What is your medication history?
Have you been taking any specific medication?
Did you notice the pain on urination and frequency after taking NSAIDs? (medication origin)
Is the heartburn relieved by ingesting viscous lidocaine (Xylocaine viscous)? (peptic oesophagitis)

ENDOCRINE/REPRODUCTIVE/SEXUAL HEALTH

Endocrine

Do you experience visual field loss, blurred vision and impaired night vision? (diabetic neuropathy)
Do you have regular pap smears and breast checks?
Has your weight fluctuated?
Have you noticed a swelling or rash around your neck? (goitre)
Did you notice your goitre and neck swelling develop rapidly? (thyroid cancer, acute viral thyroiditis, thyroid cyst)
Did you notice your goitre and neck swelling develop gradually over time? (hypothyroid, Graves' disease)
Do you experience heart palpitations along with increased heat intolerance and tremors? (hyperthyroidism)
Have you noticed any urinary symptoms and was the appearance of your face change associated with the arm and leg weakness? (Cushing's syndrome)
Have you experienced increased heart palpitations and an intolerance to heat while experiencing the muscle weakness? (thyrotoxicosis)
Have you noticed a change in hat, glove or shoe size? (acromegaly)
Have you noticed a thickening around your lower neck, along with dry skin, hair, puffy eyes and lack of concentration? (hypothyroid)
Have you noticed increased sweating and tremor in the hands? (Addison's disease, hyperthyroidism, Parkinson's disease)
Have you been unusually thirsty? (diabetes, Addison's disease, hyperthyroidism)
Have you been passing large amounts of urine? (diabetes)
Have you experienced weight gain, intolerance to cold, depression and lack of appetite? (hypothyroid)
Is the itchy skin associated with no visible rash and glucose in the urine? (diabetes)

Reproductive

Do you experience a delay before beginning to urinate or dribbling at the end? (prostate)
Did the pain on urination come on gradually and have you been experiencing it for a long time? (chlamydial infection)
Do you experience testicular pain? (epididymitis, chlamydia infection)
Do you experience urinary abnormalities with pain in the rectum, testicles, penis, lower abdomen, back and on ejaculation? (prostatitis)
Do you experience painful lesions on your genitals that ulcer? (genital herpes)
Do you ever have blood in your sperm discharge? (prostatitis)
Do you experience any vaginal itching? (*Candida*/vaginitis)
Has your vaginal discharge and itching been associated with pregnancy, taking the oral contraceptive pill, tetracycline or antibiotics? (candidal vaginitis)
Do you wipe from the perineal region (back) to front when going to the toilet? (recurrent vaginal infections spread from anus to vagina)
Had you been doing a lot of horseback or bike riding when you developed the symptoms of pain on urination and minimal discharge? (mechanical urethritis)
Have you used any vaginal sprays, douches or had bubble baths recently? (chemical vaginitis, vulvovaginitis)
Do you experience vaginal discharge when you wear nylon panties? (vulvovaginitis)
Do you experience internal vaginal itching that is also external? (vulvovaginitis, *Candida*)
Is the itching you are experiencing predominantly on the external parts of the vulva? (vulvodermatoses)
Is the vaginal itching worse after using soaps, bath oils, bubble baths, douches, perfume, lubricants or antifungal creams? (vulvodermatoses)
Is the vaginal itching worse after vaginal secretions, retained sweat, using sanitary pads, wearing tight clothing, synthetic underwear, excessive cleaning of genitals and shaving of pubic hair? (vulvodermatoses)
Do you use tampons when you have your period and do you change them regularly? (vulvar discharge and itching from hygiene concern)
Is the vaginal discharge and pain on urination associated with rectal infection, pain on walking or climbing stairs? (gonorrhoea)
Is the discharge you have experienced from your vagina/penis severe, heavy and contain pus? (gonorrhoeal urethritis)
Did the thick/purulent discharge from your vagina/penis develop 1–3 weeks after sexual intercourse? (gonorrhoeal urethritis)
Have your urinary symptoms coincided with an increase in ejaculation? (prostatitis)
Is your lower back pain associated with vaginal discharge? Is it worse or better after menstruation? (gynaecologic cause)
Is your back pain associated with burning urination, difficulty urinating or fever? (prostatitis)

Menstruation

Are you experiencing hot flushes, irregular periods, low libido, vaginal dryness, aches and pains, mood swings, weight gain or depression? (oestrogen deficiency)
Do you experience any pain when menstruation begins? (primary dysmenorrhoea)
Does the pain radiate to the front of the thighs and/or lower back? (primary or secondary dysmenorrhoea)
Does the pain you experience at menstruation occur at any other time during the month? (endometriosis)
Does the pelvic pain occur before the menstrual bleeding has begun? (secondary dysmenorrhoea)
Is the pelvic pain relieved by the menstrual flow? (secondary dysmenorrhoea)
Do you experience spotting or light blood flow at ovulation and is there any associated pain? Is the length of your menstrual cycle regular? Do you experience symptoms such as bloating, mood changes, sore breasts and period pain prior to your period? (ovulatory bleeding)
Do you experience irregular menstrual cycles and bleeding not associated with ovulation pain, premenstrual symptoms or period pain? (anovulatory bleeding)

▶ *Is your menstrual bleed unexpected and without pain?* (anovulatory bleeding)
Is your menstrual blood volume excessive/heavy and irregular? (polymenorrhagia, anovulatory bleeding)
Have you experienced any milk production from your breasts while having missed periods and negative pregnancy tests? (hyperprolactinaemia)
Is your menstrual blood volume excessive/heavy and is your cycle regular? (menorrhagia, tumours, fibroids, cancer, polyps, endometriosis, salpingitis, IUDs)
Is the pelvic pain continuous, dull or cause back pain? (secondary dysmenorrhoea)
Is the itchy skin associated with no visible rash and loss of menstrual period? (pregnancy)

AUTOIMMUNE DISEASE

Endocrine

Have you developed a rash around your Adam's apple? (Hashimoto's disease)

Integumentary

Does your skin rash worsen in sunlight? (systemic lupus erythematosus, phytophotodermatitis, polymorphic light eruptions, photosensitive eczema, solar urticaria)

STRESS AND NEUROLOGICAL DISEASE

Digestive system

Do you experience more diarrhoea during times of emotional stress? (nervous diarrhoea with no presence of blood or mucus in stools)

Urinary system

Is the incontinence volume small to moderate and associated with abdominal pressure? (stress incontinence)
Did the incontinence begin after menopause? (stress incontinence connected with oestrogen deficiency)
Are you able to voluntarily inhibit the incontinence when you are aware of it? (stress incontinence)
Do you feel a loss of urine when coughing, lifting, exercising or changing position? (stress incontinence)
Is the incontinence/passing of urine immediate and sudden? (stress incontinence)

Respiratory system

Does your cough improve at night? (psychogenic, habit cough, Tourette's syndrome)

Eyes

Did you experience a sudden onset of double vision, floaters, stars or light flashes in your vision with pain around the eye or in the head? (third-nerve palsy, aneurysm)
Do you experience pain in the eye without visual changes? (neurologic origin)
Do you experience an obscured region in your vision that seems translucent or dark and shimmering? Does this begin in the centre and move out in your visual field? (negative scotoma in migraine headaches)
Do you experience bright, shimmering, shooting lights that begin in the centre and move out to the whole visual field? (positive scotoma with migraine headaches)
Did you lose the central vision in one eye suddenly with pain and redness in the eye? (optic neuritis)
Does the visual blurring vary when looking in different directions? (ischaemic neuropathy, giant-cell arteritis)
Do you experience double vision? (weakness in one or more ocular muscles caused by conditions such as trauma, cerebrovascular lesions, MS, thyroid disorders, myasthenia gravis, brain tumour)
Do you only experience double vision in one eye when the other eye is covered? (monocular diplopia, lens opacities, dislocated lens, Marfan's syndrome, hysteria)
Is the double vision constant in both eyes? (head trauma, extraocular muscles or nerve disorder) ▶

Ears

Does your ear pain become aggravated by eating hot or cold foods? (dental pathology)
Have you experienced any sensations of nausea or feel as if the room in spinning? (inner ear vertigo)
Do you experience short bursts of a low-pitched roaring sound in your ears with nausea and vertigo? (Ménière's disease)
Is the sound only in one ear? (Ménière's disease, acoustic neuroma, diabetic neuropathy)
Does the world seem to turn around? (vertigo)

Headache

Do you need to stop moving when you have headache pain in one eye? (migraine headache)

Fatigue

Does the fatigue improve during the day? (depression)
When you cannot sleep during the night do you experience an uncontrollable urge to move your legs? (restless leg syndrome)

Depression

Do you experience associated symptoms such as decreased appetite, weight loss, lack of energy, lack of interest in daily activities, decreased libido and vague aches and pains along with disturbed sleep? (depression)
Has your sense of low self-esteem been associated with a reactive mood change to a specific event? (minor depression)
Have you experienced episodes of feeling low for more than two years? (dysthymia)
Has your sense of low self-esteem been associated with a lack of concentration and a sense of not being able to think clearly for more than two weeks? (major depression)

Anxiety and fear

Do you experience associated symptoms such as headaches, chest pain, palpitations, dizziness, diarrhoea, bloating, abdominal discomfort, feelings of nervous foreboding along with sleep disturbance? (anxiety related)
Is the fatigue you are experiencing associated with restlessness, irritability, increased sweating or heart palpitations? (chronic anxiety)
Is your fatigue not aggravated by effort? (anxiety)
Have you experienced a traumatic event recently or in the past that left you feeling very frightened? (PTSD)
Have your symptoms developed within six months of the traumatic event? (PTSD)
Have you been experiencing any flashbacks to a particular event? (PTSD)
Do you experience symptoms only when in a particular situation? (phobia)
Have you begun to avoid any particular events or situations? (phobia)
Do you believe your response to a particular event or object is excessive? (phobia/panic disorder)
How long did the episode of intense fear last? (panic disorder)
Is there a family history of panic attacks? (panic disorder)
Are there any particular thoughts that keep bothering you and you wish you could stop? (OCD)
Do you wash or clean or check things a lot? (OCD)
Do your daily activities take a long time to finish and if so why? (OCD)
Would you consider yourself a perfectionist? (possible OCD tendencies)
If you do see yourself as a perfectionist, are there any other family members that share this tendency? (possible OCD genetic tendency)
Do you worry about the way you look? (body dysmorphic disorder – BDD)
On a typical day, how many hours would you think about your appearance? (BDD, more than one hour considered excessive)
Do you ever have the sensation of being 'outside' of your body? (depersonalisation)

▶
Musculoskeletal

Is the back pain sharp, radiating and associated with numbness or muscle weakness (nerve root compression)
Do you feel shoulder-tip pain with restricted movement, a tingling hand and stiffness in the local area? (brachial neuralgia)
Do you feel restriction of movement without significant pain? (increased muscle contraction, soft tissue rather than joint, and with increased tone can indicate upper motor neuron disease)
Do you experience weakness in the upper arms and lower legs with tingling and numbness that is progressing over time? (postinfectious polyneuropathy)
Do you experience upper arm, leg or shoulder weakness associated with muscle wasting? (motor neuron disease)
Is the weakness in your fingers or feet associated with numbness? (peripheral neuropathy)
Do you experience nocturnal pain in your hands and numbness or pain in wrist, hand or forearm? (carpal tunnel syndrome)
Do you experience any tingling in the arm or hand with the pain in the fingers? (ulnar nerve entrapment)
Do you feel tingling and sensory loss, weakness and muscle wasting in your little finger and ring finger? (ulnar nerve entrapment)

EATING HABITS, ENERGY AND EXERCISE

How much exercise do you do in a week?

Diet

Open-ended questions
What is your typical daily diet?
Describe a situation when you would not feel like eating.
Do you eat regular meals? If not, what do you think would happen if you ate regularly?
Describe how you cook your main meals.
Where do you like to shop for your food?
Tell me about your appetite.
What are your favourite foods?
What foods do you dislike?

General questions
Can you tell me what you would usually eat for breakfast, lunch, dinner, dessert and snacks? Asking clients to complete and return a food diary after one or two weeks is very helpful to give more accurate dietary details. This is helpful to both clients and practitioners to better understand their eating patterns and foods/drinks consumed (see Appendix F).
How much fresh fruit do you usually eat each day?
How many different types of vegetables do you eat each day?
Do you usually eat salads or cooked vegetables?
How do you cook your vegetables?
Can you describe the size of the food portions you eat at each meal?
What percentage of your plate does your serve of vegetables usually cover?
What percentage of your plate does your serve of protein usually cover?
What percentage of your plate does your serve of starch (potato/pasta/rice) usually cover?
Do you snack between meals or in the evenings? If so, what and how much do you usually eat?
What is your water intake?
What drinks do you like to have? Soft drinks, juice, coffee/tea? How many cups/glasses/ bottles would you consume per day?
Do you experience any food cravings or aversions?
Do you know if you have any food allergies or intolerances?
Do you experience difficulties preparing food?
Do you experience difficulties eating or chewing food?

▶

▶ *Do you enjoy cooking?*
What are your cooking abilities and skills like?
Do you have difficulties accessing shops to buy food?
Do you have any significant physical disability that affects your ability to purchase or prepare food?
Do you eat out regularly?
When you eat out, what type of food do you usually eat?
Do you eat any organic food?
Have you been on any diets recently or in the past?
Is the weight gain you are experiencing unusual for you?
Do you ever experience weight fluctuations?
What times of the day do you have sugar cravings?
Tell me about your drug, alcohol and cigarette intake.
Do you use any recreational drugs?

When you have built up rapport
Does eating food seem to dominate your daily activities?
Do you ever find yourself eating certain foods in secret?
Do you think you may have an eating problem?
Are you satisfied with your eating patterns?
What is your ideal weight?
Do you worry excessively about your weight?
Do you ever make yourself vomit because you feel uncomfortably full?
Do you ever worry that you have lost control over how much you eat?
Do you eat to make yourself feel happier?
Do you ever feel guilty about how much you eat?
Have you recently had a weight fluctuation or lost more than 6 kg within three months?
Do you think you are fat when other people keep saying you are thin?
Have you ever thought you might be drinking/eating too much? [8]
Have people annoyed you by criticising your alcohol consumption?
Have you ever felt bad or guilty for drinking alcohol?
Have you ever needed a drink first thing in the morning to steady your nerves or improve your mood?
If you drink alcohol, can you tell me what you drink? [7]
It would help me if I could go over the past week with you and get an idea about how much alcohol you have had [7].

Specific questions – condition related
Do you experience heartburn that has become worse since having any of these in your diet – caffeine, spearmint, peppermint, garlic, onions, chocolate, fatty foods, alcohol or carbonated drinks? (reduced oesophageal pressure and influence reflux)
Have you taken steroids, NSAIDs, antidepressants, lithium, anabolic steroids or oestrogen-based medication? (all can cause weight gain)
Does your mood improve after you have eaten carbohydrates? (seasonal affective disorder, diabetes, low blood-sugar levels)
How much do you eat in one sitting for your evening meal or before going to sleep at night? (cause of insomnia)
Do you drink tea or coffee, cola drinks or eat chocolate prior to going to sleep at night? (caffeine-induced insomnia)
Has the feeling of depression been associated with gastrointestinal upsets? (folate deficiency anaemia)

Referral flag symptoms
Unexplained loss/gain of body weight
The client has lost interest in eating
The client has physical disability that impedes food preparation
Excess drug and alcohol intake that influences appetite
The client has financial difficulties with purchasing food

Specific body system questions

Digestive system

Open-ended questions

Can you tell me more about the circumstances that bring on your abdominal pain?
Describe the pattern of your bowel motions during the week.
Describe the physical sensation of passing a bowel motion.
How long have you experienced the abdominal pain?
Can you describe a situation when you experience constipation?

General questions

Do you experience nausea or fatigue?
Has your appetite changed?
Have you experienced any weight changes?
If you do experience diarrhoea, what volume do you pass?
How often do you pass a bowel motion?
What is the colour of your bowel motion?
What is the odour of your bowel motion?
Do you ever have bloating and a visibly swollen belly?
Do you take laxatives or enemas?
Do you experience any flatulence/wind/burping?
Do you ever develop mouth ulcers or have dental concerns?
Do you experience indigestion, bloating, constipation and have a lack of exercise? (intestinal gas)
Do you experience loud rumbling sounds when needing to or while passing a bowel motion? (upper GI)
Do you experience an urgent need to pass a bowel motion? (colon)
Is the abdominal pain relieved by passing a bowel motion or flatus? (colon)
Is the abdominal pain better after belching? (stomach)
Do you notice any blood in your stools or on the toilet paper after passing a bowel motion? (cancer, inflammation)
Do your eyes or skin ever appear yellow? (jaundice)
Do you experience episodes of indigestion or persistent abdominal symptoms related to eating? (dyspepsia)
Is the heartburn relieved by nitroglycerin? (angina or oesophageal spasm)
Do you experience alternating constipation with diarrhoea? (irritable bowel syndrome, bowel cancer, diverticulitis)
Has the diarrhoea lasted more than three weeks and/or happens in a reoccurring pattern? (chronic disorder that could be infection, inflammation, absorption defect, systemic disorder or drug induced)
Do you experience a sensation of burning, warmth and heat in the midchest that can radiate to your jaw or arms (rare)? (heartburn)
Do you experience upper abdominal pain, feeling full quickly after eating, have a lack of appetite, nausea, belching, vomiting, bloating or a burning sensation in the chest or abdomen? (dyspepsia)
Is there a large volume of diarrhoea, which is watery, pale yellow or green, smells offensive, is fatty or floating and contains undigested food? (sign of organic diarrhoea of upper GI tract)
Are your stools small in volume, frequently passed, vary in consistency, brown in colour and/or show signs of bright blood or mucus? (colonic disease of GI tract)
Is the bleeding from the bowel a bright red colour and mixed in with the stools? (haematochezia from lower in the GI tract)
Is the bleeding from the bowel a tarry black colour and mixed in with the stools? (melaena from higher up in the GI tract)
Have you experienced any vomiting and if so how much?
Is vomiting linked with nausea or does it occur without warning?
Is vomiting associated with indigestion or abdominal pain?
Does vomiting relieve your indigestion or abdominal pain?
Is vomiting related to meal times or any specific time of the day?
Did the vomiting commence before the abdominal pain? (less probability of acute condition)
Did the vomiting commence after the abdominal pain? (more often acute)

▶

▶
Abdominal pain

Peritonitism – progressive distension and worsening pain described as constant and sharp. Rebound tenderness, pain aggravated by movement.
Somatic (from the wall of the body cavity, skin, muscles, joints) – aggravated by posture/movement, after trauma or injury, the pain is accurately localised and severe. Skin will have very defined pain, muscles and joints less defined as have less nerve endings.
Visceral (organs) – aggravated by genitalia, abdominal and pelvic organs. Intermittent pain, poorly localised, generalised, often referred pain, pain difficult to tolerate. Sharp, well localised, predictable, muscle spasm, dermatome impact, colic pain when involved with hollow muscular organs, gnawing, burning pain. Often associated with vomiting, diarrhoea and constipation, sweating, nausea, heart rate changes.

Pain characteristics
Severe abdominal pain not eased by analgesics (more often vascular event or rupture)
Severe abdominal pain eased by potent analgesics (acute pancreatitis or peritonitis)
Severe abdominal pain eased by parenteral analgesic (biliary or renal colic)
Dull, vague and poorly localised pain in abdomen (more often inflammatory or low-grade infection)
Moderately severe pain of sudden onset (more likely to be renal, biliary, acute pancreatitis, small bowel obstruction)
Slowly progressive abdominal pain and gradual onset (inflammation, infection such as salpingitis, appendicitis, diverticulitis)
Abdominal pain that is constant and made worse by movement such as coughing (more often inflammation)
Abdominal pain coming in waves of 6–10 minutes and is moderate (large bowel)
Abdominal pain coming in waves of 3–5 minutes and is severe (small bowel)
Abdominal pain very severe and constant for 20–360 minutes (biliary conditions)

Referred abdominal pain

Somatic:
Central and peripheral diaphragm – subcostal region (upper part of the third lumbar vertebra, transverse colon, the lower ends of the kidneys, and the upper limit of the transverse – third – part of the duodenum)
Pelvic peritoneum – perineum
Posterior abdominal wall below transverse colon – pain at the front of the abdomen
Posterior abdominal wall on right side of transverse colon – umbilical region, navel
Posterior abdominal wall on left side of transverse colon – lower abdomen and pubic area

Visceral:
Pain from lower oesophagus, stomach, duodenum, liver, gallbladder, bile duct, pancreas – referred to above the navel and upper abdomen
Pain from small intestine, Meckel's diverticulum, terminal ileum, appendix, cecum – referred to midgut, navel and associated with vomiting, loss of appetite and nausea
Pain from large bowel, sigmoid colon and rectum – referred to lower abdomen, pubic region and associated with blood, mucus and alternating bowel motions
Pain from pancreas, kidney/ureter, genital tract and aorta, central upper abdominal – lower back
Pain from spleen and gallbladder, irritation of the diaphragm – shoulder
Kidney and urinary tract – loin to groin, tip of the penis

Vomiting

Severe vomiting without abdominal pain (can be proximal small-bowel obstruction)
Persistent vomiting small in volume (feature of peritonitis)
Faeculent vomiting (late feature of colonic obstruction)
Have you experienced any vomiting and if so how much?
Is vomiting linked with nausea or does it occur without warning?
Is vomiting associated with indigestion or abdominal pain?

▶

▶ *Does vomiting relieve indigestion or abdominal pain?*
Is vomiting related to meal times or any specific time of the day?
Did the vomiting commence before the abdominal pain? (less probability of acute condition)
Did the vomiting commence after the abdominal pain? (more often acute)
Is the vomit that comes after the abdominal pain light in colour? (digestive juices and bile – gastritis, cholecystitis obstruction)

Indigestion

Younger clients are more likely to have functional causes of indigestion
Older clients more often have serious organic causes of indigestion

Referral flag symptoms
The client experiences abdominal pain followed by vomiting (surgical intervention may be needed)
Severe back pain associated with severe abdominal pain (ruptured or dissecting abdominal aortic aneurysm)
Abdominal pain with palpitations
The client experiences bloody stools or bloody diarrhoea that is black and tarry in colour
The client experiences diarrhoea associated with severe abdominal pain
The client describes a new onset of constipation, or stools that look darker than normal
The client is vomiting blood that looks like coffee grounds
There is a history of extreme alcohol use
The client experiences vomiting or pain that is limiting ingestion of regular medications
The client has abdominal pain that is associated with fever, vomiting, diarrhoea or lack of appetite
The client experiences abdominal pain that becomes worse after meals
The client experiences abdominal pain in the presence of chronic ibuprofen (or any other NSAID drug) or aspirin use
The onset of abdominal pain is sudden
The client experiences abdominal pain that doesn't resolve and lasts more than four hours
The client experiences abdominal pain that disturbs sleep
The client experiences constipation plus pain and/or vomiting for over 24 hours
Duration of diarrhoea has been more than three months
GI symptoms are associated with extreme weight loss
The client is at risk of dehydration due to excess vomiting or diarrhoea
Family history of colorectal carcinoma
The client experiences weight loss and indigestion (in an older client)
The client experiences indigestion, weight loss and lack of appetite
The client aged over 45 years has symptoms of significant dyspepsia
The client experiences daily symptoms of dyspepsia
The client experiences reflux with symptoms such as nocturnal coughing, vomiting blood or difficulty swallowing
The client experiences indigestion with pain radiating to the back
The client experiences indigestion with signs of jaundice, abdominal mass, bleeding and recurrent vomiting

Digestive questions for children [16]
Does the pain feel like there are butterflies in your tummy?
Does the pain feel like needles in your tummy?
Does the pain in your tummy go away when you lie down?
Does the pain in your tummy go away when you poo?

To the parent:
Has your child experienced three episodes of abdominal pain over three or more months? (recurrent abdominal pain)
Does your baby cry for more than three hours a day, more than three days a week and for more than three weeks? (commonly infantile colic)

▶

▶ *Does your child's abdominal pain begin with a stressful event, is it central (without radiating) and does not wake them up during the night?* (functional abdominal pain)
Did your child's abdominal pain start with a gradual onset of cramping? (intestinal cause)
Did your child's abdominal pain have a sudden onset that was not cramping pain? (torsion, intussusception, perforation)
Is there guarding of the abdomen for the child only present when experiencing pain? (mesenteric adenitis)
Does your child not want you to touch their abdomen all of the time (not only when experiencing pain)? (appendicitis)
Is the cramping abdominal pain relieved after eating meals and/or after a bowel motion? (constipation)
Did the cramping abdominal pain begin for your child with diarrhoea, nausea and vomiting? (gastroenteritis)
Does your baby scream with pain and suddenly pull up their legs to help relieve the pain? (intussusception)
Does your baby have sudden and severe abdominal pain every 15–30 minutes and seem very lethargic or sleepy in between? (intussusception)
Do your baby's bowel motions look like red currant jelly? (blood and mucus mixed with stools, common in intussusception)
Is the pain central in the middle of abdomen and made worse by eating? (chronic gastritis, *Helicobacter pylori*, food allergy/intolerance)
Is diarrhoea usually associated with the abdominal pain the child is experiencing? (surgical intervention rare)
Does your child usually experience abdominal distension along with the pain? (surgical emergency more common)
Did the vomiting begin before the abdominal pain for the child? (a cause other than abdominal origin often the cause)
Did the vomiting begin after the abdominal pain? (cause is usually abdominal origin)
Has the child had a respiratory tract infection recently, experienced nausea and vomiting but still had a good appetite throughout the abdominal pain? (mesenteric adenitis)
Is the abdominal pain not associated with symptoms of fever but began at a time of stress for the child? (psychosomatic causes)

Children referral flag symptoms
Abdominal pain with rectal bleeding, weight loss, anaemia, loss of appetite, fever, pain relieved by eating, pain on movement, pain that disturbs sleep and similar symptoms in the child's family health history

Genitourinary

Open-ended questions
Describe your menstrual cycle.
Can you tell me about your mother's and sister's menstrual pattern and history?
What is your pregnancy history?
Describe the pain you feel on urination.
Over the past month, how often have you felt the sensation of not emptying your bladder completely?
Over the past month, how often have you needed to urinate again less than two hours after your previous urination?
Over the past month, how many times did you get up to urinate during the night?
If you were to spend the rest of your life with the urinary problems you are facing now, how would you rate this as a problem? (scale 1 to 10)

General questions
How often do you urinate?
What is the volume of your urine, what colour is it and how does it smell?
Have you had any previous urinary tract infections?
Have you experienced any decrease or increase in urination?
Has the stream of urination changed?

▶

▶ *Is your abdominal pain intense and radiate from loin to groin every 10 minutes?* (renal)
Do you experience split stream, slow stream, dribbling or straining when urinating? (voiding symptoms)
Do you experience incomplete emptying and end dribbling? (postmicturation symptoms)
Do you experience increased frequency of urination in day/night time, urgency or incontinence? (urine storage symptoms, rare to have nocturia, urgency and frequency with stress incontinence)
How many times do you need to get up in the evening to urinate? (nocturia, detrusor muscle instability)
Do you need to pass urine more than 3–4 times a night? (nocturnal polyuria)
Have you noticed any leaking of urine? (incontinence)
Do you experience dripping of urine? (partially incompetent outlet, overflow, congenital or acquired anomalies)
Did your urinary symptoms develop gradually? (less likely to be urinary retention)
Have you experienced pain on urination recently? (dysuria)
Do you notice the discharge on waking or after a long period of not urinating? (urethral discharge)
Is the discharge you have experienced from your vagina or penis clear or whitish? (urethral discharge)

Women:
Have you had any previous pregnancies?
What age were you when your period first began?
On what date did you have your last period?
What volume of blood do you experience with your menstruation?
How many sanitary pads or tampons do you use during your menstrual cycles?
How long does your menstrual bleed last?
Do you experience any spotting or bleeding in between your periods?
Is your menstrual cycle less than 21 days? (abnormal bleeding)
Does your menstrual bleed last more than eight days? (abnormal bleeding)
Do you have clots in your menstrual blood? (abnormal bleeding)
Does your menstrual flow have a heavy, light, heavy flow pattern? (abnormal bleeding)
Do you experience any pain with your menstrual bleed?
Do you often experience unusual vaginal discharge that burns or has an odour?
Do you experience thrush?
Do you use contraception and if so, what type?
Have you experienced hot flushes or excess sweating?
Do you have regular breast checks?
Do you have regular pap smears?
Have you felt breast lumps, swelling or tenderness?
Have you noticed any bleeding or discharge from your breasts?
Were you taking any specific medication, such as penicillin, ampicillin or sulfa drugs, while you experienced vaginal itching? (medication causes of vulval itching)

Men:
Do you have regular prostate checks?
Have you experienced any surgery or trauma/accidents to your testicles?
When you have developed rapport

Sexual health

It would help me figure out how to help you if I could understand more about your sexual relationships. Do you mind if I ask you some more personal questions about your sexual history? [7]
Are you sexually active?
Have you previously had sexual relationships with a man or woman?
Have you experienced any changes in libido or pain on intercourse?
Do you experience difficulty maintaining an erection?

▶

▶ | *Have you ever had a problem gaining an erection or ejaculating?*
Do you experience any bleeding after intercourse?
Do you have a history of sexually transmitted diseases?
Have you ever had a test for HIV before or any investigations for sexually transmitted diseases?
Do you have a history of sexual dysfunction?
Have you had any experience of sexual abuse?

Referral flag symptoms

Symptoms of delayed urination, weak urine stream, prolonged stream of urine, straining when urinating, urinary retention, incontinence, urgency, increased frequency, nocturia, pelvic pain (prostatism)

Male client experiences pain on passing urine

Painless macroscopic blood in urine at any age

Unexplained microscopic blood in clients aged over 50 years

Male client has experienced complications with urine flow

All urinary symptoms are accompanied by low back/loin pain

Female clients with cystitis recurring more than three times

Children who present with a urinary tract infection

Persistent urinary tract infection in clients over 40 years of age

Client experiences increased need to pass urine without increase of fluid intake

Bladder wall inflammation and oestrogen deficiency (detrusor muscle instability)

Females over the age of 18 who fail to menstruate when all secondary sexual characteristics are normal

Female client describes non-menstrual vaginal bleeding (intermenstrual, postmenopausal, or at any time in pregnancy)

Pregnancy complications may present at any age in menstruating women

Female client describes vaginal bleeding with pain in pregnancy or after having missed a period

Female smokes and/or has excess caffeine and alcohol while trying to conceive

Males are taking cannabis or cocaine while trying to conceive

Males are exposed to metal fumes, solvents and/or pesticides while trying to conceive

Female has a menstrual history of oligo- or amenorrhoea and would like to try to conceive

Female has a history of PID, past malignancy and would like to try to conceive

Male history of undescended testicle and would like to try to conceive

Intermenstrual bleeding

Irregular menstrual bleeding

Sudden change in volume of menstrual blood

Painful intercourse and/or bleeding after intercourse

Pelvic pain in men and women

Premenstrual pain for women

Drug reaction

Drugs that can affect male fertility: sulfasalazine, tetracyclines and allopurinol

Drugs that can alter menstrual bleeding

▶

COMMON DRUGS THAT MAY ALTER MENSTRUAL BLEEDING [17]	
GROUP AND GENERIC NAMES	**TRADE AND COMMON NAMES**
*Amphetamines	*Desoxyn, Obetrol
Anticoagulants	Coumadin, heparin
*Benzodiazepines	
Diazepam, oxazepam	*Valium, Serax
Benzomide derivatives	
Procainamide, procarbazine	Pronestyl, Matulane
*Butyrophenones	*Haldol, Inapsine
Cannabis	Marijuana
Chlordiazepoxide	Librium
*Cimetidine	Tagamet
Ethyl alcohol	Whisky, wine, beer
*Isoniazid	*Isonicotinic acid hydrazide
*Methyldopa	*Aldomet
Monoamine oxidase inhibitors	Eutonyl, Nardil
*Opiates	*Morphine, heroin, methadone
*Phenothiazines	*Compazine, Thorazine, Phenergan
Prostaglandin inhibitors	Motrin, Indocin
Rauwolfia	Raudixin
*Reserpine	*Serpasil
*Spironolactone	*Aldactone
Steroids	
Gonadal	
*Oestrogens	*Premarin, oral contraceptives
*Progesterones	*Provera, oral contraceptives
*Testosterone	*Android
Thyroid hormones	Synthroid, Cytomel
*Thioxanthenes	*Navane
*Tricyclic antidepressants	*Elavil

*May also produce galactorrhea

COMMON DRUGS THAT MAY CAUSE AMENORRHOEA [18]	
GENERIC NAME	TRADE AND COMMON NAMES
Amphetamines	Desoxyn, Obetrol
Benzodiazepines	
Diazepam, oxazepam	Valium, Serax
Benzomide derivatives	Pronestyl, Matulane
Butyrophenones	Haldol, Inapsine
Calcium channel blockers	
Nifedipine, verapamil, diltiazem	Adalat, Cardizem, Calan
Cannabis	Marijuana
Chemotherapeutics	Cytoxan, Myleran, Leukeran, Platinol
Cimetidine	Tagamet
Isoniazid	Isonicotinic acid hydrazide
Methyldopa	Aldomet
Monoamine oxidase inhibitors	Eutonyl, Nardil
Opiates	Morphine, heroin
Phenothiazines	Compazine, Thorazine, Phenergan
Rauwolfia	Harmonyl, Raudixin
Reserpine	Serpasil
Spironolactone	Aldactone
Steroids	
Gonadal	Ingredients of oral contraceptives
Estrogens	
Progesterones	
Thyroid hormones	Synthroid, Cytomel
Thioxanthenes	Navane
Tricyclic antidepressants	Elavil

DRUGS THAT PRECIPITATE OR AGGRAVATE STRESS INCONTINENCE

Methyldopa, prazosin, phenothiazines, diazepam, caffeine, diuretics

DRUGS THAT PRECIPITATE OR AGGRAVATE URINARY RETENTION

Adrenergic agents, calcium channel blockers, anticholinergics, androgens, antihistamines and sympathomimetic agents such as ephedrine and pseudoephedrine.

DRUGS THAT MAY PRECIPITATE URINARY INCONTINENCE

Psychotropic and sedative agents

DRUGS THAT MAY PRECIPITATE OR AGGRAVATE NOCTURNAL POLYURIA

Digoxin, phenytoin, lithium, diuretics and excess vitamin D

Urine colour [1]

Red urine – haematuria, haemolytic anaemias, beetroot, purple cabbage
Dark yellow-brown – jaundice, riboflavin ingestion
Brown smoky urine – nephritis, due to red blood cells mixing with acidic pH, malignant melanoma
Black urine – alkaptonuria, melanuria
Green urine – pseudomonas infection, copper ingestion

Respiratory

Open-ended questions
Describe how it feels to experience shortness of breath.
Describe a situation when you would experience difficulty breathing.
Can you tell me if you bring up sputum when you cough?

General questions
Have you experienced a cough or excess mucus?
If you do experience mucus, what colour, volume and consistency is the mucus?
Do you experience persistent coughing?
Do you have a history of asthma?
Do you experience any chest pain?
Did the cough begin suddenly along with a fever? (viral infection is a common cause)
Did the cough resolve within three weeks? (acute cough is most often due to viral upper respiratory tract infection, bronchitis, laryngitis, seasonal allergies and postnasal drip)
Has the cough lasted longer than three weeks? (chronic cough most often due to chronic bronchitis, bacterial infection, postnasal drip, asthma, gastro-oesophageal reflux, chronic obstructive pulmonary disease – COPD, heart failure, tuberculosis, lung tumour, habit)
Has your child experienced a recurrent cough? (recurrent viral upper respiratory tract infection, reactive airway disease, asthma, viral bronchitis, allergies)
Have you experienced any significant shortness of breath?
Do you ever experience wheezing when you are short of breath? (bronchospasm)
Do you experience shortness of breath when lying flat? (orthopnoea)
Do you know if you snore loudly?
Is your fatigue associated with headaches and upper respiratory complaints? (sick building syndrome)
Do you experience these respiratory symptoms when you are working in a modern building with inadequate ventilation? Do these symptoms improve when you leave the building? (sick building syndrome)
Does the mucus production change with different body postures? (lung abscess, foreign body, gastro-oesophageal reflux)

▶

Referral flag symptoms
Client experiences any difficulty breathing
Breathing difficulties that worsen when lying flat or on exertion
The client is breathing faster than usual and having difficulty talking
The client experienced a change in voice over time (laryngeal concern)
The client describes difficulty breathing that starts suddenly
The client has shortness of breath along with fever
Use of ACE inhibitor with a chronic cough
Unexplained nocturnal cough in elderly clients (suggestive of congestive heart failure)
The client is a smoker and there has been a significant change in character of chronic cough (possible bronchogenic carcinoma)

The client is coughing up blood

Rusty coloured blood (pneumococcal pneumonia)
Pink and frothy sputum (pulmonary oedema)
Blood that appears like red currant jelly and is associated with unusual weight loss (bronchogenic cancer)
Weight loss with large volume of blood in sputum (TB)
Dark blood in sputum with acute respiratory distress (pulmonary embolus)
Blood-flecked mucus with persistent coughing (bronchitis, URTI)
Large volume of blood with fingernail clubbing (bronchiectasis)

Persistent cough – age reference

Infant (< 1 year) – congenital malformations, viral pneumonia, rubella, cytomegalovirus, aspiration (milk, saliva, gastric contents), cystic fibrosis, asthma
Preschool (1–5 years) – inhaled foreign body, chronic atelectasis, bronchiectasis, cystic fibrosis, bronchitis with upper respiratory disease, asthma
School age – cigarette smoking, mycoplasma pneumonia infection, nervous or psychogenic cough, cystic fibrosis
All ages – recurrent viral bronchitis, asthma, pertussis, cystic fibrosis

Eyes, ear, nose and throat

Open-ended questions
Describe what is happening when you have difficulty chewing your food.
What are the taste changes you are experiencing?
Describe any additional sensations you may feel when experiencing nausea.

General questions
Do you experience any ringing in the ears?
Do you experience sensitivity to light or blurred vision?
Do you experience nearsightedness? (myopia)
Are the visual changes experienced only in one eye? (unilateral)
Do you see two separate objects either side by side or one above the other? (diplopia, double vision)
Do you only experience double vision in one eye when the other eye is covered?
Do you ever experience cross-eyed vision? (strabismus)
Do you experience areas of totally obscured vision? (scotomas)
Are the visual changes constant or do they come and go?
Do you experience near or distant vision or both?
Did the visual changes happen gradually or come on suddenly?
Have the visual changes become better or worse since you first noticed them?
Have you had excess mucus in sinuses or experienced changes in your ability to smell?
Have you had a sore throat or swollen glands?
Are your tongue or teeth sore?
Do you have any fillings, dentures or grind your teeth?

▶

▶ *Do you suffer from bleeding gums?*
Do you have any difficulty chewing your food?
Have you experienced any changes in your sense of taste recently?
Have you experienced any dizziness or sensation of the room spinning?
Have you experienced any nausea?
Do you experience scanty mucus, dry scratchy throat or nasal pain? (URTI)
Do your visual changes occur prior to getting a migraine? (scintillating scotoma)
Is your visual blurring associated with grittiness or warmth in the eyes? (dry eyes, common in older women)
Is your ear pain usually bilateral? (otitis externa due to diabetes, dermatitis, ear pickers, swimmers, impacted ear wax, serous otitis media)
Do you experience itching in the ear? (otitis externa)
Did you experience hearing difficulties prior to having earaches and infections? (birth injury, trauma, degenerative disease, occupation hazard, tumour, infection such as meningitis, measles or mumps)
Do you experience an intermittent scratching sound that is made worse by pressing on the ear? (external auditory canal disorder)
Does the ringing in the ear have a clicking or banging sound? (middle ear and eustachian tube)
Do you hear a blowing sound in your ears that is synchronised with your own breathing? (middle ear and eustachian tube)
Does the tinnitus disappear when you are lying down or resting your head? (middle ear and eustachian tube)

Referral flag symptoms
Client has experienced double vision, blurry vision or loss of vision (even if transient)
There is a personal or family history of glaucoma
There is a personal or family history of diabetes, high blood pressure or atrial fibrillation
Client experiences changes in vision along with severe eye pain, headache, scalp or jaw pain
Common visual symptoms: refractive errors, PVD, migraine, glaucoma, cataracts, dry eyes, drug side effects, transient ischaemic attacks (TIA)
Visual concerns for young people are usually due to refractive error (myopia)
Visual concerns for clients aged over 40 are usually due to accommodation problems (presbyopia)
Distance blurring in elderly people is most frequently due to cataracts
Sudden onset visual blurring in one eye is usually more serious and of ocular origin
Visual blurring in both eyes that has developed gradually over several months, with no other health signs evident, is usually a refractive error
Redness in one eye is usually more serious than redness in both eyes
Extraocular redness in both eyelids with a white eyeball and restricted eye movement may indicate orbital cellulitis, which requires immediate referral
Ear pain with purulent, mucoid or blood-stained ear discharge (perforated tympanic membrane, leaking CSF, trauma)
Earache is severe, sudden and persistent in pain
Earache with facial paralysis
Persistent unilateral tinnitus present for more than three months
Unilateral and asymmetrical sensorineural deafness
Tinnitus that interferes with daily activity
Tinnitus with hearing loss that would benefit from a hearing aid
Tinnitus associated with anxiety or depression
Objective tinnitus

▶

▶

Cardiovascular
Open-ended questions *Describe the chest pain you have been feeling.* *Where exactly do you feel the chest pain?* *What is happening to the chest pain now?* *How do you feel emotionally when you experience the chest pain?* *Can you explain what you feel when you say 'light headed'?*
General questions *Have you experienced a recurrent cough?* (can be an early sign of heart failure) *Does coughing and sneezing aggravate the headache?* (vascular origin) *Have you experienced any swelling in your extremities such as the hands or ankles?* *Have you had difficulty putting rings on your fingers?* *Have you suffered heart palpitations?* *Have you noticed an irregular heartbeat?* *Have you experienced any chest pain?* *Do you experience hot or cold extremities?* *Do you have cold or blue hands?* (peripheral cyanosis) *Do you have a tendency for high or low blood pressure?* *Do you have varicose veins?* *Do you bruise easily?* *Have you experienced blackouts, fainting or dizziness?* *Have you experienced shortness of breath when you are lying down or on exertion?* *How many flights of stairs can you climb before experiencing shortness of breath?* *Have you had rheumatic fever?* *Have you had your cholesterol checked?* *Do you suffer from headaches?* *Can you tap out the beat of the palpitations on the desk for me to hear?*

CARDIOVASCULAR READINGS
BLOOD PRESSURE READINGS

	SYSTOLIC	DIASTOLIC
Optimal BP	120 mmHg	80 mmHg
Normotension	< 140 mmHg	< 90 mmHg
High normal	130–139 mmHg	85–89 mmHg
Definite hypertension (mild)	140–160 mmHg	95 mmHg
Moderate hypertension	160–179 mmHg	95–109 mm Hg
Significant hypertension	(adult) > 180 mmHg	> 110 mmHg
	(18-year-old) 142 mmHg	92 mmHg
	(15-year-old) 136 mmHg	86 mmHg
	(10-year-old) 126 mmHg	82 mmHg
Isolated systolic hypertension	(grade 1) 140–159 mmHg	< 90 mmHg
	(grade 2) >160 mmHg	< 90 mmHg

Note: readings can be affected if the client is anxious, stressed, in pain, in dis1comfort while having blood pressure taken, cold or has engaged in recent exertion. Changes in posture can affect readings in those who are elderly, pregnant, on medication or who have orthostatic hypotension.

PULSE READINGS:		
Regular pulse	60–100 beats/min	Normal
Regular pulse	< 60 beats/min	Sinus bradycardia
Regular pulse	> 100 beats/min	Sinus tachycardia
Rapid pulse	Irregular pulse/sudden onset	Atrial fibrillation/ventricular tachycardia (fibrillation, flutter), multiple ventricular extrasystoles/heart block

Referral flag symptoms
The client experiences a discomfort that feels like squeezing, pressure or heaviness on the chest
The client experiences shortness of breath, pain down the left arm and tingling in the fingers of the left hand.
The client describes symptoms of breathlessness, nocturnal dyspnoea (left ventricular failure)
Abrupt onset of high blood pressure
The client has high blood pressure with symptoms of nausea, severe headache, disturbed speech and vision with paralysis or numbness in extremities (malignant hypertension, hypertensive encephalopathy)
The client has hypertension and protein detected in urinalysis (renal impairment)
The client has hypertension and visual impairment (hypertensive retinopathy)
The client is a child or teenager and presents with high blood pressure
The client experiences chest pain and sweating, nausea and is feeling fearful about their symptoms
The client experiences chest pain frequently and there has been a change in pattern and frequency
The pain or pressure is worse with exertion and improves with rest
The client experiences chest pain associated with feelings of light-headedness or passing out
The client describes chest pain or shortness of breath with a swollen or painful leg
The client describes a feeling of the heart fluttering or beating quickly
The client has headache pain that prevents sleep
The client experiences an isolated and very severe headache
The client experiences a change in usual headache pattern
Headache that has persisted for more than 24 hours
The client experiences headache with neurological symptoms including speech difficulties, blurred vision, lack of coordination, feelings of numbness or lack of concentration
The client is experiencing headaches with vomiting
The client experiences chronic and progressively worsening headache
The client is aged over 55 and has experienced a new and severe, acute and unrelenting headache
The client is experiencing headaches and has unequal pupil size
The client experiences a headache that is worse on waking in absence of neck discomfort (intracranial pressure)
Headache pain that is made worse by exertion, bending, stooping, coughing, straining at stool and sneezing (intracranial pressure)
The client has a rapid pulse of 200 beats/min
The client has a slow pulse of 50 beats/min
The client has a pulse of 120 beats/min at rest
The client experiences dizziness and the feeling of fainting along with palpitations
The client's systolic pressure is 90 mmHg or less
The client passes a large volume of urine after having heart palpitations and has a heart murmur (organic heart disease)
The client experiences palpitations with chest pain that radiates to neck/arm (myocardial ischaemia)

▶

►| *Drugs that can cause headaches*
Resperine, vasodilators, H_2-receptor blockers, indomethacin, angiotensin-converting enzyme (ACE) inhibitors, nitrates, beta-blockers, calcium channel blockers, sildenafil, oral contraceptives, withdrawal from ergot drugs
Stroke or transient ischaemic attack (TIA)
The client experiences weakness, numbness or inability to move any part of their body
The client experiences any changes in vision, including double vision, blurry vision or loss of vision
The client unable to speak a simple sentence
The client appears confused
The client describes and displays feelings of dizziness, loss of balance, unsteadiness or difficulty walking
The client experiences a recent head injury, stroke or seizure
The client is unable to smile
The client has a crooked tongue (if they can still stick it out)
The client is unable to raise both arms

Nervous system

Open-ended questions
Describe what the headache feels like.
How does the headache feel now?
Describe your moods recently.
Sometimes symptoms can be brought on by periods of feeling stressed; can you relate to that?
Describe the episode of intense fear you have experienced.
Describe a situation where you have felt relaxed recently.
How many hours of sleep do you expect to have each night?
Describe your routine two hours before trying to go to sleep each night.
Can you describe what effect the insomnia is having on your daily life?
Can you identify anything in particular that is keeping you awake?
What do you do if you cannot get to sleep?

General questions
How many days do you think you have worried excessively during the past 3–6 months?
Have you felt low most of the day and nearly every day for the past two weeks?
(depression)
Have you had less interest in your usual activities? (depression)
Would you like to tell me more about how you feel?
What are your sleep patterns like and do you ever experience insomnia?
What do you think about before falling asleep and when you wake up in the morning?
Do you go to bed at the same time every night?
What is the quality of your mattress and pillow?
Are you uncomfortable in your bed?
Are you ever hungry when trying to sleep at night?
Are you ever too hot or too cold when trying to sleep at night?
Have you experienced headaches?
How would you describe your concentration and memory?
Have you experienced any mood changes that are unusual for you?
Have you experienced pain, weakness, numbness or tingling in your limbs or on your skin?
Have you experienced a lack of physical coordination?
Do you have difficulty walking, sitting or running?
Have you experienced any dizziness or fainting?
Have you ever experienced a fit or blackout?
Are you under a lot of stress?
Have you experienced any mood changes, irritation or sadness?
Have you been more self-critical than usual lately?
Has there been a change in your self-esteem and how you view yourself?   ►

▶ *Have you experienced any loss of libido?*
Have you experienced extreme fatigue?
Have you experienced any visual disturbances?
Do you experience any difficulty swallowing?
Are you able to breathe in deeply?
Do you feel compelled to do certain things when feeling stressed?
Have you experienced a loss of interest in usual or routine activities?
Have you experienced feelings of fear as if awful things are about to happen?
Do you feel frightened for a particular reason?
Do you experience sudden feelings of panic?
Do you ever feel the need to use alcohol or sedatives to ease the worry or fear?
Do you experience the sensation of having a dry mouth or being excessively thirsty?
Have you experienced worrying thoughts racing through your mind?

When rapport with the client has developed, if necessary

Open-ended questions
I am wondering how low you have been feeling. Are you feeling up to telling me? [1]
Some people feel like they cannot go on when they feel very depressed. Have you ever felt like that? [1]
Have you ever made any plans to hurt yourself or someone else? [1]
I can imagine many people in your situation would get quite depressed (wait for the client to respond) [3].
You indicated you felt your life was not worth living. Can you tell me how often you feel this way?
Describe a situation when you've felt like hurting yourself.
You indicated something awful happened to you when you were a child. Would you like to share more with me about that with me?
Can you tell me who the people are who you're seeing at the window? What are they saying? [1]
I can understand why you would be so upset because you believe you are being poisoned. I can't tell you for sure that someone is poisoning you, but I can tell you that I am not harming or poisoning you. I would like to listen and help you if I can [1].
That must have been very frightening. Do you feel like talking to me about that today or should I come back to what you just shared later? [19]
What do you think it would feel like to hurt yourself?

Closed questions
Do you have suicidal thoughts?
Have you ever wished you would not wake up the next morning?
Have you thought of how you would kill yourself?
How long have you thought of killing yourself?
When do you want to kill yourself?
Have you told anyone else you have thoughts of dying and/or hurting yourself?
Do you ever feel like you are losing control?
It may be necessary to ask direct questions regarding possible suicide intent if the client has opened up about this rather than avoid the issue. Other people may need gentle open-ended questioning to feel ready to disclose that information if you think this could be an underlying issue that needs to be raised for immediate referral [1, 4].

Referral flag symptoms
Insomnia in children (usually caused by psychological stress)
Fainting, blacking out or light-headedness
Fainting associated with chest pain, palpitations, abdominal pain, shortness of breath or headache
Fainting without preceding warning symptoms
Fainting during exercise

▶

▶
Extreme headaches
Headache that begins suddenly and the client can describe the exact moment it started Headache that the client may describe as unusual for them or the worst they have ever experienced Headache that is connected with symptoms of confusion, fever, stiff neck, vomiting, seizure, weakness, numbness, visual changes or pain with chewing Headache after a recent trauma or fall
Depression
The client feels they want to hurt themselves or someone else The client has a history of abuse The client feels persistent sadness There is a lack of motivation and self-care The client shows no interest in daily activities Increased use of alcohol or substances The client has suicidal ideas The client describes hearing voices The client demonstrates inconsistent behaviour A child as the following behaviour: hyperactivity, withdrawal, eating problems, school troubles, sleep disturbances, vague physical symptoms Adolescents show signs of substance abuse or sexual misconduct
Fatigue
Use of antihistamines, psychotropics, tranquillisers, antihypertensives (reserpine, methyldopa, clonidine, beta-blockers) Sleep disturbance is associated with the use of or withdrawal from pyschotropics, beta-blockers, bronchodilators, sympathomimetics, diuretics, hypnotics, appetite suppressants, amphetamines, cocaine, alcohol or caffeine
Musculoskeletal
Open-ended questions *Describe where you are feeling the muscle tension.* *How is the muscle tension feeling now?* *Tell me about the history of your back pain.* *How does the rest of your body feel when you have back pain?* *What kind of sensation do you feel when experiencing back pain?* *Describe if there is anything in your daily living that this back pain has prevented you from doing.*
General questions *Have you experienced any specific body pain?* *Is your pain constant in all positions?* (inflammatory, infectious, tumour of spine) *Do you have a history of physical trauma or accidents?* *Do you feel tension in your body?* *Do you have postural deviations or deformities that you know of?* *Have you experienced any muscle wasting, tremors, tics, spasms or tingling sensations in your extremities?* *Have you experienced unusual weakness in muscle strength?* *Have you experienced any cramps or stiffness in your limbs?* *When you feel stiffness do you feel a restricted range of movement?* *When you feel stiffness do you experience difficulty moving but with normal range?* *When you feel stiffness do you experience painful movement?* *Is the stiffness localised to a particular joint or is it more generalised?* *Have you experienced any swelling in your body?* *Does the pain take your breath away at times?* *Does the pain affect you bathing yourself, dressing yourself, going to the toilet, cutting food or eating food, driving or managing medications?*

▶

► *What is the layout of your house? Does the pain affect your daily activities around the house?*
Do you experience a restricted range of movement and painful movement? (stiffness)
Does the pain improve with exercise/movement? (inflammatory/degenerative causes)
Do you experience your joint pain at night? (arthritis)
Is the joint swelling localised with warmth, redness and local pain? (arthritis)
Does the pain become worse with physical activity and improve with rest? (mechanical causes)
Is the pain variable, diffuse or does it feel like intense pressure? (not often organic disease, referred joint pain)
Is the muscle weakness becoming progressively worse and do you have a family history of similar symptoms? (muscular dystrophy)
Is the joint motion impaired and do you experience pain when the joint tries to bear weight or undergo physical stress? (mechanical joint pain)
Did the pain at the base of your thumb become worse after menopause? (osteoarthritis at base of the thumb)
Do you experience any shoulder stiffness or pain with the sore hands and fingers? (referred arthritis pain)
Does your finger and hand discomfort last for more than one hour in the mornings? (RA)
Have you experienced hand pain and stiffness in more than three joints in the mornings for more than six weeks? (RA)

Referral flag symptoms
When back pain is associated with incontinence or retention of stool or urine
The client feels weakness or numbness of the legs or groin area
The client feels unsteady and has weakness in the extremities
The client experiences persistent back pain and has no history of falls or other trauma
The client has a personal or family history of osteoporosis
The client has a personal or family history of cancer
The client has back pain associated with fever
The back pain is associated with burning or painful urination
The client experiences back pain and neck stiffness with a fever
When back pain is associated with weight loss, IV drug use, prolonged use of corticosteroid, being over 50 years of age, and it is not improved with rest (cancer or infection)
When back pain is associated with acute urinary retention, incontinence, loss of sphincter tone or weakness in the lower limbs (cauda equine syndrome)
Acute musculoskeletal pain in a person under the age of 20 years or over 55
Recent history of violent trauma
No relief of pain from bed rest
Intensely painful frozen shoulder with red, swollen joint (septic arthritis)
Morning stiffness with morning pain and swelling of joints and hands for more than six weeks (RA)
The client has joint pain accompanied by weight loss, fever, skin rash or extreme fatigue

Immune system/endocrine

Open-ended questions
Describe your energy levels.
Describe how you feel about being in the heat or the cold.
Tell me about the recent fever you have experienced.

General questions
Have you experienced any fever or chills?
Have you experienced a recurrent infection?
Have you noticed any lumps under your arms, in your neck or groin?
How would you rate your energy levels?
Have you been troubled by fatigue?
Do you have depleted energy and feel weary or weak? (fatigue)

►

▶ *Do you experience daytime sleepiness, decreased alertness and a propensity to fall asleep?*
(drowsiness)
Have you felt unusually anxious?
Have you noticed a change in your appearance or change in weight, hair, skin, nails or voice?
Are you sensitive to environmental temperature fluctuations?
What season do you prefer?
Have you noticed a change in appetite?

Fatigue

Have you experienced a viral or bacterial infection along with your increasing tiredness?
(acute fatigue, heart failure, anaemia)
Is the fatigue not present in the morning? (organic origin)
Is the fatigue worse as the day progresses and relieved by rest? (organic origin)
Has the fatigue been gradually progressing rather than fluctuating? (organic origin)
Is the fatigue associated with periods of prolonged physical or mental activity, inadequate rest, poor sleep, dieting, sedentary lifestyle, pregnancy or mental stress? (physiologic fatigue)

Referral flag symptoms
Client experiences unexplained persistent and recurrent fever
Client presents with a goitre
Goitre presents with a firm single nodule, hoarse voice and swollen lymph nodes (thyroid cancer)
Client has lost weight rapidly for an unknown reason

Skin and nails

Open-ended questions
Describe how the skin rash feels.
What kind of sensation does the skin rash have?
Describe a situation when your skin would bruise easily.

General questions
Do you experience excess sweating? If so, what part of your body sweats more?
Have you experienced hair falling out, if so, how much?
Do your nails break easily? Do your nails have any spots or lines on them?
Do you bruise easily?
Have you experienced any skin rashes?
Have you noticed any moles that have changed?
Have you had any lumps or frequent skin infections?
Is the skin rash associated with fatigue, weight loss or fever? (systemic origin)
Have you noticed any rashes or lumps on your genitals? (STI)

Referral flag symptoms
The client has a skin rash and is taking aspirin, an NSAID or steroid medication
The client has experienced an allergic reaction to an insect bite or food
The client experiences swelling of lips, face, tongue or throat
The client experiences redness, rash or hives over the body
The client has a skin lesion that is not healing or is changing shape and colour
Scaly patches with sandpaper texture
Nodules with central ulceration
A velvet hyperpigmented nodule in the armpit, neck or groin (may be adenocarcinoma)

Possible allergens in contact dermatitis

Tools, musical instruments, machinery, photograph materials, ceramics, glues, eyeglass frames, jewellery, paints, inks, fertilisers, cosmetics, deodorants, shampoos, medications, wood, rubber gloves, hair dyes, fungicides, nail polish, utensils, money, food colouring/flavouring, toothpaste, contraceptive lubricants, topical antibiotics, topical anaesthetics

Core

CORE QUESTIONS [1, 7–9]
Analogy: The core of the apple with the seed of ill health Using the mnemonic 'SEEDS OF HEALTH'
Core: Holistic assessment to understand the client; unique contributing emotional, mental, spiritual, metaphysical, lifestyle and constitutional factors for the individual
SUPPORT SYSTEMS
What would you like in an intimate relationship at this time in your life? *Are you in an intimate relationship?* *Do you have a regular partner?* *Do you have a religion or spiritual practice yourself?*
EMOTIONAL HEALTH
Is there anything from your own background that may affect how you are thinking about your health right now? [1] *Do you have any significant fears or anxieties at the moment?*
ENVIRONMENTAL WELLNESS
How much television or computer work do you do? *Is a mobile phone or TV or computer switched on near where you sleep?* *Have you been travelling recently?*
DAILY ACTIVITIES
Describe your lifestyle. *Do you feel balance with social, family and work life?*
STRESS RELEASE
Have you lost interest in things you usually enjoy? *Do you need to take any mind-altering substances to feel happy?*
OCCUPATION
Tell me about your current work environment and where you have worked in the past. *Do you get on well with people at work?*
FAMILY AND FRIENDS
Do you have a support network of friends and family? *Would you say you have a large number of friends?* *Do you have time to relax with family or friends?* *Can you talk about how you are feeling towards any of your friends or family?*
HOME LIFE
How would you describe your relationships and living arrangements? *Are you happy where you are living at the moment?*
EDUCATION AND LEARNING
What personal hobbies or interests do you have?
ACTION NEEDED TO HEAL
How do you want me to help you feel healthy again? *What do you think is the most important aspect of your life that needs changing?* *How much exercise do you do?*

▶

►

LONG-TERM GOALS
If you could snap your fingers and have anything you wanted in your life, what would be your wish list? *How do you feel about the future?* *Describe an ideal state of health.* *Do you feel like there is anything missing in your life?*

TIME TO HEAL
Can you describe your childhood and school days?

HAS NOT BEEN WELL SINCE
What was happening in your life when you first developed [the complaint]? *Describe a situation when you felt extremely healthy.* *What was happening in your life when you felt extremely healthy?* *Describe the last time you felt happy.* *Sometimes clients have their own explanations for why they may be unwell and it helps to understand each individual perspective, would you like to share yours with me?* [1] *Have you experienced a major life change?*

CORE QUESTIONS FOR CHILDREN
Are the parents living together and if not how often do they see their child? *Who else makes up the household where the child lives?* *How many siblings does the child have?* *Are there any childcare arrangements during the week?* *Is the family being restricted due to the child's illness?* *Are there any issues with the housing?* *How many bedrooms does the house have?* *Are there safe rooms for children to play in?* *How many smokers are in the house where the children live?* *Does the child have any pets?* *How is the child enjoying and performing at school?* *Has the child ever experienced behaviour or bullying issues at school?* *Has illness affected day-to-day activities for the child and ability to play with their friends?*
Referral flag symptoms The client has a lack of social support The client does not feel in control of the choices they are making for themselves The client feels overwhelmed with life The client does not make time for themselves The client has no particular personal interests or hobbies There is a lack of creative energy or personal life goals The client has experienced a significant trauma, shock or grief The client is questioning their own spiritual, religious or personal meaning of life

References

[1] J. Silverman, S. Kurtz, J. Draper, Skills for Communicating with Patients, second edn, Radcliff Publishing, Oxford, 2000.

[2] S. El-Hashemy, Naturopathic Standards of Primary Care, CCNM Press, Toronto, 2008.

[3] R. Neighbour, The Inner Consultation; how to develop an effective and intuitive consulting style, Radcliff Publishing, Oxon, 2005.

[4] R. McCabe, et al., Engagement of patients with psychosis in the consultation; conversation analytic study, BMJ 325 (2002) 1148–1151.

[5] R. Berkow, A.J. Fletcher, M.H. Beers, The Merck Manual, sixteenth edn. Rathway, NJ: Merck Research Laboratories, 1993 (later edition).

[6] D. Peters, L. Chaitow, G. Harris, S. Morrison, Integrating Complementary Therapies in Primary Care, Churchill Livingstone, London, 2002.

[7] M. Lloyd, R. Bor, Communication Skills For Medicine, third edn, Churchill Livingstone Elsevier, Edinburgh, 2009.

[8] N.J. Talley, S. O'Connor, Pocket Clinical Examination, third edn, Churchill Livingstone Elsevier, Australia, 2009.

[9] G. Douglas, F. Nicol, C. Robertson, Macleod's Clinical Examination, Twelfth edn, Churchill Livingstone Elsevier, London, 2009.

[10] P. Kumar, C. Clark, Clinical Medicine, sixth edn, Elsevier Saunders, London, 2005.

[11] P. Glasziou, Evidence-Based Diagnosis in Primary Care, Churchill Livingstone Elsevier, Philadelphia, 2008.

[12] R.H. Seller, Differential Diagnosis of Common Complaints, fifth edn, Saunders Elsevier, Philadelphia, 2007.

[13] R.D. Collins, Differential Diagnosis in Primary Care, fourth edn, Lippincott Williams and Wilkins, Philadelphia, 2008.

[14] J. Jamison, Differential Diagnosis for Primary Care, second edn, Churchill Livingstone Elsevier, London, 2006.

[15] L. Chaitow, E. Blake, P. Orrock, M. Wallden, P. Snider, J. Zeff, (Eds.) Natropathic Physical Medicine: Theory and Practice for Manual Therapists and Naturopaths, Churchill Livingstone Elsevier, Philadelphia, 2008.

[16] Al. Lake, Chronic abdominal pain in childhood: diagnosis and management, Am Fam Physician 59 (7) (1999) 1823–1830.

[17] J.N. Murata, Abnormal genital bleeding and secondary amenorrhea: common gynecological problems, J Obstet Gynecol Neonatal Nurs 19(1990) 26–36.

[18] J.N. Murata, Primary amenorrhea, Pediatr Nurs 15(1989) 125–129.

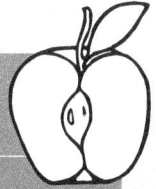

Case-taking forms – initial consultation

Section 1: Forms for the client to complete prior to consultation

DO YOU HAVE OR HAVE YOU EVER HAD:	YES	NO
Cardiovascular disease (heart attack, heart trouble, heart murmur, coronary artery disease, angina, high blood pressure, stroke, palpitations?)		
Lung disease (asthma, emphysema, chronic cough, bronchitis, pneumonia, tuberculosis, shortness of breath, chest pain, severe coughing?)		
Seizures, convulsions, epilepsy, fainting or dizziness?		
Bleeding disorders or anaemia Do you bruise easily?		
Liver disease (jaundice, hepatitis)?		
Kidney disease?		
Diabetes?		
Thyroid disease (goitre)?		
Arthritis?		
Cancer		
Are you pregnant?		

LIST ANY PHARMACEUTICAL MEDICATIONS YOU ARE CURRENTLY TAKING		
MEDICATION	**DAILY DOSE**	**HOW LONG HAVE YOU BEEN TAKING THIS MEDICATION?**

LIST THE NUTRITIONAL/VITAMIN/HERBAL SUPPLEMENTS YOU ARE CURRENTLY TAKING		
SUPPLEMENT	**DAILY DOSE**	**HOW LONG HAVE YOU BEEN TAKING THIS SUPPLEMENT?**

HEALTH SYSTEMS CHECK

TICK IF YOU EXPERIENCE ANY OF THE FOLLOWING SYMPTOMS

Head	**Skin, hair, scalp, nails**	**Ears, nose and throat**
— Headaches	— Acne	— Deafness
— Migraine	— Eczema	— Ear noises
— Dizziness	— Psoriasis	— Wax, earaches
— Fainting	— Hair loss	— Sinusitis
Eyes	— Dandruff	— Loss of sense of smell
— Eyestrain	— Excess sweating	— Blocked nose
— Light sensitivity		— Frequent colds
— Blurred vision		— Hay fever
— Double vision		— Allergies
— Watering		— Sneezing
— Red eye		— Swollen glands
— Painful eye		— Nosebleeds
Mouth, teeth and gums	**Neck, shoulders and arms**	**Chest**
— Toothache	— Aching	— Pains
— Lost or loose teeth	— Tension	— Tightness
— Abscesses	— Arm pain	— Breathing difficulty
— Ulcers	— Tingling	— Coughs
— Cold sores	— Cold hands	— Wheezing
— Mercury fillings	— Joint pains	— Palpitations
— Bleeding gums	— Numbness	
— Grinding teeth		
— Taste change		

▶

HEALTH SYSTEMS CHECK		
TICK IF YOU EXPERIENCE ANY OF THE FOLLOWING SYMPTOMS		
Digestive system — Acidity — Burning — Bleeding — Indigestion — Nausea — Vomiting — Bloating — Constipation — Diarrhoea — Haemorrhoids — Fissures — Change of stool colour — Flatulence — Excess belching	**Urinary system** — Thirst — Frequency day or night — Burning — Infections — Restricted flow — Change in urine colour or smell — Blood in urine	**Female system** — Menstrual irregularities — Cramps — PMT — Menopause — Hot flushes — Loss of libido — Discharges — Infections — Infertility — Breast lumps — Breast tenderness
Male system — Erection concerns — Lower back pain — Sciatica — Joint pains — Change in urine stream	**Nervous system** — Weakness — Poor coordination — Loss of balance — Memory loss — Difficulty concentration — Numbness — Coldness	**Emotional health** — Depression — Anxiety — Restlessness — Excess worry — Nightmares — Insomnia — Mood swings

ENERGY RATING SCALE

Energy levels:
Morning 1 2 3 4 5 6 7 8 9 10 Afternoon 1 2 3 4 5 6 7 8 9 10 Evening 1 2 3 4 5 6 7 8 9 10 Rate: 1(as bad as could be) to 10 (as good as could be)

ENERGY RATING SCALE

DO YOU EAT THE FOLLOWING FOODS? (CIRCLE IF YOU DO)	
Bread/wholegrain/wholemeal/wheat	Legumes
Cereal	Red meat
Rice/pasta/noodles	Chicken
Fruit/fruit juice	Fish
Dried fruit	Eggs
Vegetables	Biscuits/cake
Cow's milk/skim/whole	Chips/crisps
Soy milk	Lollies/chocolate
Rice milk	Jam/honey
Sheep's/goat's milk	Peanut butter/honey
Cheese	Salad dressing/mayonnaise
Yoghurt	Oil
Ice cream	Gravy/sauce
Tofu	

DIETARY QUESTIONS				YES	NO	
Do you have any specific dietary requirements? Please specify:						
Have you experienced any weight loss or weight gain recently? Please specify:						
Do you frequently skip meals?						
Do you have a healthy appetite?						
Do you drink milk regularly? If so, is it mainly: skimmed / semi-skimmed / full cream / soy / other (please circle)						
Do you use mainly butter or margarine?						
What is the main oil you use for cooking?						
Do you have any known food allergies or intolerances?						
How much of the following do you add to your food/drink? (teaspoons)	**Salt**		**Sugar**	**Sweetener**		
How many cups/glasses per day?	**Tea**	**Coffee**	**Juice**	**Soft/fizzy drinks**	**Water**	
Your weekly alcohol intake:	**Beer (glasses)**	**Wine (glasses)**	**Spirits (shots)**	**Other (glasses)**		

FOOD QUALITY AND TYPE
PLEASE GIVE AN ESTIMATED PERCENTAGE OF THE FOLLOWING QUANTITIES OF FOOD
0 = NONE / 100 = ALL

How much of your food is ...	**Prepared at home**	**Fast food/takeaway**	**Delicatessen/ sandwich shop**

▶

How much of the food you cook with is ...	Fresh	Frozen	Tinned	Pre-cooked	Reheated
How much of your fresh vegetables are ...	Organic		Unprocessed		Supermarket prepared
How much of the foods you eat a home are ...	Raw (salads, etc.)			Cooked	
How much of the cooked food is ...	Baked	Stir-fried	Fried/ deep fried	Microwaved	Steamed

Section 2: Forms for use by the practitioner during a consultation

Date:				
Preferred name:	Title	First	Surname	Initial
Address:	No. Street Suburb Postcode			
Contact phone:	(H)	(M)	(W)	
Emergency contact: Relation:	(H)	(M)	(W)	
GP contact details: Name: Address: Phone:	Does your GP know you have consulted a natural therapist? Y/N	Do you give permission for us to contact your GP if necessary? Y/N	Are you seeing any other health care professionals? Y/N	
Date of last blood tests or physical examination for any health concern:	Date:	Where did you have the investigations?	Result of investigations:	
How did you hear about our complementary therapies clinic?	Have you seen a complementary therapist prior to this consultation? Y/N	Has your experience with natural therapies been helpful for you? Y/N	Are you happy for communication to remain open with other complementary therapists regarding your health care management? Y/N	

Complaint

Define the *presenting* complaint

> **O**nset
> **U**nderstanding of cause (client)
> **T**iming (duration, frequency)
> **E**xacerbating factors
> **R**elieving factors
>
> **L**ocation and radiation
> **A**ccount and description
> **Y**our practitioner impression
> **E**xamination and inspection
> **R**ating scale

Context

Put the presenting complaint into context to *understand the disease*

Family health
Maternal
Paternal
Siblings
Allergies and irritants – current and past history
Trauma and pre-existing illness
Recreational drug use
Surgery and hospitalisation
Vaccinations
Occupational toxins and hazards
Supplements and side effects of medications

Further questions arising from *Health systems check* form

HEAD	
EYES	
SKIN, HAIR, SCALP, NAILS	
EARS, NOSE AND THROAT	
MOUTH, TEETH AND GUMS	
NECK, SHOULDERS AND ARMS	
CHEST	
DIGESTIVE SYSTEM	

URINARY SYSTEM	
FEMALE SYSTEM	
MALE SYSTEM	
NERVOUS SYSTEM	

DIETARY EVALUATION OF A TYPICAL DAY		
On rising:	Breakfast:	Mid-morning:
Lunch:	Mid-afternoon	Dinner:

DIETARY EVALUATION OF A TYPICAL DAY		
Dessert:	Snack/supper:	Bedtime:

Core
Holistic assessment to understand the client

AREAS OF INVESTIGATION	CLIENT RESPONSES
SUPPORT SYSTEMS	
EMOTIONAL HEALTH	
ENVIRONMENTAL WELLNESS	
DAILY ACTIVITIES	

AREAS OF INVESTIGATION	CLIENT RESPONSES
STRESS RELEASE	**Stress levels:** **At work:** 1 2 3 4 5 6 7 8 9 10 **At home:** 1 2 3 4 5 6 7 8 9 10 **Rate:** 1(as bad as could be) to 10 (as good as could be)
OCCUPATION	
FAMILY AND FRIENDS	**Relationship status:** **Children:** **Ages:**
HOME LIFE	
EDUCATION AND LEARNING	

AREAS OF INVESTIGATION	CLIENT RESPONSES
ACTION NEEDED TO HEAL	
LONG-TERM GOALS	
TIME TO HEAL	
HAS NOT BEEN WELL SINCE	

PHYSICAL EXAMINATION		
Skin • Dry, scaly, oily, pale, red • Hyperkeratosis (on arms and thighs) • Stretch marks • Bruises • Atopic eczema, dermatitis, psoriasis • Wounds • Hyperpigmentation	**BP**	**Pulse rate per minute**

PHYSICAL EXAMINATION

Tongue

KIDNEY
BLADDER
INTESTINES

GALL
BLADDER

STOMACH

SPLEEN

LIVER

LUNGS

HEART

Colour:

Coating:

Cracks:

Teeth marks:

Tremor:

Temperature	Weight
Respiratory rate per minute	**Height**
BMI	**Waist circumference**

Nails

• White spots/streaks

• Brittle

• Soft

• Corrugated

• Spooned

• Yellow

• Bitten

• Transverse ridges

• Peeling

• Splitting

Mouth

• Cheilosis or cheilitis

• Mouth ulcers

• Gum recession, bleeding gums, periodontitis, mercury amalgams

• Tonsils – size, colour, crypt inspissations

PHYSICAL EXAMINATION	
Hair	**Face**
• Dry	
• Dull	
• Shiny	
• Thinning	
• Dandruff	
• Coarse	
• Brittle	
• Grey	
URINALYSIS RESULT:	
Protein	
Nitrates	
Blood	
Urobilinogen	
Bilirubin	
Ketones	
Ascorbic acid	
Ph	
Specific gravity	

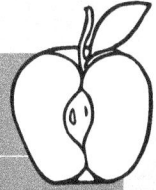

Referral letter templates

Referral letter to a GP/between therapists

Dear Dr [insert name],

Re:

DOB: **Clinic ref**:

I am a [CAM] practitioner at [insert clinic name]. Your client, Mrs [insert name], came to my clinic on [insert date] for advice about natural medicine. Mrs [insert name]'s presenting complaint included symptoms of pain in the right side of the body that moves in location, which she has experienced since [insert date], pain in the right inguinal area followed by vaginal bleeding that is not consistent with a typical menstrual cycle, green vaginal discharge and swollen right mandible lymph nodes. I noted her repeated non-attendance for laparoscopic investigation of lower abdominal pain and a history of anaemia. Her blood pressure was 150/90 on the date of the consultation. As these symptoms require further investigation to exclude serious illness, I have urged Mrs [insert name] to consult you again to ensure adequate clinical follow-up on these matters.

I appreciate your professional opinion and have suggested to Mrs [insert name] that she make an appointment with you to discuss this.

If you have any queries regarding this request please do not hesitate to contact us on [insert clinic number].

Yours sincerely,

[insert name]

Letter to client explaining cross-referral

Dear [insert name],

I am writing to advise you that I am unable to offer you [CAM] treatment at this stage. I apologise if this causes you upset or inconvenience; however, it is not a decision I make lightly. In seeking to offer client-centred care, I am careful to carry out an initial assessment to determine whether I am able to meet the needs of clients within the scope of my professional expertise. During your consultation it became evident that your needs would be better met by a direct relationship with an experienced _____ professional who can offer you continuity of care.

I appreciate your desire to pursue natural therapies, so with your permission I can write to your GP with regard to the possibility of referral to _____. I suggest you make an appointment to see your GP to discuss the options for your ongoing care. I am also attaching a list of qualified _____ who may be able to offer treatment.

I wish you well for the future.

Your sincerely,

[insert name]

These letters were inspired by a template published in: Howard-Kemp N 2008 Homeopathy clinic, University of Westminster Polyclinic, London.

Collaborative/cross-referral form

COLLABORATIVE/CROSS-REFERRAL FROM [INSERT PRACTITIONER'S NAME, CLINIC AND SPECIALITY]
Referred to: [insert practitioner's name, clinic and speciality]
Date:
Client's name:
Clinic ref:
Summary of case:
Summary of treatment to date:
Any cautions:
Desired/expected results in collaborative/cross treatment:

This form was inspired by Hal Andrews, Clinic Manager, University of Westminster Polyclinic, London.

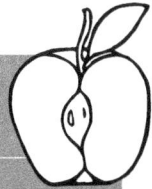

Helpful contacts

The following list contains information about Australian-based support and information organisations. Readers from countries other than Australia are encouraged to find out about similar organisations operating in their own country.

ORGANISATION	CONTACT	WEBSITE	DETAILS
Alcoholics Anonymous	(02) 9599 8866 National office	www.aa.org.au	Support for families and individuals with an alcohol problem
Alzheimer's Australia	1800 100 500	www.alzheimers.org.au	Provides support and advocacy for people living with dementia
Arthritis Australia	1800 111 101	www.arthritisaustralia.com.au	Support for people with arthritis
Asthma Australia	1800 645 130	www.asthmaaustralia.org.au	Support for people with asthma
Australian Breastfeeding Association	1800 686 2686	www.breastfeeding.asn.au	National breastfeeding helpline and website
Autism ACT Autism Northern Territory Autism Queensland Autism South Australia Autism Tasmania Autism Victoria Autism Association (WA)	1300 300 182 (08) 8947 4800 (07) 3273 0000 1300 288 476 1300 288 476 1300 308 699 1800 636 427	autism.anu.edu.au www.autismnt.com.au www.autismqld.com.au www.autismsa.org.au www.autismtas.org.au www.autismvictoria.org.au www.autism.org.au	Support and information for individuals and families dealing with autism spectrum disorders

▶

beyondblue	1300 224 636	www.beyondblue.org.au	Support for people with depression
The Butterfly Foundation	(02) 9412 4499	www.thebutterflyfoundation.org.au	Providing support for people with eating disorders
Cancer Council of Australia	13 11 20	www.cancer.org.au	Advocates for the rights of cancer patients for best treatment and supportive care; advises the Australian government and other organisations on practices and policies
Coeliac Society of Australia	1300 458 836	www.coeliacsociety.com.au	Support and information for people with coeliac disease
Diabetes Australia	1300 136 588	www.diabetesaustralia.com.au	Support and information for people with diabetes
Domestic Violence Resource Centre		www.dvirc.org.au/whenlove/servicestxt.htm	Providing information about domestic violence support and advocacy services throughout Australia
Eczema Association of Australia	1300 300 182	www.eczema.org.au	Support and information for individuals and families suffering from eczema
Anaphylaxis Australia	1300 728 000	www.allergyfacts.org.au	Providing support and information about allergies and anaphylaxis
Gamblers Anonymous	(02) 9628 7803	www.gansw.org.au	Support for families and individuals with a gambling problem
Headache Australia	1300 886 660	www.headacheaustralia.org.au	To provide support, education and research into headache disorders
Heart Foundation	1300 362 787	www.heartfoundation.org.au	Support and information for people with heart disease

Kid's Help Line	1800 551 800	www.kidshelp.com.au	Telephone counselling for children and young people
Lifeline	131 114	www.lifeline.org.au	Telephone counselling for family and relationship issues, mental health concerns, suicide prevention and support, abuse and violence, loneliness and life direction
ME/CFS Australia		www.mecfs.org.au	Providing support and information to individuals with ME/CFS
MS Australia		www.msaustralia.org.au	Providing information, support and advocacy for people with multiple sclerosis and their families
Narcotics Anonymous	1300 652 820	www.naoz.org.au	Support for families and individuals with a narcotics problem
National Association of people living with AIDS	1800 259 666	www.napwa.org.au	Support for people living with HIV/AIDS
Quitline	131 848	www.quitnow.info.au	A federal government initiative to help people quit smoking
Relationships Australia	1300 364 277	www.relationships.com.au	Provides relationship support services
SIDS and Kids	1300 308 307	www.sidsandkids.org	Providing bereavement support for people who have lost a child through SIDS or another condition
Vision Australia	1300 847 466	www.visionaustralia.org.au	Providing services and facilities for the visually impaired

Useful web-based information resources

The following web-based resources provide a range of information on both conventional and complementary medicine. Some are open access and others require a paid subscription. Readers may be able to access some of these resources via their institutional library service.

ACP (American College of Physicians) Journal Club	www.acpjc.org
Agency for Healthcare Research and Quality (AHRQ)	www.ahrq.gov
Alternative Medicine Review	www.thorne.com/practitioners/alternative_medicine_review.jsp
British Medical Journal	www.bmj.com
Cambridge Journals	journals.cambridge.org
The Cochrane Library	www.cochrane.org
The Database of Abstracts of Reviews of Effectiveness (DARE)	www.crd.york.ac.uk/CRDWeb/Home.aspx?DB=DARE
EBSCO Host	www.ebscohost.com
Family Village	www.familyvillage.wisc.edu
Free Medical Journals	www.freemedicaljournals.com
Hardin Metadirectory of Internet Health Resources	www.lib.uiowa.edu/hardin/md
Healthfinder	www.healthfinder.gov
Informaworld	www.informaworld.com
Journal of Medical Internet Research	www.jmir.org
Mary Ann Liebert	www.liebertpub.com
Medical World Search	www.mwsearch.com
MEDLINE	www.nlm.nih.gov/databases/databases_medline.html
Medscape	www.medscape.com
National Guideline Clearinghouse	www.guideline.gov
Natural Standard	www.naturalstandard.com
New England Journal of Medicine	www.nejm.com
NHS Evidence – complementary and alternative medicine	www.library.nhs.uk/CAM/ViewResource.aspx?resID=306601&tabID=290
NorphCAM	www.norphcam.org

▶

OMNI (Organising Medical Networked Information)	www.omni.ac.uk
Ovid	www.ovid.com
Oxford Journals	www.oxfordjournals.org
Pharmacognosy Journal	www.phcogj.com
Phytotherapist Perspective	www.mediherb.com.au
ProQuest Digital Dissertations	proquest.umi.com
PubMed	www.ncbi.nih.gov/pubmed
Royal College of Pathologists of Australasia online manual	www.rcpamanual.edu.au
SAGE journals online	online.sagepub.com
ScienceDirect	www.sciencedirect.com
SpringerLink	www.springerlink.com
Textbook of Natural Medicine online	www.naturalmedtext.com

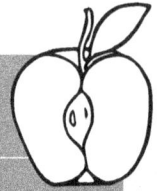

Non-orthodox investigative tools commonly used by CAM practitioners

In additional to utilising information obtained from orthodox Western medical investigations, CAM practitioners may also obtain information from one or more sources not commonly used by conventional medical practitioners. The following list provides basic information about some of the investigative tools more commonly utilised by CAM practitioners. This list is by no means exhaustive and the authors make no claims regarding scientific validity or accuracy. Readers wishing to find further information on any of the listed tools are encouraged to investigate the suggested websites and/or texts. Please note that information about investigative tools not listed in this appendix is also available from some of the listed websites. Websites listed are mostly Australian based, and readers from other countries are encouraged to seek organisations in their own country that offer similar investigative tools.

INVESTIGATIVE TOOL	FURTHER INFORMATION
Hair tissue mineral analysis Hair tissue mineral analysis measures the mineral composition of hair; it can provide insight into exposure to heavy metals as well as mineral stores in the body; mineral levels in the hair are considered to reflect mineral levels in other body tissue	**Websites** www.interclinical.com.au www.healthscopepathology.com.au www.australianbiologics.com.au www.metametrix.com **Books** • Watts DL 1995 Trace elements and other essential nutrients: clinical application of tissue mineral analysis, Publisher Meltdown International, ISBN: 1885676247 • Tabrizian I 2003 Practitioners guide to reading a tissue mineral analysis, NRS Publications
Salivary hormone testing Salivary hormone testing provides information about the non-protein bound fraction of hormones at a given point of time; the unbound fractions are considered to be more readily available to body cells and salivary hormone testing is considered by proponents to best reflect a client's hormonally related symptoms when compared with bound hormone levels measured in serum	**Websites** www.healthscopepathology.com.au www.pathlab.com.au www.australianbiologics.com.au www.metametrix.com

▶

Adrenal hormone profile Used to assess adrenal function in clients presenting with anxiety, depression, mood swings, insomnia, headaches, low energy, stress, hormonal imbalance and poor immune function; the levels of cortisol and DHEA-S are monitored over the course of a day	www.healthscopepathology.com.au www.metametrix.com
Melatonin hormone profile Levels of melatonin in the body are measured at midnight and 6:00 am. Low levels may be observed in those with sleep disturbances, poor immune function and mood disorders	www.healthscopepathology.com.au
Live blood screening Utilises dark field microscopy to screen living blood; high contrast and clarity of blood cell membranes and certain cellular and plasma contents provides the trained practitioner the opportunity to detect early changes in blood parameters and screen for a range of health-limiting processes such as inflammation, poor liver function, oxidative stress, reduced nutritional status, reduced digestive integrity and impaired immune performance	http://www.wsu.edu/~omoto/papers/darkfield.html www.metagenics.com.au www.australianbiologics.com.au
Thyroid hormone profile To assess levels of unbound free thyroid hormones TSH, FT4 and FT3, which are from tissues in the body reflecting true metabolic rate	www.healthscopepathology.com.au
Thyroid antibodies To assess thyroglobulin and thyroid peroxidase antibodies in conditions such as Hashimoto's disease, thyroid carcinoma and Graves' disease	www.healthscopepathology.com.au
Essential fatty acids (EFAs) To determine blood levels of essential fatty acids; can help practitioners determine the quantity and type of essential fatty acids to prescribe	www.healthscopepathology.com.au www.metametrix.com
Stool analysis Stool analysis may be performed to determine the presence and/or levels of a range of fungi, parasites and bacteria as well as providing information about digestive function, intestinal permeability, inflammation and nutrient absorption	www.metametrix.com www.healthscopepathology.com.au www.pathlab.com.au
Complete digestive stool analysis (CDSA) Provides an overview of digestion, absorption, intestinal function and microbial flora plus identification of pathogenic bacteria, parasites and yeasts	www.healthscopepathology.com.au www.metametrix.com

▶

Three-day parasitology (3DP) Assesses the presence or absence of parasitic infection (commonly *Blastocystis hominis, Giardia lamblia, Entamoeba histolytica, Dientamoeba fragilis, Endomilax nana* and *Cryptosporidium parvum*)	www.healthscopepathology.com.au
***Helicobacter pylori* stool antigen (HpSA)** Assesses the presence or absence of *Helicobacter pylori*	www.healthscopepathology.com.au
Functional liver detoxification profile (FLDP) To assess phase I and II liver detoxification; useful for clients with allergies, chemical sensitivities, chronic fatigue syndrome, 'leaky gut' and hormonal imbalance	www.healthscopepathology.com.au www.pathlab.com.au
Intestinal permeability (IP) Used to assess gastrointestinal mucosal integrity ('leaky gut'); the IP is a challenge test using lactulose and mannitol	www.healthscopepathology.com.au www.pathlab.com.au
Secretory IgA (sIgA) Assesses secretory IgA levels in saliva and can give information on the functional status of the entire mucosal immune system	www.healthscopepathology.com.au
Urinary amino acids Provides information on metabolic and nutritional imbalances for conditions such as chronic fatigue, frequent headaches, chronic digestive function, intolerances to foods and chemicals, depression, learning disabilities, malnutrition, neurological disorders and degenerative diseases	www.healthscopepathology.com.au www.metametrix.com
Urinary iodine Provides information about dietary iodine intake	www.healthscopepathology.com.au
Optimal nutritional evaluation (ONE) Helps assess a client's overall nutritional status and assess the functional need for vitamins and minerals	www.healthscopepathology.com.au www.metametrix.com
Urinary organic acids (metabolic analysis profile and cellular energy profile) Assesses organic acids and provides information on gastrointestinal function, cellular energy, neurotransmitter metabolism, amino acid/organic acid balance	www.healthscopepathology.com.au www.metametrix.com
Comprehensive urine elements profile (CUEP) Assesses urinary excretion of nutrient elements and toxic metals, acquired through either chronic or acute exposure	www.healthscopepathology.com.au www.metametrix.com

Osteoporosis risk assessment (NTx) Measures the risk of osteoporosis by detecting the rate of bone resorption (breakdown) long before significant changes are obvious on bone density scans	www.healthscopepathology.com.au
Bioimpedance analysis Bioimpedance analysis utilises a small electrical current that flows through the body to assess the electrical conductance properties of different body tissues to aid in determining body composition	www.metagenics.com.au **e-Document** Bioimpedance monitoring for physicians: an overview. Antoni Ivorra, 2003. Available from www.ldteck.com/1PDF/7.%20%Bioimpedance_for_physicians_rev1.pdf

TRADITIONAL CAM INVESTIGATIVE TOOLS	FURTHER INFORMATION
Iridology Iridology is an investigative tool used by many CAM practitioners to gain information about the health, strength and condition of body systems and organs; this information is determined by interpreting the markings and colouration in the iris; while iridology does not medically diagnose disease, in conjunction with a thorough case history and other investigative techniques it can provide valuable insights into a client's health and vitality and indicate which body systems require support	www.johnandrewsiridology.net www.iridologyonline.com **Books** • Bodeen DV, Jensen B 1992 Visions of health: understanding iridology, Avery, division of Penguin Putnam Inc., New York • Jensen B 1952 The science and practice of iridology, Bernard Jensen Products, Publishing Div. • Jackson-Main P 2004 Practical iridology,Carroll and Brown Publishers Limited, London
Kinesiology Kinesiology practitioners use muscle feedback to identify imbalances in structural, chemical, mental and emotional energy systems; using kinesiology muscle testing techniques, practitioners evaluate normal and abnormal body function, and may also gain information about environmental, chemical and food sensitivities	www.kinesiology.net/kinesiology.asp www.library.yorku.ca/ccm/rg/im/kinesiology www.kinesiologyfederation.org www.icpkp.com **Books** • Frost R 2002 Applied kinesiology: A training manual and reference book of basic principles, North Atlantic Books, Berkely CA • Valentine T, Valentine C 1987 Applied kinesiology: Muscle response in diagnosis, therapy and preventative medicine, Healing Arts Press, Rochester, Vermont
Pulse diagnosis Pulse diagnosis is an integral part of traditional Chinese medical practice, and is also used in Ayurvedic medicine; the pulse provides information about the blood and qi to help determine the health of internal organs and whether there are problems with the flow of energy through the meridians	http://pulsediagnosis.com http://orientalharmonicmedicine.com/articles/Chinese PulseDiagnosis.php **Article** • Rosen R, Stickley B 2007 An introduction to contemporary chinese pulse diagnosis, *Chinese Medicine Times*, 2(6):1–8. Available from <http://www.dragonrises.org/articles/article-ccp.pdf> **Books** • Hammer L 2003 Chinese pulse diagnosis: a contemporary approach (revised edition), Eastland Press, Seattle • Flaws B 1995 The secret of chinese pulse diagnosis, Blue Poppy Press, Boulder CO

Diet diary template

DIETARY EVALUATION OF A TYPICAL DAY

Please list all foods and beverages consumed in one day.

Strictly confidential

ON RISING	BREAKFAST	MID-MORNING	LUNCH	MID-AFTERNOON	DINNER	DESSERT	ON RETIRING

DIETARY PRESCRIPTION FOR ONE WEEK

Please follow these dietary and supplement recommendations.

	MONDAY	TUESDAY	WEDNESDAY	THURSDAY	FRIDAY	SATURDAY	SUNDAY
Breakfast Remedies/medication							
Mid-morning snack Remedies/medication							
Lunch Remedies/medication							
Mid-afternoon snack Remedies/medication							
Evening meal Remedies/medication							
Dessert Remedies/medication							
Fluids							

WEEKLY FOOD DIARY

Please list all food and drinks consumed, and note any relevant comments or symptoms in the last column.

	ON RISING	BREAKFAST	SNACK	LUNCH	SNACK	DINNER	EVENING	COMMENTS/SYMPTOMS
Monday								
Tuesday								
Wednesday								
Thursday								
Friday								
Saturday								
Sunday								

Index

Page numbers followed by 'f' denote figures; those followed by 't' denote tables